The Flying Vet's

Pigeon Health & Management

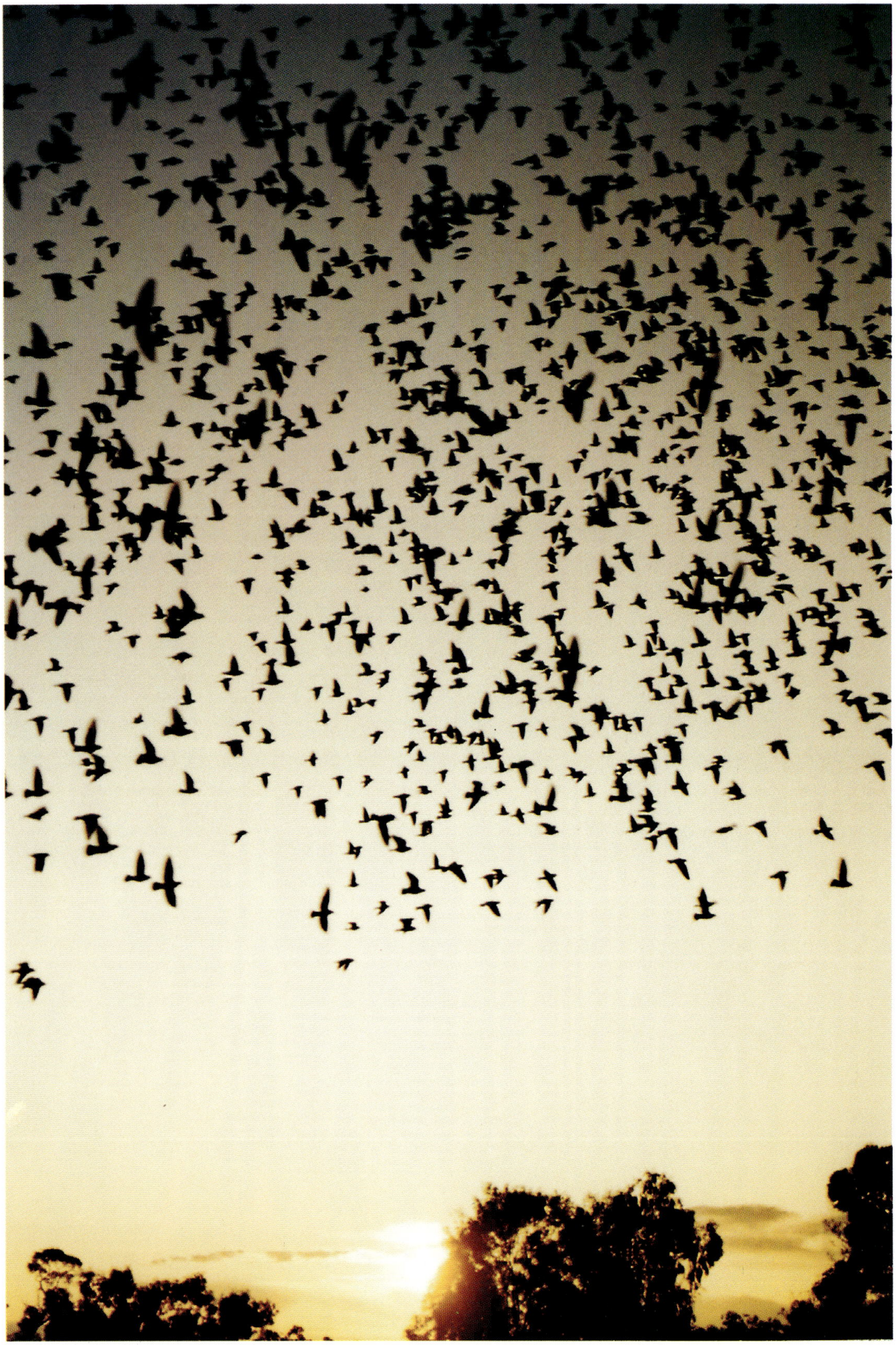

500 miles from home. A sunrise release for the 3500 birds competing in the V.H.A. 500-mile race of 1993 from Bourke to Melbourne. The winning birds took 10 hours to complete the journey.

The Flying Vet's
Pigeon Health & Management

A veterinary guide to health control, medication use and the development of race fitness for the competitive fancier

Dr Colin Walker

B.V.Sc., B.Sc., M.R.C.V.S.

I would like to thank my wife, Meredith, for her computing and editing skills and also for her patience and clear thinking in the production of this book.

Published by Dr Colin Walker
Pigeon Veterinarian
Knox Veterinary Clinic
2 Lynne Avenue
Wantirna South
Victoria 3152

First published 2000

The National Library in Australia Cataloguing-in-Publication data:

Walker, Colin, 1954- .
The flying vet's pigeon health & management : a veterinary guide to health control, medication use and the development of race fitness for the competitive fancier.

ISBN 1 876677 91 0.

1. Racing pigeons - Health - Australia. 2. Racing pigeons - Diseases - Australia. 3. Racing pigeons - Diseases - Treatment - Australia. 4. Racing pigeons - Australia. I. Title.
636.5960994

Designed by Tom Kurema
Produced by Publishing Solutions
Printed in Singapore

CONTENTS

ABOUT THE AUTHOR

Colin Walker was born in 1954 in Melbourne, Australia. He started racing pigeons in 1969 and graduated as a veterinary surgeon in 1979. He operates a bird-only veterinary clinic in the Melbourne municipality of Knox and flies with the local Knox club, affiliated with the Victorian Homing Association, which has approximately 400 members. Over the last 10 years, he has placed more and more emphasis on obtaining high positions in the Association's distance races. He has won the Association's championship twice (1985, 1995) and has been runner up twice (1990, 1991). He has won a total of 13 open Association races, with between 2000 and 10,000 birds competing. In 1995, he had birds placed in the top 30 in all but two of the Association's old bird races and, in fact, had he clocked one more bird in the Association's last five longest races, then fully 10% of all birds placed in the top 30 would have been his. That year, in the Association's 500-mile race, 30 birds homed on the day (all

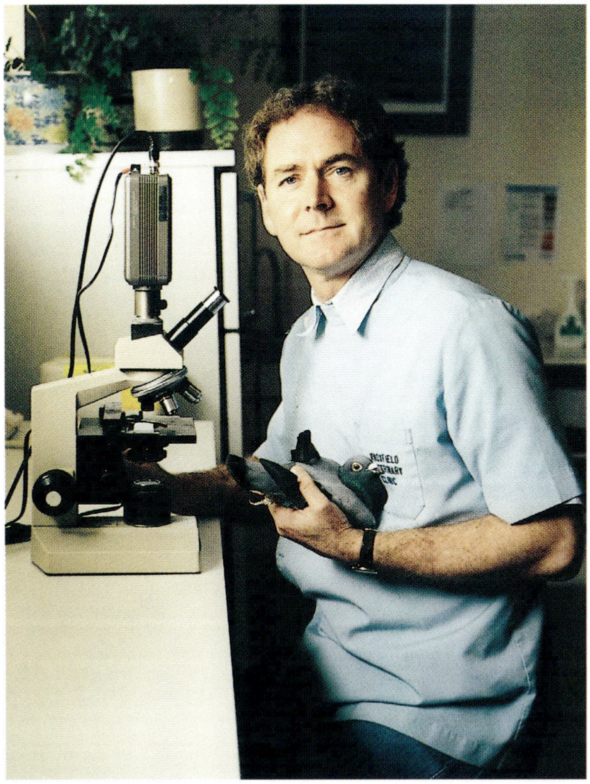

The author in front of his racing lofts, his team for the year 2000 exercising overhead.

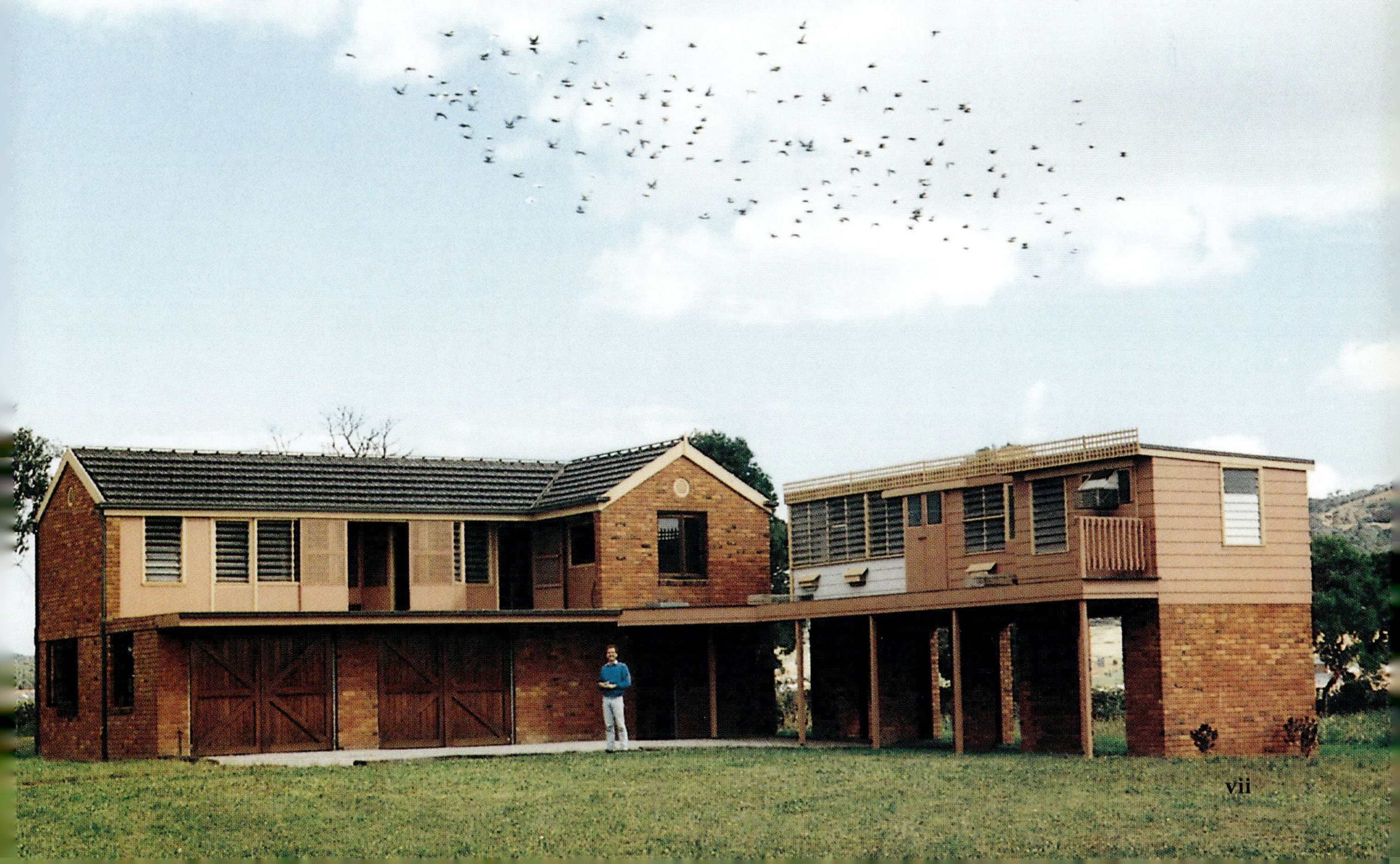

after sunset) out of 2500 sent, with Colin clocking two at 8:10 p.m. (14 hours 10 minutes on the wing) and a third at 8:12 p.m. to be 18th, 19th and 20th Federation. The next week in the 600-mile race, he was 3rd, 8th and 11th Federation, with approximately 1500 birds competing. In 1992, he was 1st Federation 400 miles (2856 birds), 1st Federation 500 miles (3444 birds), 1st Federation 600 miles (2634 birds), and 4th Federation 700 miles (2090 birds), a result never achieved before in the history of the Victorian Homing Association. He is the current holder of the record for the largest number of Association positions (bird placed in top 30) ever gained by a single member in one year (24 positions in 1991). His loft is one of only two in any Victorian federation to have won more than one Open National, winning the 1990 600 miles Collarenebri National (5342 birds) and the 1992 400 miles Langwell National (9300 birds). In the 1992 Langwell National, three birds arrived together to win and the velocity of his sixth bird was equal to the bird that gained 23rd National. In the 1992 V.H.A. 600-mile race (approx. 2000 birds competing), he clocked the Federation winner at 7:36 p.m. (13 hours 6 minutes on the wing), his second bird at 7:51 p.m. (to gain 9th Federation), with further birds arriving at 8:20, 8:30 and 10:45 p.m., to record a total of five on the day when less than a third of competing members were able to produce a clock. In the 1992 700-mile race (approx. 2000 birds competing), he was 4th and 20th Federation, and had a further five birds within 2 hours of clocking, with a total of nine on the winning day (34 sent). In the 1991 700-mile race, he was 7th Federation (clocking the only cock in the first 40 birds home) and also had nine on the winning day (23 sent). In 1998 and 1999, the birds continued on their winning way with the loft again having birds placed in the Association's top 30 in the 500-, 600- and 700-mile races.

The active competition of racing has lost none of its excitement for Colin, which, together with the fact that much of his professional time is now spent dealing with pigeons, places him in an ideal position to help fanciers with health problems associated with their birds.

In 1994, Colin established the Australian Pigeon Company, a company that manufactures medications and health supplements specifically for pigeons. The company is dedicated to provide the best veterinary supplements at an affordable price to fanciers. These products are now widely used in Australia and New Zealand, with distribution to other countries world-wide a plan for the future. It is hoped that fliers in other countries find these products of value in managing their birds' health.

FOREWORD

For the pigeon racer, nothing is more exciting than, after an expectant wait, catching sight of a home-coming bird in the distance. The sight of the rapidly enlarging dot in the sky, with its head down, working its way rapidly towards him, knowing it has come from so far, represents the culmination of not only the bird's but also his efforts. He has been involved from the original pairing of its parents, its hatching, weaning and initial flights, through to its development as a mature, competitive bird, able to return independently from hundreds of miles.

For those not involved in this activity, it can seem, at best, unusual. If the sport is to maintain its current popularity and ideally to grow through the development of a favourable public image, it must, I believe, achieve a degree of professionalism found in other sports. One way of doing this is to increase knowledge and awareness in both the public and the fancier.

Although this book's primary aim is to pass information on to active pigeon fanciers, it is hoped that veterinary surgeons looking for up-to-date avian knowledge, lay people with no prior experience of the sport, and various authorities and students looking to clarify matters regarding pigeon racing will also find valuable information within it.

Some older practices are still common in our sport, largely, I believe, through a lack of knowledge dissemination. And yet, new knowledge and medication become available each year. My aim is to present up-to-date veterinary knowledge regarding pigeon disease, medication and management, so that not only can the fancier's enjoyment of the sport increase but also, through the implementation of modern practices, the health of the birds can improve and with it the quality of racing. I have aimed to relate all veterinary information directly to management and present this in a usable and easy-to-read format.

I wish all fanciers on-going enjoyment and success with their birds.

Section I

INTRODUCTION

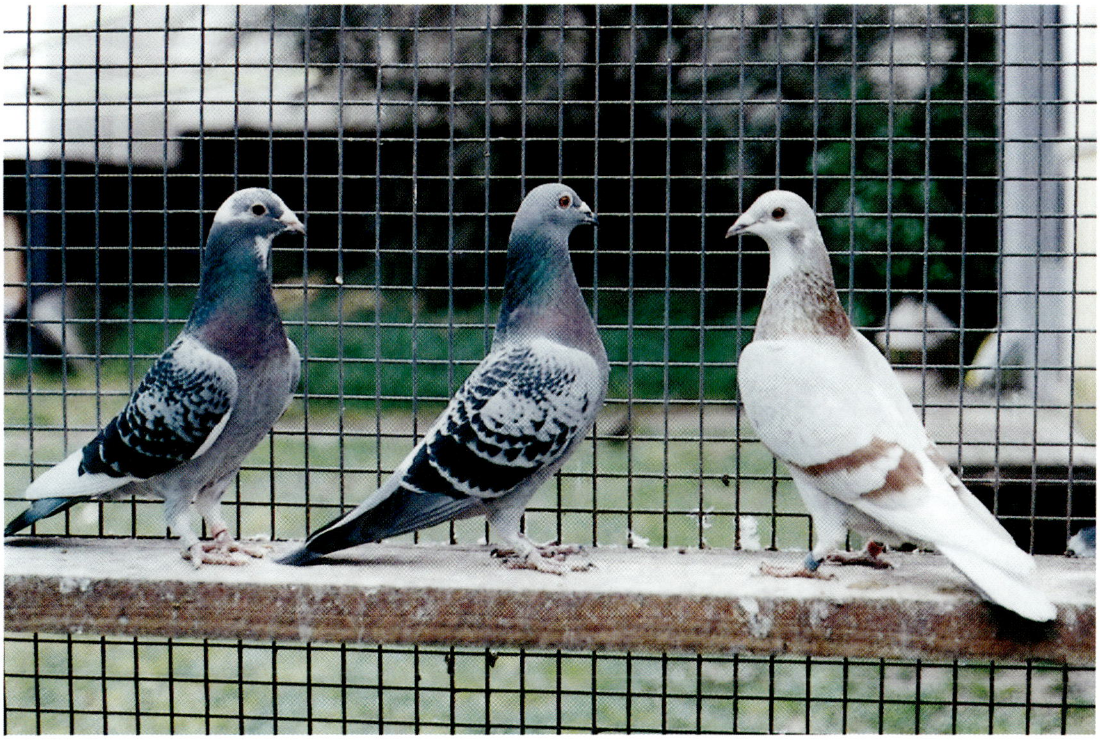

Three racing hens.

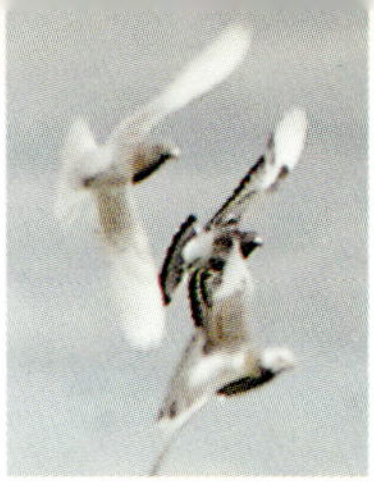

Chapter 1

THE AMAZING PIGEON

Racing pigeons have the potential to be highly strung birds and at times lead extremely stressful lives. They only weigh 400 grams and yet at times find themselves alone and vulnerable to predation, hundreds of miles from home with nothing to eat or drink. At this point, they must orientate themselves and, despite fatigue, head for home, at all times being on the look-out for hazards, in particular, birds of prey. However, in birds with the correct genetic make-up, who are adequately trained and sent to race in fit condition, it is unusual for them not to reach their lofts and usually at speeds in excess of 40 miles per hour.

In Australia, most races are 300 to 400 miles, with the longer races being 800 miles. Beneath the birds' wings pass hundreds of miles of Australia's red sandy deserts, open forests and sometimes the sea. And yet their desire and ability to return are such that, at times, they appear to do it with ease.

The modern racing pigeon must be regarded as a thoroughbred animal that is the end result of centuries of selection. The ancestors of the modern pigeon originally bred in rocky cliffs, with their food source at a distance. It was, therefore, essential for them to navigate their way home.

Man has long been aware of this ability, with even the early Egyptians using pigeons to carry messages short distances. Through the 18th and 19th centuries, selective breeding progressively capitalized on this innate ability, with the birds returning from the furthest distances and at the fastest speeds most valued. By the mid-19th century, this had progressed to the point where clubs had formed and formal racing competitions held. Today, pigeon racing is a popular sport world-wide,

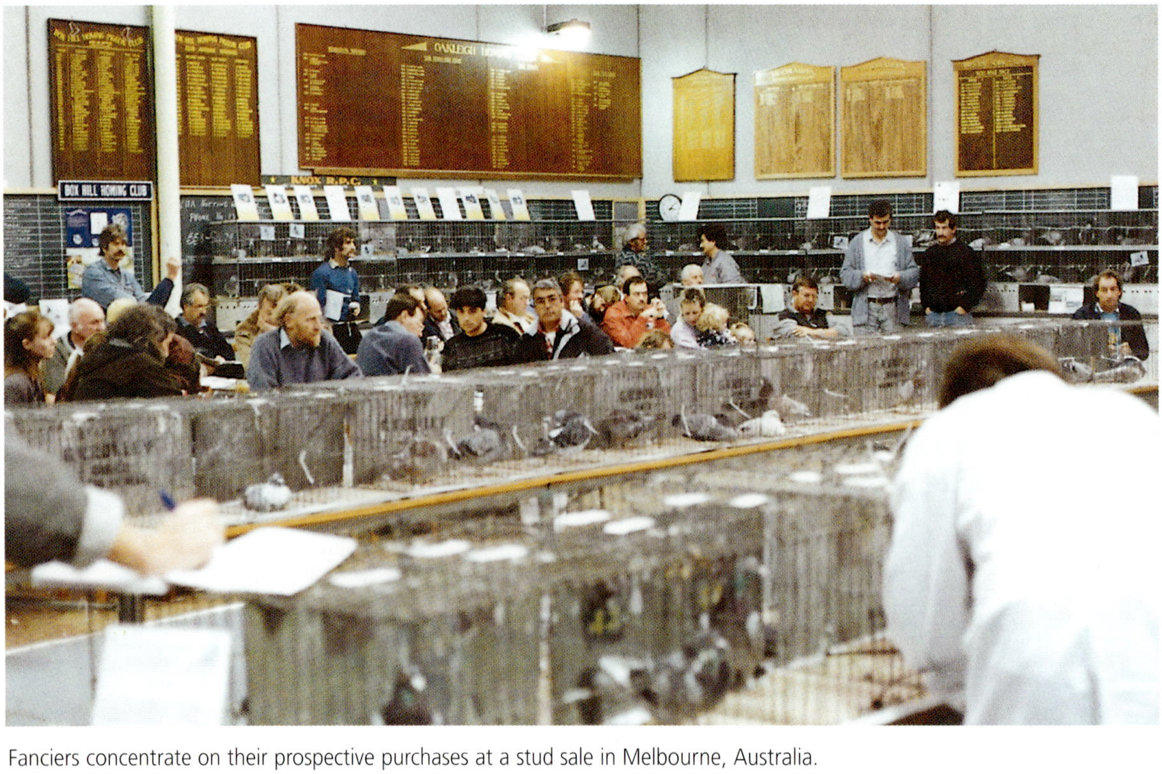

Fanciers concentrate on their prospective purchases at a stud sale in Melbourne, Australia.

particularly in countries such as England, Holland, Belgium, France, America, Japan, Germany, China and Australia.

The method by which pigeons home is basically understood but there are still gaps in our knowledge. They have an inbuilt chronometer and appear to be able to use both the sun and the earth's magnetic field. Being able to tell the time of day, they can compare the position of the sun in the sky at a release point with that at home and thus calculate the direction home. This sounds complex but experienced birds can do it remarkably quickly.

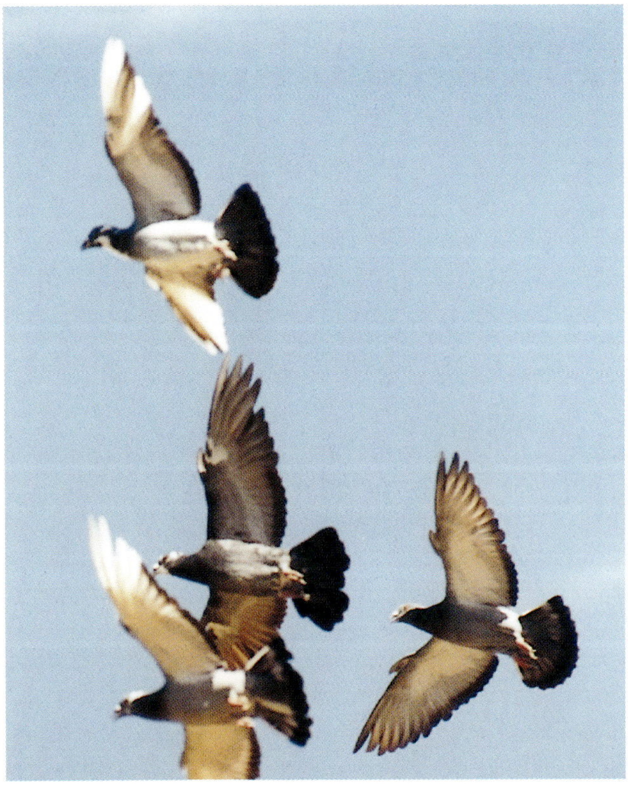

It is not uncommon for a race convoyer's report, in a 700-mile race from Queensland to Melbourne, to say that the birds upon release flew around, then grouped together and headed south in less than 1 minute. However, on overcast days, when the sun is not visible to them, they use the earth's magnetic field. In an interesting experiment, birds were temporarily blinded by placing dense plastic discs over the eyeball and under the eyelid, taken 80 miles from their loft and released. The birds flew off erratically as individuals, rather than forming a normal flock, and it was feared that all would be lost. At the home loft, 2 hours after release, birds started appearing in the sky. As they became fatigued, they hesitantly hovered down, with their feet extended, most landing on the ground around the loft but some actually landing on the 2-m x 2-m loft roof. Even though blind, they were able to pinpoint their home with this degree of accuracy. Vision is necessary, it seems, only for the final approach to the loft.

Today, pigeon racing is a popular pastime that knows no cultural or political barriers. Pigeons have adapted to and are raced in climatic conditions as diverse as those found throughout Asia (with in excess of 300,000 fanciers in China alone), Saudi Arabia, South Africa, Canada, Malta, U.S.A., and both eastern and western Europe. It seems that the innate fascination of this remarkable bird affects a proportion of the population no matter where they live.

There are about 10,000 active pigeon racers in Australia, racing their birds many weekends at different locations around the country. Although this may seem a large number, this is small compared to many other countries, in particular those in western Europe, notably Holland and Belgium, where the bigger races attract entries of tens of thousands of birds from many lofts. Here, prize money and the value of the winning birds run into tens of thousands of Australian dollars, with many individuals and studs vying for the honour of having birds with the leaders.

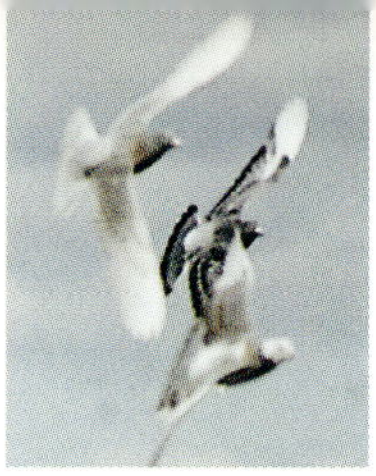

Chapter 2

PIGEON MEDICINE, THEN AND NOW

– A Veterinarian's Perspective

I first started racing pigeons in 1969 when I was 15. Like most of us, I had kept pet pigeons for several years before actually starting to race. As is the case when you keep a number of animals for a length of time, after a while one of the birds got sick. I took it to the local family veterinarian to whom we took our dog. He explained that his experience with, and knowledge of, pigeons was limited, and suggested that I take the bird to a bird 'specialist'. This I duly did. In hindsight, and after practising as a veterinarian for 20 years myself, thinking back on his advice I now realize that the knowledge available to him and the help that he could give me was rather limited.

Since that time and even since my graduation in 1979, the level of knowledge has increased tremendously. Avian medicine is, at the moment, a particularly interesting area to work in as the level of knowledge, new drugs and diagnostic tests available advance every year.

Most things that happen regarding the health of a pigeon happen for a reason. Infectious disease and other problems do not come from nowhere. In the past, the emphasis has been on the treatment of the individual sick bird, which is still important, but the fancier with the sick bird in his hand must, after diagnosis of the illness, think why it has become sick and how to stop further birds developing the same disease. A pigeon veterinarian can obviously help him with this.

As a veterinary surgeon actively involved in racing, I can easily understand how the average fancier can be confused by the information available. However, as the skill of the better fanciers and the knowledge of the pigeon veterinarians advising them increase, it is important, I feel, for the modern fancier to develop some knowledge of the factors that affect the health of our birds.

Unfortunately, in the pigeon fancy there persists a lot of backyard medicine and 'old wives' tales'. There are fanciers who not only use drugs that are 10 years or more out of date for common diseases like canker, coccidiosis and *Salmonella*, but, amazingly, some that follow advice written over 50 years ago (at a time when not even penicillin had been invented). Some of the articles written in current pigeon magazines are little different from articles on the same topic published years ago.

And so what can the modern fancier do? It is important to remember that the racing pigeon is naturally a fairly robust bird and, as a species, disease in it is relatively uncommon provided the basics of hygiene and management are met. However, in even the best-managed lofts, because of the very nature of pigeon racing where birds from many different lofts are in intimate contact, disease will occasionally occur.

With some of the common diseases, e.g. pigeon pox, the appearance of the lesion is diagnostic. However, with most diseases, diagnosis of the problem simply by examining and handling the bird is impossible. The fancier when faced with the sick bird with non-diagnostic symptoms, e.g. diarrhoea and weight loss, has three alternatives:

1 **Kill it** – The immediate problem is eliminated by killing the ill bird. However, a diagnosis is not reached and therefore the way to prevent further cases and the potential of the problem to affect racing and breeding are not evaluated.

2 **'Stab in the dark' diagnosis –** Sometimes a problem can be diagnosed by response to treatment with a particular drug, e.g. a diarrhoea and weight-loss problem responding to worming. More often than not, I am confronted by a fancier who tells me that he has treated the birds with several prescription medications, a multivitamin and then wormed them and they are still not well! Such a regime usually makes the birds sicker, wastes time and interferes with subsequent test results.

3 **Accurate diagnosis and correct treatment –** Accurate diagnosis enables the biology of the infective organism to be known. This means that not only is the cause determined and correct medication given but preventive measures can be taken to avoid it happening again. This is the preferred strategy to adopt.

For a racing loft to be successful, it must have good pigeons in a good loft under good management. When reviewing his own poor performance, the unsuccessful flyer must try to identify in which area he is lacking. Unsuccessful flyers can spend a lot of money acquiring new birds from winning lofts that are, in fact, not superior to their own but simply managed better.

Many older flyers who achieved success in the past and now whose winning performances have become less frequent blame a variety of reasons for this and, wary of modern medicines, do nothing. Often performance can lift dramatically with the introduction of improved health management.

Many flyers state that the 'good old days' of racing pigeons on good food and clean water are over, and for one to achieve consistent success this is probably true. On the other hand, some flyers

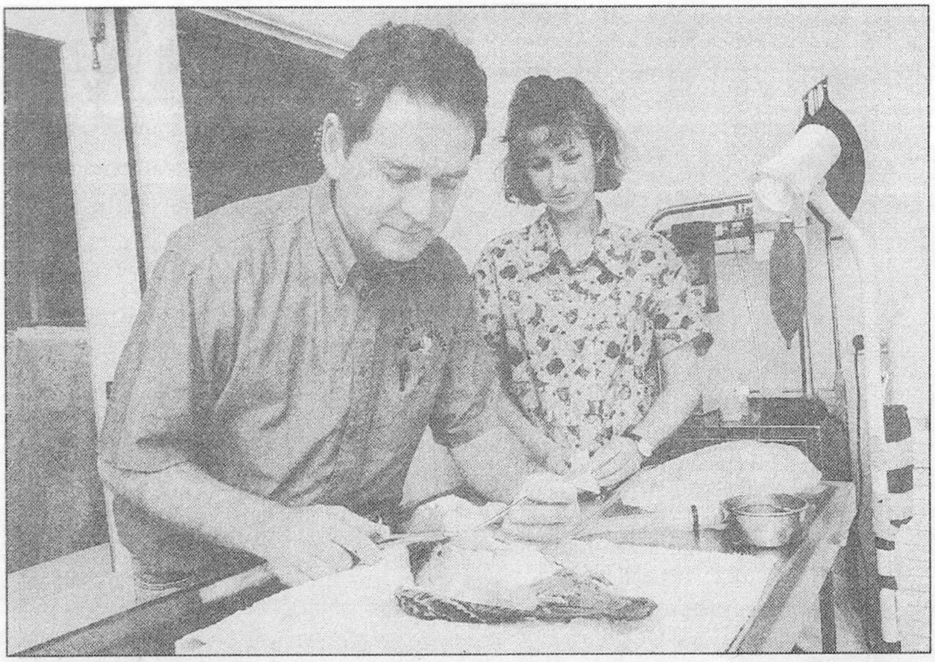

Flighty patient: *Nurse Michelle helps Dr Colin Walker with the avian operation. 008js317*

RACING PIGEON MAKES PIT STOP BEFORE NEXT FLIGHT

A RACING pigeon was back on her feet within hours of a delicate operation at Knox Vet Clinic to remove a tumor.

When the eight-year-old blue check hen arrived at the clinic with a growth on her chest, avian veterinarian Colin Walker took her straight into surgery.

"I see about 50 birds a day and cancerous tumors are as prevalent among birds as they are among other animals, or probably humans," he said.

Once the bird had been fully anaesthetised, via a gas mask, and later an oral tube, the growth was removed in a 20-minute operation. The bird was taken into recovery and went home the next day.

Dr Walker said pigeons usually lived for about 15 years.

Giving pigeon racing publicity. Clipping from a local newspaper.

believe that success can be found in a bottle and this is certainly not true. There is a place for correct medical control of identified problems but not for the indiscriminate use of medication. Medications in themselves cannot make a pigeon fly faster. They can, however, enable good birds to achieve their genetic potential by controlling health problems that affect form.

Fliers often say to me that years ago they never had any problem with disease and yet at times it can now seem a constant battle to keep the birds healthy. We now not only have to deal with very active strains of canker and *Mycoplasma* but, in addition, there are new diseases such as Circo virus that we were not aware of years ago. It is important that fliers do not become disenchanted with the effort involved in getting the birds healthy, but it does mean that fliers today have to make themselves aware of such matters to be successful.

Dr Wim Peters in his excellent book 'Fit To Win' (p. 10)describes well the changing attitude to pigeon medication. He describes how –

> *"In previous times the modern practice of treating for disease was frowned upon. Before treatment became more popular, birds in the most hygienic environment and with the strongest natural resistance, remained healthiest and were the best racers. Now that medication is aiding pigeons with less natural resistance, speedier birds often end in front, though they might naturally possess a lower resistance to disease and would possibly not have been able to compete successfully 50 years ago. Compare the donkey and the horse. The donkey's natural resistance to disease is far superior to that of the horse and it can outlive it's more favored cousin under the harshest conditions – yet not one of us would bet a penny on the outcome if it came to racing.*
>
> *Together with more refined racehorse breeding, comes a decreased resistance to disease and more dependence on management and medicine to keep health at a peak. Breeding thoroughbreds thus becomes a matter of selection for more and more speed; health becomes a function of hygiene and management – and rightfully so. Our feathered racers are no different."*

I regard the diagnosis and correct management of pigeon disease as being relatively straightforward compared to the attainment of race form. To win, the individual bird must be motivated, have genetic quality and be fit and healthy. Not only must medical problems be correctly handled, but

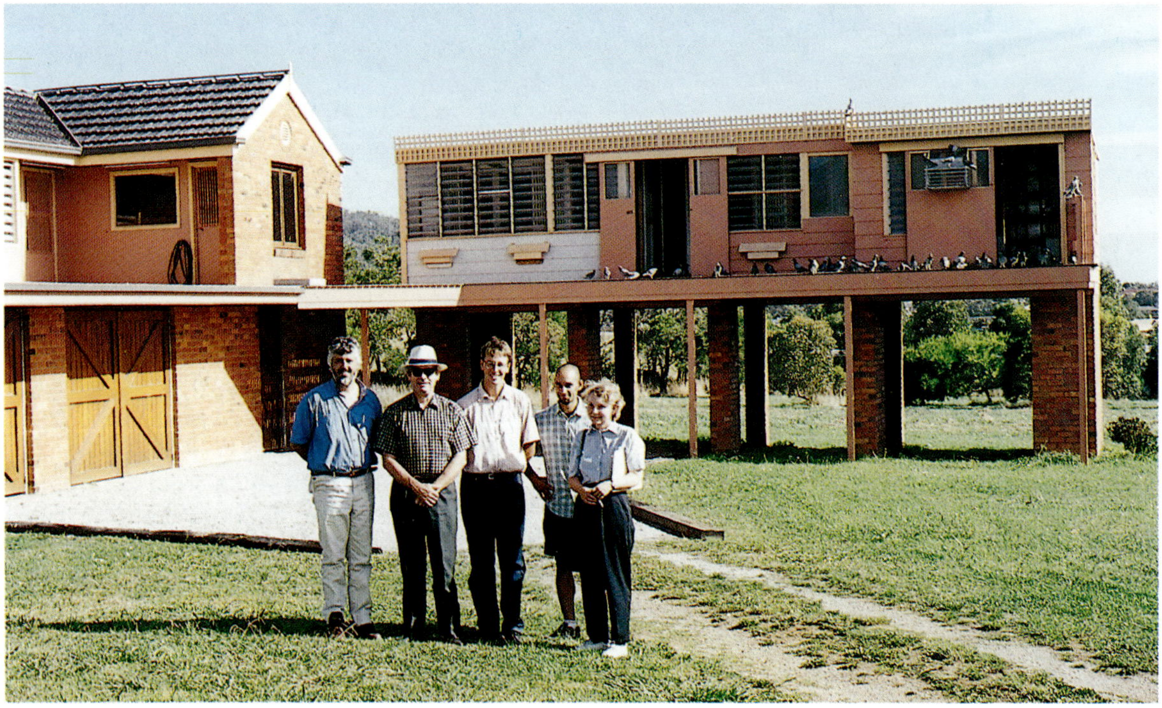

Group of Australian avian veterinarians at the author's lofts.

A case study

A young Janssen/Van Loon hen was presented with a history of being quiet in the loft and off her food. On handling, it was noticed that the pulse of her heart radiated into the abdomen. As the heart is surrounded by airsacs, which, when full of air, cannot transmit the movement associated with the beat of the heart, this indicated that material, most likely fluid, was in the airsac. Further examination revealed increased resistance to digital pressure over her right abdominal airsacs, indicating that these were likely to be the airsacs involved. The bird was behind in its moult compared to other birds its age, indicating a longer-term problem. A crop flush was performed, which contained large numbers of heterophils, indicating inflammation, with the likely source being the respiratory system. However, a faecal smear revealed no abnormalities. A tentative diagnosis of an airsac infection was made and a course of Baytril commenced, 3 drops twice daily. Within 24 hours, the bird was noticeably improved, being brighter, and had resumed eating. An x-ray taken at this time clearly showed fluid sitting in the right abdominal airsacs (see below). The bird continued to improve with the Baytril and after 5 days the owner reported that the bird was now well and treatment was stopped. Although well in herself, a bird that has had a severe airsac infection is usually left with residual damage and so the possibility of racing the hen was ruled out. However, she had considerable potential in the stock loft and was retained to trial as a breeder.

This approach, although not practical for every bird, is realistic for individual birds of value, particularly if they have potential at stock. This approach not only gave the fancier the option of breeding from his Janssen/Van Loon hen but alluded to an underlying respiratory problem within the loft, which may indicate that a flock treatment would be a wise idea. If needed in this case, a needle could have been inserted into the inflamed airsac to aspirate material for diagnosis or blood could have been collected for testing. However, as the hen was now well, this was deemed unnecessary.

Years ago, many fanciers would simply have killed this bird and today, if the rest of the birds are well and the unwell bird has no further value to the fancier, this may still be appropriate. However, if an unwell bird is the first of several or has a value, effective diagnostic measures and treatment are now available.

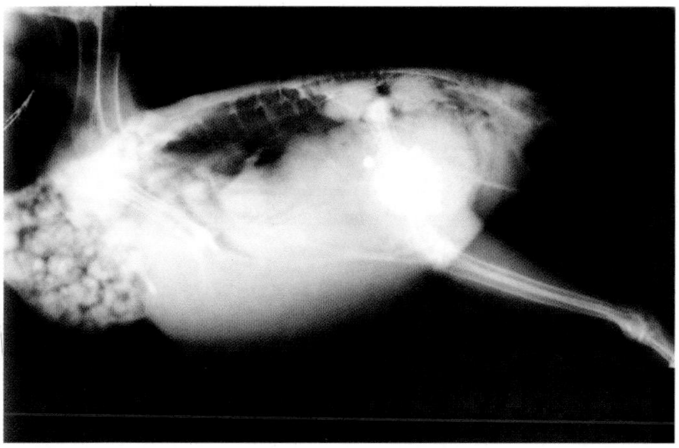

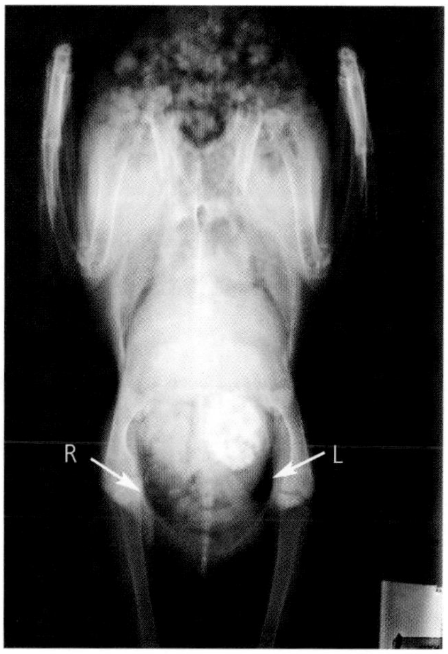

Airsacs are filled with air and should be black like the air around the bird. Fluid is denser than air and gives the airsac a light grey appearance. Compare the offending right airsac with the normal (black) one on the left.

the pigeon racer must be skilled in getting his birds fit. Race form is, in fact, superhealth and can obviously only be attained if all factors affecting health, including disease control and nutrition, are dealt with in the best possible way.

Everyone has experienced the team that is unbeatable for part of or a whole season. Why do some fanciers 'hit form', race well for a number of weeks and then lose form? Factors that are beyond the fancier's control, such as weather, affect all lofts within a given Federation. Therefore, the factors that make one loft win over another are controlled by that loft's manager. Why then should it not be possible for that manager to identify the factors associated with the development of form and manipulate them so that form is achieved? Too often a fancier at the end of a winning run wonders, "What did I do right?" Tossing and feeding regimes can be repeated, but it is more involved than that. Correct use of medications and supplements, such as multivitamins, grits and pick stones, and modification of exercise regimes and seed mixes to suit the prevailing conditions are all involved.

During racing, the average team of racers have coccidial counts of one egg on every fourth x100 microscope field, but winning teams always have coccidial counts of absolutely zero. In the same way, parasitic, chlamydial and trichomonad levels fluctuate through the season. It is possible to monitor these counts and to use medication to keep these counts minimal so as to enhance the chance of a team coming into form.

Over the last ten years, world-wide avian veterinary knowledge has undergone a quantum leap forward. Following closely have been improved diagnostic capabilities and an ever-increasing range of effective medications. As only healthy birds can become fit and only fit birds can win, to me the successful management of the birds' health is just another challenging aspect in the overall preparation of the birds for successful racing.

And so it seems that in recent decades, we have gone from having trouble in identifying and treating the common diseases to not only accurately monitoring and treating but manipulating health factors to achieve the maximal performance from our birds. It is up to the astute pigeon racer to avail himself of this modern knowledge and technology.

Section 2

THE COMMON DISEASES

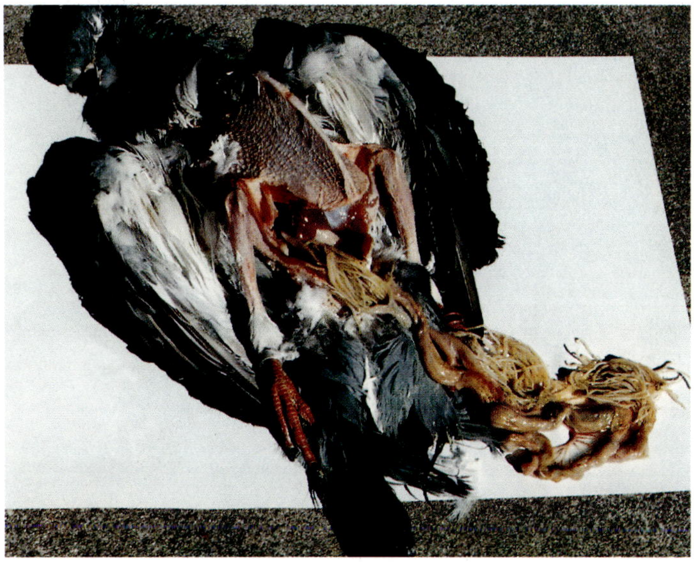

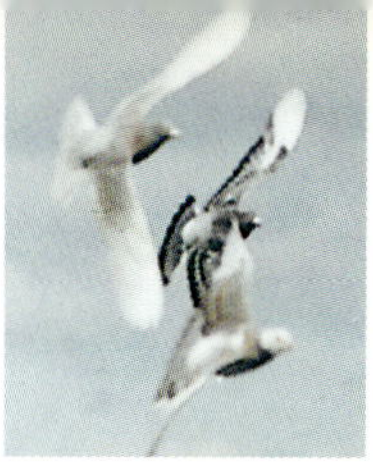

Chapter 3

INTRODUCTION

One of the aims of this book is to present an holistic approach to the development of winning form. Part of this involves the maintenance of health and so it becomes necessary to present to the fancier a basic outline of the common diseases so that he can familiarize himself with them. For those looking for a complete list of all diseases and detailed medical information, they will not find it here. Although of interest to some readers, the presentation of such information is considered beyond the need of most fanciers and could run the risk of this book becoming a veterinary text. A book that is of interest to and presents relevant information primarily to the active competitive fancier is my intent. As such, a summary of the common diseases likely to be encountered by fanciers and their effect on the form of their birds is presented so that a practical working knowledge of them can be obtained.

The important diseases during the rigours of the race program and during breeding are canker, the parasitic diseases, respiratory infection, bacterial infections such as *Salmonella* and *E. coli*, fungal infections such as thrush and *Aspergillus*, and viral infections.

In order to make the advice real for fanciers, I do mention the actual drugs used. Some of the drugs are known by their active constituent, e.g. Moxidectin. However, other names are simply brand names. Some of these brand names are used world-wide, e.g. Baytril. However, other drugs such as ronidazole are sold under different brand names in different countries, e.g. Ridsol-S and Turbosole. All drugs mentioned, both their brand names and active constituents, are listed in the Medication Guide at the end of this book. Fanciers can consult this to ensure they obtain the appropriate medication in their country, even if the brand names are different.

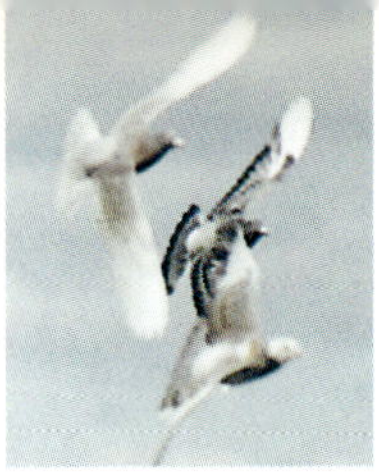

Chapter 4

CANKER –

Its prevention, control and treatment

Nature of the disease

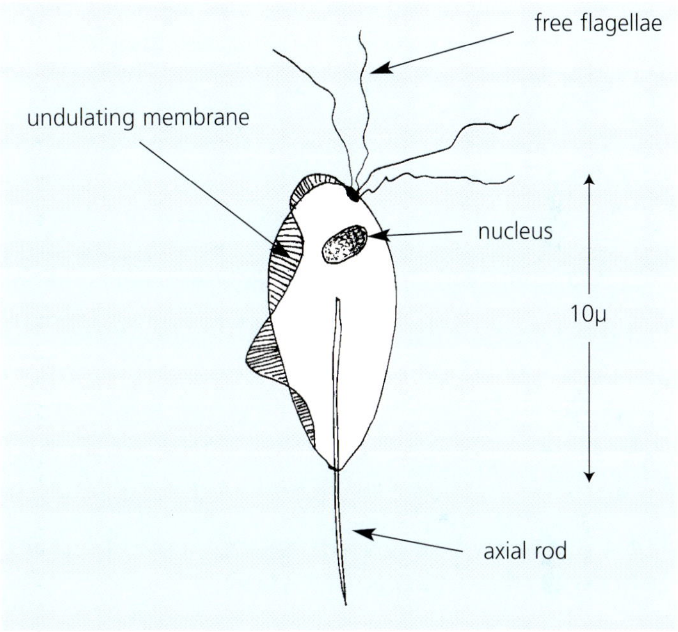

The disease canker is caused by a protozoan *Trichomonas columbae*. This is a microscopic single-celled organism. It lives within the digestive tract of pigeons, in particular the throat and crop, and can also involve associated areas such as the bile duct. The organism is fragile in the environment, only surviving for a few minutes once outside the bird. This helps with control of the disease and means that the birds cannot become infected from the loft or immediate environment as happens with other diseases such as worms and paratyphoid. The organism (trichomonad) requires intimate contact between birds to be spread and is usually transmitted by saliva or pigeon milk. Saliva contaminates food and water. As a pigeon drinks, the organism swims away from its beak and, when another pigeon comes to drink, it not only drinks the water but also the trichomonads there. When a pigeon sorts through grain, each dropped grain contains a small amount of saliva. In this way, the disease can also be spread through a feed hopper. Adult birds 'billing' can transmit the organism, as do parents when feeding their nestlings.

Control of canker during the breeding season

Correct medication is vital during the breeding season so that the level of natural immunity in the weaned youngster is as high as possible. Because the severity of the disease varies in different lofts, there is no single blanket program that is best for all lofts. There is no drug that by itself will cure canker in a loft. It is a matter of using medication correctly so that the birds can establish a strong natural immunity to the disease. It is this natural immunity that, in the longer term, protects them from the disease.

What causes canker to appear during the breeding season?

In health, every time the feeding stock bird feeds its youngsters, it passes on some of its own trichomonads to them. This gives the youngsters a controlled gradual exposure to the organism, which in turn allows them to establish their own natural immunity. Clinical disease appears in the babies when the stock birds shed too many trichomonads over a given period of time to their youngsters. Increased rates of trichomonad shedding will occur if:

- **The stock birds are stressed for any reason –** Anything that stresses the stock bird will lead to an increased rate of trichomonad shedding and includes such things as a poorly designed loft, poor management practices, incorrect feeding, and other concurrent diseases.
- **The stock birds' natural immunity is not high –** Stock birds are likely to shed higher numbers more readily when breeding if their own natural immunity to the strains present in the loft is not as yet solid. This can occur if new stock birds carrying different trichomonad strains have been introduced to the loft during the non-breeding time. All birds carry some immunity to the resident trichomonad strains in their loft. When birds from different lofts mix, they exchange their trichomonad strains. Adult stock birds during the non-breeding season are not stressed and so exposure to any new strains brought in by introduced birds is unlikely to lead to disease. They are not moulting, not breeding, and have plenty to eat, and therefore no sign of canker occurs. However, when paired, if their natural immunity to the new different strains is not solid, the stress of feeding will cause them to 'break down' and shed larger numbers of trichomonads. In the same way, the introduced birds need to establish an immunity to their new loft's resident strains. This is why canker is more of a problem in lofts that are still establishing with birds coming from a variety of other lofts. As the years roll by, fewer new birds are introduced and so the chance of new trichomonad strains getting into the loft decreases. The birds' immunity to resident strains becomes solid and the effect of the disease is less marked.

Many fanciers are frustrated when canker appears in the stock loft. With excellent care in a good loft, they wonder just how it is that the disease can come. Certainly they are on the right track with this approach because in a good loft under good care it is less likely that the stock birds will shed large numbers of trichomonads. However, some strains are so active that problems will arise no matter how well the birds are cared for.

How to manage an outbreak of canker during the breeding season

When canker does appear during breeding, its management is twofold. It is a matter of:

1 **Treating the sick youngsters –** In lofts with a canker problem, all youngsters should be checked daily. If a sick youngster is noticed, it can be successfully treated, and such youngsters can go on to become champions. Either Spartrix or Flagyl tablets* can be used, however, Spartrix is more convenient to medicate the nestlings. The dose of Spartrix is one tablet per adult bird. Estimate how big the youngster is compared to the adult and give it this proportion of the tablet once daily until well. Usually, one to four doses are required. It is often good to also medicate both the nest mate and parents for 2 days. If the unwell youngster is slow to respond, it is usually best eliminated. Individual pairs that breed youngsters with canker are best mated to different birds for subsequent rounds.

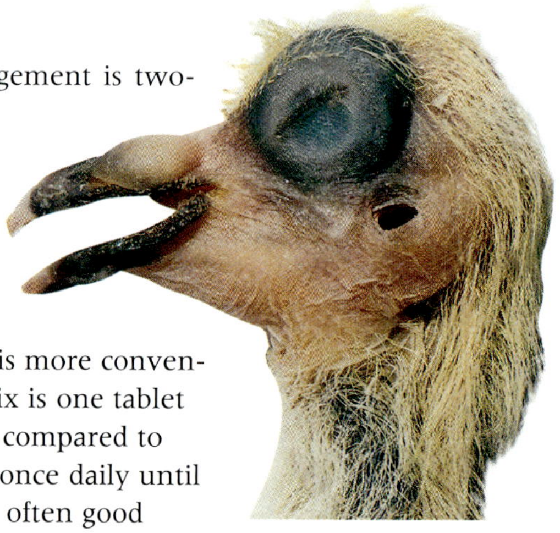

Nestling with throat canker. The skin of the throat is visibly stretched over the canker lesion.

* For details of medications, refer to Medications Available at the end of this chapter.

At the same time, it is important to:

2. **Decrease the number of fresh cases** – This is done by checking the number of trichomonads that the stock birds are shedding. This is achieved by giving 2 days Turbosole* periodically. The exact frequency depends on the incidence of canker but usually every 1 – 3 weeks is appropriate. One needs to give sufficient 2-day courses to limit the number of new youngsters with the disease, but at the same time to avoid overuse of the drug so that the developing youngster is still getting an on-going exposure to the organism. It is a matter of working between these two extremes.

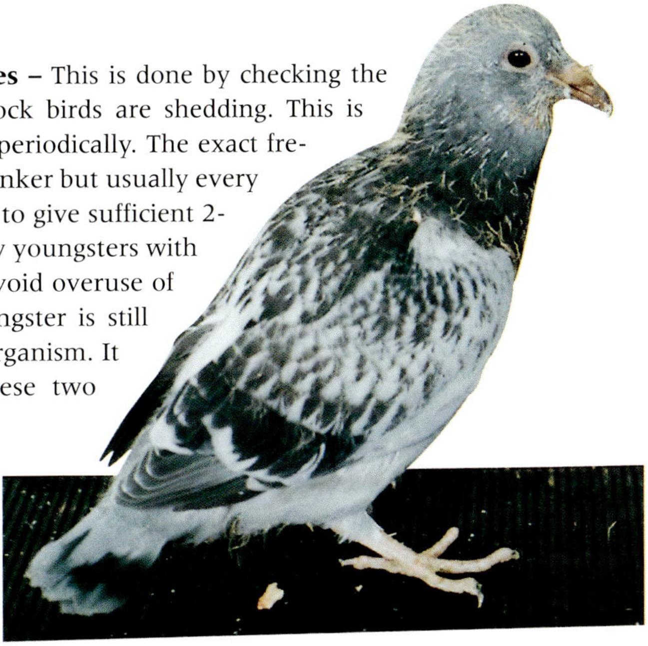

A 3½-week-old youngster with a canker nodule in its throat, showing throat distention and generally unwell appearance. The generally good condition of the bird's feathering indicates how quickly some of these infections can develop.

The important thing to always remember with canker during the breeding season is that the disease can never be controlled through medication alone. It is the development of a strong natural immunity that protects the birds in the longer term. It is important that medication is used to keep the birds well but used in such a way as to not interfere with the development of this immunity.

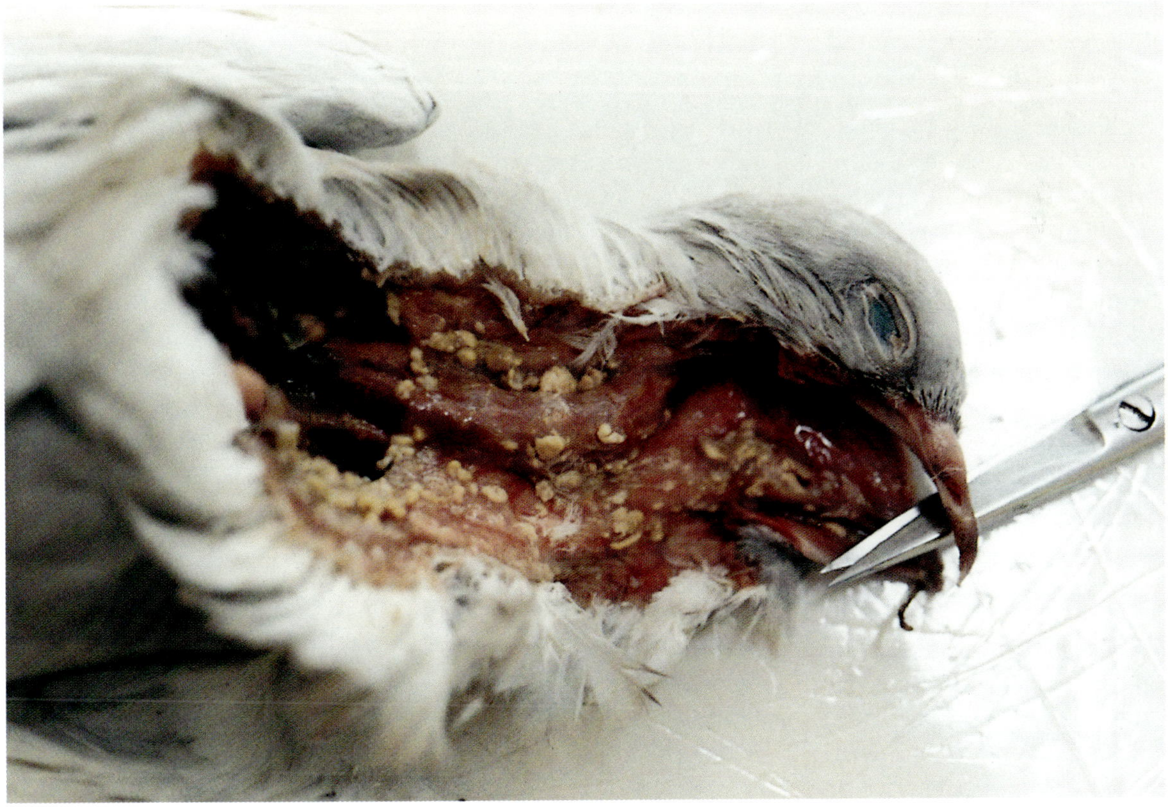

Severe generalized canker such as this is more common in young birds, which have not had a chance to develop a natural immunity to the disease.

---

* For details of medications, refer to Medications Available at the end of this chapter.

Preventive programs for the breeding season

In the stock loft that had canker last season

Treat all stock birds for 5 – 7 days before pairing and then for 2 days every 1 – 3 weeks once paired. Frequency of treatment depends on the severity of the problem and the control achieved. Try and coincide these 2-day treatment periods with the time of hatching when trichomonad shedding is highest. If canker is still a problem in certain pairs, try to only medicate these pairs. This can be achieved by breeding from them in individual runs and only medicating their water with Turbosole for 2 days as required or alternatively leaving them in the loft and just treating them with Spartrix or Flagyl tablets for 2 days when needed. Splitting the pair and remating each to other birds for the next round may help.

Stock birds can be crop flushed before pairing to identify those birds carrying large numbers of trichomonads. These birds are not only more likely to shed large numbers of trichomonads more readily once paired but also to pass on their genetic susceptibility to canker. In the longer term, it is best if these birds, when identified, are eliminated. The problem is that they may, in fact, be the winners and here lies the challenge for the fancier – to breed birds less susceptible to the disease that are also winners.

In the stock loft that had no canker last season

No treatment is required. If there was no problem with canker in last year's nestlings, then it is best not to medicate for canker. Any medication will stop the paired bird shedding trichomonads and therefore interrupt the on-going exposure of the growing youngster to the organism. This leads to a lower natural immunity and may in fact create a vulnerability to the disease in the postweaning period.

In the stock loft that had no canker last season but to which new stock birds have been introduced

As discussed earlier, all birds carry in their systems the resident trichomonad strains of the loft and usually have a strong natural immunity to them. A newly introduced stock bird brings these strains with it. These strains may not have been encountered by your own birds and the new birds may not have encountered yours. Both lots of birds in time must, through exposure, become immune to the other strains. If introduced in the non-breeding time, when the stock birds are not under any stress, i.e. not moulting and in a good loft with plenty to eat, no clinical disease will be seen. However, with the stress of breeding, any immunity already developed will be put to the test. If immunity is not solid at the time of breeding, excessive trichomonads will be shed and the youngsters may develop canker. For this reason, new birds, especially if introduced immediately before pairing, should ideally be mated in individual runs and the youngsters monitored. If youngsters in the main loft begin appearing with canker, the loft should be managed as discussed under the section How to Manage an Outbreak of Canker During the Breeding Season.

Control at weaning

In lofts with a canker problem, all youngsters can be treated with Turbosole for 2 – 3 days at weaning, to avoid any check in their development through this stressful time. In the longer term, however, the important thing during this time is that only youngsters with the disease should be treated so as not to interfere with the developing natural immunity of the flock as a whole. Affected birds should be separated and treated with either one-quarter of a Flagyl tablet (200 mg) or one whole Spartrix tablet once daily until well. This usually takes 1 – 3 days. Alternatively, the unwell youngsters' water can be medicated with Turbosole (1/2 teaspoon to 1 litre of water). It is important, however, to ensure that any unwell youngster is still able to drink. Turbosole can also be mixed

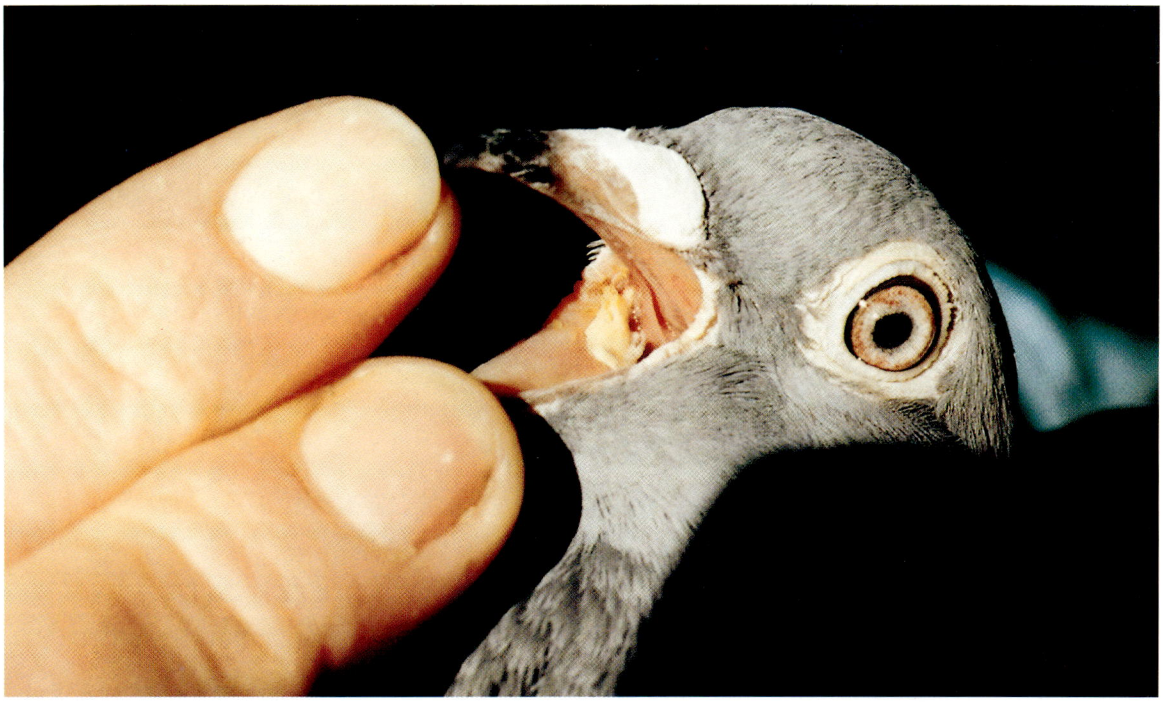

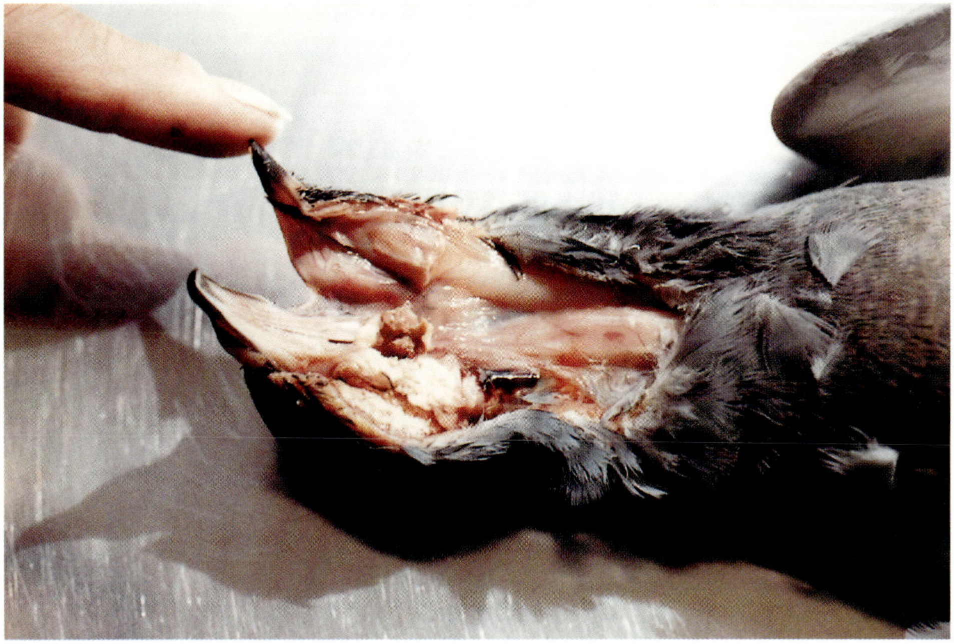

Resolving canker lesion in an older youngster with some natural immunity.

Canker nodule extending into the soft tissues of the throat.

into a paste and the youngster's throat painted with this using a cotton bud. The group of youngsters, as a whole, should only be treated if more than 10% of youngsters are showing signs, usually with Turbosole for 2 – 3 days. However, in this situation it is best to seek veterinary advice.

Control during the race season

If canker was a problem during the breeding season, this tells us that the birds have the potential to have trichomonad flare-ups in response to stress and that canker is likely to be a problem during racing. However, through good management and the correct use of medication, it is hoped that most birds have developed a reasonably strong natural immunity by the start of the race season. The stress of racing will put any immunity that the birds have formed to the test. Depending on what stresses the birds are under, trichomonad levels will rise and fall. When high, they have a typical parasitic effect, weakening the bird, in the process creating a vulnerability to secondary infection (particularly respiratory infection) and compromising race performance. They also produce a toxin that makes the birds feel unwell. Birds with elevated trichomonad levels are said to have 'wet canker'. Signs of infection can be subtle and quite varied. Typical signs that would alert the fancier to its possible presence include:

- **'Penguin' posture –** Associated with proventricular (glandular stomach) and crop pain. Birds will lean back on their tails and gulp. Noticed particularly after eating and drinking.
- **'Dry feather' –** Due to lack of down feather drop and bloom production.
- **'Leady' feel –** Affected birds will not come into condition and feel heavy in the hand.
- **Wet dropping –** Inflammation in the digestive tract creates a thirst, leading to elevated water intake and urine production. This produces a clear watery rim around the dropping.
- **Green droppings –** Due to digestive tract irritation and in some birds decreased food intake.
- **Inflammation in the throat –** Tonsillitis and increased clear to grey bubbly mucus.
- **Interference with crop function –** Delayed crop emptying and sometimes vomiting.
- **Increased food consumption by team as a whole.**
- **Dry yellow canker –** In birds of any age, this tells you that many other birds have elevated trichomonad levels, which have not yet passed the threshold for yellow material to form.
- **Indirect signs –** Poor loft flying, poor tossing, respiratory problems that respond poorly to medication or quickly relapse, a dramatic improvement in the birds' general vigour in response to anticanker medication are all suggestive.

Definitive diagnosis, however, depends on microscopic examination of a crop flush. Microscopic changes that are suggestive of the problem also develop in the dropping. These changes are associated with the stress of the disease and include elevated *E. coli* and yeast levels. These changes, however, do not occur in all birds.

Race lofts are divided into one of two groups for the purposes of canker management:

1. **Those without resident wet canker strains –** Since the rapid spread of wet canker strains through the racing pigeon fraternity since the early 1990's, not many lofts now fit into this category. In these lofts, canker is unlikely to be a problem during breeding and crop flushes done on members of the race team will be repeatedly negative. Here, an effort is made to prevent the introduction of these strains with returning race birds. In races where the birds are provided with drinkers, returning race birds are medicated with Turbosole (1/2 teaspoon to 1 litre of water) for 24 hours upon return. Often the single big drink that returning race birds have, although not sufficient to treat an active infection, will clear the trichomonads picked up from a recent exposure.

2. **Those lofts with resident wet canker strains –** In these lofts, canker is likely, but not always, to be a problem during breeding, and crop flushes done on individual race birds, particularly following stress, will contain large numbers of trichomonads. Here, attention focuses not on treating returning birds, because the strains are already in the loft, but on keeping the numbers of trichomonads low so that they cannot affect race form. This is achieved by giving periodic 2-day courses of Turbosole. The length and frequency of each treatment is variable from one loft to the next, being affected by a number of factors intrinsic to that loft. In most lofts, however, 1 – 2 days every 1 – 3 weeks will keep trichomonad levels low. In the absence

of testing, treatment 2 days every third week is advised. This is usually given on the Monday and Tuesday. Preferably, however, the use of Turbosole within a loft is based on the results of testing birds from that loft. If trichomonads are detected in a crop flush, an initial 2-day course of Turbosole is given. Follow-up crop flushes are then done every few days so that the exact time that trichomonads start to reappear is detected. Once this interval is known for that loft, then, given a constant set of loft parameters, the trichomonads will repeatedly and predictably reappear at this time. Follow-up 2-day Turbosole treatments at this interval will ensure the trichomonad levels are always low and therefore not given a chance to affect race form. The main loft parameters are the genetic make-up of the birds, the strain(s) of trichomonad present, the loft environment and the management practices. If these change, the use of Turbosole may also need to change, e.g. increased tossing combined with cold weather may stress birds, leading to premature trichomonad flare-ups and a shortening of the treatment interval for one or two treatments. Generally, however, as the season progresses, the need for medication declines as the birds get older, both their level of fitness and natural immunity rise and, in particular, in Victoria, as the weather becomes warmer.

Other sites of canker

As fanciers would be aware, most canker lesions are found in the bird's throat and are often associated with their tonsils here. However, canker can affect a variety of other sites.

Navel canker

If pigeon milk is spilt into the nest bowl and this, in turn, contaminates a nestling's navel that has not fully healed, a canker nodule can develop on the navel. Treat the nestling with the correct dose of Spartrix daily (usually 1 – 4 days). Antiseptics (such as Betadine) can be applied to the navel daily until the area has dried. After several days, the nodule can be 'popped' like a scab and separated from underlying healthy tissue. The condition must be caught early for treatment to be successful and for the youngster to be of value racing. The condition is more likely to occur when nest conditions are poor, leading to delayed navel healing, and is therefore often associated with 'wet nests' and with inappropriate nesting material. The condition is also more likely to occur if the parents are shedding large numbers of trichomonads. A suggested course of treatment is:

- Treat youngster and both parents daily with Spartrix.

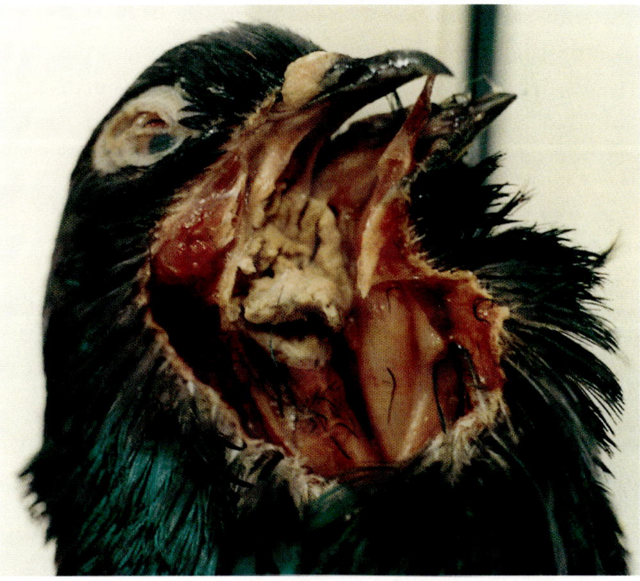

Pigeon's throat opened to show canker lesions involving the tonsil area.

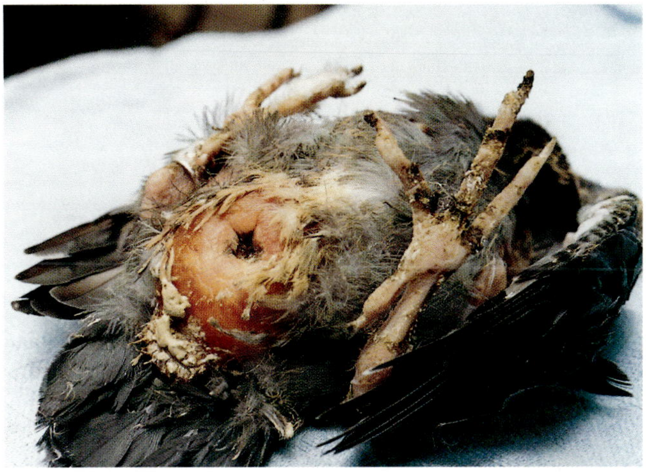

Canker nodule in the navel.

- Dab navel daily with Betadine.
- Clean nest.
- Treat parents for 'wet nest' if appropriate (PVM Powder and Probac).
- Improve nest conditions.

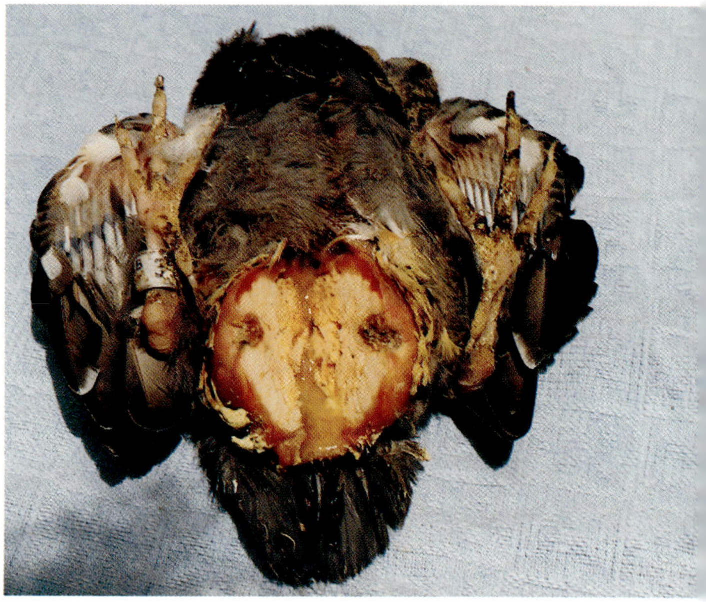
The same nodule, open to show its extent.

Sour crop

In pigeons with sour crop, at least 90% have an internal canker nodule located at the base of the crop or within the glandular stomach (proventriculus). As the nodule increases in size, it squashes the windpipe, making breathing difficult and blocking the crop outlet. This interferes with crop emptying, leading to bacterial infection of the crop and secondary starvation and dehydration due to the crop contents not being able to pass into the bird's system. Usually by the time the bird is noticed to be unwell, the condition has passed the point where it will respond to treatment. Deaths often occur due to the nodule growing through the stomach wall, leading to stomach contents leaking into the chest. Alternatively, the nodule can damage the heart or large blood vessels within the chest, causing sudden and severe bleeding. Such birds are often found dead on the floor with blood coming from the mouth. It is always worth attempting to treat valuable birds and I suggest :

- Manually empty the crop.
- Give electrolytes in water.
- Treat bird with 3 drops Baytril twice daily.
- Treat bird with 1 tablet of Spartrix or a 1/4 Flagyl tablet or 0.5 ml Flagyl syrup once daily.
- Separate unwell bird from loft mates.

Pigeon with 'sour crop'.

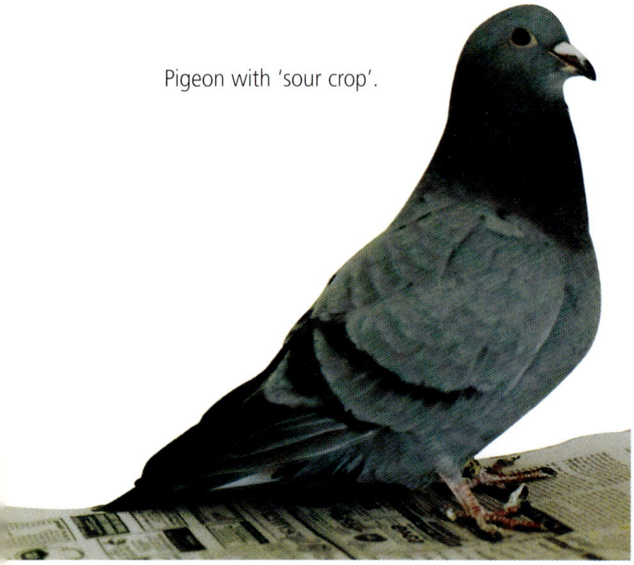

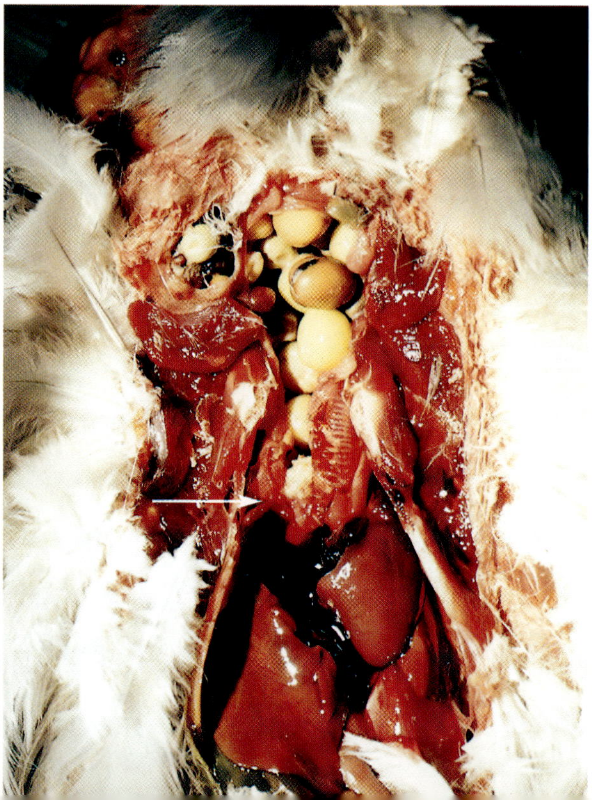
A pigeon during autopsy with the front of the chest removed, exhibiting the three complications experienced with a proventricular canker nodule, i.e. breathlessness, delayed crop emptying and internal bleeding. In the centre of the photo can be seen a canker nodule (arrowed) growing in the wall of the glandular stomach (proventriculus). Stretched over this is the bird's windpipe, which is why many of these birds develop difficulty breathing. The nodule has physically obstructed the stomach so that ingested food is accumulating in front of it in the crop. The nodule has also caused internal bleeding and an organizing blood clot can be seen sitting around the liver below it. Treatment must commence very early in these cases to be successful.

Cloacal canker

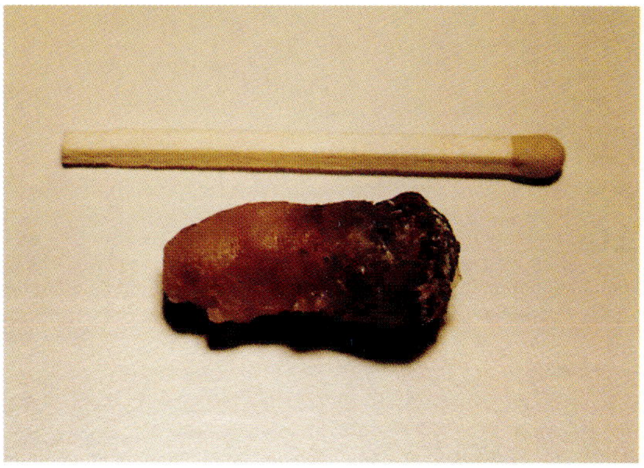

Canker nodule expressed from the Bursa of Fabricius.

The cloaca is the pigeon's bottom. Within its wall is a gland called the Bursa of Fabricius. This gland is an important part of the youngster's immune system. It shrivels up and disappears during puberty. If pigeon milk containing trichomonads contaminates the nest bowl, the trichomonads can cause a trichomonad nodule to develop in the cloaca. Affected birds are usually noticed to be a bit quiet or their growth is slightly retarded compared to others of their age. On examination of the cloaca, a firm lump can be felt in the skin above it. Sometimes these lumps do not become apparent until the postweaning period. Affected birds should be treated daily with either Spartrix or Flagyl, usually for 3 – 4 days, by which time the nodule has usually localized and can be expressed by gentle but firm pressure through the cloaca.

Canker nodule in throat or crop

Older youngsters or mature stock birds with a reasonably strong natural immunity will often try and localize a canker infection, leading to nodule formation. If in the throat, these nodules can usually be seen or if in the crop wall can usually be felt as firm mobile lumps ranging in size from 0.5 cm to 4 cm in diameter. Affected birds are treated daily with Spartrix or Flagyl tablets. Once localized (usually 1 – 4 days), throat lesions can usually be teased free with a cotton bud or crop lesions pinched free into the crop. Occasionally, surgical removal is necessary. Premature attempts at removal usually result in excessive bleeding.

Internal canker

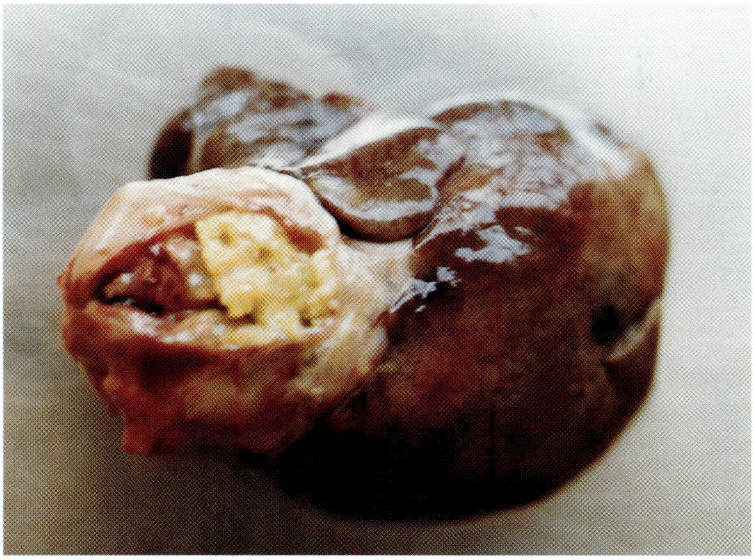

Canker nodule growing in the bile duct.

Canker can infect internal sites associated with the digestive tract, notably the bile duct, which drains bile from the liver into the bowel. Birds with internal canker nodules usually display non-specific signs of illness, including weight loss, lethargy, reluctance to eat and green diarrhoea. The final diagnosis is often made at autopsy. In lofts with a canker problem, it is usually best to include a daily Spartrix or Flagyl tablet in the treatment regime of an unwell bird in case this is the problem.

Sinus canker

Sometimes canker organisms can invade the sinuses through the slot in the roof of the mouth and form a canker nodule here. The birds present with a firm swelling across the forehead between the

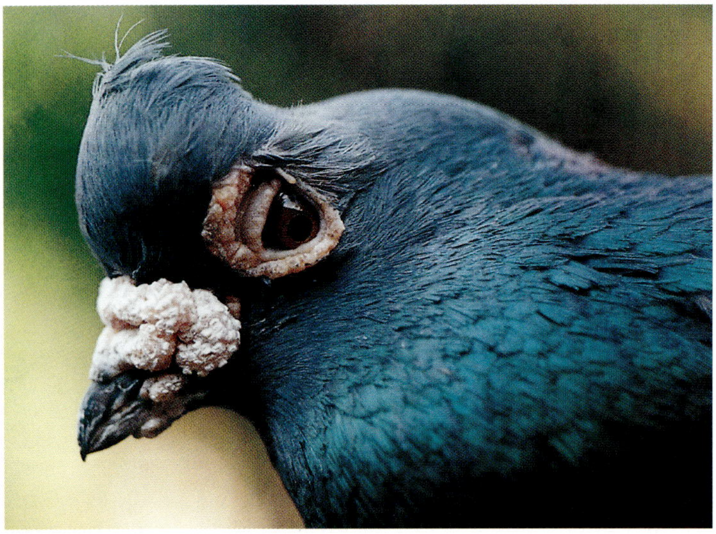

base of the cere and the eyes. Anticanker medication is given for 4 – 5 days to kill the active infection. After this, lancing the area by making an incision in the skin over the most prominent area of the nodule enables the canker nodule to be expressed. Once the nodule is removed, it is best to continue with anticanker medication for several days. Healing is usually uneventful.

A pigeon with a canker nodule in its sinus, before surgery.

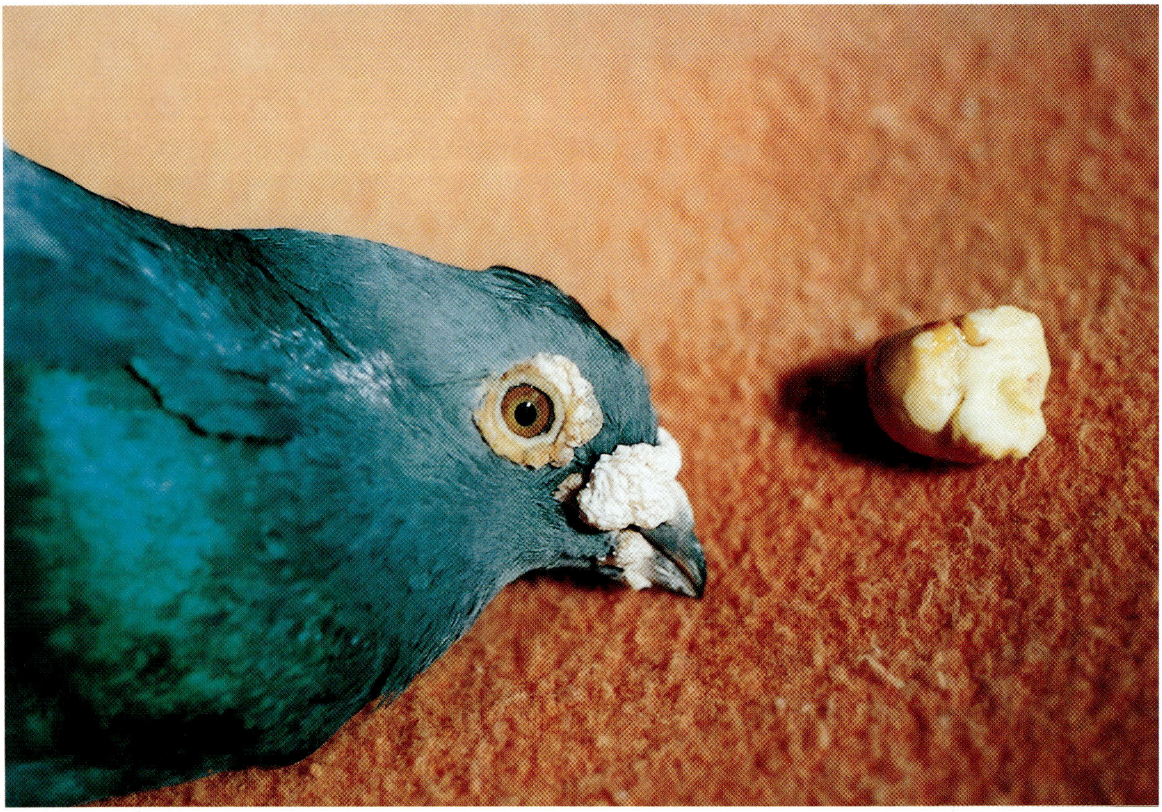

The same pigeon after surgery.

Other sites

It is important not to confuse infection in other parts of the body with canker. Trichomonads, partially because of their fragility, can only infect the digestive tract and associated structures. Pigeons are very restricted in their response to infection. Their white blood cells lack many of the enzymes (called lysosomes) that are normally found in mammals and therefore cannot produce pus. For this reason, no matter where the site of infection, the resultant reaction often looks like a canker infection. Bacterial (or other) infections of the skin, feet and eye, etc. for this reason are often confused with canker because of their appearance.

Medications Available

Any one of a group of medications called nitro imidazoles are effective against trichomonads. There are four commonly in use:

1 **Dimetradazole –** The common brand name here is Emtryl, available as a water-soluble powder. Dimetradazole was the first nitro imidazole available and is still an effective drug, although trichomonad resistance to it in some areas is a problem because it has been used for the longest. It must be used with care as it has a narrow safety margin. Overdose leads to a reversible loss of balance and coordination and, in high doses, death. The medication can interfere with sperm production in cocks, leading to a temporary infertility, and so is not recommended for use during breeding. The usual dose is 1 teaspoon (3 grams) to 4½ – 8 litres of water. Lower dose rates should be used in stock birds feeding youngsters and during hot weather when water intake increases and evaporation occurs from drinkers, increasing the concentration of the medication.

2 **Carnidazole –** The common brand name here is Spartrix. It is only available in tablet form. It has a wide safety margin and is very useful for individual bird dosing, particularly youngsters in the nest. The dose is one 10-mg tablet daily.

3 **Metronidazole –** The common brand name is Flagyl. This is available as a water-soluble syrup and as tablets in a variety of strengths. It is very economical, with the tablets being useful to dose individual birds. Individual birds are given ¼ of a 200-mg Flagyl tablet once daily. Flagyl syrup is water-soluble and is given at the dose of 5 – 10 ml per litre but is very sugary and not very palatable to the birds.

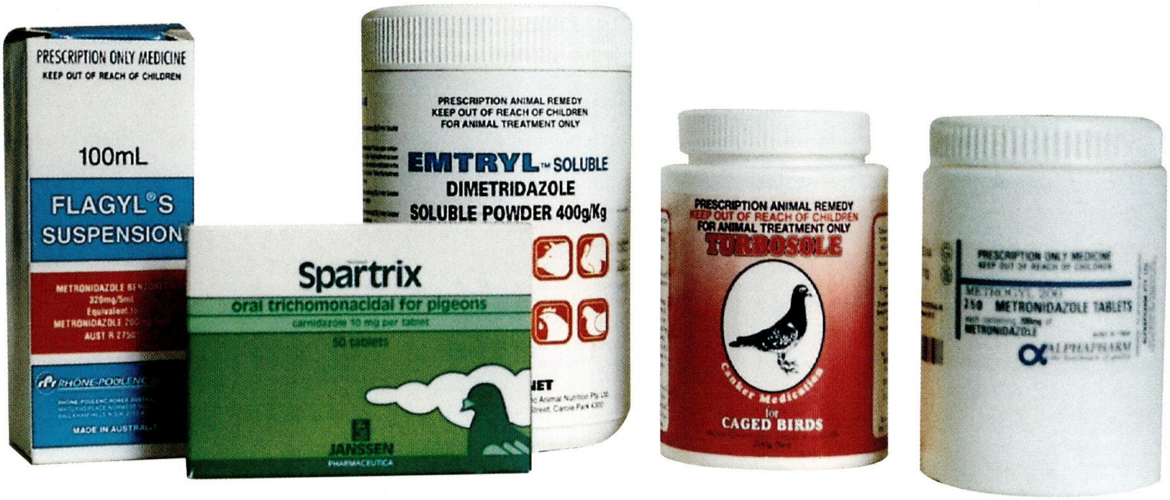

Canker medications as dispensed in Australia. From left to right, Flagyl suspension, Spartrix tablets, Emtryl powder, Turbosole powder and Metronidazole tablets.

4 **Ronidazole –** This is available as a water-soluble powder under a number of brand names world-wide, including Ridsol-S, Turbosole, Tricho-Plus and Ronivet. The usual strength used is 10%. The dose at this strength is ½ teaspoon per litre. Weaker preparations are available but the birds need to be treated longer with these. The drug is very bitter so preparations stronger than 10% tend to be unpalatable to the birds. It has a very wide safety margin and is safe to

use during breeding, racing and moulting. World-wide, ronidazole is the current medication of choice to treat canker. However, in some countries it is not available for use in pigeons, authorities being concerned that resistant organisms may develop. As the drug is used in food-producing animals such as pigs, its use is reserved for these.

In any canker-control program, it is often best to rotate between at least two of these medications in order to decrease the chance of a resistant trichomonad strain developing. Currently, ronidazole-based preparations are used as the primary treatment because of their effectiveness and wide safety margin, but it is a good idea to swap to one of the other available drugs every third or fourth treatment.

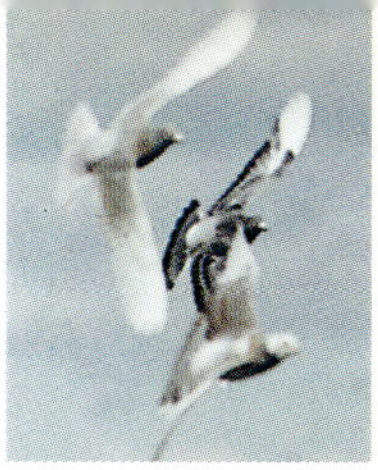

Chapter 5

THE PARASITIC DISEASES

There are many parasites that infect pigeons and I feel that it is beyond the scope of this book to discuss all of them in detail. The most important and most commonly encountered parasites are roundworm, hairworm, tapeworm, lice and mites and Coccidia.

Worms

Worms are a primary and serious parasite and it is important that they are completely eradicated for the birds to perform at their best. They weaken the bird, meaning that race performance cannot be optimal, and also increase vulnerability to other secondary diseases, such as canker and respiratory infection. There are three common intestinal worms – roundworm, hairworm and tapeworm.

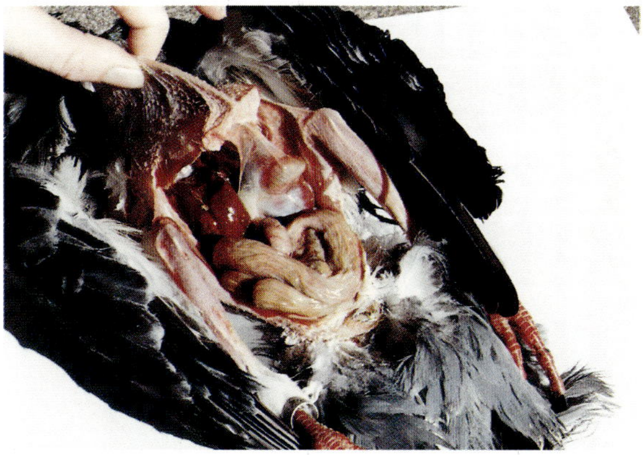

Above: Autopsy of a pigeon with a heavy roundworm burden. More than 300 roundworms were removed from this pigeon's bowel at autopsy and were the obvious cause of its emaciation. Here the thin-walled bowel can be seen stretched around the worms.

Roundworm and hairworm

These worms live in the digestive tract of the pigeon and release eggs, which are passed with the bird's droppings. After several days in the environment, these eggs become infective and, if then accidentally ingested by a pigeon, hatch inside it and grow into the new worm. In the loft, there is no easy way for the fancier to tell whether his birds have these parasites as the adult worms are only rarely passed in the droppings and indeed hairworms are microscopic. They are usually diagnosed by microscopic examination of a dropping sample, in which their eggs can be seen.

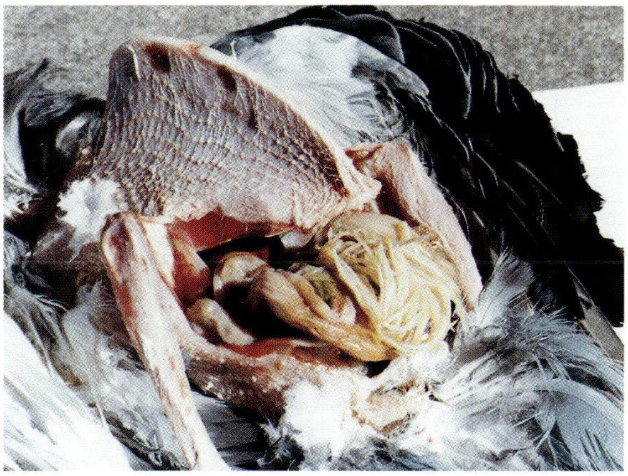

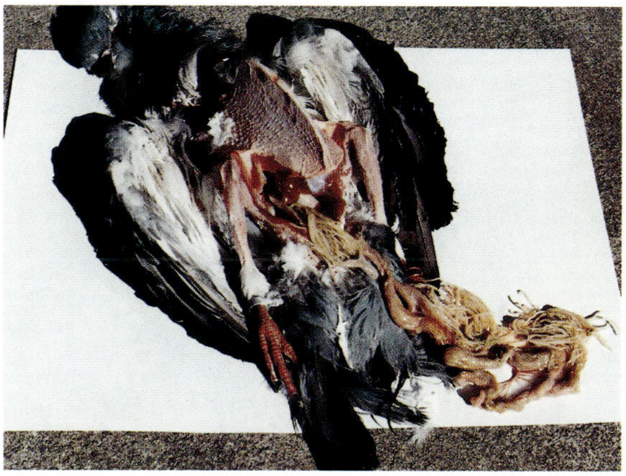

Above left and right: The bowel of the pigeon has been opened, revealing the worms.

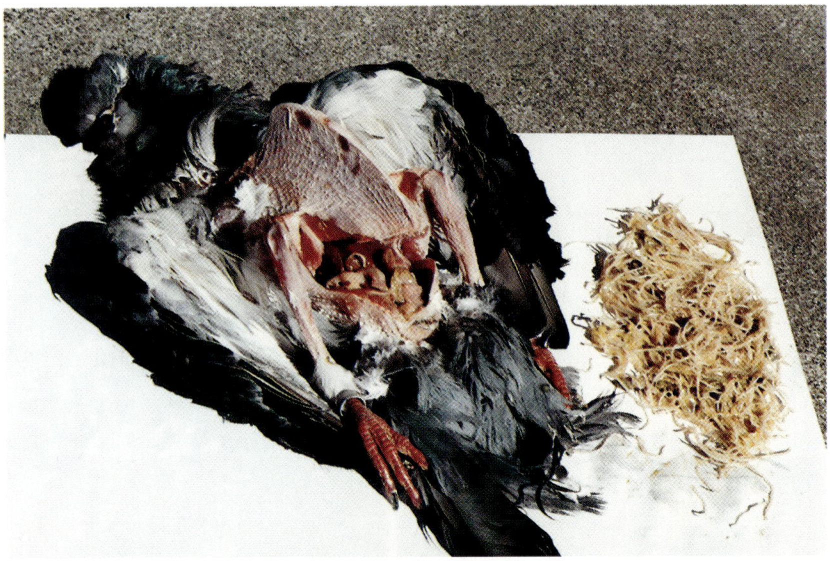

Left and below: When most worms are removed from the bowel, the full bulk of the worms is readily apparent. As few as six roundworms are sufficient to make a pigeon look unwell on the perch. None should be tolerated in a competing race bird.

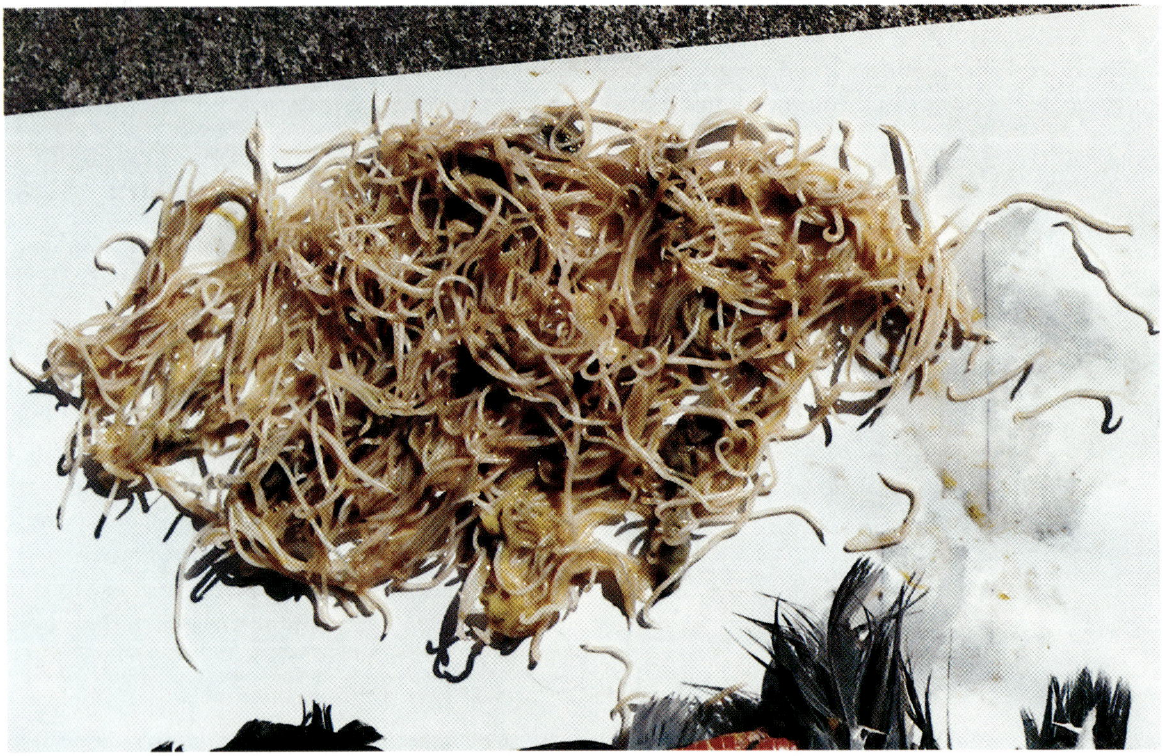

Treatment

I recommend Moxidectin to treat hairworm and roundworm. Moxidectin (2 mg/ml) is a clear fully water-soluble liquid that, when diluted in the drinking water, is readily taken by the birds. The dose is 5 ml per 1 litre of water for 24 hours. It has a wide safety margin and is perfectly safe to use during racing, breeding and, in particular, moulting. Moxidectin does not cause nausea and vomiting as many older worming preparations do and so the birds can be fed and loft-flown quite normally. Moxidectin also has the added advantage that it eliminates any external parasites that feed off body fluid. Mites in pigeons live off blood and so these are all cleared with Moxidectin. Lice live off feather debris and bloom and so in theory this drug should have no effect on them but in practice, during the 3 weeks following Moxidectin treatment, most lice also disappear. Moxidectin is also a safe and effective treatment for airsac mites at the usual dose given above.

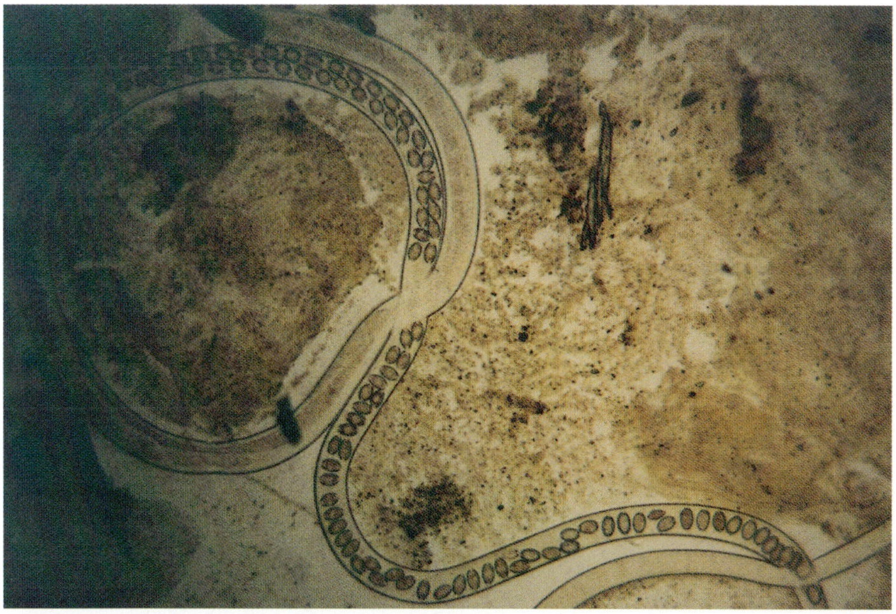

Pregnant hairworm, its body packed with eggs, magnified 40x under the microscope.

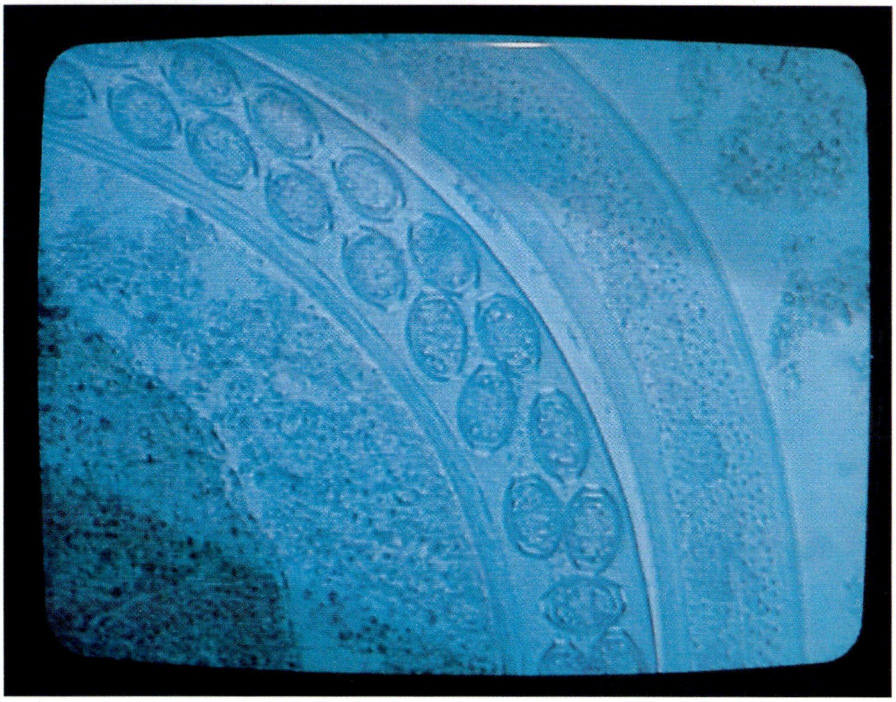

Same hairworm, magnified 100x. The characteristic hairworm eggs with their bipolar plugs are clearly visible in two rows in the parasite's body.

Control in the stock loft

The stock loft should be completely free of worms. The roundworm lifecycle can be completed in 3 – 4 weeks and so a single worming before breeding (or racing) will improve things for that period of time only. Eradication can be achieved by using Moxidectin twice at a 3-week interval, followed by a superthorough clean after each treatment. This removes droppings passed before medication, which may contain infective parasite eggs with the potential to reinfect the birds. It is a good idea to have the droppings rechecked 3 weeks after the second worming to ensure that the parasite has been cleared. Once these parasites have been cleared, worming any new bird before it goes into the stock loft should prevent reintroduction of worms. The dose of Moxidectin for a single bird is 0.25 ml of the neat liquid. If it is not possible to completely and thoroughly clean the loft, Moxidectin can be repeated every 3 weeks over a 6-month period as the longest that eggs can remain infective in the environment is 5 – 6 months. Worms can also re-enter the stock loft if the droppings of pigeons or doves outside the loft can enter. To prevent this, any external flight should either have a grid or suspended floor.

Control in the racing loft

It is important that the race team is free of worms before racing. The need to treat can be determined by a dropping analysis. In the absence of testing, it is better to assume that the birds are infected and treat twice at a 3-week interval followed by a thorough clean before the commencement of racing. With the commencement of Thursday night basketing, race unit reinfection can occur and so it is important that the droppings are regularly checked during racing to monitor this. If a positive result is returned, worming is usually done on the Sunday or Monday (when racing is on the Saturday). In the absence of testing, it is a good idea to give the birds 1 day Moxidectin every fourth week (usually on a Monday) to clear any roundworms or hairworms that might have been picked up in addition to any lice or mites that they might be carrying.

Tapeworm

Tapeworms also live in the pigeon's digestive tract. They have a head or scolex, which is embedded deeply into the lining of the pigeon's bowel. Behind this head mature segments, called proglottids, which are essentially packets of eggs. New segments are continuously forming behind the head, pushing maturing segments further and further away until eventually ribbons of segments trail behind the head down the bowel, with the most mature ones at the end. When fully mature, these egg packets snap free either singly or several at a time in ribbons before passing down the bowel and out with the droppings. The fancier will notice either a segmented white ribbon hanging from the pigeon's cloaca or, alternatively, as the segments are motile when passed, he may see small white segments wriggling within the droppings shortly after being passed or air-dried segments stuck to the surrounding perch. Tapeworms are therefore not a microscopic diagnosis because these segments can be seen with the naked eye. Different types of tapeworm vary in size. The small ones look like white pieces of cotton trailing through the dropping, larger ones look like pieces of rice stuck on the surface of the droppings, while the largest ones appear as whitish squares up to 0.5 cm x 0.5 cm. Once in the environment, the eggs inside these segments are ingested by insects. These eggs hatch into infective larvae in the insects. Pigeons become infected by eating these insects.

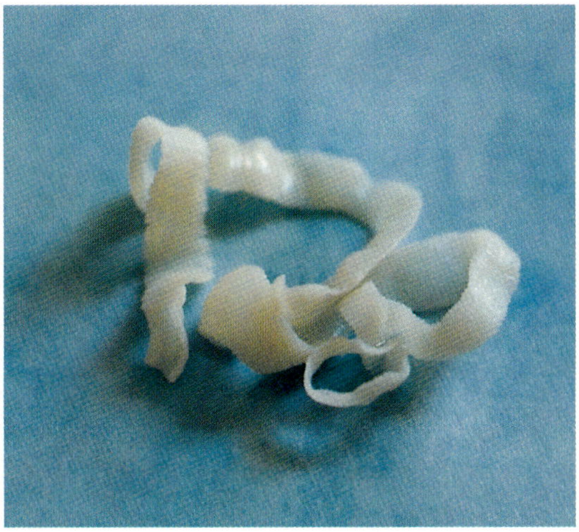

Above: Tapeworm.
Below: A tapeworm as passed with a bird dropping.

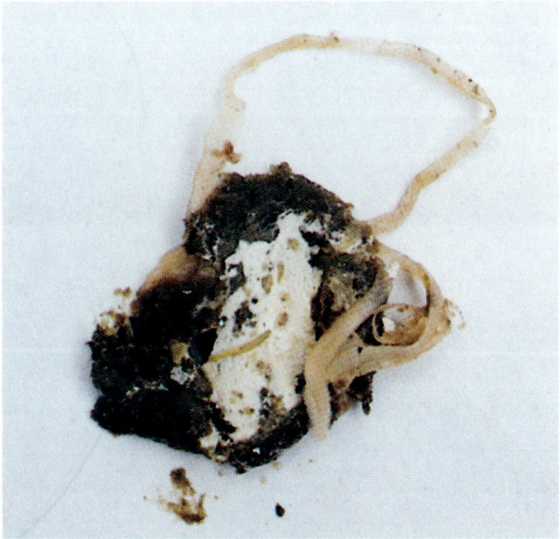

Treatment

For tapeworm eradication, I recommend Prazivet Solution. This is a new preparation that has many advantages over previously available treatments. It is fully water-soluble, meaning that birds do not have to be picked up individually and given tablets. It only needs to be made available for 24 hours, unlike other water-soluble preparations. It can also safely be given during racing, breeding, and, in particular, moulting. There is no need to remove food and the birds behave quite normally so that feeding and loft training can continue uninterrupted. It is also very cheap, costing less than 4 cents to treat each bird. The dose is 5 ml to 1 litre of water. Alternatively 0.25 ml of of the neat solution can be given to each bird. It's active constituent is praziquantel. Praziquantel tablets (Droncit) are also available for those fliers preferring to give tablets to individual birds.

A tapeworm's lifecycle can be completed as quickly as 21 days. This means that if a pigeon swallows an insect the day after worming, within 21 days it will have tapeworms again. It is therefore important to minimize the birds' exposure to insects. However, in the warmer northern areas of Australia where tapeworms are common, Prazivet can be given for 1 day every 3 – 4 weeks. Weevils are one of the insects that can carry tapeworm and so seed that either has or has had weevils in it (look for the little bored holes) must be avoided. Within the loft, slaters are the most common insect carrying tapeworm. When disturbed, slaters roll themselves into balls, which I think pigeons mistake for peas, because these balls are a similar size and colour. To prevent reinfection, it is therefore best to spray out the loft with Permethrin Solution simultaneously with a Prazivet treatment. Permethrin has a residual effect for 4 months.

Lice and mites

The two most common external parasites of pigeons are lice and mites. Lice live their entire lifecycle on the bird, dying quickly once they are off the bird. They live off feather debris and bloom. Mites, on the other hand, drink blood and other body fluids and not only live on the pigeon but also in cracks and crevices throughout the loft and, in particular during the breeding season, below nest bowls and within nesting material, only moving onto the birds and nestlings at night to feed.

These differences mean that, to control mites, the loft must be sprayed at the same time as the birds are treated, while this is not necessary with lice.

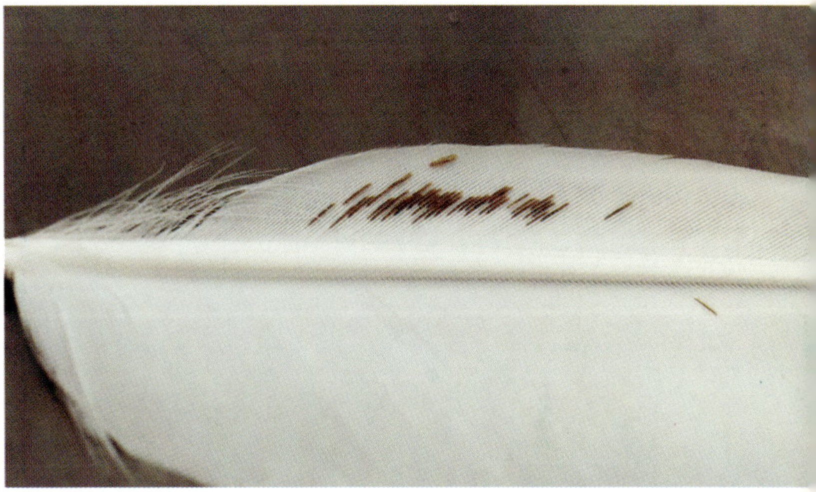

Above: Common pigeon lice clustered on the vane of a flight feather. *Below left and right:* Lice and mites on the flights of a pigeon. The cigarette-shaped lice are visible in the vanes of the feather. Lice and mites are clustered against the quills.

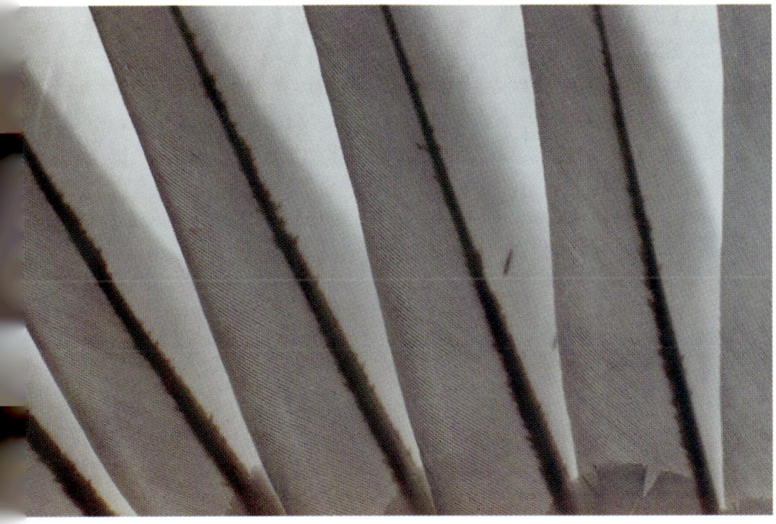

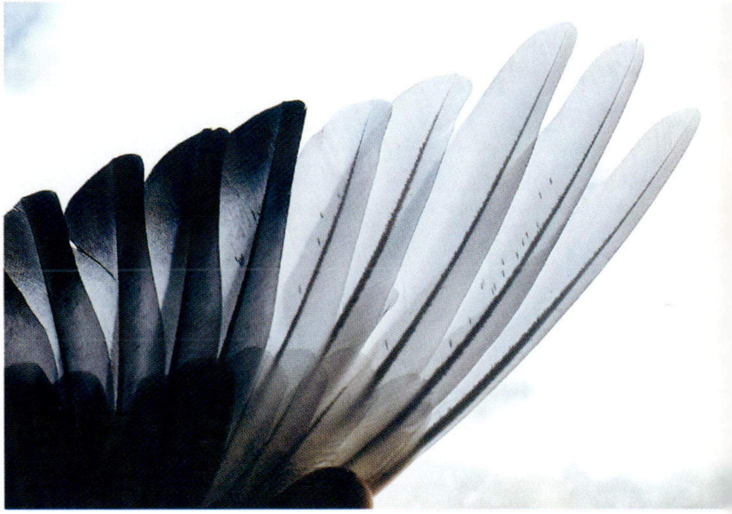

These differences also mean that avermectins, like Moxidectin, will work well against mites but only have limited action against lice. An insecticide is used to dip or spray the birds when lice are a problem and also to spray the loft for mites.

Treatment

Permethrin is the insecticide of choice. Permethrin is a synthetic pyrethroid and is used to treat lice and mites. Pyrethroids are plant-origin insecticides, which are very effective but very safe for use in pigeons. Permethrin Solution is used in the following three situations:

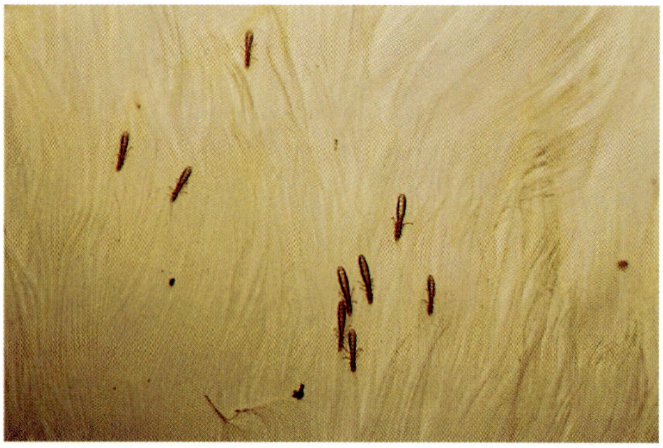

Lice on the surface of feathers.

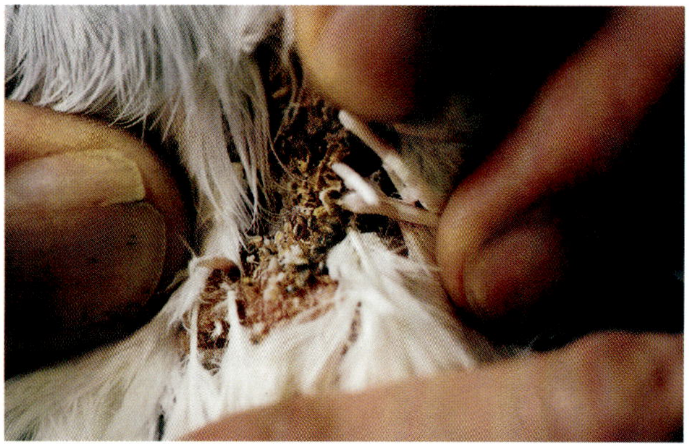

Golden or Large body lice grouped on the skin of a pigeon's abdomen. Their presence and the irritation they cause leads to dried skin flakes and discharge accumulating on the skin.

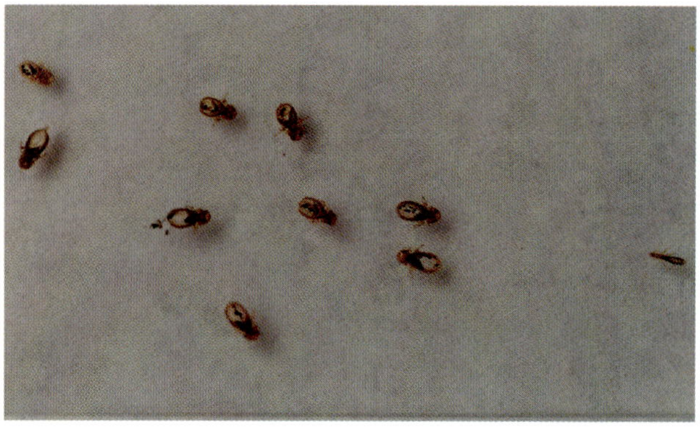

Close-up of nine Golden body lice on the left and a single Common louse on the right.

1 **To dip birds to eradicate lice –** Fill a bucket, diluting 10 – 20 ml Permethrin to 1 litre of water. Use warm water and treat the birds in the morning of a warm day. Add half a teaspoon of soap flakes to act as a wetting agent. Immerse birds up to their neck, fanning their wings and tail through the solution. Momentarily dip their heads below the surface. Addition of the wetting agent enables complete penetration by the Permethrin. Immediately after being dipped, the birds are completely drenched, with the feathers collapsing on themselves to expose their skin, but within 2 hours return to normal appearance. Permethrin does not remove the birds' bloom and has a residual effect for up to 4 months.

2 **To spray the loft –** This is done in conjunction with Prazivet treatment to kill any insects in the loft that might be carrying any tapeworm and also to eradicate mites in conjunction with a Moxidectin treatment. It is also done before breeding to eliminate mosquitoes, flies and, in particular, red mite. Birds are removed from the section, which is then scraped clean. Permethrin is diluted 10 – 20 ml to 1 litre and sprayed onto the clean scraped surfaces and into any nooks and crannies. The loft will dry in 1 – 2 hours and the birds allowed to re-enter.

3 **To treat individual birds –** It is a good idea to have some diluted Permethrin mixed and ready to use in a spray bottle. Any introduced birds can be quickly sprayed before being placed in the loft as can any late returning race birds. The usual dilution used is also 10 – 20 ml to 1 litre.

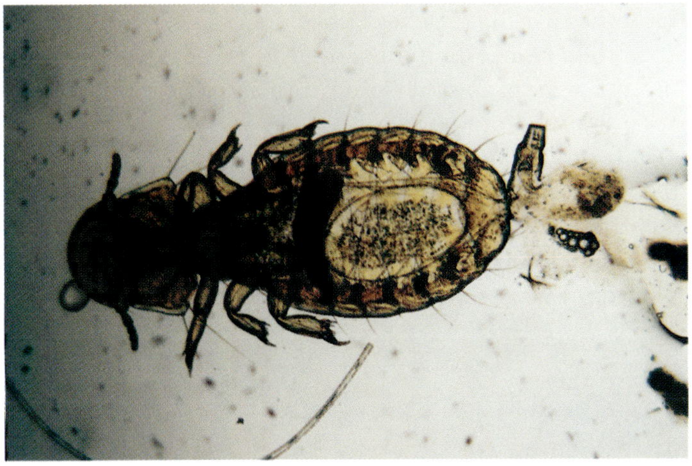

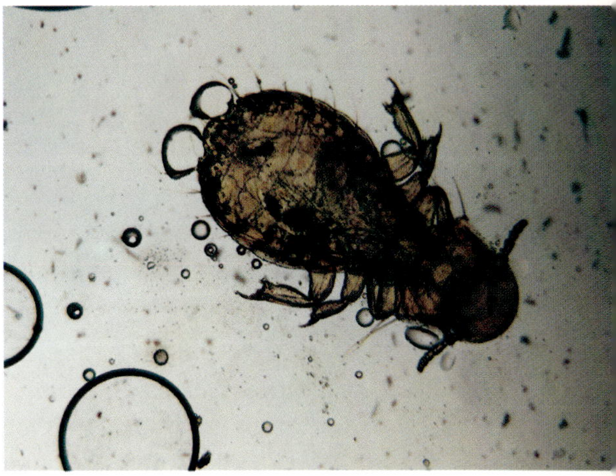

Above left and right: Microscopic picture of Golden body lice. The larger of the two is pregnant, containing a single large egg.

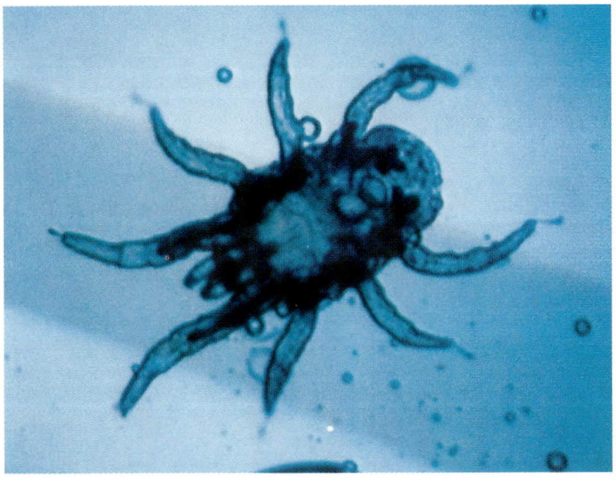

Left: Microscopic picture of a mite. Adult lice and mites are easy to distinguish. Lice are true insects and have six legs, whereas mites are actually 'little spiders' and have eight legs. It is important to distinguish between the two because, for mites, easy-to-use oral avermectins such as Moxidectin are effective, whereas heavy lice infestation requires spraying or dipping of the birds. Also, mites can live in the birds' environment where lice cannot, and so to control mites, the loft also has to be treated (i.e. sprayed).

In summary, for mites either treat the birds with Moxidectin or spray or dip them with Permethrin and at the same time spray the loft, while for lice just dip or spray the birds.

Coccidia

Coccidia are fascinating organisms. They can infect not only pigeons, and in fact all birds, but also dogs, cats, sheep, pigs, cows and a range of other animals. They are, however, very species-specific so that it is only pigeon Coccidia that can infect pigeons and, for example, only sparrow Coccidia that infect sparrows. There are, however, several types that can infect each animal. The most common Coccidia type in pigeons is called *Eimeria* spp.

Animals become infected by swallowing the organism's eggs. All Coccidia once swallowed replicate in the cells of the host, in the process causing extensive damage. In pigeons, this occurs in the lining of the bowel. After multiplying here, the newly produced eggs are passed in the droppings. When initially passed, the eggs (oocysts) are thin-shelled and contain a spherical body, which looks granular, called a sporoblast. The sporoblast is an amorphous blob of protoplasm. Once in the environment, the sporoblast within the bigger egg develops into several smaller eggs called sporocysts (there are four in *Eimeria*), which in turn each contain a number of structures called sporozoites (there are two in *Eimeria*). Once this has happened, the egg is said to be sporolated. It is not until this has happened that the egg is infective if swallowed. This process usually takes 4 – 5 days but depends on temperature and humidity. Once an infective (i.e. sporolated) egg is swallowed, the sporozoites hop out and burrow into the wall of the bowel. They at first multiply asexually in the bowel cells but then develop into the equivalent of male and female gametes, which then 'mate' to produce further eggs (oocysts), which rupture back through the bowel lining before being passed in the dropping, thus completing the lifecycle.

The significance of Coccidia for us as pigeon racers is that, as the Coccidia multiplies in the bowel lining, it damages it, interfering with it doing its job of digestion properly. This is complicated by the fact that each time an egg ruptures back into the bowel from the lining, it causes a microscopic 'pin prick', allowing the bird's blood, electrolytes and protein to be lost.

This weakens the birds and interferes with the absorption of vital nutrients. Severely affected birds develop greenish diarrhoea, are lethargic, thirsty and lose weight. Race birds with even the slightest infection are not able to give of their best.

In most lofts, a low level of infection is present and out of the racing season is regarded as normal, serving to maintain the flock's level of immunity. In two situations, the organism can increase in number and cause clinical problems:

1 **As a primary disease, where there are flaws in loft management or design that lead to high exposure to the organism –** The loft must be clean and dry. A build-up in the loft is prevented by regular cleaning with particular attention to the drinkers and hoppers. There is no place for wetness in a healthy loft; it not only enables the Coccidia egg to become infective more quickly, but promotes bacterial infection.

2 **As a secondary disease, where other factors weaken the bird, enabling the Coccidia to increase in number and cause clinical disease –** Such factors may be other concurrent disease, such as worms, or alternatively overcrowding, excessive tossing, poor nutrition, etc.

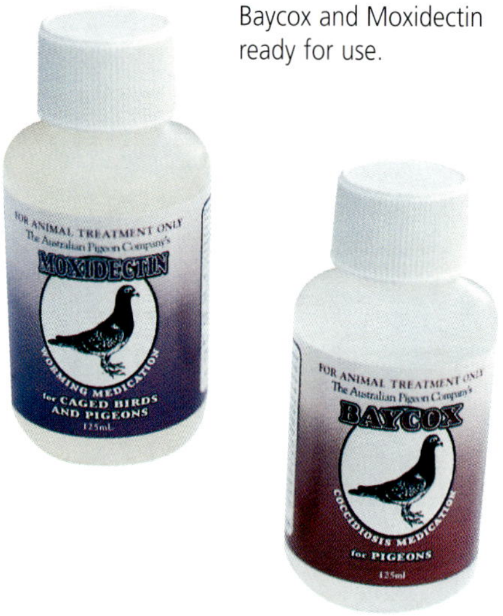

Baycox and Moxidectin ready for use.

Treatment

Coccidia should always be suspected where loose droppings appear, particularly in young birds or following wet periods or heavy training. Diagnosis is through faecal examination under a microscope. The best drug to use is Baycox, which acts entirely within the bowel. It does not interfere with race form and can therefore be safely used during racing. It can also be used safely during breeding and moulting. The dose is 1 ml per 2 litres of water for 2 – 3 days. Avoid medicating if you believe your birds do not have coccidiosis.

Monitoring of coccidial counts by faecal examination (I suggest every 4 weeks) through the race season is a good indicator of the team's form. Birds with elevated counts will benefit from a course of Baycox. In faecal samples from perfectly fit birds, no coccidial eggs are seen.

Other parasites

Other less common parasites that the fancier might encounter are pigeon flies, scaly leg mites and *Hexamita*.

Pigeon flies

Have you ever seen a row of holes on a pigeon's flight feather? These are caused by a special type of fly called *Pseudolynchia canariensis.* The adults live on the body of the bird, scurrying between the feathers. They are blood suckers, with their bites causing pain, irritation and restlessness. They will insert their feeding tube into a blood-filled growing feather follicle to feed. As this feather unfurls, the tunnel created by the feeding tube unravels into a series of holes.

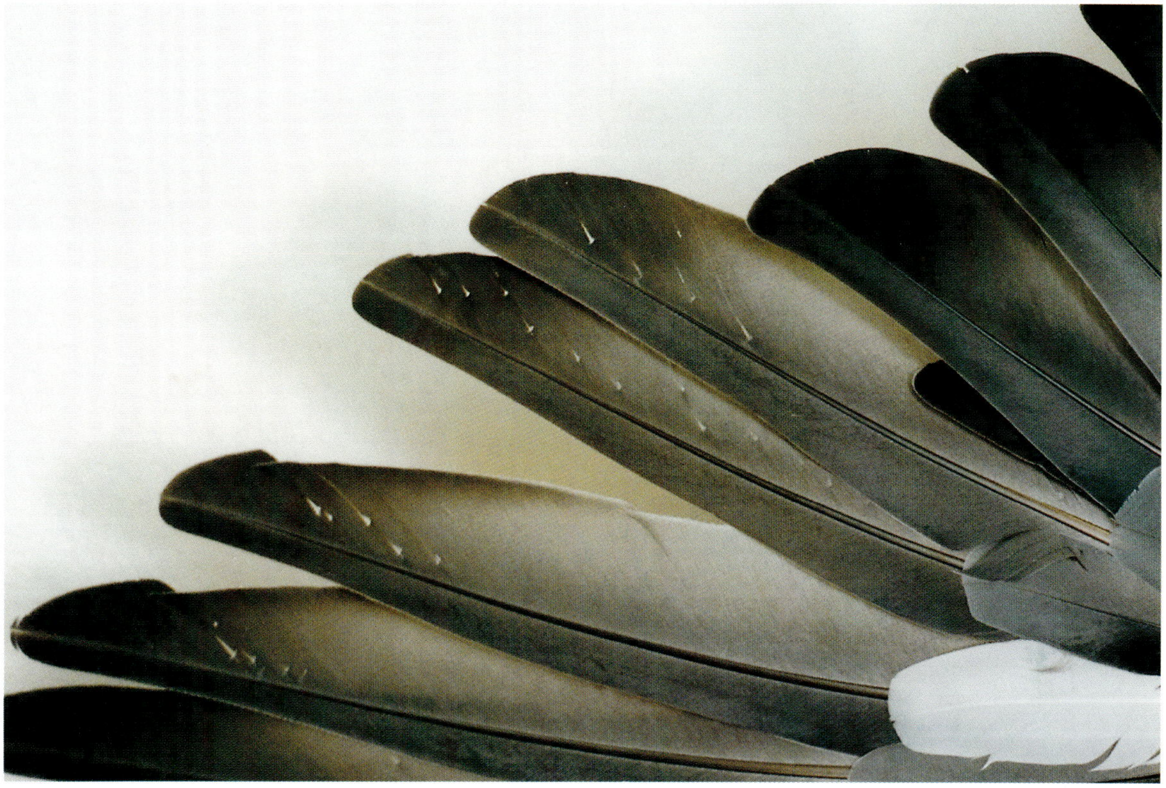

Above: Damage to flight feathers caused by pigeon fly.

Left: Pigeon flies. Note their long wings.

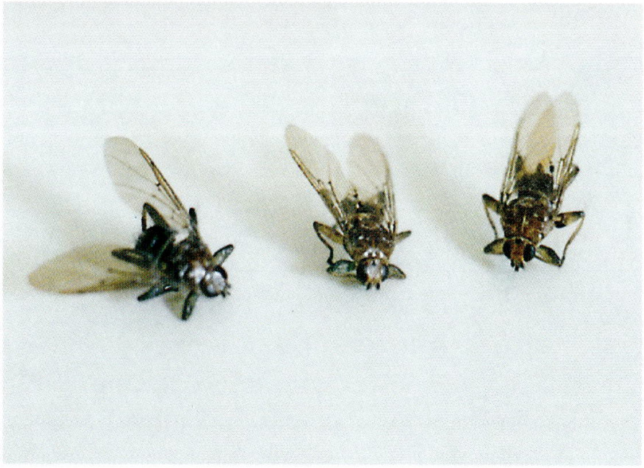

The flies lay their eggs on accumulated pigeon droppings and their maggots develop here. Fly numbers are highest during the warmer months when the birds are breeding when they can bite nestlings and breed in the droppings around nest bowls. Interestingly, the saliva of the adult flies gives the nestlings diarrhoea, which makes it easier for the maggots to survive.

Treatment

On-going hygiene and efficient disposal of droppings (remembering that accumulated droppings below a grid floor or piled in the garden near the loft can serve as breeding grounds) will do much to control the problem. However, if necessary, any flies on the birds can be killed by either spraying the birds with Permethrin or treating them with a 24-hour course of Moxidectin. Coupling this with spraying the loft with Permethrin, particularly before breeding, will solve the problem.

Scaly leg mites

Some mites, e.g. *Cnemidocoptes mutans*, will actually burrow into the skin of a pigeon's feet. They lay their eggs in the tunnels they create and leave little breathing tubes connected to the surface. This irritation causes the skin of the feet to become thickened and scaly. At any one time, the mites can also be found on other parts of the body, in particular on the wing butts, around the face and on the skin over the abdomen. Even though the mites are infectious, only certain birds seem vulnerable so that not all birds in the team will be infected.

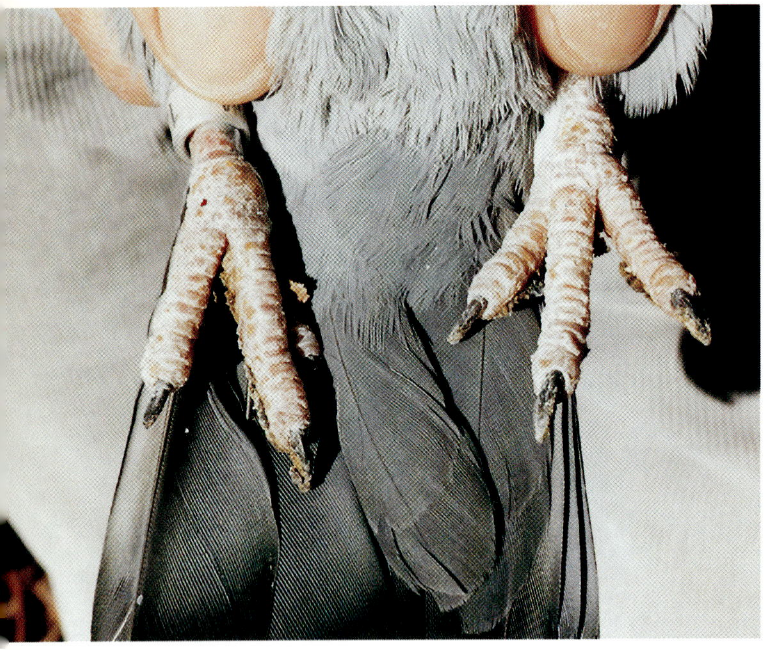

An early case of scaly mite infestation.

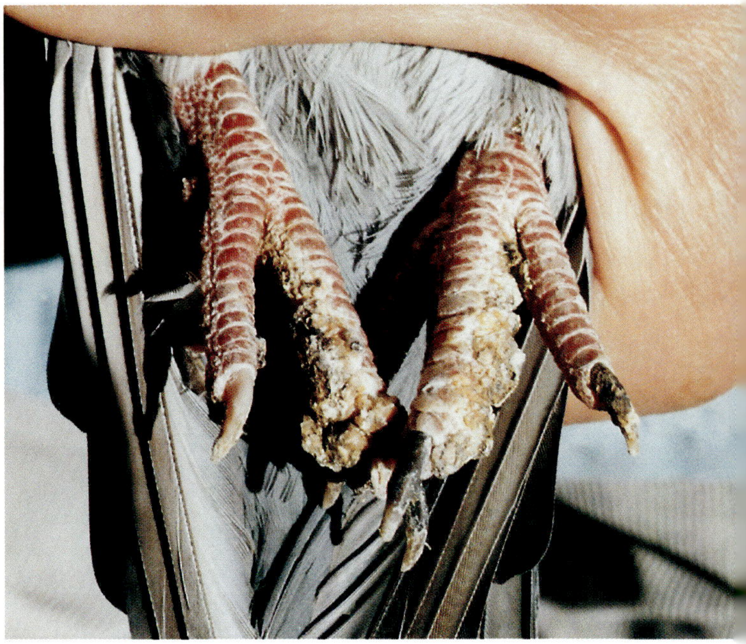

A more advanced case of scaly mite infestation.

Treatment

The best treatment is to give all birds a simultaneous 24-hour course of Moxidectin. It is important not to confuse scaly leg mite infestation with the thickened crusty growths that occur on the feet of some birds with age.

Hexamita

Hexamita is an organism closely related to the organism that causes canker. It lives primarily in the bowel and in high numbers can cause diarrhoea. It is diagnosed by microscopic examination of a fresh faecal smear, in which it looks just like a canker organism but appears slightly more elongated and moves faster and more purposefully. Well-cared-for, non-stressed pigeons can carry low-level infections asymptomatically. However, *Hexamita* should be totally eradicated in any racing pigeon loft to ensure that the birds give their best.

Treatment

Any medication that kills canker also kills *Hexamita*. However, *Hexamita* needs to be treated for longer. Usually, a continuous 7-day course of a drug such as Turbosole is given simultaneously to all birds in the loft. The organism cannot survive in the environment and so reinfection from the loft is not a concern. Treating all birds simultaneously for 7 days therefore ensures eradication. It is always worthwhile doing a follow-up dropping test to ensure its removal.

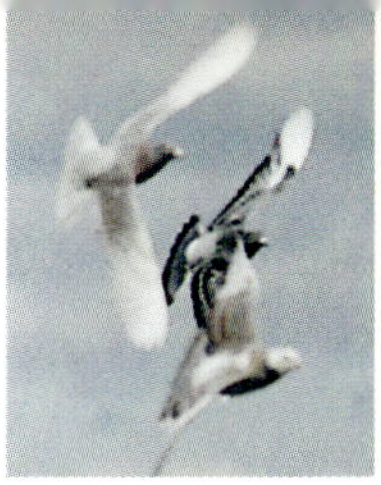

Chapter 6

DID YOU KNOW?

- The average weight of a racing pigeon is 400 grams.
- Pigeons drink on average 45 ml of water per day (range 20 – 60 ml).
- Cocks have two testicles but hens have only one ovary.
- Pigeons eat on average one-tenth of their body weight in grain daily, i.e. 40 grams (range 20 – 100 grams).
- Pigeons have several kidneys on either side of their abdominal cavity.
- Pigeon milk is not actually milk at all but is mainly composed of superficial cells, packed with fats and other nutrients, that flake from the surface of specialized areas of the crop lining.
- Pigeon feet resemble reptile feet because, like all birds, pigeons are direct descendants of the dinosaurs.
- Plucking a feather is more painful for a pigeon than cutting the skin.
- Pigeons have special glands in their eyelids that produce a mucus that makes their tears stick to the front of the eye. This means that they can fly at the speeds they do even in hot conditions without the surface of the eyes drying. This would be analogous to us having our head outside the car while it was going at 60 km/h, facing the breeze and not blinking.

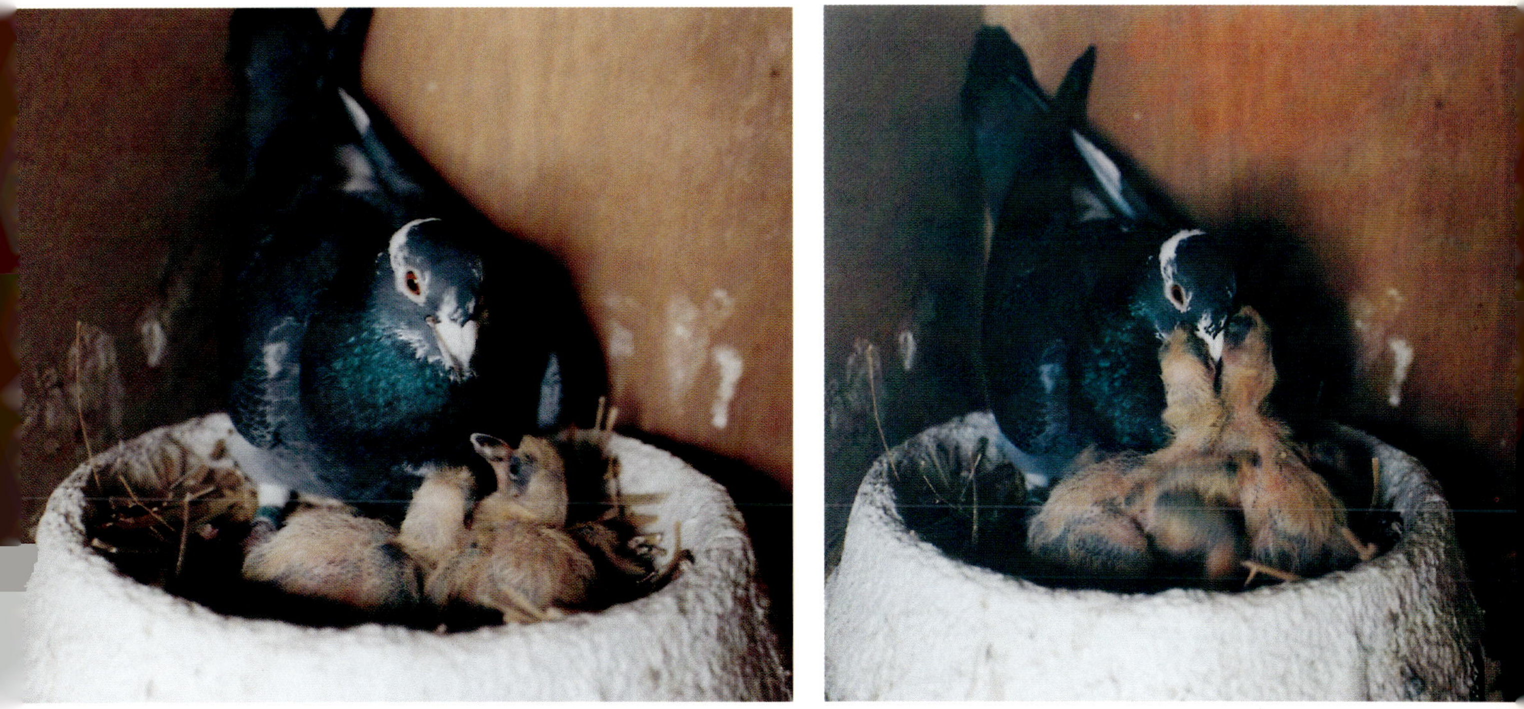

Race cock feeding his nestlings.

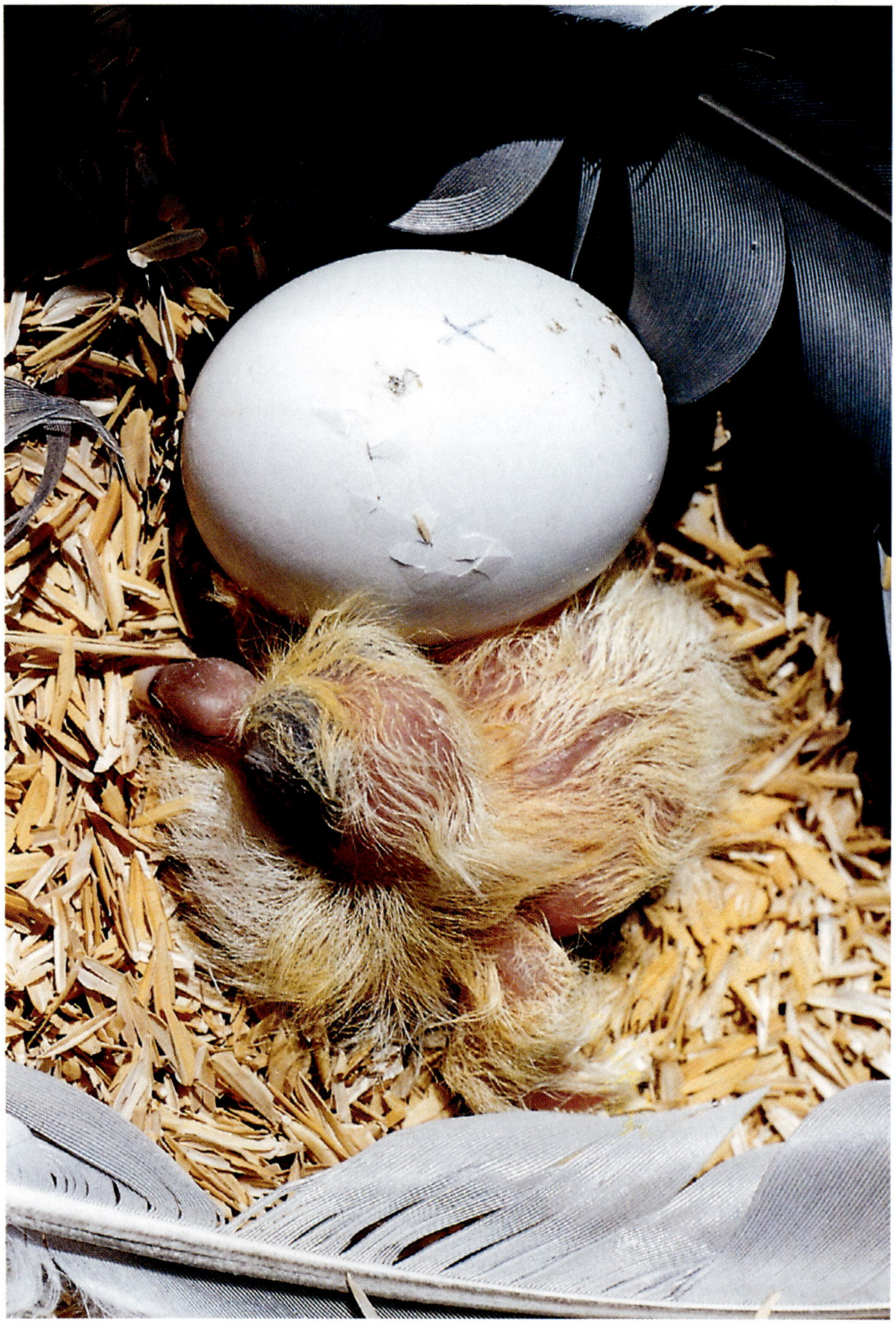

The moment of hatching. One youngster has hatched and the second egg is 'pipping'. The cross on the egg is an identification marker.

- A pigeon's body temperature is 41.8°C.
- With age, some hens behave and look like cocks because the outer hormone-producing layer of their ovary wastes away.
- A pigeon's blood volume is on average 32 ml.
- Pigeons only have muscles in the lower of the two main eyelids.
- If you shine a light in one eye of a pigeon, it will come out the other eye – only a fine bone plate separates the two eyes.
- A pigeon's pulse rate is 140 – 400 beats per minute.

- Blind pigeons can still find their way home. In experiments in which pigeons were temporarily blinded by putting black discs over the surface of the eyes, the birds still homed from 80 miles. It seems that vision is only necessary for the final approach to the loft.
- The bright colour of the iris in the eye is due to tiny fat droplets, which reflect light. When the bird is ill, these fat droplets are absorbed and the colour becomes duller.
- A pigeon's eyelashes are actually little feathers.
- Pigeons, like other birds, have a unique and bizarre structure called the pecten, which sits on the top of the optic nerve in the back of the eye. It is thought to improve vision clarity or to aid in long-distance navigation.
- Testicle size is not constant. Testicles increase up to tenfold in size at the start of Spring in preparation for breeding.
- Fresh air enters a pigeon's lungs when it both breathes in and breathes out. When a pigeon breathes in, some air goes into its lungs and some air goes into its back airsacs. When it breathes out, the air in the lungs moves into the front airsacs while the air in the back airsacs, which is still fresh, moves into the lungs. This makes for an extremely efficient respiratory system and is part of the reason why pigeons can out-exercise horses, greyhounds and men, with fit birds being able to beat their wings for hours without fatigue.
- The yolk, which is essentially a ball of yellow slime with a single cell sitting on its surface, develops into a chick in only 18 days.
- In pigeons, the lungs connect with the cavities of some bones, including the bones of the wings, legs, shoulders, spine and ribs. If a pigeon's wing is broken and the broken bone sticks out through the skin, it can breathe through this if its mouth and nose are taped shut.
- When a pigeon breathes in, the top of its windpipe moves up and almost sucks onto the slot (choana) in the roof of the mouth.
- If a pigeon can't move its ribs, as can happen if held too tightly, it will suffocate in under 1 minute.
- A pigeon's vision is very sensitive to colour and movement. When we look at the face of a watch, we can only see the second hand moving, while experiments have shown that pigeons can also detect the movement of the hour hand. Similarly, experiments have shown an amazing sensitivity to colour. If people are shown the colour purple and also the colour pink, and then a gradation of intermediate shades from purple to pink and from pink to purple, eventually a midpoint is reached where the two mixtures are perceived as identical. At this point, pigeons can still detect six more changes in tone.

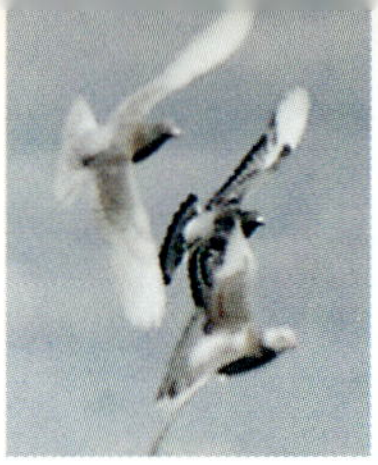

Chapter 7

RESPIRATORY INFECTION

If you ask any experienced flier what health problem he fears the most, then if it is the breeding season he will probably say canker, but if it is the race season he will probably say respiratory infection. Respiratory diseases are very common in pigeons. They are the major cause of poor performance and pigeon loss during the race season. Young birds under stress are most at risk of contracting respiratory diseases, although healthy old birds can fall ill when exposed to respiratory diseases in the race basket. Race birds with respiratory infection can be difficult to detect and yet, like a human athlete with flu, cannot compete. When some fanciers talk about respiratory infection, they give the impression that they are discussing a single problem and, yet, several organisms can be involved and often simultaneously. Clinical respiratory infection in pigeons is the end result of the interplay of a number of factors but, in particular, the type of infective organism and the vulnerability of the birds to infection are important. The respiratory system can be infected by *Chlamydia*, *Mycoplasma*, bacteria (in particular *E. coli*), fungi, viruses and mites. The control of some of these starts, in certain lofts, not only before racing and not even during breeding, but right before the stock birds are paired.

Stress is always a big factor. The vulnerability of the pigeon is affected by what stress it is under. Stress weakens the bird, enabling infective organisms to cause clinical disease. The control of respiratory disease is therefore two-pronged.

1 **Control of any predisposing stress factors –** These can take the form of :
   - **(a)** Environmental triggers, e.g. dampness, overcrowding, low hygiene,
   - **(b)** Management triggers, e.g. poor feeding, excessive tossing, or
   - **(c)** Concurrent disease, in particular parasitism. This includes wet canker. The combination of either worms or elevated trichomonad levels and respiratory disease is very common.

The fancier must establish a healthy loft environment, otherwise respiratory disease will continually recur, despite medication.

2 **Correct use of appropriate drugs to either eradicate or keep the organism level low so that disease does not occur.**

The organisms that infect the respiratory system and how they are controlled are set out below.

Chlamydia

Chlamydia is a microorganism that is found within the system of many pigeons all the time. There are many strains, which vary tremendously in their capacity to cause disease. Lofts tend to have resident strains to which those birds, often through their on-going exposure, have developed an immunity. In such lofts, it is only when the birds are stressed that the *Chlamydia* is able to flare up and cause disease. It is through contact with other birds (strays, in race units, new introductions) that new and potentially nastier strains gain entry to the loft. Control of *Chlamydia* is, therefore, double-barrelled and involves the control of stress to avoid resident *Chlamydia* strains flaring up together with the prevention of new chlamydial strains entering the loft.

Control of stress to avoid chlamydial strains, already in the loft, flaring up

A subsequent chapter deals with what constitutes stress and how to avoid it, but essentially this involves on-going good care with good management practices, a good loft environment and control of other diseases, notably the parasitic diseases. Any problem that weakens the birds makes them vulnerable to a chlamydial flare-up. Sometimes, however, despite the best possible care, because the strain of *Chlamydia* in the loft is virulent or the family of pigeons is particularly vulnerable (as with some European strains), it becomes necessary to medicate the birds through stressful times to prevent chlamydial flare-ups and the resultant clinical disease. The particular times when these flare-ups are more likely to occur are during breeding, after weaning and during the racing season.

Breeding

Stress for a stock bird is breeding. Stressed stock birds will shed the organisms in their droppings, saliva and eggs. If the *Chlamydia* is in the egg, the developing embryo is weakened and can either die during incubation, during the hatching process or as a nestling or, if it survives, be a retarded youngster. In a nestbox heavily contaminated with *Chlamydia*, the developing youngsters become weakened and die. If these things have happened in earlier years, and breeding has commenced, it is too late to treat the stock birds. However, medication (usually doxycycline) can be given before mating to decrease the level of *Chlamydia* in the stock birds' system. This means that they will then require more stress before they start to shed the organism.

The length of treatment depends on the need, usually 7 – 30 days. If your loft has a history of chlamydial problems during breeding, a prebreeding doxycycline course is a good idea. *Chlamydia* can be completely cleared with a 30 – 45-day course of doxycycline. However, this is rarely done because the weaned youngsters will be exposed to the organism later in life and may in fact be more vulnerable to illness through this lack of exposure and the resultant low level of natural immunity. Doxycycline, like other antibiotics, causes disruption of the normal bowel bacteria, interfering with vitamin metabolism and calcium absorption. It is therefore important that preventive courses are completed several

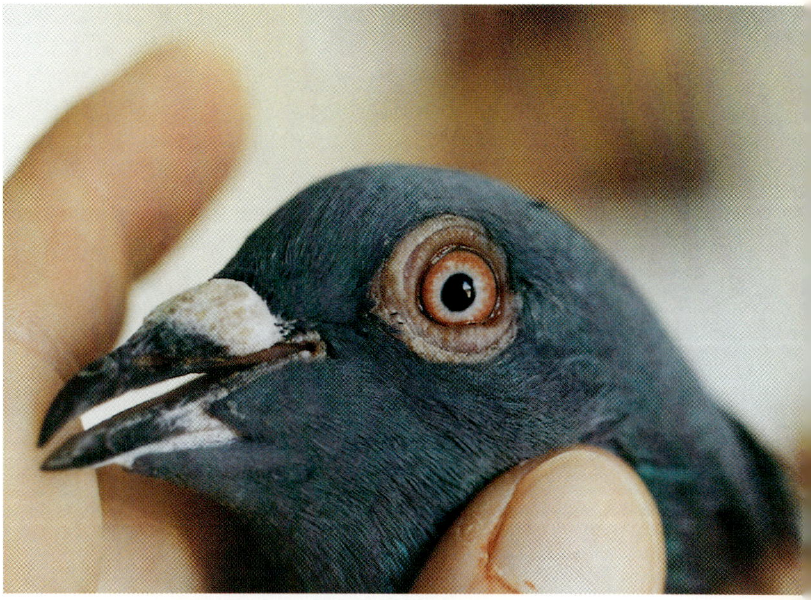

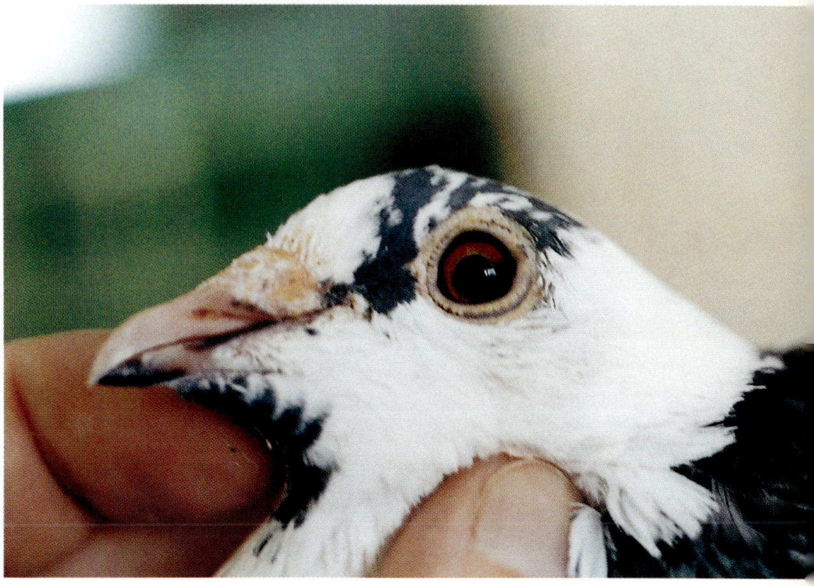

Birds with mild respiratory infection, with discharge from sinuses staining the cere. Inflammatory material from the sinuses flows under the cere through the slot in the roof of the mouth into the back of the throat. As it does this, the cere acts a bit like a sponge, absorbing material and becoming stained.

weeks before pairing and there is benefit in giving the birds probiotics, vitamins and calcium supplements following them.

After weaning

The next vulnerable time is the postweaning period, when both weaning and moulting are the underlying stresses. In Victoria, Australia, January to May are the respiratory months. Most lofts contain large numbers of young birds having just had the stress of weaning and now having the stress of moulting, coupled with young bird tossing and racing. It is a time of high humidity and fluctuating temperature, conditions that favour respiratory disease. Between 1 December and 1 March (the usual time that the last youngsters are weaned in many lofts in Australia), fanciers must monitor the youngsters, in particular, for signs of 'one-eye cold', dirty wattles or sneezing. However, green watery droppings, failure to thrive, shortness of breath and a reluctance to fly may also be indicative of the problem.

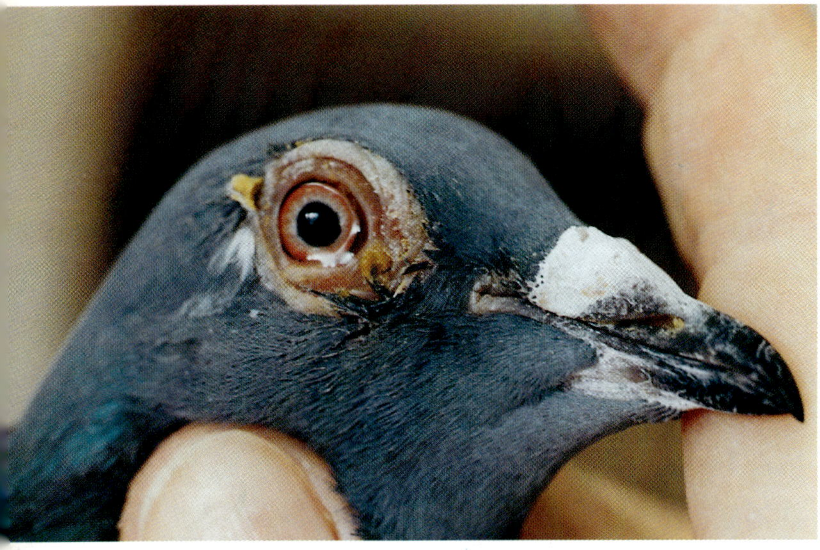

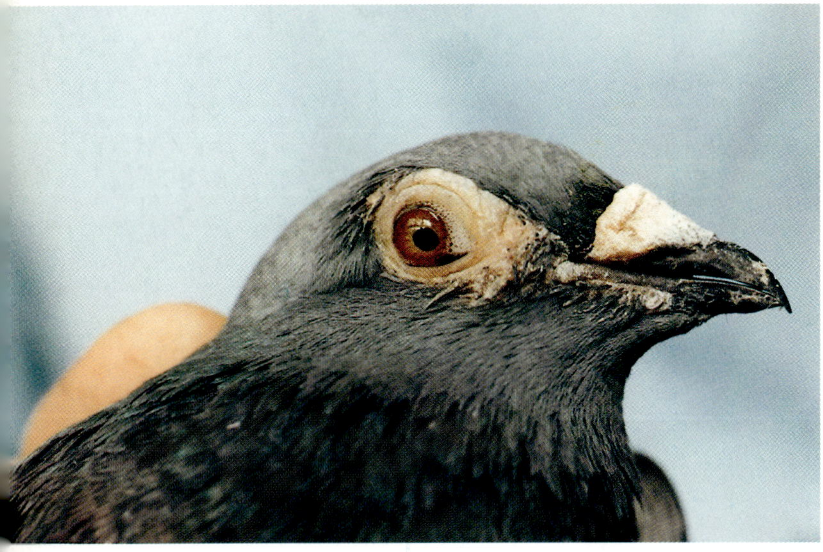

Birds with more severe respiratory infection. The eye has become involved. With irritation, excessive tears are produced, more than can flow down the tear duct, leading to 'wet eye'. The continual blinking action sometimes whips this fluid into a froth, as in the bird in the second photo. Some tears overflow the eyelid margin and dry to form yellow material stuck to the feathers around the eye.

Because of the disruption to normal bowel bacteria caused by the antibiotics, which can compromise feather quality and check development, and also because of the interference with development of a natural immunity, it is important that only the birds that need medication should receive it. If only a small number are affected, they may be treated individually with doxycycline (Vibravet 50 mg, 1/2 tablet once daily) or Baytril (3 drops twice daily). Once on medication, they stop shedding the organism and so there is no need to isolate them. If one bird has become unwell while the others are okay, it is often a reflection on its vigour. If such a bird fails to respond quickly or relapses, it is unlikely to go on and make a competitive race bird and is often best eliminated. If more than 5 – 10% of young birds are affected, with fresh cases daily, then all should be treated. Usually doxycycline 12% (1/2 teaspoon per litre for 3 – 5 days) is used. However, such a situation represents a major flaw in the birds' environment or management and the longer-term solution is not going to be drugs but identification and correction of the underlying cause. In young birds, this is often overcrowding. A faecal examination and a crop flush are a good idea to check for any concurrent disease in addition to reviewing other loft factors.

After 1 March in Australia, as the youngsters get older, fanciers look for signs of poor loft flying, excessive panting after training, and sneezing within the loft. Even in the most healthy lofts, there can be occasional outbreaks of respiratory diseases. It is important to recognize that more than three sneezes within 5 minutes from 100 birds is a significant indicator of early respiratory disease. One would expect two to three sneezing outbreaks between January and May, even in the best-managed loft. If there is doubt as to whether a sneezing outbreak is due to chlamydial respiratory infection, a test called a chlamydial antigen test can be done on the droppings by an avian veterinarian. Medication is used during this time as it is from 1 December to 1 March. However, provided the birds are well, medication is best avoided. With on-going good care, the birds are likely to fix themselves and the level of natural immunity they form as a result will be much higher.

More than three sneezes within 5 minutes from 100 birds is a significant indicator of early respiratory disease.

During the racing season

As mature race birds, it is racing itself that provides the stress, testing the level of immunity formed by the birds. In a well-managed loft where drugs have been used correctly, this immunity should be relatively solid by the start of the season. Racing puts this immunity to the test. In race birds, signs of *Chlamydia* flare-ups are considerably more subtle. The birds are older, their natural immunity is higher and their response to disease is different. The signs observed have been modified by these factors. Birds with respiratory infection have lost their zest for life and this is reflected in their race results. However, many things can lead to disappointing results and, as antibiotics have the potential to make a race team worse, I, like most fanciers, have to be convinced that respiratory infection is present and that their use is warranted. Birds that are reluctant to fly, quiet in the loft and with dry feathers (no bloom) are suggestive of respiratory infection. Sneezing (more than three times in 5 minutes from 100 birds), scratching at the nose, yawning, and wiping the nose on the wing butt all indicate irritation of the upper airways. On opening the beak, the tonsils may be inflamed, a thick white mucus may be extending into the throat from the windpipe or from the slot in the roof of the mouth, which may be closed due to swollen edges, the top of the windpipe may be red and inflamed, the beak at the nostril opening may be wet, the cere may be slightly discoloured or there may be a slightly mucous component to the birds' grunt while the gums or the muscles may be bluish. Chronically infected birds show delayed recovery after a race and will develop green droppings after stress because of damage to the liver. Testing of the droppings usually confirms the diagnosis.

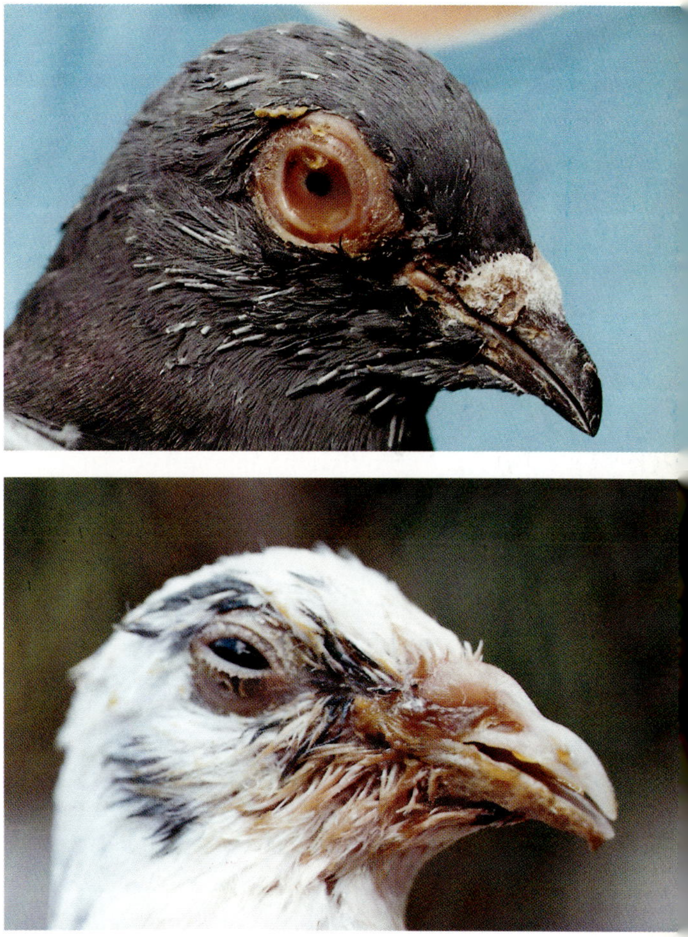

Birds with severe respiratory infection, with heavy eye and nose discharge.

If the loft has not had respiratory problems in previous years, I feel it is best to try and avoid antibiotic medication but monitor the birds closely and treat for 3 – 4 days if respiratory infection occurs. If respiratory infection during racing has been a problem in earlier years, preventive courses of antibiotics can be given before racing in the same way that they are given to stock birds to decrease the level of *Chlamydia* in the birds' system so that they are less likely to break down with the stress of racing ahead. Depending on the severity of the problem in earlier years, these courses are usually 7 – 20 days in length. In such lofts, follow-up periods of medication may be necessary during the season, and a common recommendation is 3 days treatment every third week, with Monday, Tuesday and Wednesday usually being the days to treat such a resident problem. After antibiotic use during racing, the birds should always be given a day on either probiotics or multivitamins.

Prevention of new chlamydial strains entering the loft

New strains enter the loft through exposure to other birds. Stray youngsters and youngsters bought at squeaker sales are always high risk because, due to their age and the stress they are under, they are likely to be shedding chlamydial organisms they are carrying. Strays should be removed immediately and birds introduced deliberately only from reliable sources. By far the main means of exposure is through the race unit. One stray is one exposure. Ten birds going to a race and each sharing a drinker with ten other birds is 100 exposures (i.e. like getting 100 strays in one day). In some situations and, in particular within certain clubs and areas of Australia, it becomes necessary to medicate returning race birds to guard against infection picked up in the race unit.

All lofts are continually being exposed to respiratory infection through the race unit. In the race unit, many different birds from many different lofts mix intimately in a warm humid environment, which is ideal for the transfer of disease. In addition, the confinement, different feeding patterns and time away from the loft stress the birds. As a result, the *Chlamydia* levels can rise to the point where form is affected.

Management

It can be seen that the appropriate management regime for *Chlamydia*, including use of medications, varies from loft to loft depending on each loft's earlier problems and particular loft-based factors. An example is what I do with my own birds. My own loft is based on an established Australian long-distance strain. *Chlamydia* is not a big problem. I do not medicate my stock birds before pairing because I do not have chlamydial problems during breeding. If I did, however, I would treat for 7 – 21 days before mating as the need dictated. I get three to four youngsters per year with eye colds and these are individually treated with Baytril (3 drops twice daily). To date, these have responded promptly. My race loft is very enclosed, which gives me good control over the loft environment and enables me to keep it as close to ideal as possible. Draughts, temperature extremes and high humidity can be avoided. I would like to think that I care for my birds well. Under my system of management during racing and with my loft environment, the resident chlamydial strains do not flare up during the race season and so I do not treat preventively before racing. I do, however, have intermittent flare-ups of wet canker and the birds are regularly checked and treated through racing for this. I feel that with inadequate control of this, because of the trichomonads' parasitic, i.e. weakening, effect, it is likely that the *Chlamydia* would also become a problem. I check my birds' droppings once or twice weekly and the birds are monitored closely for signs of respiratory infection. If a respiratory infection became established, the birds would be given a 3 – 5-day antibiotic course. My returning race birds are not treated for respiratory infection because, to date, this has not been a problem. However, if it was a problem, I would treat them.

If respiratory symptoms are noted during racing, all birds are treated with antibiotics (e.g. Doxy-T, Resfite) for 3 – 5 days. It is important to treat these outbreaks early before they change into the serious form of respiratory, which can involve, and permanently damage, the airsacs, thus seriously compromising race performance.

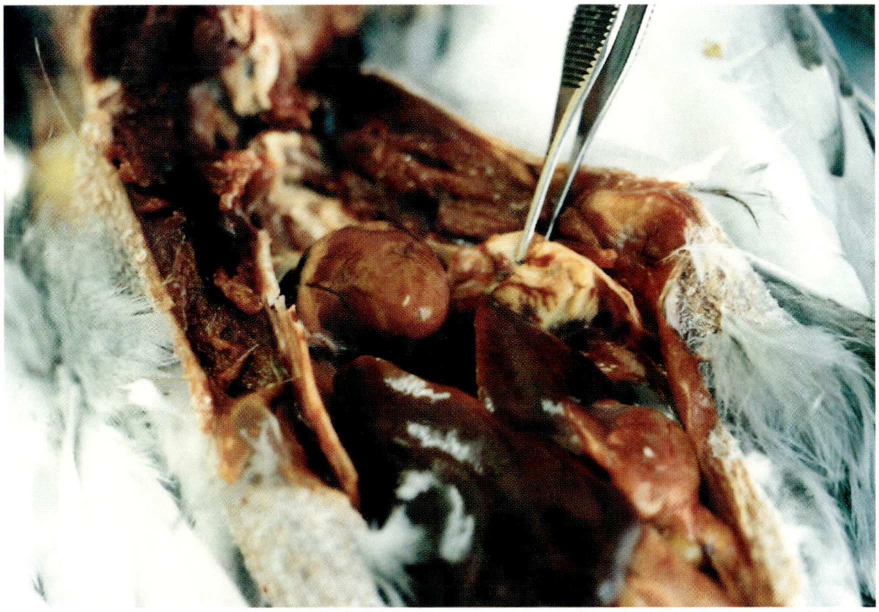

Airsac infection. The forceps are holding the bird's left thoracic airsac. This membrane should normally be tissue thin and transparent. With severe on-going infection, yellow inflammatory material has accumulated within the airsac and the fine blood vessels running across it's surface indicate an advanced inflammatory response. Treatment may save this bird's life and it may subsequently be of value for breeding, however, it's racing days are over.

'One-eye cold'

Pigeons have a number of sinuses in their head. When the lining of a sinus becomes inflamed, it secretes fluid, which accumulates in the sinus. Each sinus is drained by a series of very narrow tubes, which means that fluid often forms more quickly than it can drain away. One of the main sinuses is doughnut-shaped and runs around the eye. Because of the effect of gravity, fluid moves to the bottom of the sinus, causing a bulge to develop below the eye. Interestingly, this bulge is only visible because, unlike in mammals, where the outer sinus wall is bone, in birds it is soft tissue. Most sinus infections are due to either *Chlamydia* or *Mycoplasma*. *Chlamydia*, in particular, also inflames the membrane lining the eyelids, called the conjunctiva, causing a conjunctivitis. The associated irritation causes excessive tears to be produced, which overflow the eyelid margin and become air-dried and stuck to the feathers. Discharge drains from the sinus through ducts under the cere, staining it, before flowing through the slot in the roof of the mouth into the throat. This combination of a conjunctivitis and sinusitis is what fliers call a 'one-eye cold'. Baytril 2.5%, 3 drops twice daily, or ½ Vibravet 50-mg tablet (doxycycline) once daily usually quickly fixes these birds in 1 – 5 days.

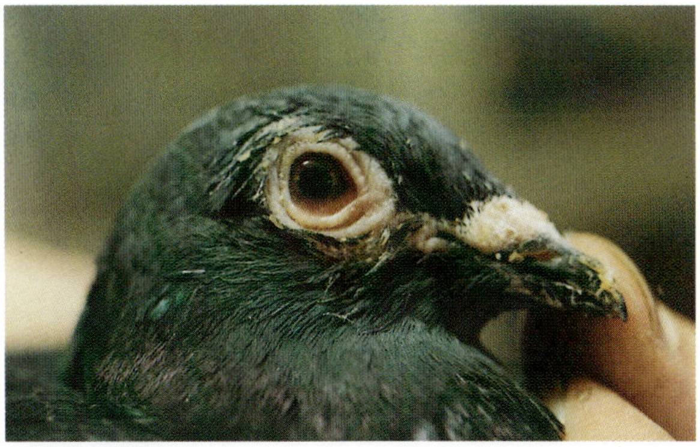

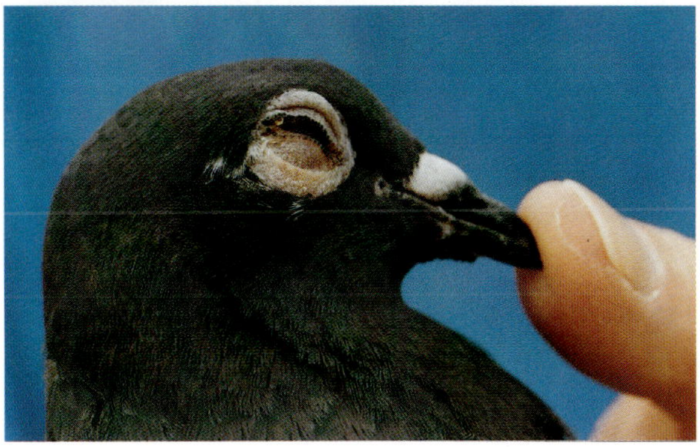

Two birds with 'one eye cold'.
Note the swelling of the sinus below the eye in the bottom lower photo.

Mycoplasma

Mycoplasma is a problem of the race season. It is what is called a primary erosive disease. Many veterinarians agree that *Mycoplasma* by themselves do not cause disease and, in fact, in experiments in which healthy pigeons have been deliberately infected, the birds have not become sick. However, the organisms do superficial injury to the lining of the respiratory system, enabling secondary organisms, notably *Chlamydia*, bacteria (such as *E. coli*) and fungi (such as *Aspergillus*), to become established. In this way, *Mycoplasma*, although not directly affecting health, has a big effect on race performance. Failure to control the problem in an affected team renders all attempts at success hopeless. Some Dutch veterinarians state that as many as 90% of teams are affected and teams are presumed to be affected unless they have been recently treated. Pigeons harbouring *Mycoplasma* organisms cannot achieve superhealth and are prevented from achieving top racing results.

Mycoplasma are primary pathogens of the respiratory system and the signs displayed by the birds depend on the part of the respiratory system affected. In the throat, nose and windpipe, signs are similar to those described for *Chlamydia* earlier. However, *Mycoplasma* notably causes inflammatory changes in the top 20 – 30% of the windpipe, causing mucus to accumulate there and birds that have a broken grunt or sound mucousy in the upper airway always make me think of *Mycoplasma*. Where the airsacs are affected, the birds cannot properly breathe and so even moderate exercise is tiring and sometimes forces the birds to land on the nearest available surface, which may be a tree or building near the loft. Because of the difficulty in breathing, the gums and muscles can turn blue and because of the inability to exercise, muscle tone and race fitness cannot come. The airsacs regulate fluid within the body by controlling evaporation of moisture from their surfaces. When diseased, excessive moisture is lost and the birds, therefore, need to drink more even after moderate exercise or run the risk of dehydration. Often, however, signs are very subtle and may simply be deteriorating performances.

Like *Chlamydia*, *Mycoplasma* are more likely to cause disease when the birds are stressed. Most lofts do have resident *Mycoplasma* strains and new *Mycoplasma* strains can enter the loft through contact with other birds. *Mycoplasma* is a difficult disease to diagnose in the live bird. Only certain labs culture *Mycoplasma*, which is an expensive procedure. Blood tests are used to diagnose the condition in chickens. There are changes at autopsy, both grossly and microscopically, that are suggestive. Changes are also found on faecal smears and crop flushes of affected birds, which are discussed in other sections of this book. A good response to a short treatment trial with Doxy-T (see Medication Guide) also supports the diagnosis

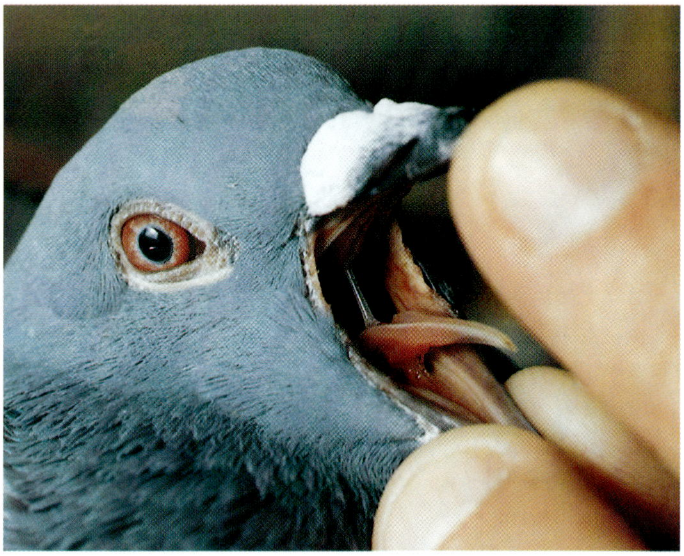

Race-age bird with thick white mucus extending from the slot in the roof of the mouth into the windpipe. This bird is likely to have a *Mycoplasma* infection. In race-age birds, signs of respiratory infection, particularly *Mycoplasma*, are often very subtle.

Management

What should the fancier do if the problem is diagnosed?

- **A health profile,** i.e. examination of the saliva and droppings, to assess any concurrent disease that may need treatment and general on-going good care to ensure a good response to medication.

- **A gradual return to exercise –** Always with respiratory infection there is an extended convalescence of usually 1 – 3 weeks. The birds must be given time to recover their fitness once medication has cleared the infection. They should not be forced to fly around the loft and once it is apparent that their vigour for flying has returned, initially short tosses only should be given (less than 1/2 hour). Observe the birds closely for signs of breathlessness on landing from these tosses and only when they are handling these well should longer tosses be given. When managing tosses of 1 – 1 1/2 hours well, it is usually safe to resume racing. In well-managed lofts with no other health problems, response to treatment can, however, be dramatic and I have had an interesting experience where two flyers both diagnosed with *Mycoplasma* in their teams succeeded in gaining 1st and 2nd Federation (3000 birds) in an all-day 500-mile race 3 weeks after treatment.
- **Good food, good care and an appropriate multivitamin supplement speed recovery.**
- **Medication –** The choice of drug is sometimes dependent on the involvement of secondary organisms such as *Chlamydia* and *E. coli.* Baytril can be used with care during racing. Other antibiotics such as doxycyline, Tiamulin or Tylan are effective. However, the current recommendation is that doxycycline and Tylan combined be given. An initial course of usually 5 – 10 days is given depending on the severity of the infection with several follow-up courses, usually 2 – 3 days every 2 – 3 weeks until one is sure that the birds are well. The usual preparation used in Australia is Doxy-T, which contains doxycycline and Tylan.

In some Federations in Australia, there is significant risk of picking up nasty *Mycoplasma* strains in the race basket. In these areas and Federations, antibiotic combination medication is given throughout the season to control the problem, usually for 2 – 3 days every 2 – 3 weeks depending on the severity of the problem and the control achieved.

Fungi

Fungi growing in the environment release spores (the fungal equivalent of seeds). If these are inhaled by pigeons, they can cause respiratory problems. The most common fungus involved here is *Aspergillus,* which is widespread in nature. Under normal conditions it is a secondary agent, causing disease only when the birds' resistance has already been lowered by some other condition. However, it can cause an acute primary disease under conditions favouring its growth, when the birds are exposed to large numbers of infected spores from their immediate environment. In this acute form, due to irritation of the respiratory system, inflammatory fluid accumulates in the lungs and airsacs. This form is most likely to affect youngsters soon after weaning. The birds appear sick, being fluffed up, are reluctant to eat and lose weight. Individual birds do get a chronic form of the disease, in which individual spores germinate and grow causing visible moulds (not unlike those seen on stale bread) to form in the airsacs. These birds are profoundly unwell, with weight loss and a breathlessness progressing to death.

Ideal conditions for the presence of fungal growth are warmth and moisture, but particularly moisture. Straw, if used as a floor dressing or for race baskets, must be kept dry. Should the straw become wet, fungi can rapidly multiply and lead to massive presence of infected spores, increasing the risk of an outbreak. In damp lofts, fungi can germinate also within the loft itself, e.g. on walls and on droppings. If lofts with high humidity are infrequently cleaned, damp droppings accumulate, which are an ideal base for fungal germination. A particular risk here is associated with grid floors. A rapid formation of mould on droppings can therefore be associated with high humidity, keeping the droppings damp and giving environmental fungal spores a chance to germinate. However, quick growth can also occur if the droppings contain a lot of fungal spores when passed. This occurs if the birds swallow them, which in turn means that their seed may be contaminated with fungal spores. Seed that is free of fungal spores at harvest is unlikely to contain fungal toxins.

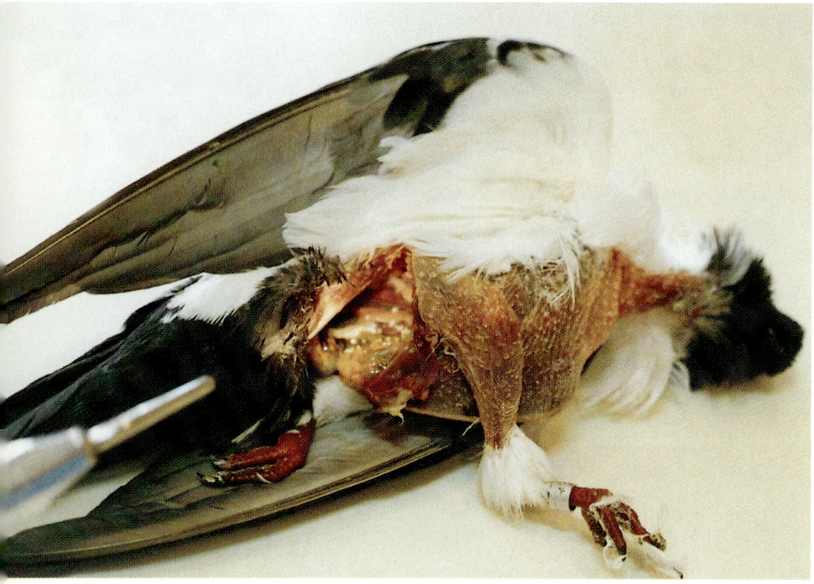

Autopsy specimen where the bird's abdominal airsac has been opened to reveal a fungal infection. The fungus can be seen as small white moulds growing on the surface of the airsac.

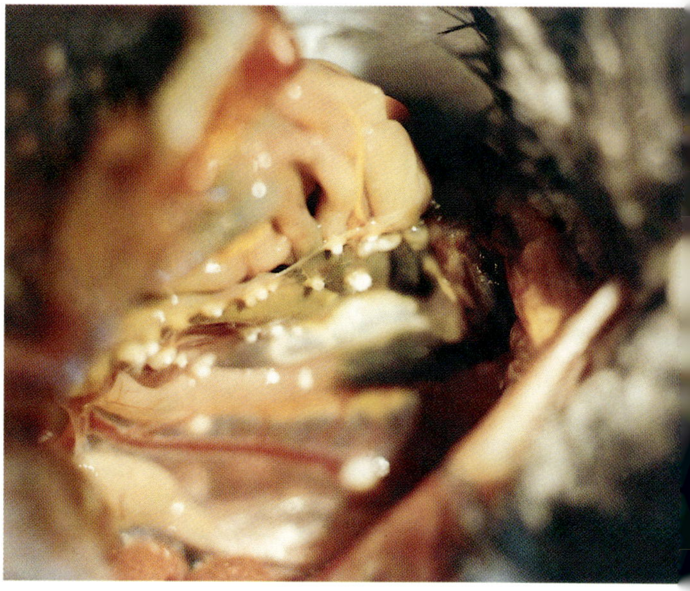

Close-up of the abdominal airsac of the autopsied bird.

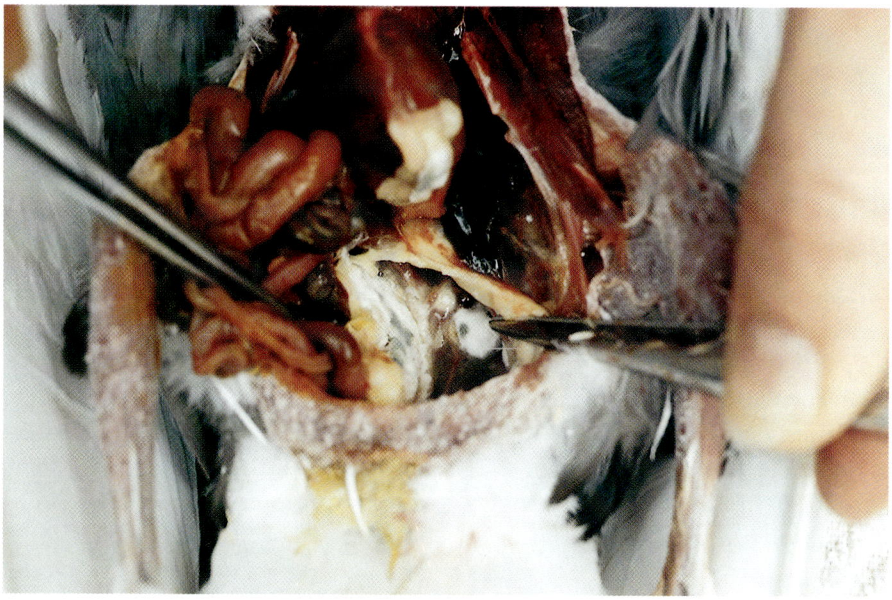

Autopsy specimen. Bird with generalized fungal infection of the abdominal airsac. The normally transparent airsac has become thickened and yellow and plaques of mould are growing across it's surface.

Conversely, heavy contamination of seed with fungal spores can be associated with fungal toxin contamination of the grain. These toxins weaken the bird generally, creating a vulnerability to secondary problems, in particular *Mycoplasma*, but also directly suppress the immune system further, making the bird vulnerable to disease. Fungi in the seed, therefore, are doubly dangerous in regard to the respiratory system, in that they predispose the bird to respiratory infection but also contaminate the birds' environment via the droppings with spores that, if given the opportunity to germinate, can infect the respiratory system directly.

Management

The treatment of fungal respiratory infection is difficult in that only a few antifungal drugs are absorbed from the bowel, e.g. Ketoconazole, Amphoteracin B, and can act throughout the body. These are best used under the guidance of a veterinarian familiar with pigeons.

Essentially, it is best to ensure that the level of care of the birds is good so that they are more able to resist infection while at the same time minimizing their exposure. This means keeping the loft dry and clean, in particular with regard to substances readily colonized by fungi such as straw and damp droppings. Loft contamination can be decreased by checking seed quality. If necessary, the loft can be sprayed with antifungal disinfectants, e.g. chloramine. This is quite safe and is a good practice to include in regular loft maintenance in high-humidity areas.

In the face of an outbreak:

- Remove the source of infection, e.g. damp straw, damp droppings below a grid floor.
- Spray loft with chloramine.
- Have a health profile done (i.e. a crop flush and faecal smear).
- Return to activity as for *Mycoplasma* recovery.
- Supplement with multivitamins.
- Medicate with antifungal drugs under veterinary guidance.

Mites

Several different types of mite infect the respiratory system in pigeons. Some live in the nasal passages, causing superficial irritation, making the birds sneeze and scratch their nose. Others live deeper in the windpipe and airsacs, causing a range of respiratory signs depending on the severity of infection. The adult mites produce eggs that are coughed up and swallowed by the pigeons. The problem is diagnosed by finding their eggs in the birds' droppings microscopically, but at times this can be difficult as they are only shed intermittently. At autopsy, the adult mites are just visible to the naked eye as little white dots but are easy to overlook. Sometimes, one can be lucky enough when opening a bird's beak to see one run across the floor of the bird's mouth and dive down the windpipe or alternatively run up and disappear through the slot in the roof of the mouth. They are effectively treated with either Moxidectin (2 mg/ml, 5 ml to 1 litre of water for 24 hours) or Ivermectin (10 mg/ml, 1 ml to 1 litre of water for 24 hours).

Viruses

Several viruses have the potential to cause respiratory infection in pigeons. Of note here are Herpes virus, Circo virus and to a lesser extent Adeno virus. Fanciers need to be aware of their existence, particularly when birds with respiratory infections are not responding to routine medication. Their diagnosis, management and treatment can be involved and if fliers are concerned, they should contact a pigeon veterinarian. (Refer to chapter Common Viral Infections.)

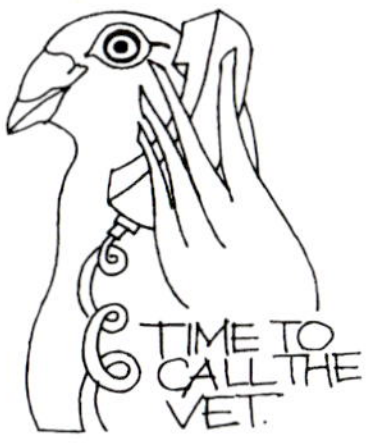

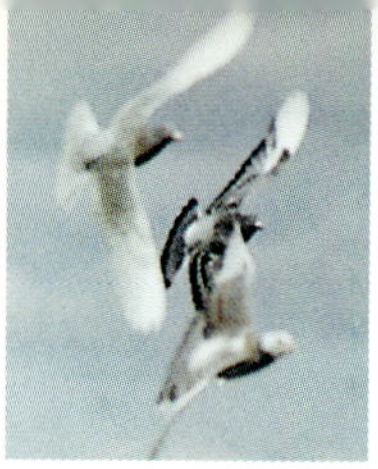

Chapter 8

E. COLI

There has been much talk over the last couple of years in the pigeon fancy regarding *E. coli* and yet before this time it was something most pigeon racers had not heard of. With this influx of information, there have been a number of misconceptions that have crept in and so, just what does it mean to have a pigeon veterinarian tell you that your pigeons have *E. coli* and what effect can it have on the birds' race results?

E. coli is one of the most widely distributed organisms on the face of the planet. There are different strains (or serotypes) of *E. coli*. These serotypes differ in their ability to cause disease. The big dilemma with *E. coli* and pigeons is interpretation, i.e. how to interpret the finding of the presence of *E. coli*. The reason for this is that *E. coli* can be found in most normal and healthy pigeons. Leading American pigeon veterinarian Dr David Marx, President of the American Association of Pigeon Veterinarians, guarantees that he can culture *E. coli* from over 90% of the best performing racers, and states that you have to interpret the finding by taking a lot of other things into consideration.

Interpretation of presence of *E. coli*

Just because *E. coli* is there doesn't necessarily mean that it is causing disease. So, how do we decide? *E. coli*, if present, usually restricts itself to the bowel. However, with some serotypes, and this only occurs with the nastier strains, they can spread from the bowel throughout the body and invade other organs, such as the liver. When *E. coli* invades the body from the bowel, it always causes disease. And so, if *E. coli* is found anywhere else in the body, then it is definitely a problem. The dilemma comes if it is just present in the bowel. If the strain in the bowel is capable of causing disease, it causes an enteritis. An enteritis is an inflammation of the bowel wall. With nasty strains, this inflammation is severe, leading to loss of fluid and interference with digestion. This in turn leads to a green watery dropping and an obviously unwell bird. With mild strains, the inflammation is also mild and changes in the dropping are less marked. The droppings may remain formed but become slightly green or have a slightly elevated water content, leading to the white component of the dropping being smeared rather than sitting distinctly and separate. Similarly, the signs of ill health displayed by the bird can be subtle, such as cessation in the drop of down feathers or a shortening in the length of time that the birds will voluntarily spend on the wing.

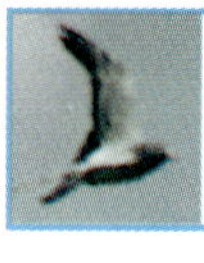

Just because *E. coli* is present doesn't necessarily mean that it is causing disease.

Nasty disease-producing strains can cause disease in their own right. As the strain becomes milder and milder, the birds have to be progressively more and more run down until a threshold is passed that tips the balance in favour of the organism, enabling it to cause disease. Many *E. coli* strains in pigeons are simply opportunists, waiting to cause disease if something stresses the birds. This can be an on-going environmental or management problem or another concurrent disease. In particular, *E. coli* often becomes involved with disease that damages the bowel lining, such as worms or Coccidia, and is often also involved as a secondary agent with viral problems, in particular, Adeno virus. As European fanciers would be aware, Adeno virus infection in pigeons has been a considerable problem, particularly in Holland over the last few years. A combined infection of Adeno virus and *E. coli* has been identified and called Adeno-coli syndrome. In bacteria-free pigeons, often Adeno virus causes little or no problem. In the presence of *E. coli*, because the Adeno virus damages the lining of the intestinal tract, the *E. coli* can invade and cause disease. Thus controlling the *E. coli* with antibiotics makes the symptoms of Adeno virus infection decrease greatly. Probably one of the reasons *E. coli* is such a common secondary invader is that it is present much more frequently. There are other bacteria that can also be opportunistic but aren't usually present. If these were present when the pigeon was run down or stressed, then they would cause disease, too.

One trap with interpretation is that, in bacterial bowel disease, the bacteria are often identified through culture. This is where the organism is actively grown in the laboratory. *E. coli* is very easy to grow, while other organisms that can cause similar signs, such as *Salmonella*, can be quite difficult to grow. This means that sometimes *E. coli* is given the blame when in fact another bacterium more difficult to culture is the real cause but is overlooked. Diagnosis can be even more difficult when the droppings are simply examined under the microscope as a fine faecal smear. Bacteria occur in two common shapes, dots (called cocci) or short lines (called rods or bacilli). Different types of bacteria differ not only in their shape but also in size, their ability to move and other characteristics. *E. coli* are mid-sized rods that are often motile (i.e. capable of movement – some types are not). The dots for the most part are normal bacteria called enteric streptococci (or enterococci). Many of the rods are also harmless and, in fact, some are beneficial, e.g. *Lactobacillus*. For those with microscopes, it is easy to be mystified by the different shapes, sizes and movement when examining a faecal smear under 400x magnification. What we like to see is a mix of bacteria and a predominance of dots. If there are many dots for every short motile rod, then everything is probably okay. When the number of motile rods increases, and certainly when these become the predominant bacterial organism present, it is time to consult a pigeon veterinarian. Always, however, what is seen down the microscope must be related to what the birds are doing, i.e. how they appear in themselves and what the droppings look like on the perch.

Although some *E. coli* strains can cause disease in their own right, usually *E. coli*'s disease-causing capability is secondary. Its presence, therefore, should not be taken to mean disease in healthy pigeons with normal droppings. The mere presence of *E. coli* should not precipitate a treatment program and it is a mistake to start to treat routinely unless there is actually a problem.

Dr Marx states in a recent article:

"Treating for E. coli which isn't causing any problem is non-productive. In fact, we know that when we treat for E. coli, we disturb all the normal bacteria too which can make the pigeon more susceptible to invasion by various things such as E. coli when it gets repopulated as well as the other bacteria in the environment that it's exposed to chronically. Treating for just the mere presence of E. coli is not productive and the birds will always start showing it again within a week or so after you stop treating. It's an unattainable goal to eliminate E. coli for all practical purposes."

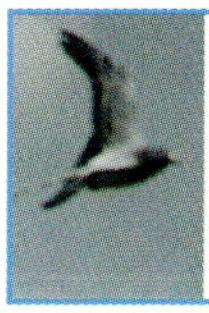

Treating for just the mere presence of *E. coli* is not productive and the birds will always start showing it again within a week or so after you stop treating.

So what parameters do we use to tell if there is a problem with *E. coli*?

- If *E. coli* is identified in parts of the body other than the bowel.
- If, at any time during the year, a bacterium fitting the description of *E. coli*, i.e. a mid-sized motile rod, is the predominant organism on microscopic examination of a faecal smear or faecal culture and the birds are either sick or the droppings are abnormal.

- If, during the race season, changes occur in the birds, indicating a loss of form, no matter how subtle, and *E. coli* levels increase in the droppings.

Management

And so what do we do if there is a problem? There is always the possibility that a nasty strain could enter the loft via the race or toss basket or in a stray but this is unlikely, and so the first thought by the fancier should be that this is probably a secondary problem. The fancier should therefore think about what has happened recently in the loft, looking for the cause of *E. coli*'s appearance. The fancier should develop a checklist, looking for factors that have put the birds under stress and triggered the *E. coli* flare-up. The reasons will vary from one loft to another and so the answer for each fancier is going to be different. In some lofts where *E. coli* is not usually present, its appearance may indicate a single management mistake or a recent hard toss, etc. Often the answer is self-evident. In cold-sensitive lofts, the problem may be intermittent and correlate with changes in weather. Here the answer may be a change in loft design. In some lofts it may be a good indicator of another disease, e.g. Coccidia or wet canker, so that in lofts with a known medical record the appearance of *E. coli* can be used to monitor the treatment and management of other problems. In one loft, the advice may be to decrease the birds' workload and to increase the energy content of the birds' food either by altering the grain mix or the use of specific supplements, such as Polyseed Oil. In another loft, the advice may be to give 2 days of an anticanker medication followed by some multivitamins. There are, therefore, many answers that are all correct to solve the one problem and the answer is not necessarily medication. If it is not possible to identify the stress factor, the *E. coli* will respond poorly to any medication or quickly return once medication is withdrawn. On the other hand, if the stress factor can be quickly identified and corrected, then the lift that the birds get in overall health will often allow them to clear the *E. coli* by themselves.

E. coli is a particularly handy health monitor during the race season. As many strains of *E. coli* are very weak and rarely cause disease, the appearance of *E. coli* in the droppings is not necessarily going to be a problem but, particularly during the race season, may well indicate that the birds are on the verge of breaking down: it indicates the potential for a problem. It is at this time that the astute fancier must use his fanciership skills and sometimes a pigeon veterinarian to head off an impending loss of form. As an example of this, I relate the following story. Recently a mixed-grain sample and droppings sample arrived at my clinic. The grain was cultured and was all normal except for the wheat, which was found to be heavily contaminated with fungi. The droppings contained a low but significant level of *E. coli*. On being told the results several days later, the fancier's reply was that he thought the wheat was the problem. I was surprised as the wheat to the naked eye looked quite okay. He stated that all he had noticed was that the birds had stopped dropping down feathers. Thinking back, he realised that the only thing he had changed was starting a new batch of wheat in his seed mix. He had already stopped feeding the wheat and feather down production had resumed. This fancier is extremely successful and his powers of observation are probably part of the reason why. Other fanciers may not have noticed this, kept feeding the wheat and wondered why form had trailed away.

And so, what do we do when we see *E. coli* in the faecal smear? Our approach differs, depending on the time of the pigeon year.

Out of the race season

If out of the race season, *E. coli* is found in the faecal smear and the birds are not ill nor do they have abnormal droppings, no treatment is indicated. One should persist with on-going good care and have the droppings monitored.

During the race season

The approach to disease is very different during the race season and I suggest the following steps be taken:

- If *E. coli* is not normally present, review recent management practice and try to identify the trigger factor and prevent it happening again.
- If *E. coli* is a frequent finding, review loft-based stresses, loft design, ventilation and management practices. The loft may be too crowded, the birds may be chronically overworked, or feed quality may be poor.
- If no problem is readily apparent, then decrease the birds' workload, increase the calorie content of the seed mix and recheck the droppings in 2 days.
- Always start the birds on probiotics. The *E. coli* might go away by itself but it is best to take no chance.
- Consider using antibiotics only if the birds are sick or the birds' droppings are poor and the above measures have not helped. Antibiotics should always be used with care, no matter what time of year. The antibiotics that kill *E. coli* also kill many of the normal bacteria in the bowel, which are necessary for nutrient absorption and vitamin production. If antibiotics are used during moulting, they can compromise feather quality. Incorrect use during breeding can adversely affect youngsters' development. During racing, most bowel-active antibiotics cause some nausea and should not be used within 48 hours of basketing.

Preventive measures in problem lofts

Most bacteria like warm damp conditions and *E. coli* is no exception. Humid conditions are not only stressful for the birds but also favour bacterial multiplication in the loft environment. Humidity and loft design are discussed later in this book. Humidity can either come from inside the loft (in moisture from expired air and droppings) or from outside the loft. When the humidity is coming from outside the loft, the answer is often to close the loft in, particularly at night. When the humidity comes from inside the loft, the answer is to alter the loft's ventilation or to decrease the number of birds kept.

As *E. coli* is passed in the droppings, hygiene within the loft, particularly regarding drinkers and hoppers, will decrease exposure of the birds to the organism.

In numerous experiments, regular probiotics have been shown to protect the bowel from bacterial invasion and their use 2 days per week, e.g. Wednesday and Sunday, can help protect the birds, particularly in lofts prone to *E. coli* problems. As *E. coli* is usually a secondary agent, good control of all other diseases will also decrease its incidence.

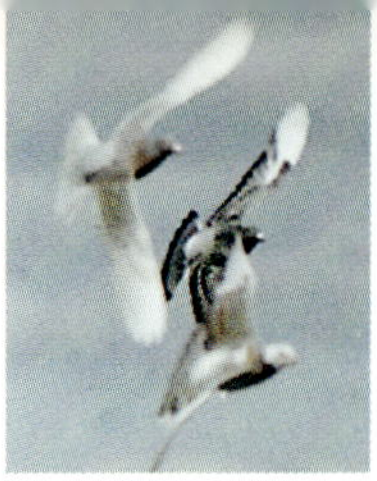

Chapter 9

PARATYPHOID

Paratyphoid is a disease caused by the bacterium *Salmonella typhimurium*. It has always been a problem with our birds. The bacterium likes warm, humid conditions and even though it is more of a problem for New South Wales and Queensland fliers, it is seen in all States of Australia. The disease seems more common and causes more severe symptoms in fancy pigeons, particularly of certain breeds, e.g. Modenas, Show Homers and high-flying breeds, in particular Doneks.

There are many different types of *Salmonella*, varying in their ability to cause disease and also in the type of disease they cause. The signs displayed by the birds also depend on their age and on their level of immunity. In pigeons, the disease can take four forms:

1 **Bowel form –** The classic 'going light', with weight loss, lethargy, green diarrhoea, loss of appetite and rapid death. This is the usual form seen in very young youngsters with no natural immunity.

Older birds with some immunity are able to localize the infection to a particular site. Often this is in the membranes around the brain (meninges) or in a joint so that we see the following two forms of the disease:

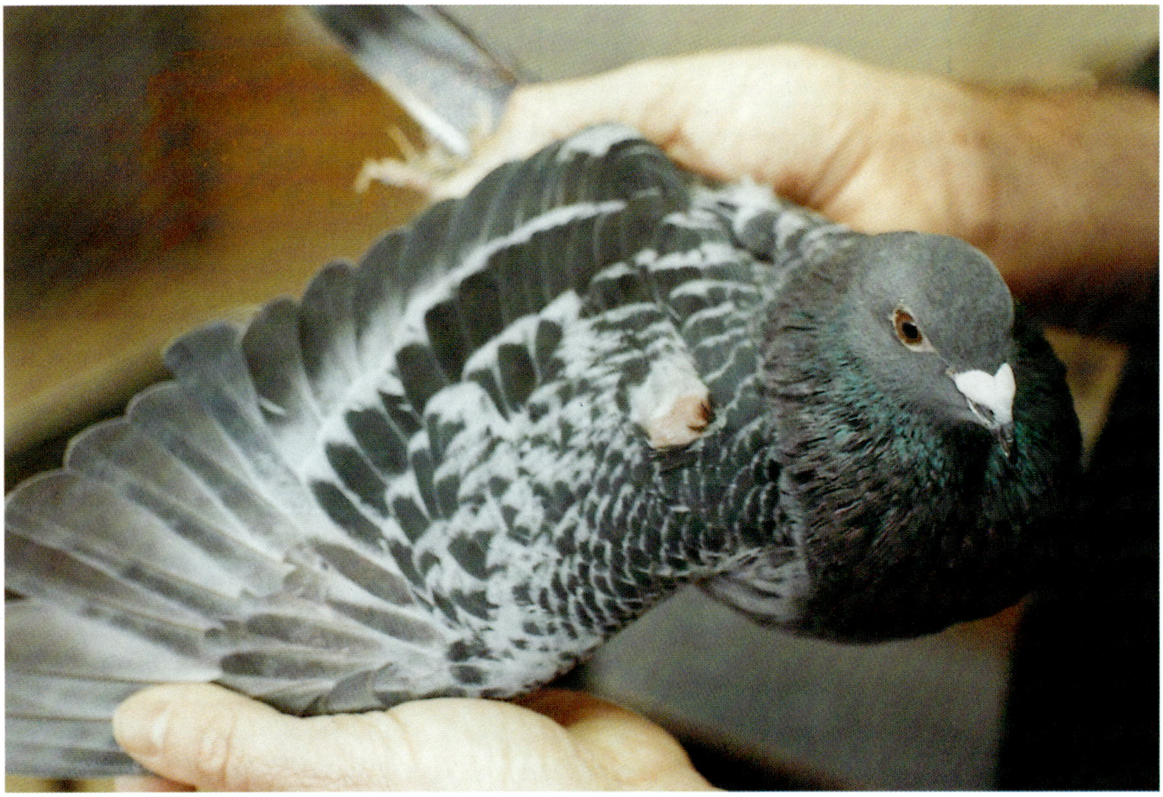

Hen with the joint form of paratyphoid. The first joint in the right wing is visibly swollen and red.

2 **Meningeal form –** The meninges are the membranes surrounding the brain; whe they interfere with the brain's function so that the bird may be poorly coordina head in an unusual position, or be paralysed.

3 **Joint form –** Swollen, red, painful joints of the wings and legs.

In birds of any age but more so in adult birds, the bacteria can penetrate the bowel wall and pass via the blood stream to a wide range of sites to cause a generalized disease:

4 **Generalized form –** Multi-organ involvement, usually seen as a very sick pigeon, rapidly losing weight, often with a short clinical course leading to death. The bacteria sometimes localize in the gonads, causing infertility in cocks and hens. Hens that continue to cycle often produce infected eggs that fail to hatch.

The disease can have a reasonably high mortality rate, particularly if young birds are involved. Upon recovery, not all birds will clear the organism from their system and these birds become what are called 'carriers' and are virtually asymptomatic. Sometimes the only signs exhibited by these birds are that they may be occasionally quiet and develop greenish diarrhoea. However, it is the droppings of these asymptomatic carriers that are the usual source of infection. Other species can also carry the organism, in particular wild birds and rodents. Once in an environment, the organism can also survive and multiply there. Birds usually acquire the infection by eating seed or drinking water contaminated by the organism. Once ingested, it can either multiply in the bowel or invade the body through the bowel wall to attack a variety of organs or joints, as mentioned above. The organism can also affect fertility and, if the ovary is affected, can actually be in the egg at the time of laying or pass through the shell of the egg if droppings containing *Salmonella* contaminate the nest box. Once in the egg, it infects the developing embryo, often killing it, resulting in a dead-in-shell youngster. Some infected embryos survive incubation but, because of their weakened state, die during hatching or in the first few days of life. Carrier birds are progressively damaged by each bout of the disease and their potential as either race or stock birds is obviously compromised.

The disease has always been difficult to control because:

- The asymptomatic carrier is common, hard to identify, and difficult to treat,
- The organism not only survives but also multiplies well within the environment, and
- It is carried by other species, including wild birds and rodents.

Factors in control

Control is based on on-going good care, strict hygiene, control of rodents, elimination of carriers, the correct use of medication, and occasionally vaccination. An attempt should be made to avoid entry of the organism into the loft.

Avoid entry into the loft

Through the very nature of pigeon racing, where many birds from many different lofts are in intimate contact in race units each week, the potential for exposure by race birds is high. In the stock loft, however, bird entry is under direct control. All new stock birds should be regarded as potential carriers of the disease. As explained, the asymptomatic carrier is common. When stressed, these carriers shed the organism in their droppings. Veterinary examination of the droppings at this time can detect the organism's presence. At other times, the bird may test negative even though it is carrying the disease. The routine testing of new birds is therefore not always reliable. Mature birds that occasionally become quiet and develop greenish diarrhoea should be suspected. Introduced birds, 2
particularly from suspect lofts, should be isolated and treated with Baytril for 10 days before loft

entry. An antibiotic, however, can only act where the blood stream carries it, and in some carriers the organism is contained in inaccessible sites, e.g. microabscess in the liver, where the organism is encapsulated and therefore not accessible to antibiotics. Consequently, there is no fail-safe way of preventing the organism entering the stock loft. However, a period of quarantine before entry, a course of antibiotics during quarantine, and testing of any birds that become sick will minimize the risk. Obviously, birds should ideally only be introduced from other lofts, including studs, known to be free of the disease. In addition, rodents should be controlled and contact with the droppings of wild birds should be avoided. If flights are provided, this can be achieved by suspending them so that any wild bird droppings can fall through the roof and through the floor of the flight.

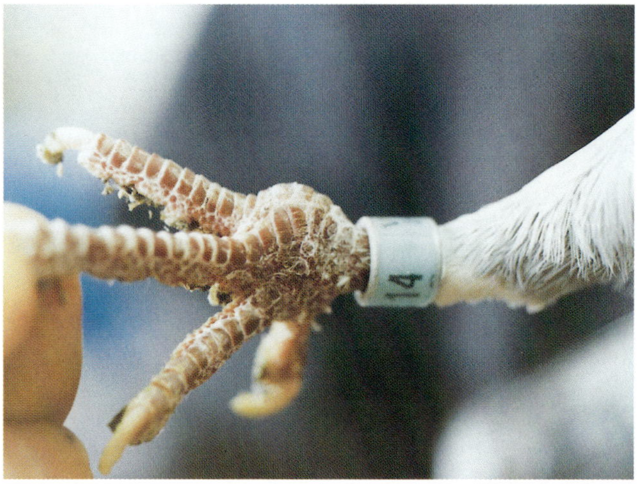

Joint form of paratyphoid. The infection has localized in the joint of the foot.

Hygiene within the loft

As explained, the organism not only survives but multiplies within the environment. The loft, food and water must be clean. A build-up of germs in the loft is prevented by regular cleaning and disinfecting. If a disease outbreak occurs, disinfection using chloramine is a good practice in all lofts. The disinfectant is sprayed onto the scraped, cleaned surfaces of the loft, using a fine mist spray, and allowed to dry while the birds are exercising. Chloramine can safely be used to disinfect the water and food dishes.

Correct use of medication

Several antibiotics have action against *Salmonella*. The usual one prescribed for unwell birds is Baytril 2.5%, at a dose of 1 ml per 1 litre of water for flock treatments or 3 drops twice daily to individual birds, both for 10 days. In most situations, only individual birds are treated. Regular courses of 'preventive' antibiotics to control *Salmonella* are debatable and should be discouraged. It has been shown that periodic short courses of antibiotics can, in fact, predispose the birds to the problem. This is because the antibiotics kill a lot of the normal beneficial bacteria in the pigeon's bowel, which serve to protect it from colonization by *Salmonella*. When antibiotics stop, there is a short time when the bowel is recolonized by bacteria from the immediate environment and during this time *Salmonella* can establish. Antibiotics given to all birds when only a few are affected can also select for resistant strains of the organism. There is, however, good evidence that in problem lofts, the regular use of probiotics decreases the incidence of *Salmonella*.

Diagnosis

The disease is sometimes tentatively diagnosed by the clinical appearance of the birds and the overall flock picture. However, definitive diagnosis is made by growing or culturing the organism in the laboratory. Swabs for culture can be taken from the blood or droppings. However, even in infected birds the organism is not always present. A better choice is an actual site of infection such as a swollen joint or a suspect organ identified at autopsy.

Management in the face of an outbreak

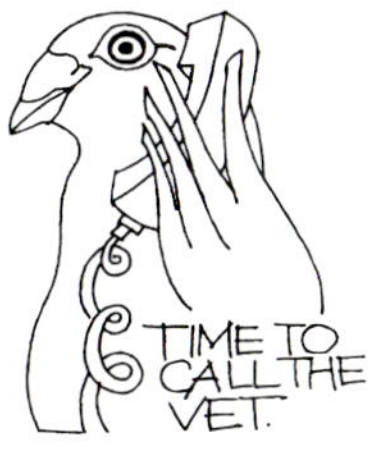

What should the fancier do if faced with an outbreak of *Salmonella*? There is no single approach that is best and what is done needs to correlate with the severity of the problem. Some strains of *Salmonella* are relatively common in the environment and are only mildly capable of causing disease. Many birds that come in contact with these strains do not in fact become unwell but rather, through this exposure, develop an immunity to them. In these lofts, problems are often sporadic and mild. If, say, only one or two of 100 birds develop an infection in the joint, these birds are separated and started on a 10-day course of Baytril. The loft is thoroughly cleaned and disinfected to decrease exposure of the other birds to the organism. If the unwell birds respond quickly and well to medication, they can be returned to the flock after 10 days. If response is slow, or the birds are not normal after 10 days, then unless they are birds of particular value for which further treatment might be considered, they are usually best eliminated as they may not be capable of clearing the organism and can serve as an on-going source of infection. In many vulnerable lofts, such as a Show Homer loft, the disease can be effectively managed this way, with only a low and manageable number of birds becoming unwell each year. With generally good management practices in place, most birds will be able to resist the disease. If the number of birds becoming unwell is too high to man age in this way, then a continuous 10-day course of Baytril to all birds may be considered. It is unlikely, however, that this would eliminate the disease as the antibiotic will not clear the organism from some carrier birds and these will later recontaminate the loft.

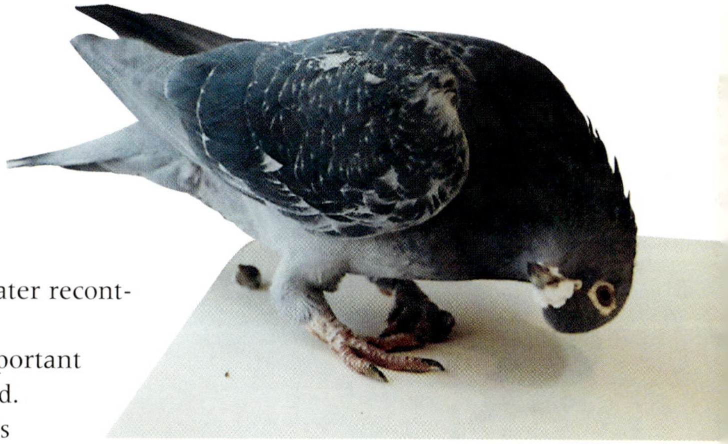
Bird with meningeal form of paratyphoid.

During a 10-day course of medication, it is important that the loft be thoroughly cleaned and disinfected. However, as it is not possible to sterilize a loft, this only serves to decrease bird exposure to the organism.

Problems are always much less likely to occur if the fancier is providing on-going general good care. Management flaws such as overcrowding, poor hygiene and poor control of parasitic diseases weaken the birds and predispose them to infection. If *Salmonella* is an on-going problem, the loft and the way it is managed must be reviewed.

Salmonella in most lofts can be managed by separating and treating unwell birds and ensuring on-going good management practices so that most birds can resist the disease. Regular probiotics can be given as needed. In the case of a more severe outbreak, a 10-day course of Baytril can be given to all birds, coupled with loft disinfection with chloramine and a review of the loft environment and management practices generally. If the disease is still a problem, vaccination can be considered.

For the purposes of management of an outbreak, I find it easiest to divide the approach into three levels based on the severity of the outbreak. These levels and their management are listed below:

1 **Most birds well, less than 3% of birds sick, good loft managed well –** Separate unwell birds and treat with Baytril, 3 drops twice daily. Very thoroughly clean and/or disinfect loft. Provide on-going good care. Use probiotics. If unwell birds respond quickly and completely, return to flock; otherwise eliminate them.

2 **More that 3% of birds affected, with fresh cases almost on a daily basis, indicative of spreading disease –** Separate and treat unwell birds as above. Thoroughly clean and disinfect loft. Cease breeding if occurring. All birds to receive 10-day course of Baytril 2.5%, 1 ml

to 1 litre of water, followed by 7 days probiotic. Probiotics 3 days per week (minimum) for as long as needed.

3 **Recurrent flare-ups of disease affecting significant numbers of birds –** Vaccination protocol as outlined below.

Vaccination

Various vaccines against *Salmonella* are available. Although vaccine use has had its problems and has at times not been fully protective, in certain lofts vaccination can be a useful adjunct to control. There are many different strains of *Salmonella,* and so, for a vaccine to be of value, it must be prepared against local *Salmonella* strains. Vaccination, in effect, gives the birds a small dose of killed bacteria, thus giving the birds exposure to the organism and enabling them to develop an immunity without any risk of developing the disease. Often two vaccinations are given initially, at a 4-week

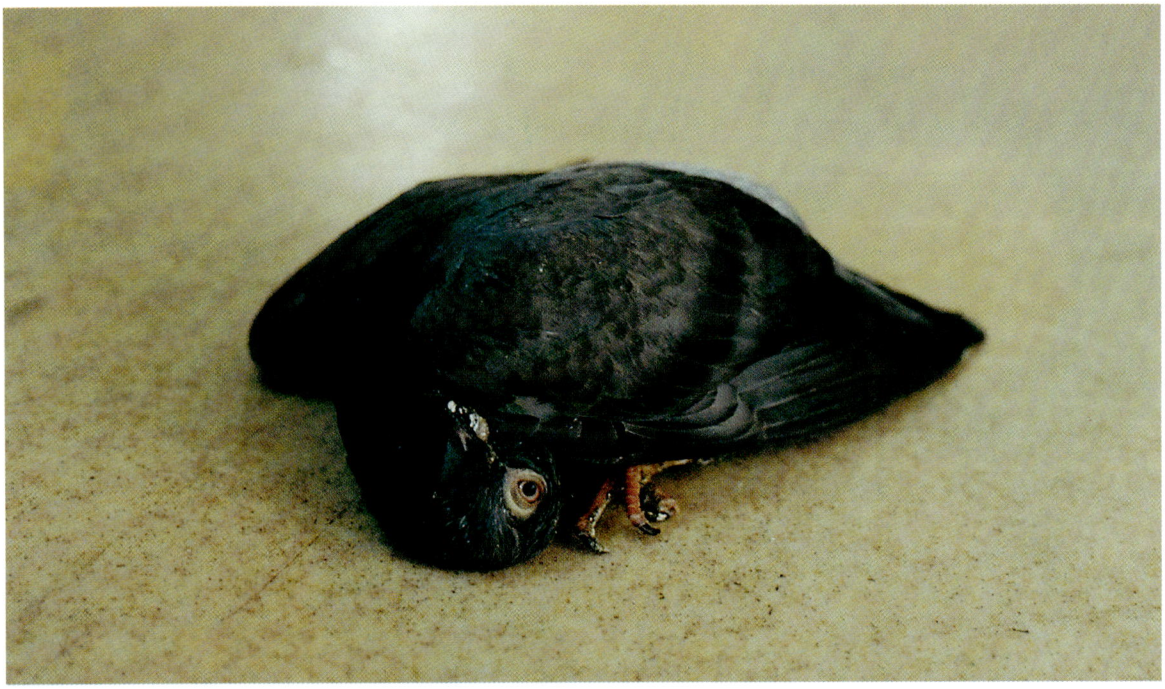

Bird with severe meningeal form of paratyphoid. Prior to the availability of fluoroquinolone antibiotics, such as Baytril, such cases were virtually hopeless.

interval, followed by annual boosters. Because vaccines contain the bacterial toxin, there is always the chance of a reaction to the vaccine and so it is suggested that several birds be vaccinated first and then start the full vaccination program 3 days later if there are no adverse reactions. Correct storage of the vaccine with its bacterial toxin is critical, and the vaccine should not be frozen as this will cause endotoxin release.

Whether to vaccinate or not is a matter of weighing up the potential for exposure, the risk the fancier is prepared to take, and the cost. In Australia, the disease in race birds is uncommon and because the vaccine is not fully protective and has the risk of side effects, widespread use of the vaccine is not recommended.

I see vaccination as having particular value in a loft that has had a problem with *Salmonella* and also as an aid in controlling the disease if an outbreak occurs.

When to vaccinate

Vaccines can cause a local reaction and can make the birds feel unwell in themselves. Only healthy adult birds should be vaccinated. The ideal time is after breeding and moulting but before racing starts. Vaccination during racing should be avoided as it will put the birds off form. Vaccinating birds while they are incubating and feeding youngsters may cause them to hop off the nest. Birds should be fed and watered before vaccination as some may be unwell for 8 – 24 hours after vaccination and may not eat and drink during this time. Birds younger than 12 weeks of age should not be vaccinated.

When an outbreak occurs and the decision has been made to vaccinate, it is important to vaccinate all apparently normal in-contact birds as soon as possible. It is best, however, to treat all birds for 2 days with antibiotics, e.g. Baytril, before vaccination. In some birds that are in the very early stage of the disease but appear normal, the vaccine may make them sicker. This effect can be decreased if all birds are initially pretreated. A 10-day course of antibiotics is usually given.

The following vaccination protocol is followed

Flock with many birds showing signs of *Salmonella*

↓

Collect samples and confirm presence of infection by testing

↓

Separate affected birds; eliminate severely affected birds

↓

Commence treatment of all birds with Baytril for 10 days; 2 days later, vaccinate in-contact birds that are still well

↓

Spray loft weekly with chloramine, and wash drinkers and waterers daily with chloramine

↓

Monitor birds closely by observation and possible testing, provide on-going good care and supplement with probiotics

↓

Second vaccination 4 weeks later

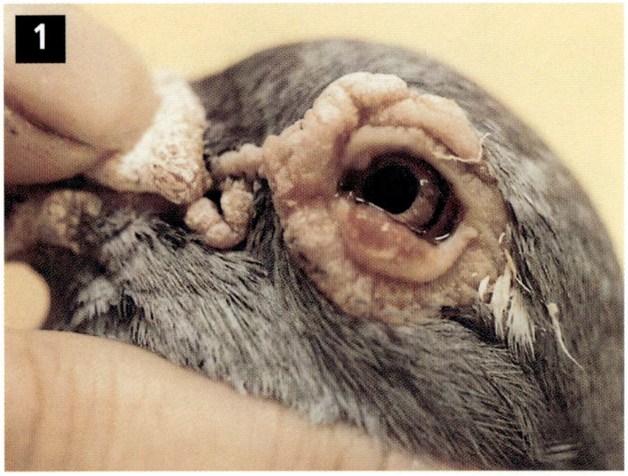

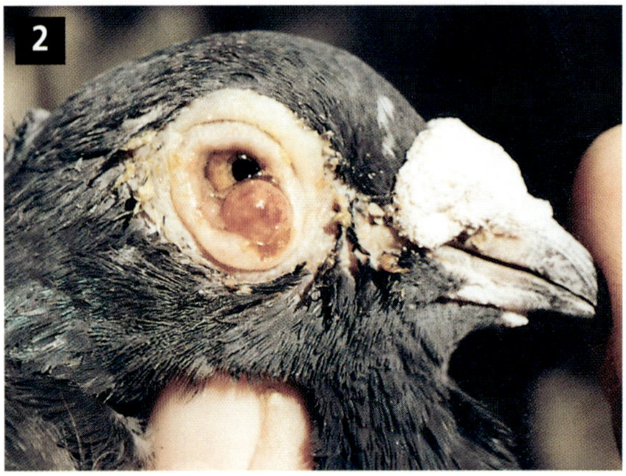

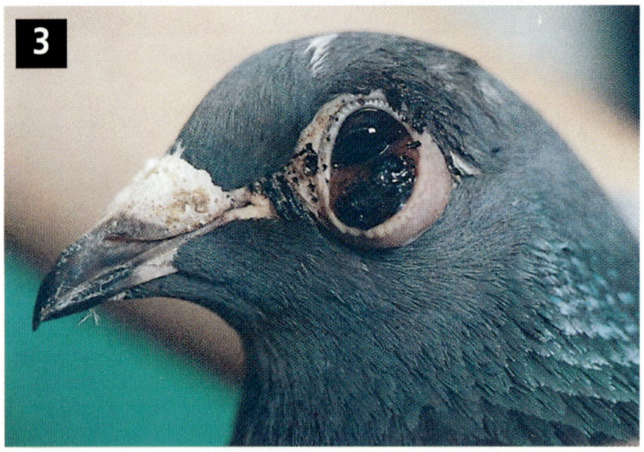

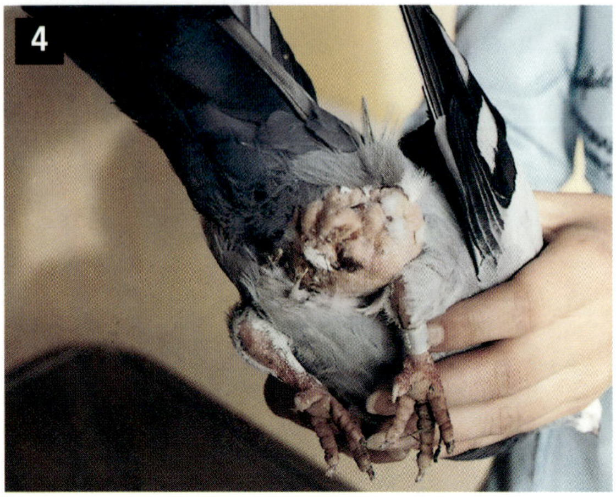

Tumours

A whole range of tumours can affect pigeons. Some of these are benign while others are malignant. Some are readily visible, occurring superficially on the skin or associated structures. Many, however, are internal. When on the exterior, their presence becomes immediately obvious. However, when inside, fanciers are often unaware of their presence until they start to affect the health of the bird. Often, affected birds develop the non-specific signs of losing weight, becoming fluffed up and less active in the loft. Treatment depends on the nature of the tumour. Benign tumours, both internally and externally, are often very amenable to surgery. However, no treatment can usually be offered for malignant tumours. Cancer tends to affect older birds more commonly and should always be thought of when an aged bird becomes unwell. Treatment is always more likely to be successful the earlier veterinary attention is sought and so birds suspected of having any tumour should be taken to an avian veterinarian promptly.

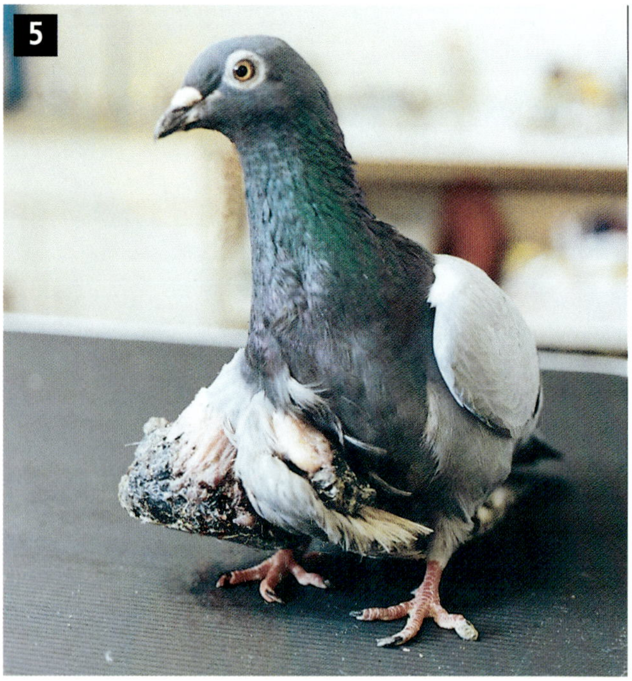

Photos 1 – 3: Three birds with tumours involving the lower eyelid. Some of these are induced by exposure to U.V. light.
Photo 4: Bird with a large fibrolipoma. These are benign, fat-based tumours that often grow in the skin over the abdominal wall or at the wing butt. Being benign, surgical removal cures the condition. However, the larger they are at surgery the more involved their removal becomes.

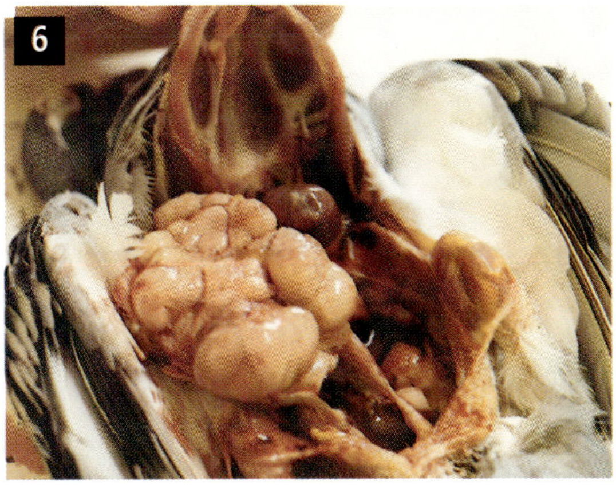

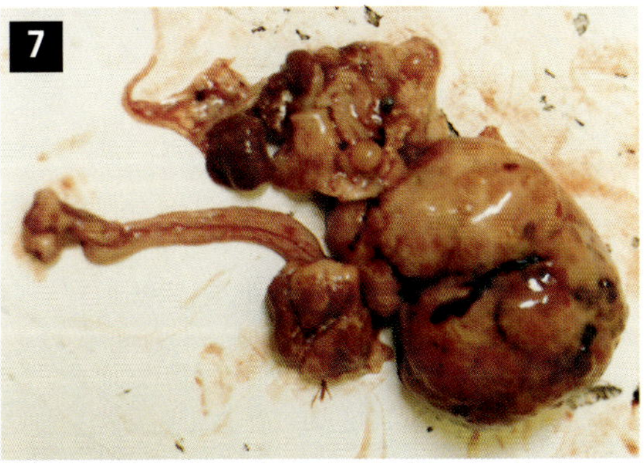

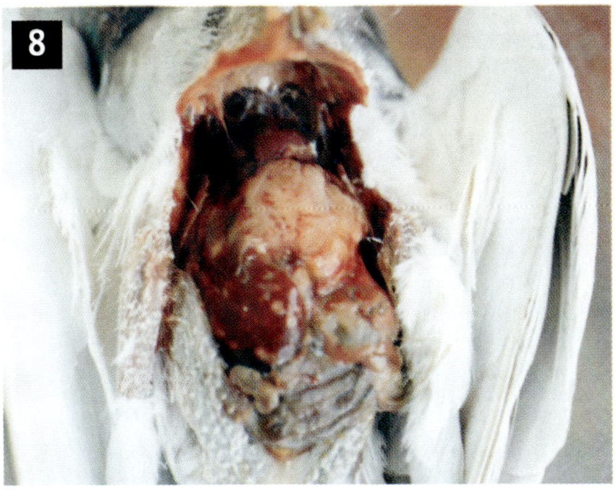

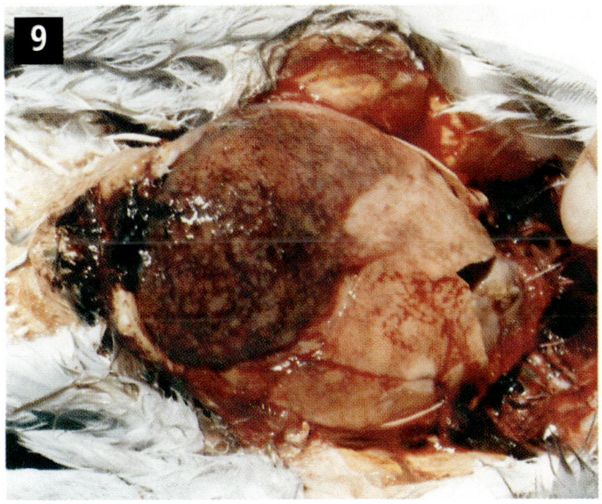

Photo 5: Bird with a fibrolipoma of the wing butt. This bird should have been presented months earlier and the only way now to remove the tumour is in fact to remove the wing. Being a benign tumour, the bird is still quite well in itself.

Photos 6: Autopsy specimen – an ovarian tumour.

Photo 7: Autopsy specimen – an ovarian tumour growing from the lower left-hand corner of the ovary. The tube extending to the top is the bird's oviduct.

Photos 8 and 9: Autopsy specimens – two birds with liver cancer.

Photo 10: Bird with an eye tumour. Treatment has been delayed and the eye has been destroyed and the tumour invaded the side of the head.

Photo 11: Pigeon with an osteosarcoma. This is a highly malignant tumour of bone, which sends secondary tumours into the system very early in the course of the disease. No curative treatment could be offered this bird.

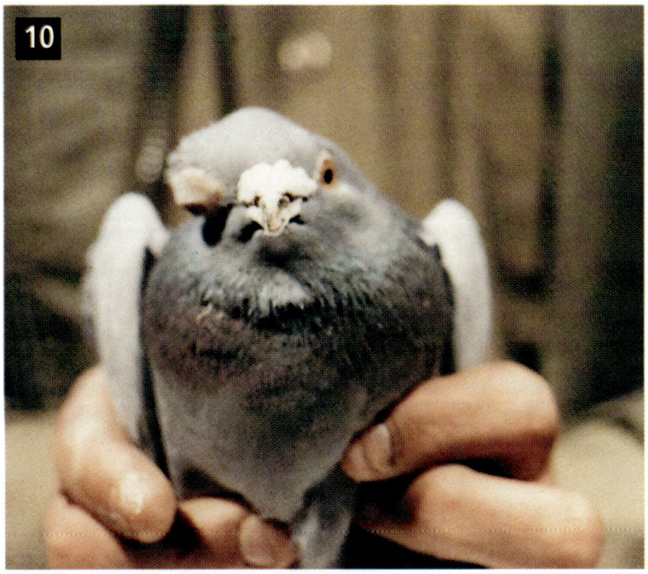

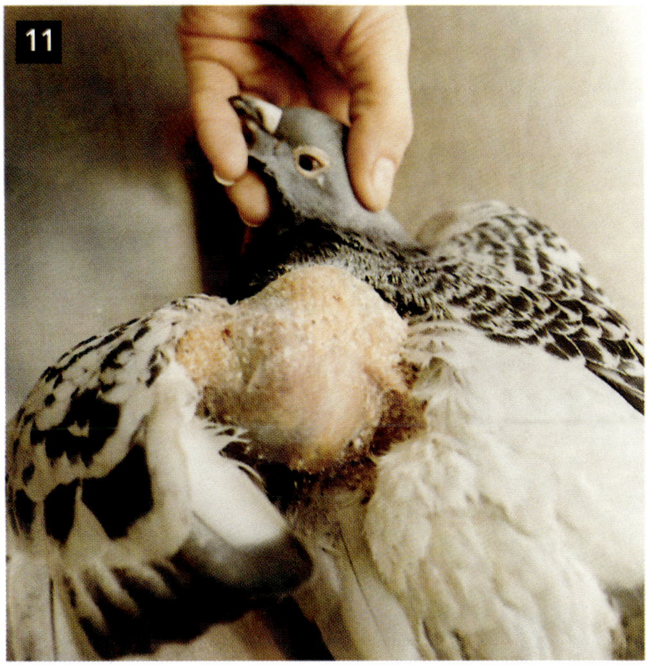

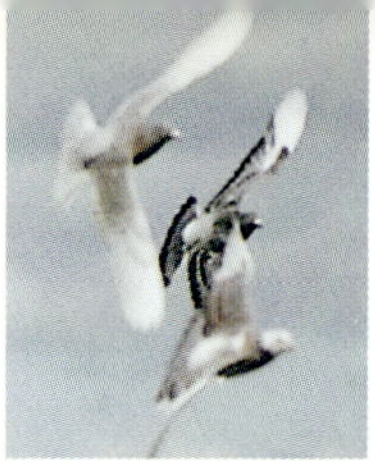

Chapter 10

COMMON VIRAL INFECTIONS

More than 14 infectious viruses have been isolated from pigeons. However, only five cause disease with any frequency. These are Herpes, Circo, pox, Adeno and paramyxovirus. In Australia, only the first four are present.

Herpes virus

Two strains of Herpes virus can cause disease in pigeons. One, Pigeon Herpes Encephalomyelitis virus, affects the brain and causes incoordination and paralysis; this has not as yet been recorded in Australia. The other causes Inclusion Body Hepatitis and is considerably more common than most fanciers would realize. At my clinic, we see approximately 50 cases between December and May each year and I regard this as an underestimate of its frequency through underdiagnosis of the disease, with many fanciers simply killing the few severely affected birds and not seeking veterinary advice. Inclusion Body Hepatitis occurs in pigeons world-wide, and there are several different strains. These strains may also cross-infect other species, including budgies, and, interestingly, even falcons. As the virus affects the bowel, throat and respiratory system, it is found in the droppings, saliva and nasal discharge. Transmission can occur through contact with contaminated food or water, as well as through direct contact between birds. Youngsters between 4 and 16 weeks of age are most susceptible, but birds of any age may catch the disease, particularly if they are run-down. When the disease appears, as many as 50% of all birds in the loft may be affected, with up to 10 – 15% of the birds dying.

Clinical course

Birds that catch the disease and recover usually fail to clear the virus from their system and act as asymptomatic carriers of the disease. These birds periodically shed the virus during their life following stress. The virus can be shed in the droppings, saliva and pigeon milk and is reasonably stable in the environment, being able to survive at 56°C for up to 30 minutes. In a race-loft situation, clinical disease usually first appears in the later-bred youngsters. No matter how well the stock birds are cared for, their general condition deteriorates with each round, and if some of these birds are carriers, then past a certain point they will start to shed the virus, in the process infecting their youngsters. The virus has an incubation period of 5 – 10 days. Clinical signs of the disease vary enormously because the virus can affect multiple sites throughout the body

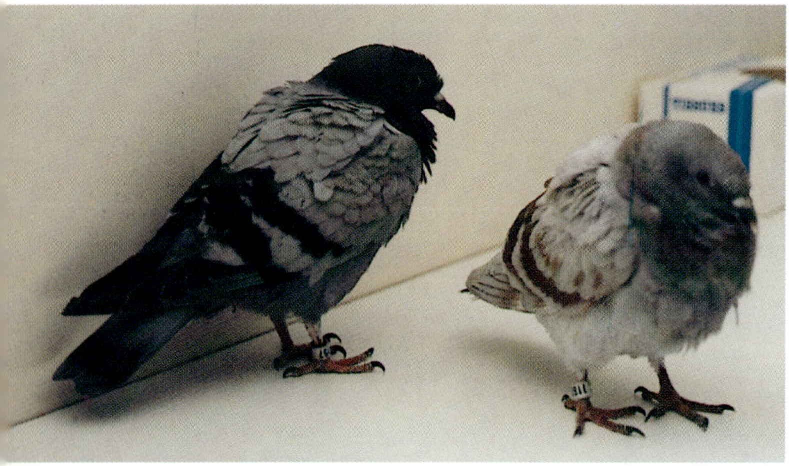

Obviously unwell youngsters, which were subsequently diagnosed with Herpes virus infection.

and affect each of these to a variable extent from one bird to another. Due to this, the disease mimics signs seen in other more common infections, such as canker, *Chlamydia* and *Salmonella*.

In individual birds, it can infect one or all of the following sites:

- The liver, leading to weight loss, poor appetite and green diarrhoea;
- The bowel, leading to dehydration, weight loss and diarrhoea;
- The crop, leading to delayed crop emptying and vomiting;
- The throat, causing mucus production and the appearance of small pale spots in the tonsillar area of the soft palate;
- The trachea, leading to shortness of breath and coughing;
- The nerves of the neck, wings and legs, leading to lameness and wobbly S-shaped necks;
- The skin.

Severity of infection varies from one bird to another, so that some become acutely sick and may die within 24 hours without living long enough to lose condition. Others may be unwell for extended periods and then die, or alternatively make a full recovery, while others still may just appear a bit quiet for a few days.

Diagnosis

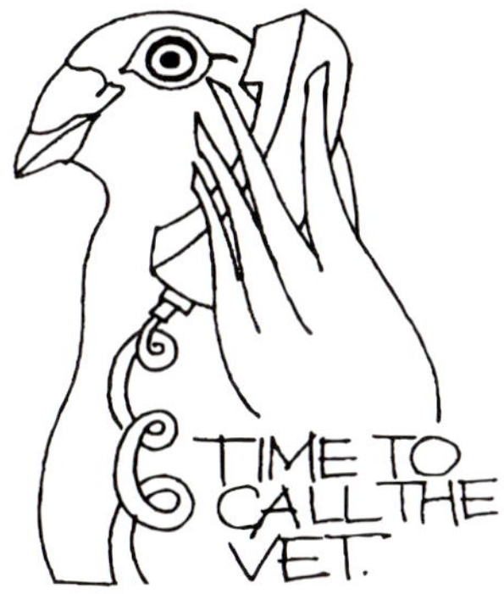

Typically, it is the flock picture that arouses suspicions that the birds are infected with Herpes virus rather than the signs exhibited by a single bird. Usually several birds are affected at any one time, showing a variety of signs as listed above, with typically the more affected birds being fluffed up, reluctant to move, underweight and with green diarrhoea. If Herpes virus is suspected, usually routine tests on the droppings and throat swabs are done initially to rule out other problems. Sometimes results here are suggestive, for example the throat mucus may contain a lot of bacteria and white blood cells. A gross autopsy usually reveals grey-green localized ulcers on the lining of the upper airway, throat, crop and intestine. The airsacs, liver, and abdomen generally, and, less commonly, the kidney, pancreas and spleen may be inflamed. For definitive diagnosis, however, tissue samples collected from a freshly dead bird (less than 20 minutes) must be examined microscopically by an avian pathologist. The virus is visible with special stains under high magnification as either red or blue inclusion bodies within the nuclei of infected cells.

How to manage an outbreak

The initial thing to do in the face of an outbreak is to establish an accurate diagnosis. With any disease problem that mainly affects youngsters that have moulted fewer than three flights and that start to show a variety of signs as described, with some dying, Herpes virus should be suspected. As these unwell birds are an on-going source of infection, they should be immediately isolated, in order to minimize the exposure of other birds and so avoid fresh cases. Of these, one or preferably two should be selected for submission to an avian veterinarian for diagnostic purposes.

No drug is available to routinely treat the disease on a flock basis. Attention must therefore focus on controlling further spread of the virus and ensuring that the pigeons' immune systems are maximally functional by providing on-going good care and controlling any concurrent disease. This not only enables them to resist infection but also to reduce virus levels as quickly as possible if they do, in fact, become infected. This involves four steps:

1 **Identify and correct any predisposing stress-based loft factors and provide on-going good care –** No overcrowding, good hygiene, free access to good-quality grain and grit, no

forced flying, provision of vitamin and mineral supplements.

2 **Control of concurrent diseases** – A health profile is essential to identify concurrent diseases, in particular parasites, so that these in turn can be treated, to prevent them prolonging the birds' recovery. Both American and Australian avian veterinarians have noted that recurring canker is common in flocks with endemic Herpes virus.

3 **Minimize exposure to the virus by further birds** – This is achieved by removing unwell birds and the maintenance of hygienic conditions.

4 **Probiotic use** – One of the ways Herpes virus enters the body is through the digestive tract. The maintenance of a healthy bowel population of bacteria will help birds resist the disease. Similarly, in unwell birds, the normal bowel bacteria are disrupted. Keeping this population as normal as possible helps speed recovery. I usually recommend that an initial course of 5 – 7 days of Probac be given, followed by a minimum of 2 – 3 days weekly until the problem has passed.

Other species of Herpes virus infect other birds, and in some of these a vaccine is available. Different Herpes viruses cause Infectious Laryngotracheitis in chickens and Pacheco's disease in parrots. Vaccine use here, however, is not without its problems, with the vaccine occasionally causing severe side-effects and sometimes failing to give immunity. At present, no vaccine is available for use in pigeons.

A drug, Acyclovir, has been shown to be effective in treating some strains of Herpes virus. The drug is expensive and not always available, but has been given to individual birds (assuming a weight of 500 grams) as a water-soluble powder at the dose of 40 mg directly into the crop three times daily. The same powder can be added to the food at doses as high as 2.5 grams per kilogram of feed. This drug can have severe side-effects, particularly involving the kidneys, and its use is far from routine. However, it may have a role in saving individual birds of particular value.

Pigeon pox

Pigeon pox is a virus that causes the development of dry crusty vesicles on the skin of pigeons. The disease is usually regarded as a mild one, with the birds displaying mild or no signs of systemic disease. Different viral strains vary in their potential to cause disease, with most strains causing only small vesicle formation. In fact, most clinically affected birds are infected by 'escaped' vaccine strains of the virus. Some strains, however, can cause severe soft tissue damage, leading to deformity of the eyelids and/or the tongue or loss of sections or all of the beak. For the average pigeon fancier, however, pox is more a disease of inconvenience rather than one through which he stands to lose birds.

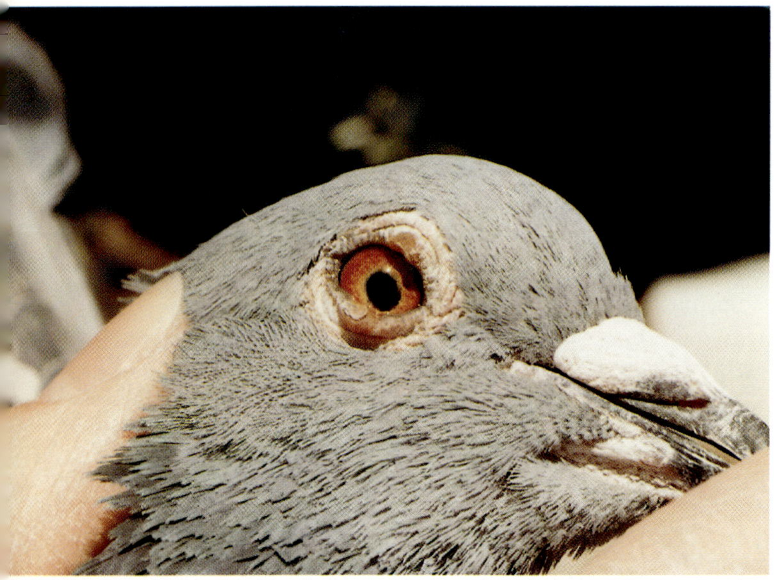

Two 'vaccine-strain' pox vesicles on the eyelids of a non-vaccinated pigeon that had been pecked by a recently vaccinated bird.

Clinical course

Birds with the disease excrete the virus in tears, saliva and sometimes their droppings. At certain times, the virus is also found in their blood. For birds to become infected, the virus needs a break in the skin or mucus membrane lining the mouth to gain entry, and so the usual mode of transmission is fighting, where the beak of an infected bird simultaneously breaks the skin and leaves a small amount of saliva behind. For this reason, most lesions are around the eyes and beak. Mosquitoes and other blood-sucking insects can also transmit the disease but can usually only gain access to the unfeathered parts of the body and so cause lesions around the head and also on the legs. The exception here is red mite, which, when transmitting the disease, can cause vesicles to develop anywhere on the body. When non-infected and infected birds share drinkers or bath water, the virus can be transmitted. When birds are sharing bath water, the virus can infect the feather follicle at the time the feather is emerging and cause vesicles to form here.

The virus runs a natural course of 4 – 6 weeks, with birds spontaneously recovering. Deaths rarely occur and when they do are usually secondary to the physical bulk of the vesicle interfering with breathing, eating or vision. Fortunately, most affected birds develop only one or two small (approximately 3 mm) vesicles and essentially remain well in themselves. Birds recovered from the disease develop a life-long immunity. No direct treatment is available. However, as lesions in the mouth often become secondarily infected with bacteria and/or trichomonads, treating these will help to dry the lesion up, minimize tissue damage and make the bird more comfortable while the virus runs its course. Usually, 1/4 of a 200-mg Flagyl tablet once daily and 1/2 a 50-mg doxycycline (Vibravet) tablet also once daily give good control of these secondary agents.

Vaccination

Pigeon pox is controlled through vaccination.

Timing of vaccination

Only well youngsters over 6 weeks of age should be vaccinated. Birds under 6 weeks of age should ideally not be vaccinated. When we vaccinate birds, we in fact give them a mild dose of the disease. Youngsters younger than 6 weeks of age are struggling to form a natural immunity to many common problems, including wet canker and *Chlamydia*, and giving them a mild dose of a live virus can severely stress them, enabling other organisms to flare up and cause disease. For this reason, it is important that only well youngsters in well-managed lofts are vaccinated, otherwise other disease problems can be expected.

Once vaccinated, birds carry a scab at the inoculation site for 4 – 6 weeks and are infectious to other birds during this time. As most Federations exclude birds with any infectious disease from race entry, vaccination must be done 6 weeks or more before the commencement of racing.

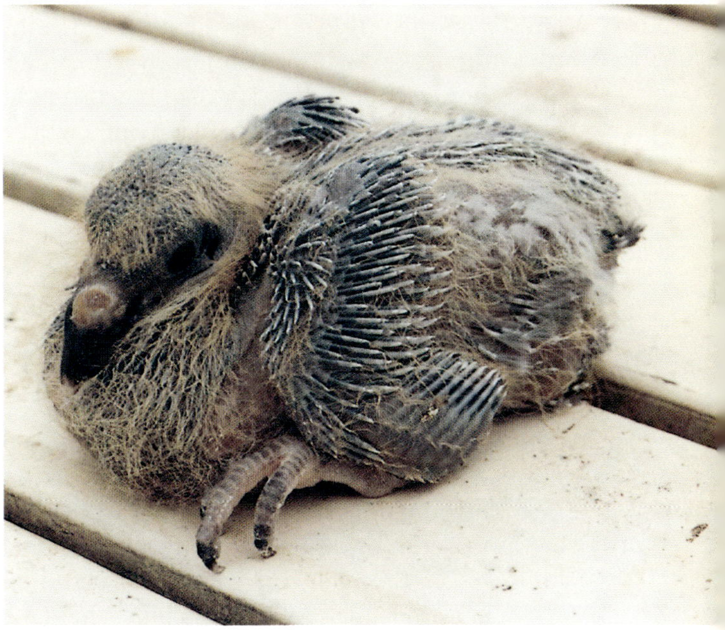

Pigeon pox vesicles on the beak of a 7-day-old youngster. For the vesicle to be this size at this age, this youngster must have become infected virtually in the first day of life.

Vaccination technique

The vaccine is supplied in two bottles, which should be kept frozen until immediately before use. One bottle contains a clear frozen diluent. The other contains an orange pellet of dried vaccine. To prepare the vaccine, remove the caps from both bottles. The diluent will thaw in approximately 1 minute and the resultant liquid is then added to the viral pellet. The cap on this bottle is then replaced and the contents shaken gently to produce an orange liquid. This is the vaccine. The aim of vaccination is not to inject the vaccine but rather to create a deep scratch so that the vaccine is

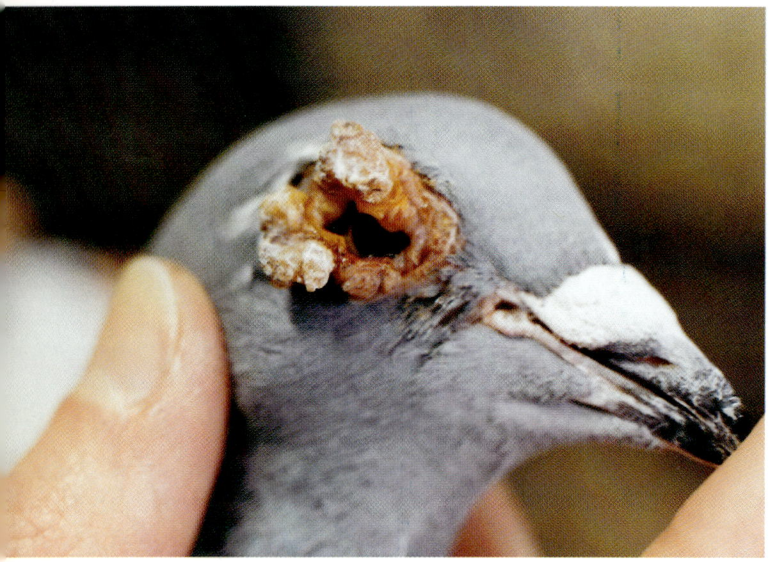

Advanced pigeon pox.

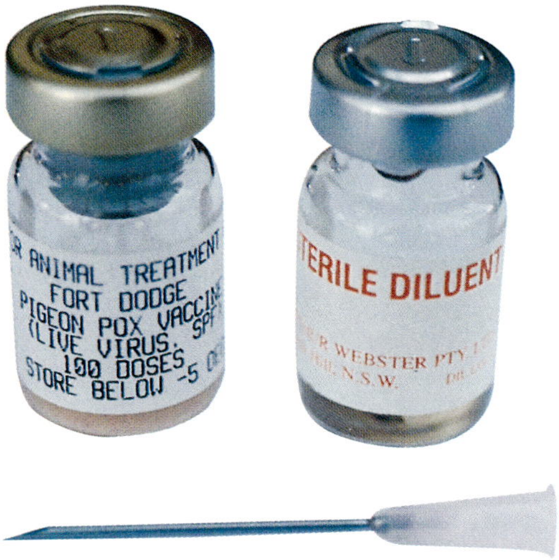

Pigeon pox vaccine.

mixed with both blood and air, mimicking the natural mode of transmission. I use an 18-gauge needle, which after dipping in the vaccine is slid parallel to the skin so that the tip runs under the skin for about 1 mm. This should result in a small amount of bleeding. The best place to vaccinate birds is on the outside of the thigh. Folding a few feathers back the wrong way will expose a narrow strip of skin, which is an ideal vaccination site. Many fliers vaccinate near the keel. However, this is not recommended. The skin here is very thin and it is very easy to insert the needle too far, in the process damaging the underlying flight muscles. This can cause some residual soreness and even if this only happens in one bird out of a hundred, that bird might have been the current year's big winner.

After vaccination, a yellow thickening should appear initially, which will develop into a crusty lump within 10 days. This crust will fall off 4 – 6 weeks after vaccination and the bird is infectious to other non-vaccinated birds until this happens. As with birds that recover from the active disease, vaccinated birds are usually immune for life.

Postvaccination care

After vaccination, birds, for the most part, may be treated normally. They can be fed and loft-flown normally and indeed, for young racers, I feel that it is important that they be kept in their loft routine. The only time to be a bit careful with them is about 7 – 10 days after vaccination as the scabs are forming. At this time, the virus is in the blood stream and the birds develop a slight fever. Some birds will appear mildly unwell, being a bit fluffed up and reluctant to exercise and may have slightly watery droppings. Also at this time, the uvea (the iris and its support structures in the eye) in some birds can become inflamed. This makes them a bit light sensitive and squinty. If flown late in the day, when the shadows are starting to get long, they can become confused and a fly-away is possible.

A common question at the clinic is whether vaccinated birds should be allowed to get wet or bathe. They can, of course, provided all birds have been vaccinated. This is only a concern if unvaccinated and vaccinated birds are mixed.

Following vaccination, healthy birds in good lofts rarely become unwell. However, because the vaccination is a stress, it can contribute to a disease flare-up in birds that are already stressed due to poor management practices or already carrying diseases. Subclinical infections of diseases such as *Chlamydia* and wet canker can flare up after vaccination because of the superimposed stress of the vaccination, and in fact can serve to notify the fancier that these diseases are present. After vacci-

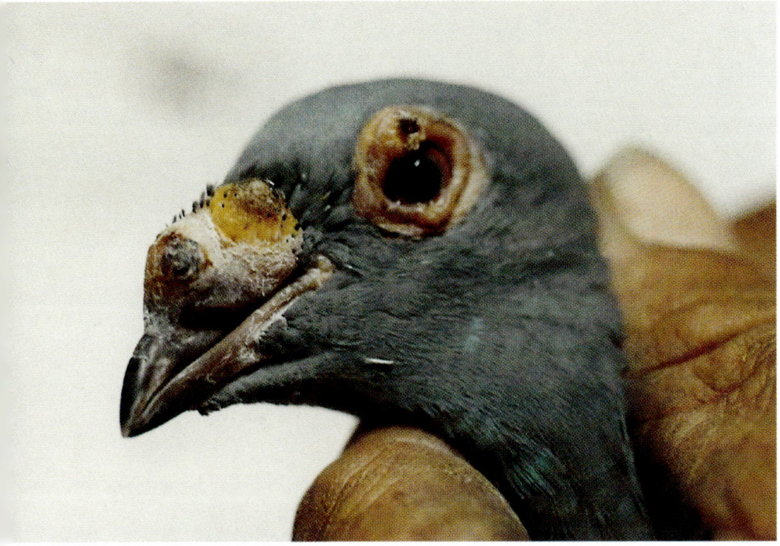

Stock cock with pox vesicles on the eyelids and the cere.

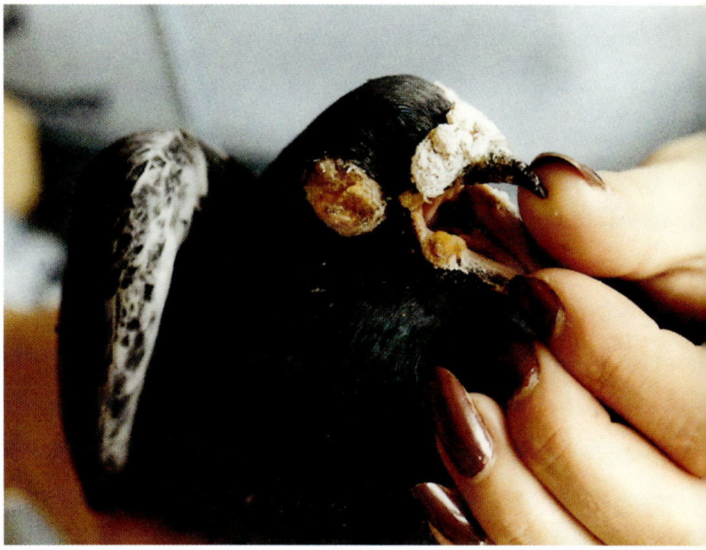

Extensive pox virus lesions on the eyelids and beak margin.

nation, it is therefore particularly important that the fancier provide on-going good care and monitor the birds for any concurrent diseases. If respiratory infection or canker appears, antibiotics and anticanker medication can be used without directly interfering with the development of an immunity to pox. However, birds that are stressed for any reason in the 4 weeks after vaccination tend not to develop as strong a level of immunity.

Management of an outbreak

Out of the racing season

If an outbreak occurs out of the racing season, provided birds are over 6 weeks of age and it is at least 6 weeks before racing, the best thing to do is simply to vaccinate the birds. If vaccinating in the face of an outbreak, birds already with the disease should not be vaccinated.

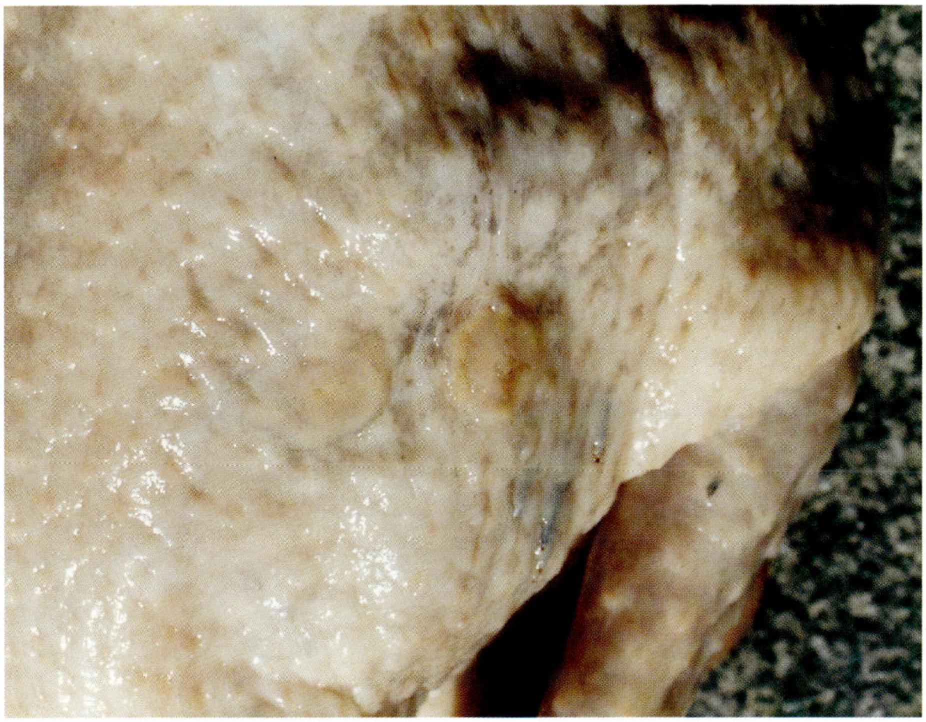

One of a batch of meat pigeons condemned for human consumption due to the pox vesicles revealed when plucked.

During racing

If an outbreak occurs during racing, the situation is not as easy. The usual reason for vaccinating is to prevent just this occurrence. As mentioned above, the disease is rarely fatal but tends to be one of inconvenience. If birds appear with pox in the racing loft during the season, the flier has one of two options:

1 **To vaccinate all birds –** This means that between 4 and 6 weeks of competition are lost and so this option is rarely taken.

2 **To separate affected birds from the rest of the team –** These birds can be fed, watered and exercised separately and when recovered after 4 – 6 weeks can be brought back into the team as fresh birds. The difficulty here comes in that the virus has an incubation period of 10 days. By the time it is realized that the bird has pox, it may have already pecked or in some other way infected several birds in the loft, which are now incubating the disease and further spreading it. Eventually, most of the team ends up with the disease. In many lofts, however, this does represent an effective means of containment and as soon as the fancier has had a 10-day break without any new cases, he knows that the outbreak is controlled. Recovered birds are competitive.

   In 1995, no pox vaccine was available in Australia. I chose this option to control the spread of the infection and won at the distance on two occasions with birds that earlier in the season had had pigeon pox and had to be spelled.

Outbreaks that occur during breeding are usually initiated by mosquitoes as there is not the same exposure to birds from other lofts as there is in the racing loft. Individual birds that become infected are usually best immediately separated in order to minimize spread of the disease. Mosquitoes can be discouraged by regular spraying with Permethrin Solution.

Conditions that look similar

The most common disease that pox is confused with is canker. When pox appears on the skin (the cutaneous form), the dry crusty lumpy appearance of the lesion is usually diagnostic. However, when it occurs in the mouth (mucosal pox), the lesion looks like a yellow plaque, which is easy to confuse with canker. Indeed, in some birds, I can only tell the difference by swabbing the lesion and looking under the microscope. Often, the fancier is alerted to mucosal pox by no response to anti-canker medication. There are two simple loft-based tests that a fancier can use to distinguish the two:

1 **The site of the lesion –** If an imaginary line is drawn through the base of the bird's beak, then any lesions between this line and the tip of the beak are likely to be pox vesicles. This area is too hostile and exposed for trichomonad organisms to survive. Conversely, lesions on the throat side of this line are likely to be canker.

2 **Attachment to surrounding tissue –** As canker lesions invade, there is often a fragile line of inflammation at the edge of the lesion, which enables separation of the canker nodule from the surrounding tissue. The pox lesion is a vesicle or blister of the mouth lining itself, and so cannot be separated from it.

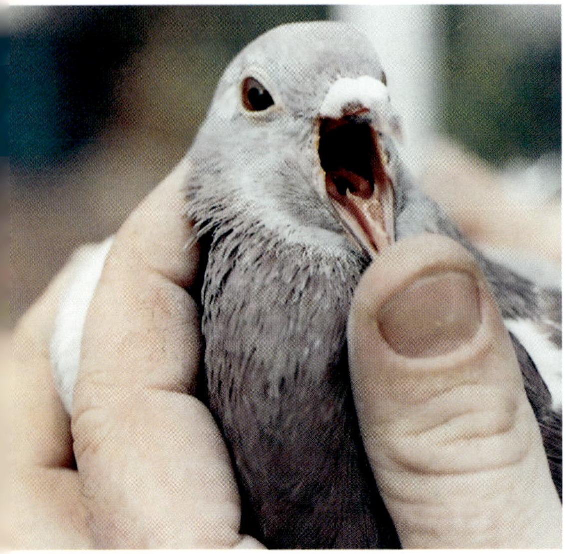

Pox vesicle on tongue. This 'mucosal' form of the disease is easy to confuse with canker. Pox causes a 'blister' to form. In this bird, the central part of the blister has gone to reveal the outer edge of the blister or pox vesicle.

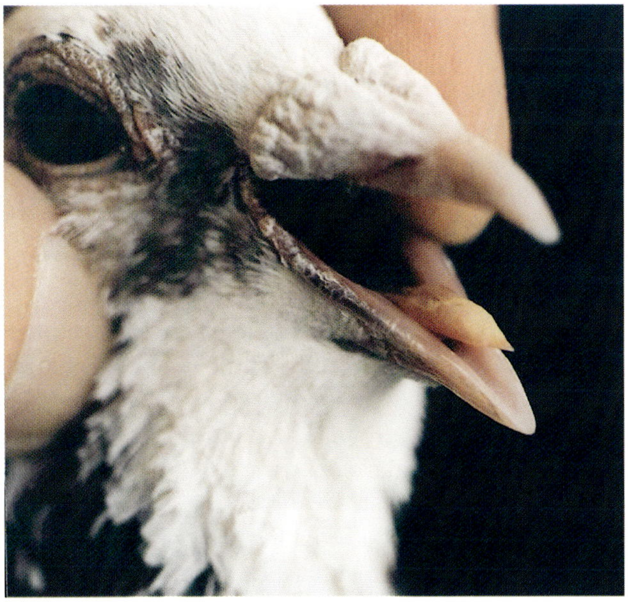

Pox vesicle on the tongue. Severe lesions can lead to the loss of part or all of the tongue.

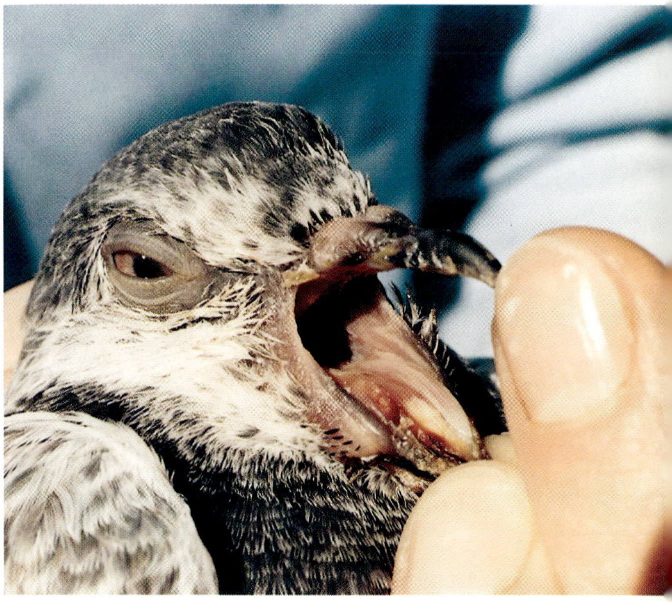

Severe pox lesion of the lower beak. Severe lesions on the beak can interfere with its blood supply, leading to loss of part or all of the beak, as in this case.

Adeno virus infection*

There are two types of Adeno virus that infect pigeons. Type 1 mainly affects young pigeons and involves the digestive tract, causing diarrhoea and vomiting. Many of these birds recover. Type 2 affects older pigeons and involves the liver, with most birds that become unwell dying within 24 hours.

A paper published in 1995 by several Belgian veterinarians described a new fatal disease of racing pigeons in that country. It began in October 1992 and was characterized by sudden death in pigeons of all ages. Some birds displayed a fluid yellow diarrhoea and vomiting before death. However, the main sign was sudden death, which occurred within 24 hours of the onset of illness, with none of the sick birds surviving longer than 48 hours. Losses from one loft to another varied but often were approximately 30%. In some cases, it reached 100%. In $1^1/_2$ years from January 1993, nearly 1000 pigeons that died of the disease were examined at the University of Gent, Belgium. These birds had a hepatitis (liver inflammation) with extensive death of liver tissue microscopically. Examination revealed that the cause was an Adeno virus.

The spread of Adeno virus in a loft was unusual in that it usually started in a single age group but then spread to birds of all ages. Other birds that had been in intimate contact with the dead birds often remained well. Even youngsters in the nest grew normally if they were able to feed themselves after their parents had died.

Subsequent testing showed that only immunosuppressed birds (i.e. those in which the immune system's function was compromised) were vulnerable to the disease. However, the exact cause of the immunosuppression was unclear. Researchers have suggested that the Adeno virus that causes a disease in chickens had mutated or changed slightly to allow it to adapt to pigeons and cause this serious new disease. Definitive diagnosis is made by microscopic examination of tissues in which, with special stains, the viral particles can been seen as inclusion bodies within the birds' cells.

This type of Adeno virus infection is rare in Australia and to date, at my clinic, I have seen only one case. In this loft, 8 birds out of 150 died within 24 hours and then there was no problem.

The disease reported in 1995 is now called Adeno Virus Type 2. The first (called Type 1) was discovered in 1976 and is associated with disease in young pigeons (compare this with the other form

* Many thanks to my veterinary colleague Dr Gordon Chalmers, of Canada, for much of this information.

of the disease). In this type there is a watery diarrhoea and weight loss. *E. coli* often complicates this Adeno virus infection and results in a more severe diarrhoea as well as vomiting and occasionally respiratory symptoms. The disease has a low death rate and some birds can spontaneously recover. Affected birds lose condition and if racing persists results are poor and there are increased losses. There is also decreased resistance to other diseases. The disease was reported in Great Britain in 1994 and 1995. Large numbers of infected birds were reported by Dutch pigeon veterinarian Henk DeWeerd in south-west Holland by the end of 1991.

Whereas Adeno Virus Type 2 infection does not respond to antibiotics, this Adeno virus-*E. coli* combined disease is usually successfully treated with antibiotics. If birds are autopsied, there is an obvious enteritis (bowel inflammation), but the liver can look normal and extensive death of liver tissue is not seen microscopically. There are, however, the characteristic viral inclusion bodies. Adeno virus Type 1 is also uncommon in Australia. Only a few cases have been seen at my clinic, the last one being in a Victorian country loft in mid-1996. Cases were managed by ensuring that the loft environment and management were good and that all secondary diseases, notably wet canker and Coccidia, were treated in order that the birds were best able to clear the virus. The concurrent *E. coli* can be treated with the antibiotics Baytril or Sulfa AVS or alternatively probiotics.

To date it seems that both types of Adeno virus infection are rare in Australia, but the introduction of birds into Australia with any viral disease is a concern. Obviously, quarantine is part of the answer. However, if there are healthy carriers of Adeno virus, preventing further entry will be difficult, particularly as the Belgian investigators found healthy pigeons in lofts where birds were dying suddenly of Adeno virus infection. A similar difficulty has been witnessed with wet canker and mycoplasmal strains in Australia since 1990 and there is concern that apparently healthy birds could also bring Adeno virus into Australia.

Circo virus*

Circo virus is sometimes called pigeon AIDS because of the way it damages the immune system and creates a vulnerability to secondary infection.

Circo virus is still a relatively new problem in pigeons. Circo virus-related disease has been identified in chickens and parrots and since 1986 Circo virus has also been shown to cause disease in pigeons. It was first demonstrated in Canada in 1986, then in Australia in 1989, and in the U.S.A. in 1990. The first confirmed case at my clinic in Melbourne occurred in 1994 and we now confirm the infection in about 50 lofts per year although I feel that the problem tends to be underdiagnosed through non-presentation of sick birds by some fanciers.

Clinical course

The virus damages a particular type of white blood cell called a lymphocyte. These are closely associated with the body's immune defences. With damage to the population of lymphocytes, the birds become susceptible to secondary infections with other viruses, bacteria and parasites. Infected birds can become very ill over a short period of time. Alternatively, the virus can lead to an on-going problem with control of diseases such as canker or respiratory infection because of damage to the immune system. This is because we rely on a low-grade exposure to disease-causing agents in the postweaning period to form a strong natural immunity in the developing youngster. In birds with Circo virus, because the immune system is damaged by the virus, they cannot respond in the normal vigorous way to this exposure, so that a good natural immunity cannot form.

Like many other infections, Circo virus infection seems to be most important in young pigeons. Birds diagnosed with the problem have ranged in age from 6 weeks to 1 year. Most commonly, however, the virus causes death in very young pigeons and then appears to strike older youngsters that

---

* Many thanks to my veterinary colleague Dr Gordon Chalmers, of Canada, for much of the this information.

have already moulted three to four flights. These birds are thin, dehydrated, reluctant to move and have a yellow discharge dried on the margins of the beak. These older youngsters die very quickly after they begin to show signs. It is unusual for youngsters that have dropped five or more flights to be affected. Presumably, older birds have an age-related resistance or have developed solid immunity as a result of earlier infection. The virus does seem hard to transmit in the loft. Typically only low numbers (less than 10% of birds) become ill and die. Other birds in the loft of the same age, even with on-going daily direct contact with sick birds, may not develop signs of disease and can remain completely healthy.

The main problem with Circo virus infection in pigeons is associated with the virus' ability to cause massive destruction of the cells that direct and coordinate the body's defences against a variety of other diseases. With the immune system compromised, other disease-causing agents such as bacteria, *Chlamydia* and canker are able to cause disease.

There may well be carrier birds in a flock, i.e. birds that appear completely normal but shed virus during periods of stress. Stress for a stock bird is breeding and so it is likely that carrier stock birds pass the virus on to a percentage of their own youngsters, which will become unwell during the postweaning period. It may be that, because the virus spreads relatively slowly in a flock, this itself may allow more birds to develop good immunity rather than outright disease. Once in the racing loft, it can spread from youngster to youngster although it appears that most youngsters exposed in this way, if in a good loft, will develop an immunity rather than become sick. The virus can be spread by droppings or nasal or oral discharges.

Interestingly, in parrots, Circo virus also damages the feather follicle. The feathers that grow from these diseased follicles are abnormal, often having persistent feather sheaths, bleeding into the pulp cavity of the feather and fret marks. In the last few years, similar lesions have been seen in pigeons. Microscopically, no evidence of Circo virus has been found in these birds. Bacterial, fungal and nutritional problems that damage the follicular lining can cause similar lesions, however, it may be that, with the advent of more advanced testing, in particular a blood test called PCR, that a Circo virus involvement will be demonstrated in these birds.

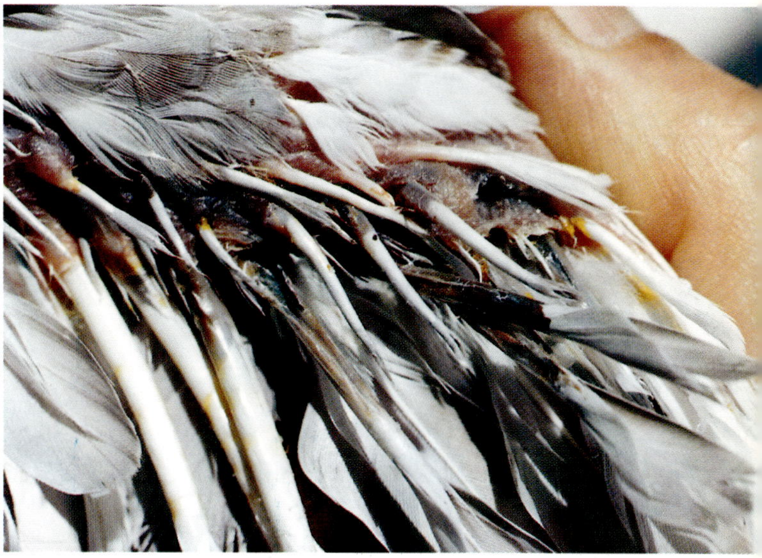

Suspect Circo virus infection of the feather follicles, leading to abnormal feather production. The feathers produced from these inflamed follicles have persistent feather sheaths and blood and other debris extending into the feather shaft and are easily removed from the inflamed follicle.

Diagnosis

Be suspicious of Circo virus infection if:

- Your pigeons, particularly the youngsters, are showing a variety of disease signs and in some birds these progress to the stage where they die, and
- There are on-going problems with disease such as *E. coli*, wet canker, or in particular respiratory infection, despite good care, good management and correct medication.

However, it is not possible to diagnose Circo virus simply by looking at the birds. The signs observed are usually those caused by the secondary infections and so can be extremely variable. Birds presented at my clinic, which were subsequently shown to be infected with Circo virus, have exhibited loss of appetite, lethargy, diarrhoea ranging from slightly sloppy to profuse and gelatinous,

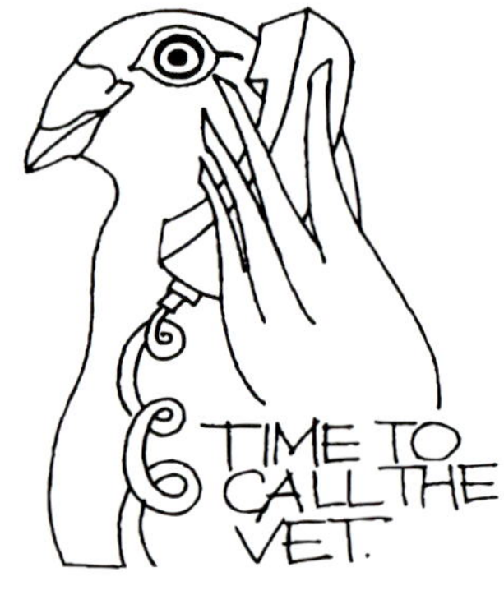

loss of weight, nasal discharge, difficulty breathing, yellow exudate at the beak margins and death. Given the different signs exhibited, it is difficult to find a common pattern of disease as a basis for suspecting a Circo virus infection. However, the occurrence of one or more outbreaks of disease in young pigeons may well provide the first tell-tale signs that Circo virus is active in your birds.

It is important to get an accurate diagnosis and not to jump to conclusions. Although finding several problems in a single youngster on routine testing (crop flush and faecal smear) and disease recurring a short time after effective treatment or a slow response may arouse suspicions, a definitive diagnosis requires microscopic examination of the bird's tissues. The Bursa of Fabricius is a gland made up of lymphoid (tonsil-like) tissue inside the cloaca; it degenerates at puberty. It is here that the virus causes the most damage and can best be demonstrated. Birds need to be presented live for diagnostic autopsy. The virus is most likely to be found if the bird is sick at the time of presentation and less than 5 months of age. Following euthanasia, sections of all organs are collected but particularly the Bursa of Fabricius. The disease produces characteristic 'inclusion bodies' in infected cells. The inclusions, which appear to contain large aggregates of viral particles, have a blue-black grape cluster appearance when tissue is treated with a common stain (H & E). Electron microscopic examination of these inclusion bodies will further reveal the characteristic appearance of the viral particles they contain.

How to Manage the Disease

Frustratingly, there is not as much that we can do for the disease as we would like. There is no direct treatment for Circo virus. However, I suggest that the disease is managed in the following way:

- **An attempt should be made to keep the virus out of the loft –** Keeping the virus out of the loft is hard through the very nature of pigeon racing where birds from many lofts mix weekly in race units. However, birds should not be introduced from lofts known to have an underlying health problem. Be particularly cautious of acquiring youngsters at squeaker sales as these are more likely to be actively shedding the virus. Stray youngsters, particularly if they look unwell, should immediately be removed. An attempt can be made to identify carrier stock birds by remating those whose youngsters appear weak or die.
- **If the virus does gain entry, try to minimize its spread –** This is achieved by removing sick birds immediately and providing on-going hygiene.
- **Provide on-going good care –** This places the birds in the best situation to resist infection and similarly gives those in which infection establishes the best chance of recovery.
- **Treat secondary diseases –** A health profile is vital to identify secondary problems so these can be effectively treated. Treating the secondary infections is important. This allows the birds to survive long enough for the damaged immune system to repair or partially repair itself. It seems that a certain number of young birds will be affected, but that, depending on the age of the flock, most birds will develop enough immunity through direct contact with sick birds to survive in good health. To quote Dr Gordon Chalmers:

> *"Circoviral infections are not likely to disappear in the near future, and as the virus spreads, there will likely be more cases of the secondary diseases mentioned earlier to indicate that Circo virus is active in a number of lofts. Forewarned is forearmed. We can help our own situations by getting accurate laboratory diagnoses of Circoviral infections and the diseases that follow it. Vigorous and rapid treatment of these secondary diseases are likely to be our main defence against losses triggered by infection with Circo virus."*

- **Use probiotics –** As one of the ways Circo virus enters the body is through the digestive tract, the maintenance of a healthy bowel population of bacteria helps well birds resist the disease. Similarly, in unwell birds, the normal bowel bacteria are disrupted. Keeping this population as normal as possible helps speed recovery. I usually recommend that an initial 5 – 7-day course of Probac be given, followed by a minimum of 2 – 3 days weekly until the problem has passed.

Although it is disappointing to find that the virus has entered the loft, the good news is that, despite being infectious, Circo virus does seem hard to transmit and it has been my experience that in well-managed lofts less than 3% of youngsters will become severely unwell and die. Also, as the level of immunity in the loft as a whole tends to gradually increase, although of great concern the first year it is diagnosed, the problem does tend to become less and less with each year so that within 3 – 4 years the virus' effect is reduced to a manageable level.

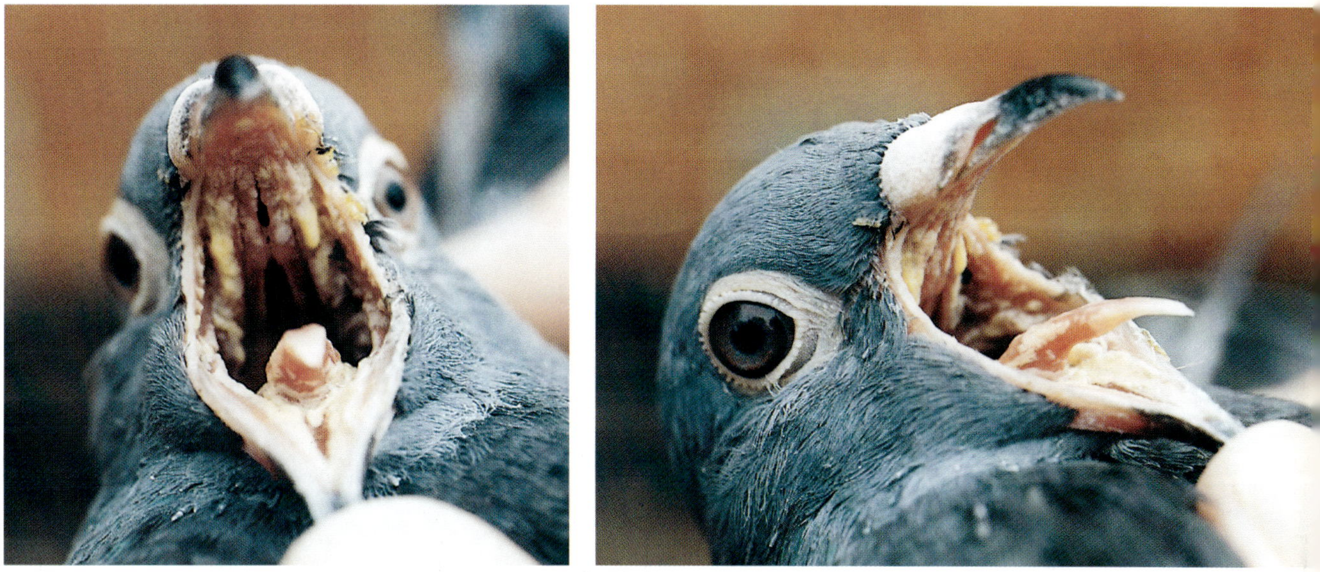

Bird with Circo virus infection with the oral viral ulcers covered by yellow discharge, found in many birds with this infection. This bird also had a secondary canker infection.

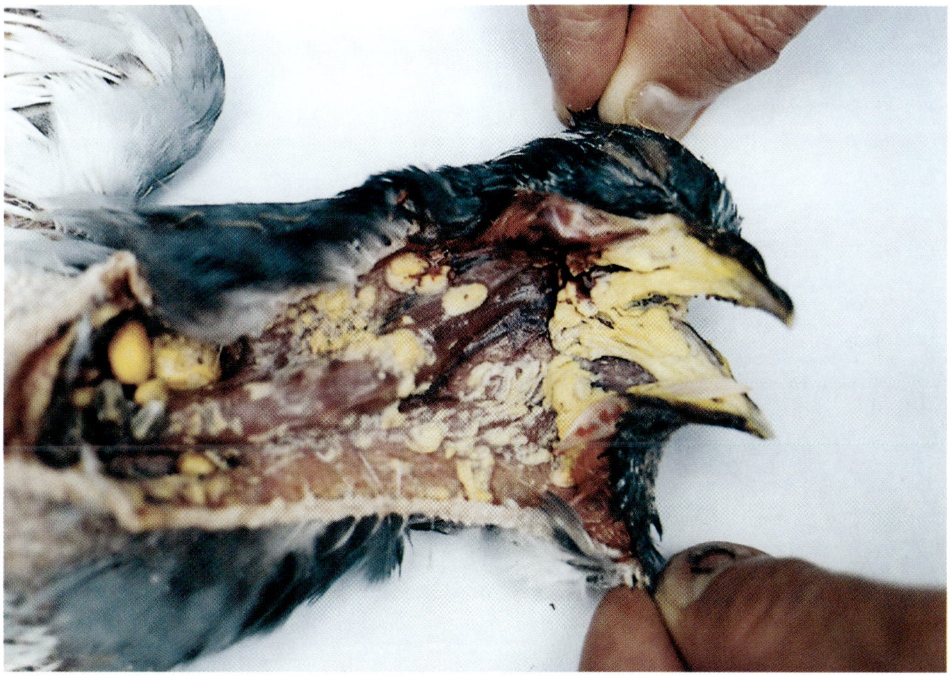

Autopsy specimen. Circo virus ulcers with secondary canker infection.

Ruptured airsacs

Often fliers ring my clinic saying that their birds seem to have filled up with air. This is usually due to a ruptured airsac. Like us, pigeons have a windpipe, which carries air down into the lungs, but, in addition, pigeons have blind sacs, called airsacs, which run from the sinuses in their head and from their lungs. There are nine main airsacs, one across the front of the chest, two either side of the chest and two either side of the abdomen. Oxygen cannot enter the bloodstream through these as it does from the lungs but they are important in temperature and moisture regulation and, as they are essentially pockets of air, they keep the body weight light, making flight easier. When inhaled, air goes down the windpipe into the lungs and out into the airsacs. If there is a tear in the airsac, air can percolate out through this and accumulate under the skin. Airsacs usually develop tears either as a result of injury, when the bird flies into something (this can even occur in stock birds that knock themselves on the corner of a perch, etc.) or secondary to a respiratory infection, when there is a perforating ulcer that erodes through the airsac. Respiratory infection can sometimes block the fine tubes that connect airsacs, leading to overinflation. If the bird has been unwell or has shown other signs of respiratory infection and then develops an accumulation of air under the skin, it can be assumed that either a rupture has occurred secondary to this infection, or a connecting tube has become obstructed with inflammatory debris. Also but rarely, a rupture can occur secondary to internal disease, such as a tumour. If a bird was well and is then suddenly noticed to have ballooned up, then a tear associated with an injury is the most likely cause. The usual airsac that is ruptured is the one that is across the front of the chest, because it is more vulnerable to injury. This leads to the neck becoming superinflated with air. If the airsacs on either side of the chest or abdomen are ruptured, air accumulates under the skin over these areas first before extending elsewhere.

To treat these birds, it is important to remove the air that has accumulated under the skin. If the air pressure continues to build up, this pressure can relay back onto the lungs and the birds can have trouble breathing and sometimes smother. To remove the air, a hypo-

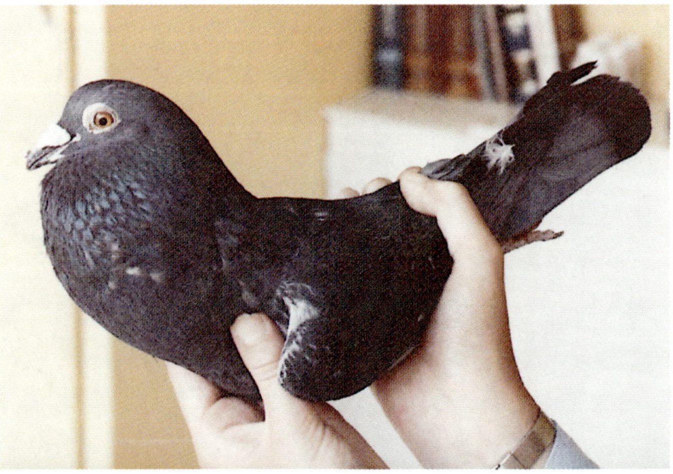

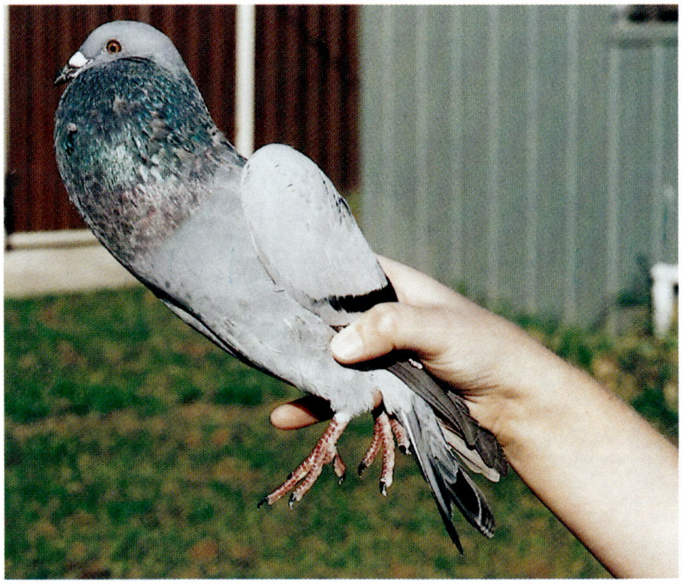

Two birds, each with a ruptured interclavicular airsac.

dermic needle and syringe are used. The tip of the needle is put just through the skin at the point where the skin is tightest with the air underneath it. While sucking with the syringe, air is drawn out through the needle. This usually needs to be done morning and night. This not only makes the bird more comfortable but allows the airsac to collapse back into position so that the tear comes into apposition and is then given a chance to heal. Small tears may heal in 1 – 3 days. More severe tears may take up to 3 weeks. I have only ever had one or two birds that never healed. In addition to removing the air morning and night, it is important that the bird is confined. It must not do any exercise that would make it short of breath or pant as this tends to reopen the healing tear in the airsac. I usually use an 18-gauge needle and a 20-ml syringe. These can be obtained from a pharmacy or a veterinarian. Where an associated respiratory infection is suspected, antibiotics are given, usually Vibravet 50 mg, ½ tablet once daily for 5 days.

Paramyxovirus

A paramyxovirus, closely related to Newcastle Disease Virus, was first recognized in pigeons in the late 1970's, probably having arisen in the Middle East. The virus reached Europe by 1981 and spread virtually all over the world except for a few places, including Australia.

There are several different types of paramyxovirus. The type that infects pigeons is called Paramyxovirus Type 1 (PMV-1). Paramyxoviruses in this group also cause Newcastle Disease in chickens and many other types of birds. However, the paramyxovirus that infects pigeons is no longer considered to be classic Newcastle Disease virus.

Paramyxovirus enters the body through the respiratory and gastrointestinal tracts. It is also thought that the virus might infect embryos, with the virus being included with the egg at the time of its formation or alternatively contaminating the egg shell after laying.

In the early stages of the disease, the virus affects the bowel. Affected pigeons show a variety of symptoms, including loss of appetite, diarrhoea, vomiting and a thirst initially. Following this, the nervous system is affected. This causes a rigid paralysis of the wings and occasionally the legs, leading to incoordination accompanied by head tremours and a twisted neck. Occasionally, a floppy paralysis also develops. The virus can also cause eyelid swelling, embryo death, and the growth of unusual feathers if birds are affected while moulting. In young birds, significant mortality can occur. Affected old birds, provided they can still eat and drink, or if force fed, can recover within 3 – 4 weeks after first becoming unwell.

Diagnosis

The signs displayed by the birds are very suggestive. However, the disease is diagnosed either directly by culturing the virus from the droppings or respiratory discharge from affected birds, or indirectly by a blood test in which antibodies for the virus are detected.

The disease can at times look similar to several other conditions including poisonings (due to organophosphates, carbamates, or heavy metals such as lead), calcium deficiency and the meningeal form of paratyphoid. Usually the overall flock picture presented, together with clinical signs displayed by several affected birds, allows diagnosis to be made. However, if needed, the above tests are done.

Vaccination

The disease is controlled through vaccination, of which several are available to fanciers in different parts of the world. Local avian veterinarians can advise fanciers as to what is available and what is best for them.

Section 3

YOUNG BIRDS

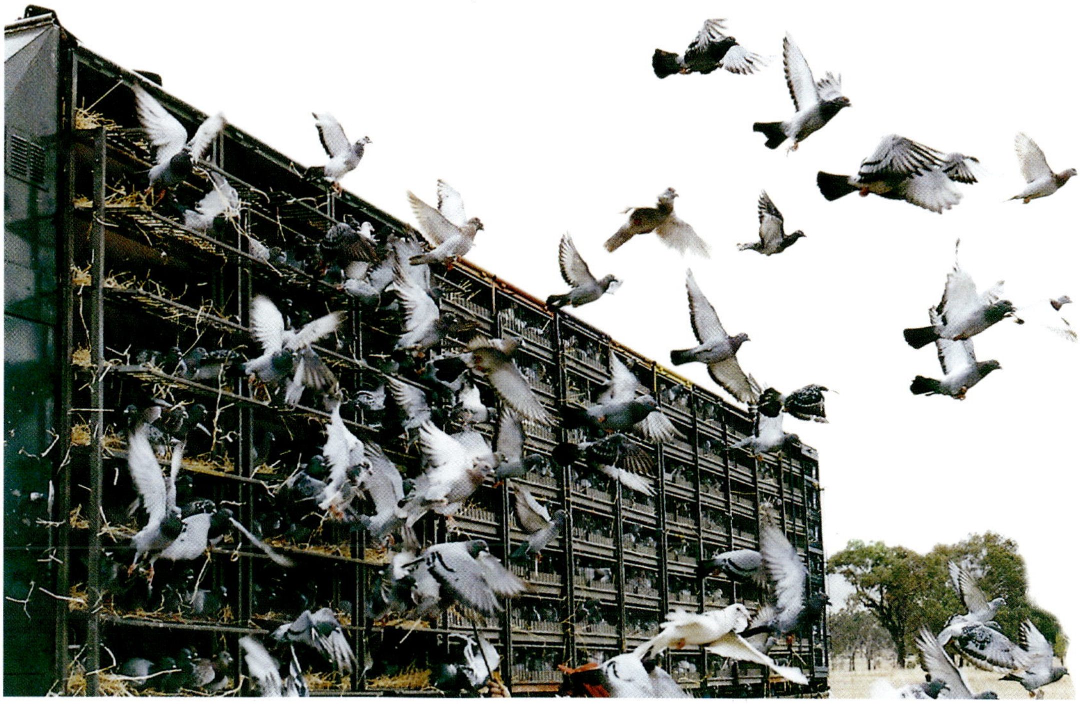

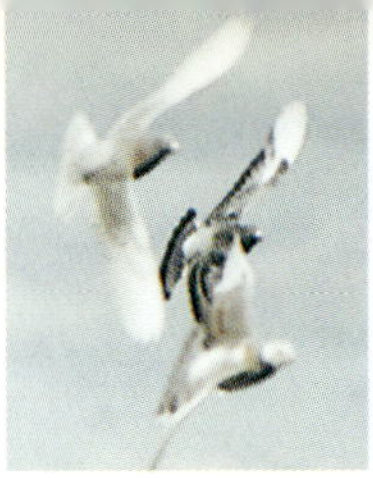

Chapter 11

WEANING

The racing life of most of our birds starts when they are weaned into the racing loft at around 28 days of age. Each youngster carries with it its own genetic code, which determines its potential. It is racing that realizes this genetic potential. It is important that we, as fanciers, give those youngsters with the genetic make-up to win the chance to do so.

Weaning and the following months are critical in this regard as it is during this time that many basic behaviours and 'the love of home' are established. A 28-day-old youngster can be viewed as the raw material that good fanciers convert into the end product of a competitive race bird. The process can occur in as short a period of time as 3 months. This reinforces how quickly a pigeon can learn and shows that there is little room for error. There is a big difference between simply breeding 100 youngsters, putting them into the race loft and ending up with an unruly mob of pigeons that do not know a routine and are scared of you to a bonded kit of young racers that are ready to start winning.

During weaning, the youngster:

- Must establish itself within the loft and develop a bond to the loft and to some extent its owner, and
- Be given the best of care and correct health management so that it has the best chance to develop physically.

The bonding of a youngster, I believe, should start in the nest. If you only put your hand in the nest box at 7 days of age to ring the youngster, then by 28 days when you go to remove them they will throw themselves around the nest box. The first chance to develop a quiet, settled race bird has been wasted. Youngsters as young as 7 days can sense the owner's presence. It is good to touch each youngster every day from ringing onwards. Touch it on its head, near its eyes to ensure that it sees you and under its beak just for a moment. Talk with the same tone that months later you will use to call it quickly into the loft from a race. By weaning, your hand, something that would otherwise be frightening, has become commonplace and familiar. By 28 days, the youngster will already be developing a confidence in you.

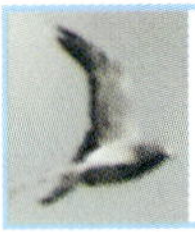

Young pigeons are creatures of habit and find security in being able to predict the pattern of their day.

Young pigeons are creatures of habit and find security in being able to predict the pattern of their day. Once the youngsters are weaned, feed them at approximately the same time each day and talk to the birds in the same tone and using the same words that were used in the nest box. Before puberty, one of the big attractions of the loft to the youngsters is that they are fed there. You should aim to also have the food associated with you, but not through keeping the pigeons hungry. Fill the feed tray by hand. Squat by the hopper and, while calling the birds in the now familiar tone, fill the tray one handful at a time. Initially some youngsters may be a bit shy but they quickly learn to associate your hand with food. Within days they will learn to pick the grain from your hand as it drops into the tray and then from your hand. They don't have to be hungry to do this. Simply putting the food down and leaving has wasted the second opportunity to bond with the birds. It is important that to mature race birds, your hand is not frightening.

Race birds later in the season will need to be caught one to four times per week. Rather than scattering away from your hand, they will just as likely peck it as it approaches, it being viewed as a non-frightening intruder onto their perch.

The weaned youngster must also bond to the loft. Preferably they should be weaned by 28 days (as a guide, the skin between the feathers should still just be visible under the wing). If this is not possible, one should be suspicious of an underlying health, dietary or management problem. If they can feed themselves earlier, then wean them earlier. At weaning they should be walking and feeding, but not flying. Always wean in batches as pigeons are basically a flock bird and feel vulnerable when not with others. This is accentuated in the youngster. Never wean into sections containing older birds as these will dominate and possibly injure the youngsters. More importantly, they will severely interfere with the bond that the youngster needs to develop with the loft. Try and wean into the section to which they will race as young birds. Often a pigeon will race for the first 6 months of its life to the perch that it first hopped onto when weaned. Their ability to recognize and how observant they are is demonstrated by the way that nestmates, sometimes, will identify and find each other, choosing adjacent perches. Youngsters must never be overcrowded as, ideally, each individual youngster should not have to continually defend its perch but be confident that it has its own place or mini-territory. It is best to wean in the morning to give the youngsters a longer time to sort themselves out before the first night.

The daily loft routine must now begin. This is one of those times when the fancier does need to be a bit cruel to be kind. The youngster must exit the loft from the first day after weaning onwards. By 5 – 6 weeks of age, a healthy youngster will be strong on the wing. If it is not familiar with the outside of the loft or the appearance of the loft from the sky, it is much more likely to get lost. It will find new things more frightening the older it is when first exposed to them. Youngsters should be allowed out of the loft at least once a day and, ideally, at the same time so they can develop confidence in a routine. For those who will not waddle out, they should be gently placed onto the loft roof, landing board or fly-in, etc. Some may scurry straight back in, but do not place them out a second time in that training session. Most youngsters within 2 weeks of weaning will recognize a daily routine and readily exit the loft and be beginning to form a loose flock. They only need to go out of the loft once per day but need to be fed at least twice daily. Youngsters will often eat hesitantly and yet need to eat quite a large amount each day because of the high nutritional requirement associated with growth. Unlike adult race birds, which can do well with a single daily feed, the developing youngster will therefore do better with several smaller meals.

The actively growing youngster should never be kept hungry and I know of no successful flier at the distance who treats his youngsters in this way. However, even though they should be given as much as they want at each meal, food should never be left lying in a tray 'in case they get hungry later' or for the slower ones. This encourages bad habits, particularly in certain headstrong birds, which eventually break the routine of an otherwise manageable group. Through familiarity, they need to become accustomed to cleaning procedures, the use of scrapers and other necessary loft procedures.

By 6 – 8 weeks, most youngsters will have a good understanding of 'the way of the loft'. They will be keen to go out for an anticipated fly and will come in to be fed when called, even if not hungry, simply because they associate your voice and that particular time of day with going into the loft. Once in the loft, they will sleep because they know they are not going to be fed or allowed out of the loft out of routine. In this way, the growing youngster eats and exercises regularly and rests well within the loft on a perch that it is increasingly regarding as its own. All of these things are conducive to good physical development and minimize stress on the youngster, which, in turn, decreases the chance of health problems. Already the better youngsters will be showing the desire to get back to their perch when removed, a natural desire that is developed during racing.

By 18 weeks, the youngster has dropped four flights and can safely start its training tosses. Always try to get them returning to the loft in these initial tosses at the normal time they would be fed.

From the youngster's health point of view, weaning is a challenging time. It presents a dilemma in that the youngster, simply through weaning, comes in contact with many environmental organisms that have the potential to cause disease and yet, because of its age, it has not been alive long enough to develop a natural immunity that is sufficiently solid to protect it from disease. What we are aiming for is a controlled gradual exposure to these organisms so that the youngster's natural immunity becomes progressively more and more solid. In the adult race bird, it is this natural immunity that protects it from much disease. It is therefore obviously vital for racing success that this immunity be allowed to form. The way we can assist in this is two-fold :

1. **Firstly, by keeping the number of organisms down to a level that the youngster can cope with –** This involves regular cleaning and maintenance of a hygienic loft environment and the provision of good-quality food and clean water. In the loft, disinfection is best avoided at this time so as to maintain a constant but low exposure to organisms. In the same way, it is important not to overuse medication.
2. **Secondly, by avoiding stress –** A healthy bird is able to cope with a significant number of disease organisms before it succumbs. On the other hand, a stressed or weak bird will succumb to a much lower number of organisms because its immune system is weakened.

Disease prevention at this time is really a combination of on-going hygiene so that the number of disease organisms is kept to a level that the birds can cope with and avoiding stress so that the growing youngsters' immune system can fight disease and form a strong natural immunity. Common sense really. The main stress for young birds is overcrowding. No more than 25 youngsters should be kept in a 2-m x 2-m x 2-m section. Correct feeding is important. Problems with the quantity, frequency and quality can all cause stress. The food must also be nutritionally balanced. Growth and moulting require mixes with higher protein levels than during racing. The mix needs a protein level of at least 11%. This can be achieved by feeding a mix containing at least 40% peas or beans (which are 20 – 25% protein) or other high-protein grains such as vetches (approximately 35% protein). Problems with loft design can also cause stress. The loft must make the youngsters feel secure and, at the same time, provide a healthy environment. Essentially, the loft must be dry without being dusty and provide adequate ventilation without exposing the youngsters to extremes of temperature or humidity. The youngsters should be allowed adequate rest. Ensure that when weaned, they all learn quickly where the water is. My own youngsters have grit, a pick stone and PVM Powder in front of them all the time. Multivite Plus is given in their water every day.

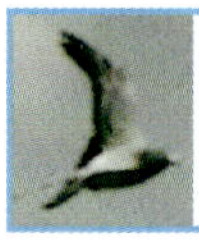

Overcrowding is the most common stress predisposing the young bird to disease.

A number of substances that stimulate the immune system can be given during this time and are used regularly by some fanciers. These include Levamisole (which at a higher dose also worms the birds). If used at a lower dose, it acts as a mild immune stimulant. It does, however, make some of the birds look a bit queasy and can cause some youngsters to vomit. I do not recommend its use. However, the herbs garlic and Echinacea are natural immune stimulants that are safe and palatable and can be used to advantage during this time. These, however, do not replace, by a long way, the basic need for a good management system and environment.

If disease does appear at this time, it is important that only sick birds are medicated so as not to interfere with the on-going exposure to organisms and the development of natural immunity in the team as a whole. Unwell youngsters should be separated, the nature of their problem identified accurately and treated. The fact that certain individuals become unwell while the team as a whole remains well does, to some extent, reflect their decreased vigour. Youngsters that fail to respond to medication quickly or relapse are unlikely to go on and make competitive race birds and are often best eliminated.

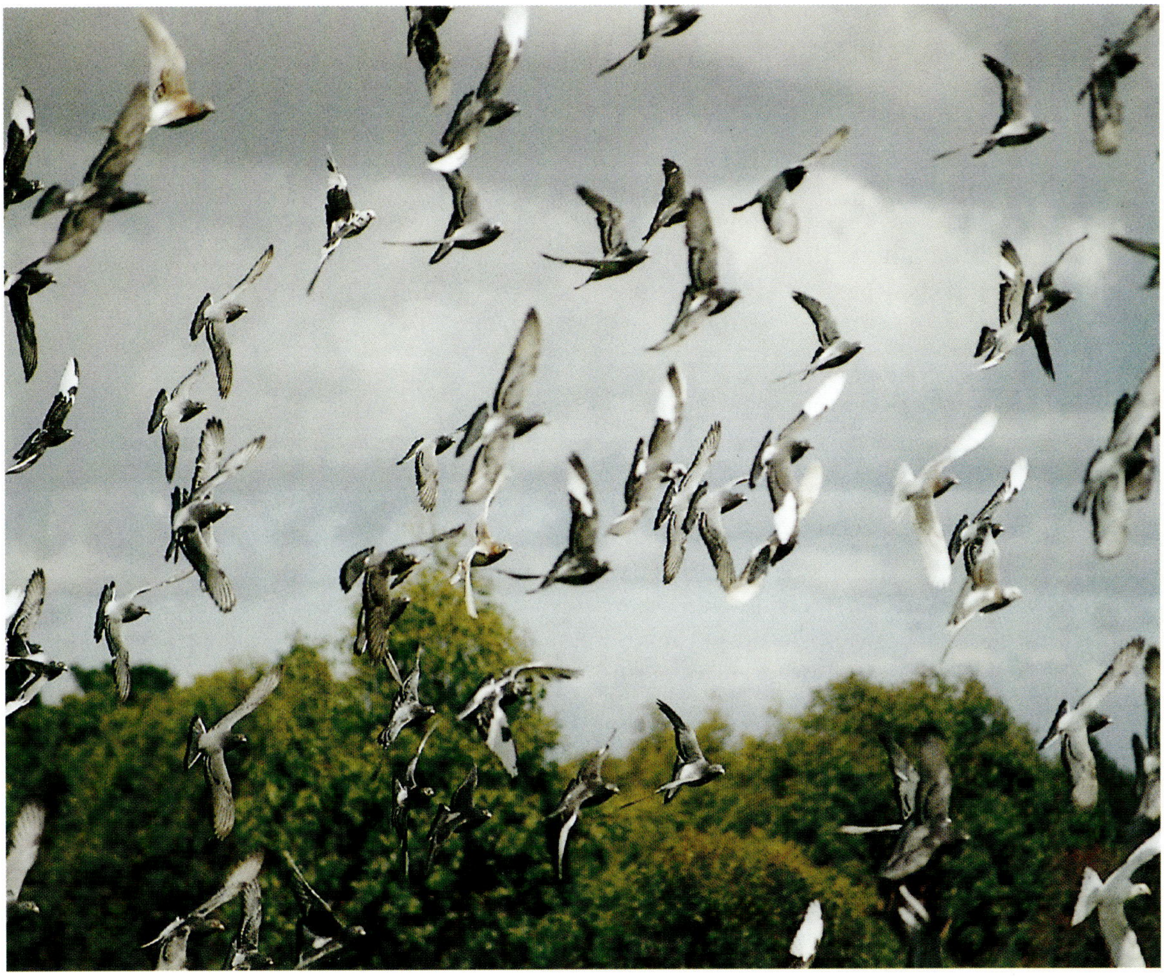

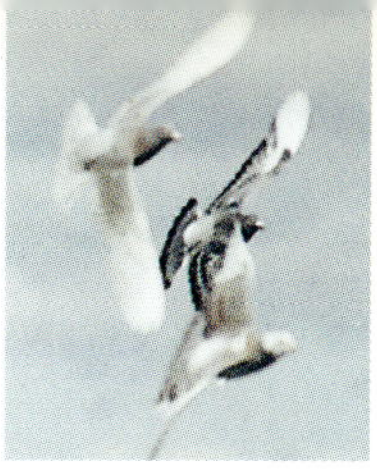

Chapter 12

YOUNG BIRD DEVELOPMENT

Within 100 days of hatching, the young racing pigeon grows into a bird that can be tossed and trained. This development occurs because of the basic instinct that all pigeons have and the inherent genetic potential that has been developed in racing birds, and relies heavily on correct management by the fancier. This is how it should happen.

Youngster development after weaning is divided into five stages.

Stage 1   28 – 32 days of age

This is the initial time away from the parents, most youngsters being weaned by at least 28 days. For the youngster, this is a time of settling and learning to look after itself in the new loft. This stage occurs quickly and in the robust youngster should be completed in only 4 days.

At 28 days of age at the latest, youngsters are removed from their parents, i.e. weaned. They should be able to walk. They can fly in a clumsy fashion to reach perches but otherwise are reluctant to fly. They prefer to stay on the loft floor and most are not able to eat properly from a hopper. They tend to eat small amounts often and tend to be messy feeders, scattering food about the floor.

By 31 days, they should be responding to the owner's voice with some youngsters sitting on the same perch each day, although they have no real sense of individual territory. They gain security from each other's company and prefer to huddle together on the floor or with other youngsters on the same perch. They already have an innate fear of birds in the sky. By the end of this stage, many should already know the basic loft routine, responding to the approach of the owner and anticipating release from the loft and feeding. Approximately 10% will know and recognize the fancier.

Stage 2   33 – 49 days

The youngsters are now settled in the loft. This is a time of rapid development and learning.

By 33 days of age, the youngsters should realize that their loft is their home. With repetition of the daily loft routine, the youngsters quickly learn, and, by only 38 days of age, the youngsters should be established in a loft routine and be starting to fly as a flock. They no longer huddle together when in the loft. Some individuals will, however, still be slow eaters so seed will need to be left for sufficient time to ensure they all get enough.

By 42 days, they should be flying well as a flock and responding well to voice commands. In the stock loft, most of the second round should now be ready for ringing. The youngsters can now distinguish their owner from other humans and with correct care will have developed a confidence in him, making them tame and easy to pick up. They prefer to eat smaller seed. Up until now, they have been reluctant to eat peas but now more youngsters are accepting them. However, when offered a variety of grains, they elect to eat the larger grains, particularly corn, last.

By 43 days of age, they should respond quickly when called into the loft. They should be flocking well and getting high when flying. They should be improving noticeably in their understanding of the loft regime every day.

By 46 days, they should be flying strongly in a crescent-shaped flock for up to 20 – 30 minutes. Territoriality will be increasing with individual birds starting to display aggression to loft mates, pecking at birds on adjacent perches. Droppings should now be those of an adult, not watery like those of a baby.

By 47 days, the flock should be ranging, just visible in the distance.

By 48 days, birds should be bonding to a perch or nest box in the loft, with the first actual fights between individual birds over perches starting to occur.

Stage 3 50 – 60 days

The young bird should now be behaving like a young adult in all ways except sexually. The normal bird should be territorial within the loft and ranging well when flying. During this time, the moult starts in earnest and the eye begins to change colour.

At 50 days of age, most will have dropped their first flight and some will have dropped two. The colour of the eye changing to that of an adult will be readily apparent, and the first shiny neck feathers will be starting to appear. The birds will be starting to make their first adult cooing sounds.

By 55 days, approximately 25% will now have shiny feathers around their neck. The youngsters should be behaving like a race team and be established in the loft routine, i.e. flying well, coming when called, and associate particular times with feeding and resting. They should know the routine of the loft, and, with correct management, be confident in it.

Stage 4 61 – 100 days

During this time, puberty occurs, and with it there is an associated change in behaviour. The moult and general development continue.

By 61 days, puberty has started in some youngsters. Some birds start to display behaviour that has a sexual basis. Some young cocks will crow around the floor and on their perch.

By 67 days, premating behaviour will occur between some young hens and cocks, such as billing, and there will be weak attempts at mating. Half of the wing coverts should by now be moulted.

Stage 5 100 days onward

Healthy birds that have been correctly managed, should now be sufficiently mature and educated to be tossed.

It is hoped that the above gives fanciers a basis of comparison with their own youngsters to ensure that their development is occurring normally. It is interesting to note that the youngsters that do well are often those that have not been drawn to the fancier's particular attention during development. This means that they have done what they should have at the right age. Youngsters that are slow to look after themselves in the loft or slow to fly, etc., and therefore do come to notice, rarely seem to end up in the clock. Nevertheless, with good management, most racing pigeons develop uneventfully from an egg to a youngster that can be trained, in the remarkably short time of 100 days.

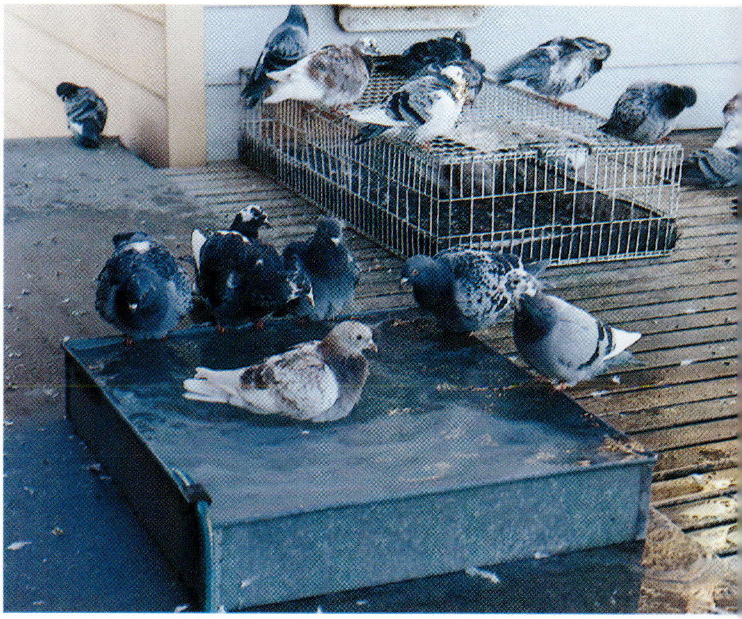

Stage-5 youngsters enjoying a bath.

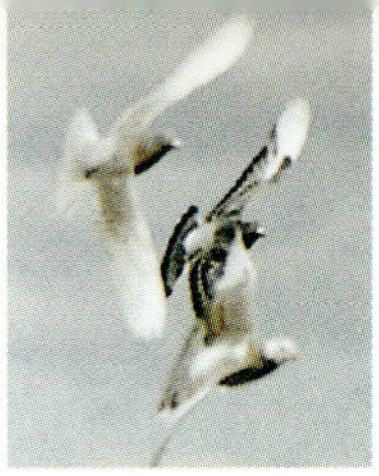

Chapter 13

MEDICAL PROBLEMS IN YOUNG PIGEONS

As indicated in earlier chapters, avoiding stress in young pigeons will do much to prevent disease in them. In Australia, most fanciers wean youngsters from early November until the end of February. In the Northern Hemisphere, this occurs 6 months earlier. During these weaning months, most lofts are progressively filling with youngsters. Many normal features of the young pigeons' existence, such as moulting and establishing their perch in a new loft, provide unavoidable stress. Most growing pigeons can tolerate a single stress but,when stresses start to overlap, opportunistic infection can take advantage of the birds' weakened immune system and the youngsters can become sick. In addition, in some areas the weather during these months is changeable and humid, conditions that favour the spread of disease.

Ways that the fancier can minimize stress in his young birds include:

- **Avoiding overcrowding –** Ideally, no more than 25 birds in a 2-m x 2-m x 2-m section.
- **Providing a seed mixture of good quality and in adequate quantity, given at regular intervals –** The seed should be clean, free of dusts and moulds, and contain sufficient levels of protein for growth and moulting. I work around a basic mix of 40% dun peas, 20% safflower, 15% corn, 15% milo, 5% wheat and 5% small seeds.
- **Providing grit and a pink mineral –** Grit should always be in front of the growing youngster. It contains the calcium that is vital for the formation of a healthy skeleton. A pigeon is independent at 4 weeks, and can reproduce at 6 months. This is analogous to a human being

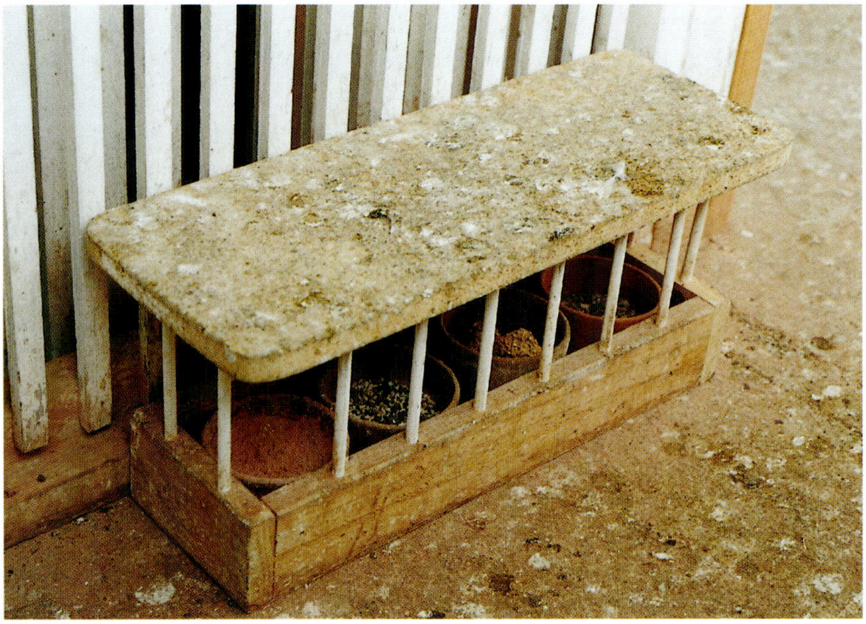

A simple, accessible but hygienic method of offering a range of grits, pink minerals and pick stones to young pigeons.

full grown at 5 months of age and sexually mature at $2\frac{1}{2}$ years. With such a phenomenal growth rate, nothing must be lacking. The bones are genetically programmed to increase in size and if calcium is lacking they will not be as strong as they should be. Pink minerals such as PVM Powder provide not only calcium but also a ranch of vitamins and minerals. Regular use of a water-soluble multivitamin is also useful.

- **Enabling adequate rest periods –** The young bird must develop a bond with the loft and a perch within it, and must feel secure when there. People tell me that pigeons get used to anything, such as backyard dogs, incinerators, and kids playing directly in front of the loft, but I think, drawing an analogy with some people that live on a busy road, that just because they get used to it does not mean they like it.
- **Providing a good loft –** Essentially, a pigeon loft must be dry without being dusty and provide adequate ventilation without exposing the birds to extremes of heat and cold.
- **Keeping the loft clean –** Regular cleaning removes germs and provides a healthier environment.
- **Keeping groups of young birds together** – Young birds will form groups within the loft as part of the pigeons' basic flocking instinct. Fanciers may note that youngsters weaned on the same day may still be sharing the same section within the loft as adults. Young birds are easily intimidated by older birds.
- **Controlling internal and external parasites –** Both internal and external parasites drain the body of nutrition that would otherwise be available to the growing youngster.
- **Correctly timing pigeon pox vaccination –** The two constraining parameters are the date racing starts and the age of the birds. Race programs in all States are different. Pigeons should not be vaccinated closer than 6 weeks to the start of racing, as usually scabs are carried for 4 – 6 weeks postvaccination. Birds carrying these scabs are infectious and therefore ineligible for competition. The pigeon pox vaccine is alive and gives the birds a mild dose of the disease. In birds facing other stresses, this may be sufficient to induce diseases such as canker or respiratory infection that were not apparent. Obviously, this is most likely to occur the younger the pigeons are at vaccination. All young birds within the loft should be vaccinated at the one time.
- **Checking the youngsters regularly for illness and ensuring that ill birds are separated, accurately diagnosed and treated –** Beware the overuse of drugs, which can interfere with the on-going natural exposure of the developing pigeon to potentially infectious organisms. Incorrect use of drugs at this time may in fact render the team more vulnerable to disease.
- **Establishing a routine that is familiar to the young bird.**

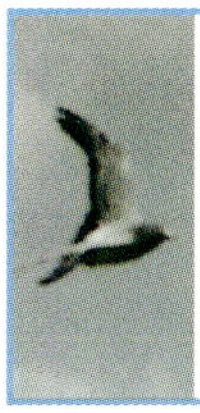

Except for parasite control, avoid flock treatments in young pigeons, only treating unwell individuals so as not to interfere with the developing natural immunity of the team as a whole.

Management of disease

Overlapping stresses in the form of environmental or management flaws, or failure to control primary diseases such as parasitism, can trigger a disease outbreak. Occasionally in the best lofts under good managers, disease will occur despite good control of young birds' stresses. I find it convenient to divide the diseases of young birds into four groups based on the signs observed.

1 **Canker –** Fanciers will be familiar with the thick yellow scum that occurs in the throat of youngsters. Affected birds should be separated and treated with either a 1/4 of a Flagyl 200 mg or whole Spartrix tablet once daily until well. This usually takes 1 – 3 days. Alternatively, the unwell youngster's water can be medicated with Turbosole, 1/2 teaspoon to 1 litre of water. It is important, however, to ensure that the unwell youngster is still able to drink. The group of youngsters, as a whole, should only be treated if more than 10% of youngsters are showing signs, usually with Turbosole for 2 – 3 days.

2 **Respiratory signs –** In young birds, this usually appears as either a dirty cere or 'one eye cold'. Affected youngsters should be separated and treated with either Vibravet 50 mg, 1/2 tablet once daily, or alternatively Baytril, 3 drops twice daily. If more cases are developing every day, or more than 10% of youngsters are affected, the flock can be given either Doxycycline 12% (1/2 teaspoon to 1 litre of water) or Resfite (1/2 teaspoon to 1 litre of water) for 2 – 5 days. However, in this situation it is likely that there is some underlying management or environmental flaw, which will need to be corrected to prevent on-going problems. I find the presence of mucus in the throat an unreliable indicator of respiratory infection in young pigeons. All pigeons have approximately 1.5 ml of mucus in the throat all the time. The level of mucus may increase with respiratory infection but this is difficult to quantitate. Similarly, I am cautious in diagnosing respiratory infection if the birds pant after exercise. Birds with respiratory disease may pant excessively but this is affected too much by other factors, such as the stage of the moult, level of fitness and heat of the day, to be a reliable indicator. More than 90% of respiratory disease in young pigeons is due to *Chlamydia* or *Mycoplasma*. The organisms are already in the systems of many young birds and an increase in their numbers is triggered by stress. When the birds are stressed, the organism increases in number and can move to several sites throughout the body, including the respiratory and gastrointestinal tracts. During these chlamydial flare-ups, it is important that the fancier provides a healthy loft environment to ensure that the birds' immune system is maximally functional in order to help bring the organism numbers down. Sources of on-going stress, such as overcrowding, must be eliminated. In addition, antichlamydial drugs are used to lower the chlamydial count before significant damage can be done. The aim of treatment in young birds is not to eliminate the organism but rather to reduce the chlamyidial count to a level where it is no longer causing problems. Even in the best-managed lofts, several flare-ups would be expected in Australia between January and May. By May, the birds are older, fitter and have finished moulting, and many problems become self-limiting. Once on treatment, birds stop shedding the organism and so recovering birds can be returned to the loft. Young birds in particular respond better to medication once back on their own perch and with other pigeons.

3 **Bowel signs –** Look for discolored droppings with a higher than normal fluid content. Affected youngsters are usually quiet and underweight. The three most common causes are Coccidia, thrush and *E. coli*, although worms are a problem in some lofts. Microscopic examination of a faecal smear is necessary to determine the actual problem. If Coccidia is involved, then the entire group of youngsters can be given Baycox (1 ml to 2 litres of water for 48 hours). This does not interfere with developing immunity. Thrush and *E. coli*, if mild, can be successfully treated with Probac (1/2 teaspoon to 2 litres) or, if advanced, Sulfa AVS (1 teaspoon to 4 litres for 48 hours). These problems can reflect loft stresses, which will need to be corrected to stop the on-going need for medication.

4 **Very sick or dying youngsters –** Here affected birds are fluffed up, reluctant to move and often underweight, with a reduced appetite. The diseases mentioned earlier can, in their most severe forms, appear like this and usually testing for these is done initially. However, the gen-

eralized form of paratyphoid, *Aspergillus* (a fungus that affects the respiratory system) and in particular the viral diseases, Herpes virus, Adeno virus and Circo virus, must be considered. Often, one or more birds need to be submitted for autopsy and the relevant tissue samples submitted for examination by an avian pathologist. In this situation, it is usually best to seek veterinary advice.

PARASITES

Both internal and external parasites can also be a problem in youngsters. However, in a well-managed loft these should not occur in the stock loft and therefore should not be present in the weaning youngsters. They can, however, enter the loft with late returning race birds, strays and youngsters deliberately introduced. Roundworms and hairworms, if present, should be totally eliminated. The best treatment is Moxidectin (2 mg per ml, 5 ml per litre for 24 hours in the drinking water). This will eliminate all mites including airsac mite and approximately 80% of lice. If lice are a problem, then to completely eliminate them the birds will need to be dipped. This can be safely done from 6 weeks of age and it is best to use Permethrin Solution. Some mites (but not lice) can survive in the cracks and crevices of the loft. In this situation the Moxidectin can be repeated at 4-week intervals or, alternatively, the loft can be sprayed with Permethrin. Pick a warm day, move the youngsters out of the section, and spray the Permethrin onto the scraped surfaces of the loft. These will dry within a couple of hours and the youngsters can be reintroduced. Permethrin is a residual insecticide and has the advantage of controlling mosquitoes, pigeon flies, and other insects (which can carry tapeworm) for up to 4 months. Tapeworm, if a problem, can be treated with Prazivet (5 ml to 1 litre for 24 hours). An alternative is Droncit ($^1/_8$ – $^1/_4$ tablet per bird, single dose).

USE OF MEDICATIONS

Many of the medications routinely used during racing can have side-effects in the growing and moulting bird, compromising feather quality and bone development and interfering with the development of natural immunity. Similarly, the appearance of disease during this time is often associated with environment or management problems, which must be corrected to avoid the on-going need for medication. Medication is usually only part of the answer to health problems in the young bird loft. However, with correct management during weaning, the fancier will find himself at the start of racing with a team of both psychologically and physically right youngsters, which will be able to realize their full genetic potential and he will be able to enjoy racing.

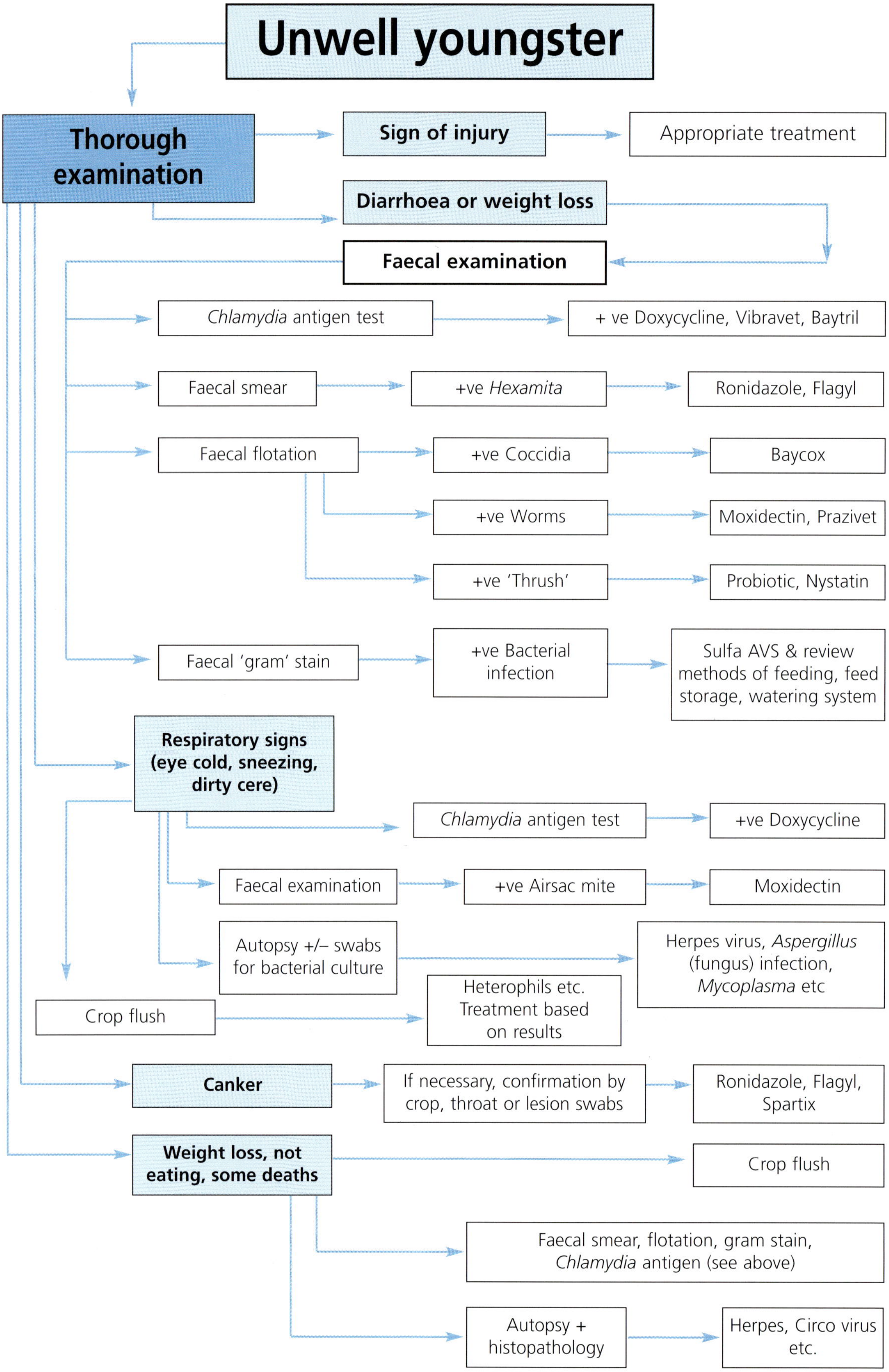
Unwell youngster
Thorough examination
Sign of injury
Appropriate treatment
Diarrhoea or weight loss
Faecal examination
Chlamydia antigen test
+ ve Doxycycline, Vibravet, Baytril
Faecal smear
+ve Hexamita
Ronidazole, Flagyl
Faecal flotation
+ve Coccidia
Baycox
+ve Worms
Moxidectin, Prazivet
+ve 'Thrush'
Probiotic, Nystatin
Faecal 'gram' stain
+ve Bacterial infection
Sulfa AVS & review methods of feeding, feed storage, watering system
Respiratory signs (eye cold, sneezing, dirty cere)
Chlamydia antigen test
+ve Doxycycline
Faecal examination
+ve Airsac mite
Moxidectin
Autopsy +/– swabs for bacterial culture
Herpes virus, Aspergillus (fungus) infection, Mycoplasma etc
Crop flush
Heterophils etc. Treatment based on results
Canker
If necessary, confirmation by crop, throat or lesion swabs
Ronidazole, Flagyl, Spartix
Weight loss, not eating, some deaths
Crop flush
Faecal smear, flotation, gram stain, Chlamydia antigen (see above)
Autopsy + histopathology
Herpes, Circo virus etc.

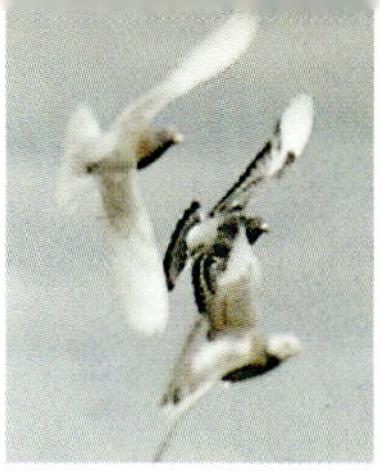

Chapter 14

YOUNG BIRD RACING

Although beyond the scope of this book to discuss the technique of young bird racing in detail, the following are general considerations.

Feeding

For many young bird fliers, particularly in Australia, food is one of the key motivational aids. Young birds have not gone through puberty and so apart from the basic love of home, which is inherent in them, food can be a major incentive. When feeding young birds, it is important to concentrate. Too little food and the birds may not grow properly, too much and the fancier has lost one of his means of controlling his birds and an opportunity to create incentive. The young bird should not feel that food is precious but feel that it is perhaps in limited supply, so that it feels that if it does not eat now it will miss out and its companions will eat all the seed. In this way, a sense of competition within the team is created. This sense of competition is extended into the sky so that, when coming to the loft on a toss or race, the birds will compete against each other in an attempt to ensure that they are in the first group home and will therefore not miss out on a feed. In attempting to beat his loft mates home, the bird is not simply homing but is in fact racing and the fancier has contributed to achieving his aim, i.e. to win. Pigeons do not, however, learn by negative evaluation. That is, if they come late and do not get fed they do not learn to home more quickly. The astute fancier must therefore ensure that every bird receives food when it returns. In this way, the bird receives what it perceives to be its reward. If this is not done, then incentive is lost.

Feeding needs to occur at regular, predictable times as regular meals not only promote sound growth but young birds in particular develop security in a predictable daily routine.

As to what to feed, the main requirement is that there is adequate protein in the diet for growth and the accompanying moult. Various authorities vary in just what level of protein is adequate but suffice to say that 40 – 50% of the diet should be made up of a mixture of protein-based grains, such as peas, beans, lupins or vetches. Protein-rich supplements such as yeasts (Brewer's Yeast, ID Yeast), which are 45% protein, are of benefit. Pigeons really like the taste of these and so they are not only of nutritional benefit but a way of providing a treat. It is important once the moult starts that some oil seeds are in the mix, e.g. safflower, rape and peanuts, to provide the unsaturated fatty acids necessary for a lustrous moult. The addition of oils, such as wheatgerm or Polyseed Oil, are useful here.

Moulting

One of the difficulties of young bird racing is that the birds are moulting while these races are on. It is not only hard to get birds into form during the moult but the flight feathers during growth are painful, restricting performance. This is particularly so with the eighth, ninth and tenth flights.

Young birds that are raced hard and fed lightly will have a slow moult. However, such management tends to compromise their long-term development. If young bird racing is managed correctly, a normal moult and growth will occur and in fact the growing youngster will benefit from the experience gained. Youngsters bred too early (before August in Australia) run the risk of having a double

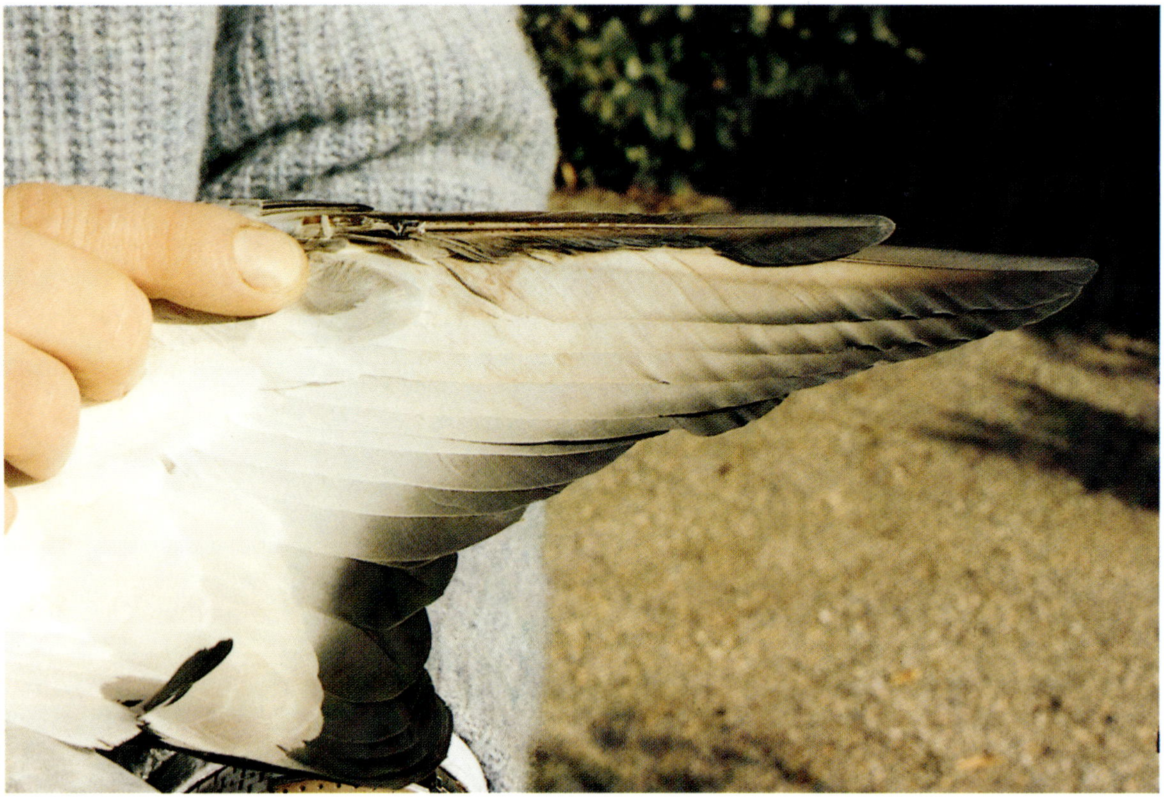

Bleeding from the growing follicle of the tenth flight in a youngster that was forced to fly in this condition. The blood-filled follicles during feather growth appear very painful in some birds, while other birds seem not to be bothered.

moult, which is disastrous for form. The only legal and apparently non-detrimental way of stopping or retarding particularly the flight moult is through the darkness system, in which the daylength is kept below 8 hours.

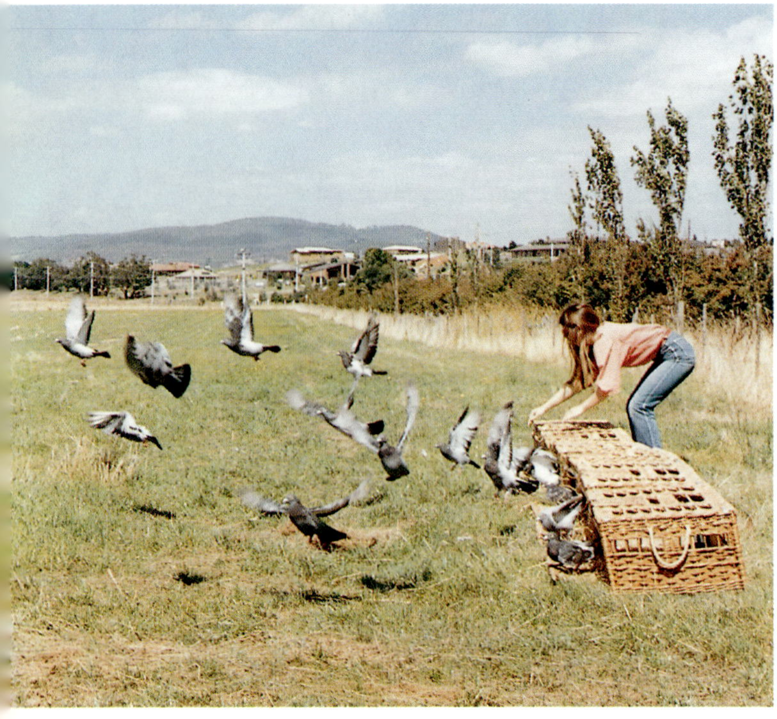

Tossing

Tossing in young birds must not only serve to educate the birds to become familiar with the basket, car travel, orientation and a reward upon return, but to develop confidence in them. Young birds are very much a flock animal and are much more reluctant to 'break' than an older pigeon. To this end, tossing with other fanciers who live nearby and tossing pigeons in smaller groups or singly is worthwhile. Some fanciers talk about establishing a 'necklace' of pigeons across the countryside, where single birds are released at a few-minute intervals. This can be difficult and dangerous in Australia because of the large number of falcons. Birds that have been attacked by falcons

Tossing a kit of young birds.

several times learn to anticipate further attacks and become 'falcon shy' and will probably never break.

For young bird races, it is a good idea to look at the map and attempt to calculate just where you think your birds will need to break to come straight home. As young birds are slower learners than old birds, it is worthwhile going to this point many times.

Motivation

In the past and still for many fliers today, young birds race simply for their love of home and to be fed. More and more, the motivation techniques used in old birds are being adapted for use in young birds. The older youngsters are paired and can be raced on the natural system. Young postpubertal hens can be teased with cocks. Some fanciers fly even young pigeons on the widowhood system, or a form of it, where both sexes are trained and run together for a short period of time after return from a race or toss, the rest of the time the two sexes being kept separate from each other. Many European breeds seem to undergo a precocious puberty and so lend themselves to this style of racing.

Interpretation of results

The results of many races are affected by loft location and wind direction on the day. Because young bird races are short, the effect of these factors is particularly marked. It is important that fliers in a good position on the day do not get an artificially inflated opinion of their birds and make a realistic assessment of their birds' ability.

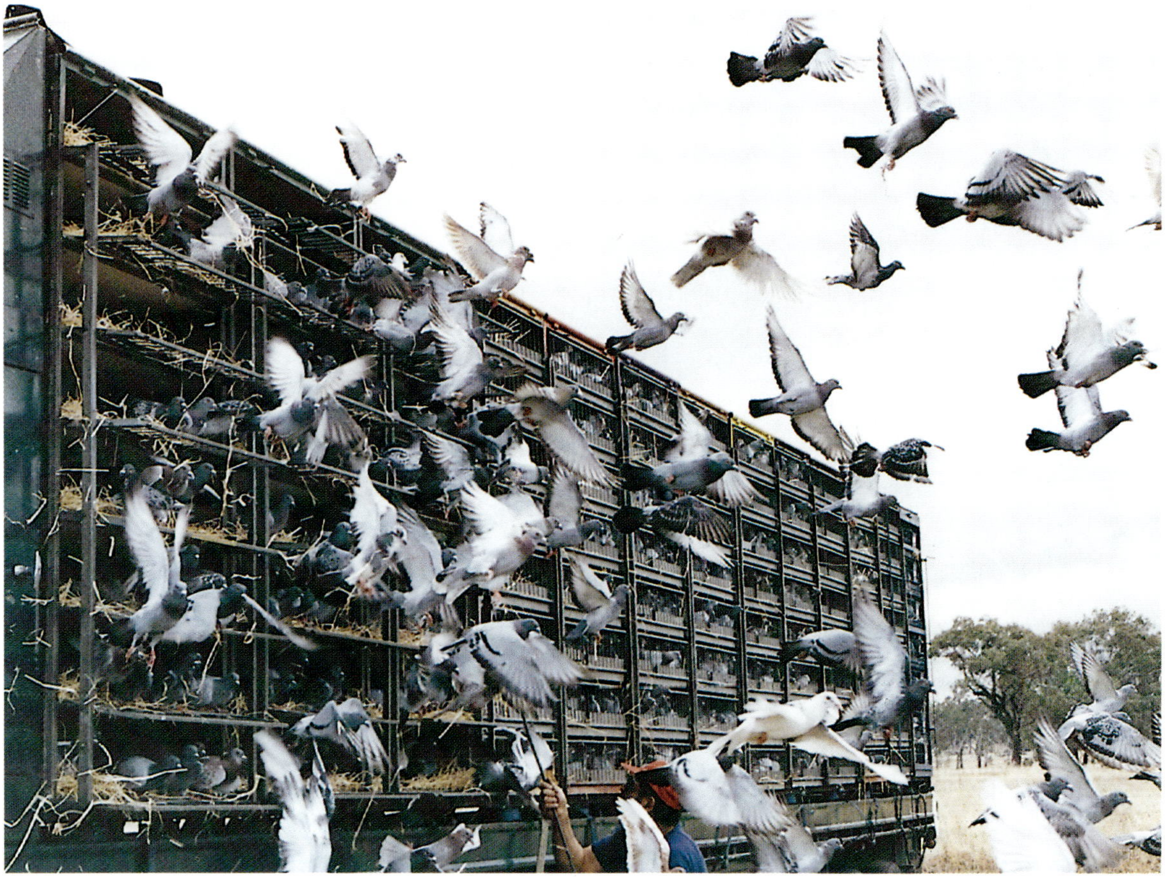

Liberation in one of the V.H.A.'s young bird races from Kyabram to Melbourne, 120 miles.

Section 4

RACING

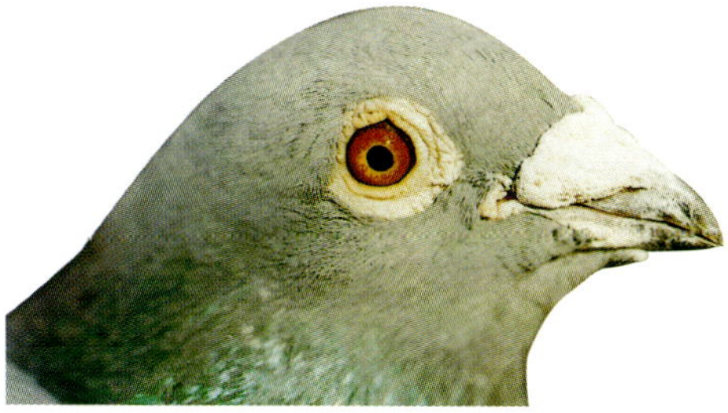

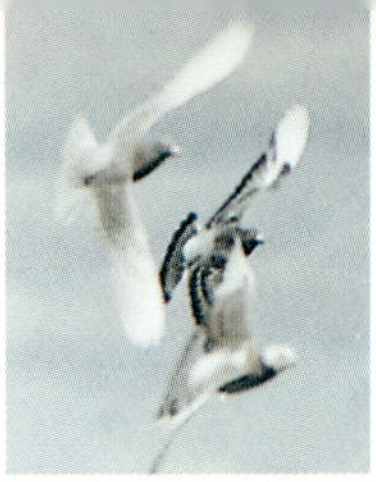

Chapter 15

HEALTH AND ITS EFFECT ON RACE FORM –

Controlling disease during the race season

What separates the team that is simply competing and achieving average results from the team that is winning? The team that is winning is said to be 'in form'. Many factors contribute to this form to varying extents, but one thing is for certain and that is that a team that is not healthy cannot be in form.

In young pigeons that are obviously sick, most fanciers are able to recognize the common diseases, e.g. respiratory infection and canker. In a mature race bird, which is a member of a team that is not in form, no sign may be visible to the fancier apart from the lack of prizes, and yet the same diseases are at work. The problem appears differently because the birds are older, have some immunity and their response to infective organisms is modified. However, as the bird matures, exposure to these germs continues and, depending on a variety of factors, the organism will be cleared at different rates. And so in race teams, the level of Coccidia, trichomonads, *Chlamydia*, etc., will rise and fall.

For the competitive race bird to be in form, the level of these organisms must be low. The race bird should therefore be not only fit but also superhealthy to be in form. As a feature of its normal life, it is under many stresses – extreme exertion, vulnerability to predation, time away from the loft – which can all make it more susceptible to disease. At the same time, because of the very nature of pigeon racing, where many birds from many different lofts are in intimate contact, the potential for exposure to infection is enormous.

Very often, a fancier will come to me during the season and say that his birds look good and are tossing well and yet their results are disappointing. We have all experienced the time when the birds are just 'not right'. What can the fancier do to try and avoid this situation and try to head off any potential health problems before they have a chance to affect race results? Obviously, in a well-designed loft that is kept clean, where the birds are sensibly managed, have been allowed to develop their natural immunity, and are generally robust, problems are less likely to occur. It is necessary to evaluate initially just what diseases are present, if any. I recommend a health check 4 – 6 weeks before racing and then repeat testing as the need dictates once racing has commenced. Usually every 4 weeks is adequate. A health check involves a thorough clinical examination of several birds, examination of a sample of the fluid aspirated from the crop, and a variety of faecal tests.

I must mention here that it is very important that any medication used during racing is used correctly. As explained in earlier chapters, the overuse of drugs can interfere with the normal exposure of the pigeon to potentially infectious organisms, and interfere with the development of its natural immunity, thus rendering it more vulnerable to disease. Similarly, the incorrect use of drugs during racing is to be discouraged. If the fancier is uncertain about the health of his pigeons, he is best to consult an avian veterinarian.

With the start of racing, it is important that the fancier has an understanding of what diseases are most likely to affect his result and the best way to manage them.

Wet canker

Up until several years ago, most fanciers, and many veterinarians for that matter, thought that canker was a disease that pigeons either did or did not have. Pigeons with the classic yellow nodule in the throat or elsewhere were said to have canker. Those without the nodules were thought not to have the disease. Our understanding of this has now altered and a wet form of the disease has been identified. More than 20 different canker strains have now been classified. Most of these do not, in fact, produce the yellow mass familiar to many fanciers unless present in very large numbers but rather cause a red, mucus-producing inflammatory condition of the throat. These invisible or 'wet' strains cause a much more insidious disease and, in fact, are much more damaging to the performance of race birds. In health, a bird is exposed to the resident trichomonad strains in its loft from a young age. The feeding stock bird passes on some of its own trichomonads to its youngsters with each feed. This controlled gradual exposure to the organism allows the developing youngster to develop its own natural immunity so that by the time it is of race age, it is less likely to be bothered by the problem. Older race-age birds usually have a fairly solid natural immunity and so it is unusual to see yellow material accumulate in them. However, the stress of racing will put any immunity the pigeon has already developed to the test, with the result that trichomonad numbers will rise and fall. Race performance has an inverse correlation with the number of trichomonads present. As trichomonad numbers rise, race performance falls, and as trichomonad numbers fall, race performance improves. When high, they have a typical parasitic effect, weakening the bird, in the process compromising race performance and creating a vulnerability to secondary infection (particularly respiratory infection). They also produce a toxin that makes the birds feel unwell. Those birds with elevated trichomonad counts of any strain with no yellow material visible are said to have 'wet canker'. To the naked eye, there is no obvious sign of infection but red inflamed throats, exaggerated swallowing, leaning back on the tail (penguin posture) and quiet fluffed-up pigeons are all suggestive.

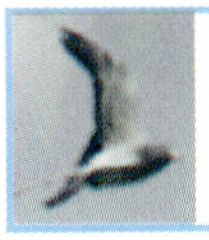

It is not possible to achieve consistent race success without good control of wet canker

Adult birds always carry a variable number of canker organisms from one or more strains in their throat all the time, the actual level being determined by the interplay of a large number of factors including the age and genetic make-up of the bird, its overall health, the natural immunity it has to a given strain and the strain itself. In the mature, stress-free bird, such as a non-breeding stock bird, problems are rare. However, the competitive race bird's life is far from stress-free and its exposure to different strains of the organism is continuous through the season.

It would not be an exaggeration to say that when checking birds by crop flush at my clinic during the race season, if it has been more than 3 weeks since any preventive medication has been given, then 90% of these teams will have wet canker. This means that 90% of untreated teams are performing below their best and yet fortunately this problem is quite easy to control with modern medication. It is unrealistic to think that any one flier's birds are going to be resistant to infection given the on-going stress of racing encountered by all birds and the sharing of drinkers that occurs in race units. I feel it is not possible to be consistently successful unless this disease is monitored and controlled.

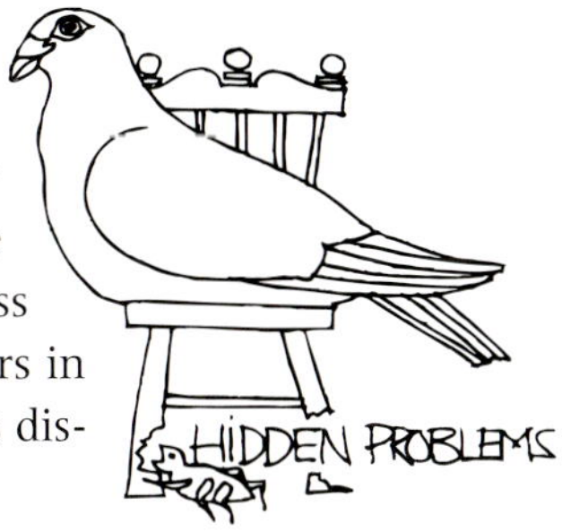

Diagnosis

The signs mentioned above and in the chapter on canker are suggestive. However, a crop flush is necessary for positive diagnosis. Changes develop in the dropping that are suggestive of the problem. Pigeons with wet canker become thirsty. This leads to the droppings becoming watery. Also, under the microscope, changes in the dropping associated with stress may become apparent, i.e increased levels of yeasts and/or *E. coli*. However, these changes are not present in all birds and they will occur in other conditions that cause stress.

The best indicator of infection is, however, the crop flush. Sometimes the number of trichomonads can be surprising and I have personally handled birds that appeared well but were from a team performing poorly with huge numbers of trichomonads. It is tremendously rewarding to see the resultant lift in performance approximately 2 weeks after treatment.

Management during racing

If canker was a problem during the breeding season, this tells us that the birds have the potential to have trichomonad flare-ups in response to stress and that canker is likely to be a problem during racing. If wet canker is not a problem in the loft, attention focuses on preventing returning race birds from bringing new strains of trichomonad into the loft with them. Providing Turbosole in their water before they mix with other birds in the loft will achieve this. However, very few lofts fit into this category now. If wet canker is already a problem in the loft, it is a matter of keeping the trichomonad levels low through periodic 2-day courses of Turbosole, usually every 1 – 3 weeks in most lofts, while at the same time avoiding any obvious stresses so that the trichomonads are less likely to flare up. Regular crop flushes will monitor trichomonad levels and determine when medication needs to be given. Given a constant training regime, this will often be predictable and repeated. Rather than wait for the associated loss of form to occur, 2-day courses of Turbosole can be given with this frequency. However, on-going monitoring is important to ensure that adequate control is achieved.

Coccidia

In many pigeons, this organism is present in low numbers. However, in teams that are in form, the coccidial count is always zero.

Coccidia is a small protozoan that lives in the wall of the bowel. Its eggs are passed in the droppings (more so in the evening). After a period of time in the environment, these eggs become infective. They become infective quicker in humid conditions. Infected eggs are then swallowed. Once in the pigeon, larvae from these eggs burrow into the wall of the bowel, undergo several lifecycle stages and then release eggs themselves, which rupture through the fine lining of the bowel wall. As they do this, they damage the bowel wall, leading to loss of tissue fluid containing protein and also blood. The damage also interferes with digestion and the absorption of nutrients. It is vital that this parasite is controlled if race form is to be achieved.

In birds that are going to get on the winner's list that weekend, no coccidial eggs are found in the droppings. Coccidial eggs will increase in number in the droppings in one of two situations:

1. Poor hygiene, particularly associated with high humidity, which leads to damp droppings accumulating in the loft, in the process exposing the birds to large numbers of the organism, or

2. With severe on-going stress, when the low numbers of parasite present in the bird can opportunistically multiply, in the process shedding large numbers of eggs.

In Australia, I have noticed a particular correlation with open lofts. In open lofts, when it is cold the pigeons are cold and when it is hot the pigeons are hot. The ideal temperature within a loft for a pigeon is 20 – 25°C and it is best if the humidity is less than 60%. The more time the pigeons spend away from these ideals, the less likely they are to come into form and the more difficult problems such as Coccidia are to control.

Diagnosis

Severely affected birds will be generally weak, reluctant to fly and anaemic. However, in mild cases, the birds may simply be just that bit off the pace. As with other diseases that inflame the bowel wall, green watery droppings will appear. Green watery droppings during the race season usually mean only one of three things: either Coccidia, *E. coli* or thrush. All are readily apparent on a faecal smear, which will quickly identify the problem.

Management during racing

Hygiene and control of dampness will minimize exposure to the parasite. Avoiding stress will minimize flare-ups. If the problem is diagnosed, the drug of choice is Baycox (1 ml to 2 litres of water for 2 days). This drug is poorly absorbed from the bowel, making it ideal for use during racing. It simply flushes through, killing the Coccidia as it goes. Because it is poorly absorbed, it does not get into the pigeons' system and there is no potential for loss of form. In most lofts, following a 2-day course of Baycox, it usually takes at least 4 weeks for Coccidia to start reappearing on faecal smears despite the on-going stress of racing.

Airsac disease (*Mycoplasma* infection)

The two principal infectious agents that cause respiratory infection in pigeons are *Chlamydia* and *Mycoplasma*. Both can infect all parts of the respiratory system but typically *Chlamydia* involves more the upper airways and sinuses, while *Mycoplasma* affects the airsacs and windpipe. *Mycoplasma* inflames the airsacs, interfering with their function. Birds severely affected with *Mycoplasma* are obviously unwell and reluctant to fly. However, in most race-age birds, the disease takes on a more insidious form so that nothing may be apparent to the fancier with the bird in the hand. It is only during exercise, which in mild cases may need to be extreme, that a decrease in exercise tolerance is apparent. In affected teams, it is often not until the first hard race of the season or the distance races start that a fancier's suspicion of a problem may be aroused. Unfortunately, there is no 'live bird' diagnostic test for *Mycoplasma* readily available. Diagnosis involves the sacrifice of a bird and an examination of the lungs and airsacs under the microscope by an avian pathologist. Typically, there are an increased number of clumps of white blood cells, called lymphoid aggregates, in the airways, which form in response to the infection.

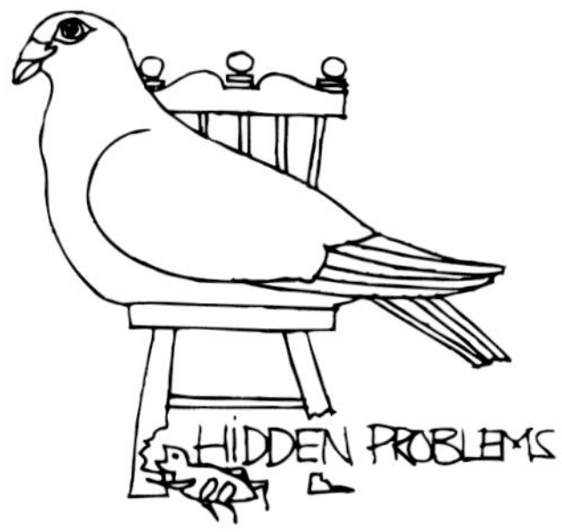

Diagnosis

Mycoplasma is a difficult problem to detect in race birds. However, late clocking, more late arrivals and heavier losses on hard days may arouse the fancier's suspicions. It is diagnosed definitively at autopsy through microscopic examination of tissues by an experienced avian pathologist. The signs shown by the birds, together with changes in the droppings (stress changes, i.e. elevated *E. coli* and thrush) are suggestive. A crop flush may reveal elevated levels of bacteria and the presence of inflammatory cells called heterophils. A good response to the appropriate medication (Doxy-T) is also suggestive.

Management during racing

If the problem is diagnosed during racing, a 3 – 7-day course of Doxy-T is given with follow-up

2 – 3-day courses every 1 – 3 weeks until the birds are well. These keep the problem under control while the birds' immunity rises and fitness gradually returns. Following treatment, a gradual return to work through loft flying and short and then long tosses over a period of weeks is necessary as the birds recover. Unless caught early, however, there is the potential for permanent damage to the air-sacs and subsequent compromise of a potentially good bird's performance.

Worms

A serious but common problem, these primary parasites have no place in the competitive racing loft. They rob the birds of nutrition, and create a vulnerability to secondary infections. There are three worms that are seen with any frequency: roundworm, hairworm, and tapeworm. The first two all have what is called a direct lifecycle, in that the adults live within the digestive tract of the pigeon, release eggs in the droppings, which after a period of time become infective. If these are then swallowed, they in turn develop into adult worms in the digestive tract. Roundworms are by far the most common. Their lifecycle can be completed as quickly as 21 days. A single 'blind' treatment for worms before racing is therefore of limited value. There is no point if the birds do not have worms and quite inadequate if they do, unless treatment is repeated and associated with hygiene measures, as any droppings passed before treatment will contain eggs and therefore have the potential to reinfect the birds. Tapeworms, on the other hand, require an intermediate host. The intermediate host, which in this case are insects, eat the tapeworm egg, which is passed in the pigeon's dropping. The egg goes through several lifecycle stages within the insect. The insect is then, in turn, swallowed by the pigeon and an adult tapeworm establishes in the pigeon's bowel. The insects can be small beetles and slaters living around the loft, but the weevils that contaminate grain can also act as intermediate hosts.

It seems that as few as six roundworms are sufficient to prevent a pigeon coming into form. At my clinic, we have seen birds with as many as 300. Because of continuous race and toss exposure to other birds' droppings, I suggest faecal examination every 4 weeks once racing has commenced so that if worms are detected their numbers are still low and have not had a chance to put a team off form. It is too late if by the 400-mile races a fancier submits a faecal sample for testing because of a poor season and large numbers of roundworm or hairworm are detected. By the time the birds are treated and have become well, the season is over.

Diagnosis

Hairworm and roundworm are readily diagnosed by examination of faecal smears. Tapeworm can sometimes also be diagnosed in this manner but the diagnosis is less reliable because tapeworm eggs are only intermittently shed. However, unlike the other worms in which adults are only rarely passed in the droppings, tapeworm segments, which break off the tail of the growing worm, will appear in the droppings periodically. These can be seen by the fancier. They are usually 1 – 2 mm x 4 – 5 mm in size and a creamy white colour, although different types vary in size.

Management during racing

The number of worms present in the loft must be absolutely zero if the birds are to give of their best. To this end, it is important that the birds are either treated before racing to eradicate any that may be present or alternatively checked to ensure that they are free of infection. There are two safe-to-use, effective wormers available for use in the racing pigeon. Prazivet (5 ml to 1 litre of water for 1 day), which kills tapeworms, and Moxidectin, which is used to kill all other worms. The dose of Moxidectin is also 5 ml to 1 litre of water for 24 hours. The birds may be fed and exercised normally while on these medications and neither affects race form. Moxidectin also kills any external parasites that are in contact with body fluids. This means that it kills mites and, over an extended period of time, some lice.

Roundworms are of particular significance with the start of Thursday night basketing (for a Saturday race), when the birds are fed and watered in the units. Typically in teams that have been free of the problem, low numbers of worm eggs start appearing in their faecal smears. It is important that these are identified and treated before they have a chance to infect more birds within the loft and start to affect the form of the team as a whole. In areas where tapeworms are a problem, it may be necessary to treat with Prazivet every 3 – 4 weeks and to spray the inside of the loft with Permethrin Solution at the start of the season to keep insects out of the loft.

E. coli

E. coli is a bacterium that is usually present in the bowel of pigeons. With stress, it increases in numbers. It can invade the bowel wall, causing an enteritis (leading to loss of tissue fluid and an interference with nutrient absorption) and the development of green watery droppings. It also produces a toxin, which makes the birds feel unwell. It is often associated with high humidity (which in itself is an acknowledged stress in pigeons), which keeps the droppings damp in the loft. If this is coupled with poor hygiene or poor watering and feeding practices, this leads to a high exposure to the organism.

Diagnosis

The appearance of green watery droppings associated with stress or high humidity should alert the fancier to a possible *E. coli* problem, particularly if it resolves with the use of probiotics (Probac) or sulfur-based antibiotics (Sulfa AVS). Tentative diagnosis is made through examination of a faecal smear, where *E. coli* appears as a mid-size motile rod. A pigeon that is going to win the Fed that weekend will often have none visible. However, levels of two to three per x400 microscope field are regarded as normal in most pigeons. Conclusive diagnosis is reached through culture of the organism in the laboratory.

Management during racing

Control of any on-going stresses, particularly high humidity, will minimize flare-ups. If possible, the humidity in the loft should be such that the droppings quickly dry out. In order to achieve this, it may be necessary to alter the loft's ventilation, close in the loft to keep out night-time humidity, or install heaters. In some lofts, through situations beyond the fancier's control, it is not always possible to eliminate predisposing factors, e.g. the loft may face south or alternatively be surrounded by tall trees (in a neighbouring property). Mild flare-ups can be controlled by the use of Probac (½ teaspoon to 2 litres of water for 1 – 2 days). More severe cases can be treated with Sulfa AVS (1 teaspoon to 4 litres of water for 1 – 3 days). In lofts with a resident *E. coli* problem, the fancier should monitor for green watery droppings and on days when significant numbers are present, use Probac for 24 hours, while at the same time avoid the circumstances that led to it flaring up, where possible.

Thrush

Not all fungi that cause disease in pigeons are caught. Some are always present in the birds' system, albeit at very low levels in healthy birds. This is so with *Candida*, which is a yeast. Yeasts are a specialized type of fungus, whose specialized spores (called blastospores) are found within the digestive tract of pigeons. Birds with elevated levels of yeast in their droppings are said to have 'thrush'. Essentially, however, the finding of elevated numbers of yeasts in the droppings of race birds during the season is a non-specific sign and simply indicates that the birds are under stress. This stress can come from concurrent disease, notably respiratory infection and wet canker. Alternatively, it can come from a recent management problem with the birds, e.g. overflying, too low a level of energy in the grain mix, rationing, overcrowding, etc. It is important that any predisposing stress factors are identified and corrected, otherwise the problem will recur.

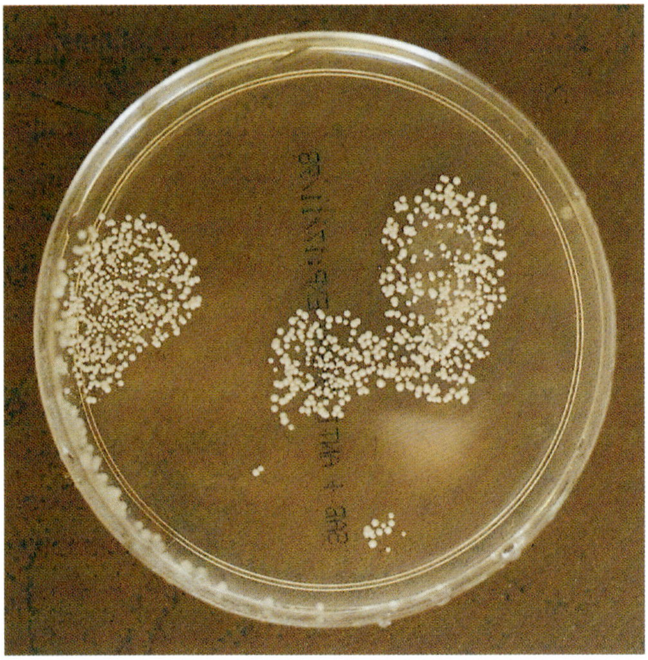

Yeast organisms that cause thrush, growing on a culture medium.

In particular, examine the birds closely for signs of respiratory infection, i.e. eye colds, dirty ceres, tonsillitis, increased level of sneezing, etc., and a crop flush to check for wet canker would be a good idea. If either of these problems is diagnosed, then medication for these should be given initially. The fancier must think about what has happened recently with the birds. In young birds, remember that they are not only growing but also moulting. Because of this, they need a grain mix that is made up of at least 40% fat- or protein-based grains, i.e. a high-energy mix. They should also be given as much as they want to eat for at least one meal a day. The yeasts themselves can be effectively treated with avian probiotics such as Probac. Green mushy droppings in race birds are usually due to one of three things: either Coccidia, thrush, or *E. coli*. If these appear, a faecal smear will identify the cause and treatment can be given. In some lofts, because of their orientation and ventilation, etc., the birds are prone to thrush and *E. coli*, the two conditions often occurring together. In this case, it is best to monitor the birds for green mushy droppings and use the probiotics for 1 – 2 days when required.

Thrush in the droppings usually simply means that the birds are stressed. It is the job of the fancier and veterinarian to figure out what is causing this stress.

Chlamydia (See also Respiratory Infection in the section The Common Diseases)

Chlamydia is an intracellular organism that is found within the system of most pigeons all the time. It is the most common cause of respiratory infection in pigeons. It can be eradicated from the birds by a 30-day course of Doxycycline. However, this is inappropriate in a race team as there is continuous on-going exposure during the race program. With stress, it increases in number and spreads throughout the body. It can affect the bowel and liver but most problems are associated with the respiratory system. In young birds, which are often under multiple stresses, such as growing, moulting, establishing a perch in the loft, etc., signs can be severe in some lofts and include eye colds and dirty ceres. In older race-age birds, signs are often more subtle, with the birds just not being right.

Diagnosis

The clinical signs observed in the birds are often sufficient to make a diagnosis. Fanciers need to be particularly observant because signs in the race team can be very subtle. Sneezing is often a good indicator, with more than three sneezes in 5 minutes from 100 birds being suggestive. Birds may

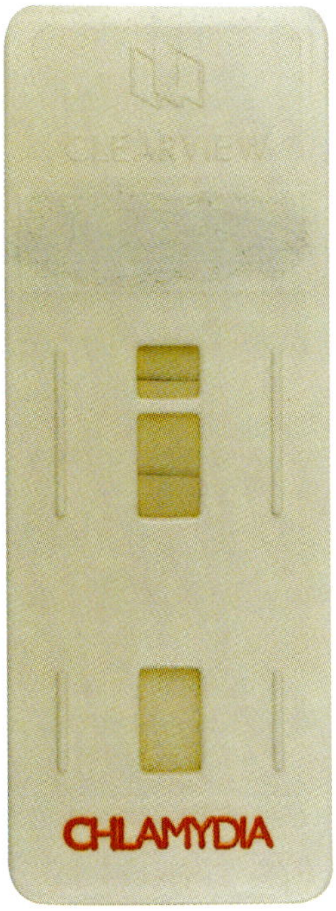

Chlamydia antigen test. When *Chlamydia* is causing disease, it is shed through the bowel wall and can sometimes also be found in eye and nose discharges. Dropping samples are heated at 80° C for 10 minutes in an extraction fluid. After cooling, five drops of supernatant are placed on the lower window. A blue line appearing in the top window indicates that the test has been done correctly, while a blue line in the middle window indicates the presence of *Chlamydia*. The test is not without its problems with both false negatives and false positives occurring. It is, however, useful in determining, for example, if an outbreak of sneezing is associated with a respiratory infection or something else irritating the sinuses, such as dust or fumes.

show a mild conjunctivitis, leading to a sluggish blink and light sensitivity. The throat may be red and contain more mucus, the tonsils may be a markedly redder colour than the surrounding tissue, with the groove down the middle being deeper or deviating. The fringe may temporarily disappear. The sinuses around the pigeon's eye may be slightly puffy. Examination of the droppings may show stress changes (e.g. elevated *E. coli* and yeasts). A specific test can be done on the droppings, called a *Chlamydia* antigen test. When the disease is active, the organism is shed through the bowel wall and is present in the droppings. This test detects it there. If a bird is autopsied, the organism's presence can be detected by an avian pathologist.

MANAGEMENT DURING RACING

Attention must always focus on avoiding the stresses that are likely to trigger a flare-up. This includes control of other diseases, in particular worms, Coccidia and wet canker, avoiding obvious management flaws, such as overtossing and underfeeding, and ensuring that the grain is free of fungal toxins.

In good lofts, with an experienced manager, respiratory infection tends to be less of a worry. Some lofts, however, do have on-going respiratory problems. Wet canker, because of its parasitic effect, often triggers a *Chlamydia* flare-up, and so the two problems are commonly seen together. In such lofts, the stress of racing is often enough to trigger these problems and it becomes necessary to regularly use respiratory antibiotics through the season to control the problem. Doxycycline-based antibiotic preparations for 2 – 3 days every 2 – 3 weeks, particularly in the early races when the pigeons are younger and the weather is still cold, can be used here. In such lofts, there is often a benefit to be gained by giving a longer antibiotic course, e.g. doxycycline 12%, 1/2 teaspoon to 1 litre of water, for 7 – 21 days immediately before racing to significantly lower the chlamydial level in the birds.

Fungal problems (See Respiratory Infection chapter in section The Common Diseases)

There are two problems relating to fungi during the race season:

1 **Contamination of the grain by certain fungi and moulds that produce toxins –** It is important that the fancier ensure that the grain is of high quality and in particular is free of mould. Many fungi that grow readily on grain produce potent toxins that are not only directly toxic to the bird's liver and kidney but are also what we call immunosuppressive, i.e. they compromise the bird's immune system, creating a vulnerability to other disease, in particular respiratory infection. A grain culture can be done to ensure that the seed is free of fungal spores. Mycotoxins, i.e. fungal toxins, should always be thought of when dealing with an unexplained illness. Mould appearing on droppings after several days in the loft can indicate that the droppings contained a lot of fungal spores when passed. This in turn may mean that

the seed contains a lot of fungal spores. Alternatively, droppings that quickly become mouldy may mean there is a problem with the loft's ventilation and humidity, allowing droppings to remain damp, in the process giving fungal spores in the environment a base on which to germinate.

2 **Inhalation of fungal spores from fungi growing in or around the loft –** Mould growing on droppings or elsewhere in the loft, for example on straw, produces spores, which, following inhalation by the birds, have the potential to infect their airsacs and thus cause a fungal airsac infection.

With monitoring and the correct use of medication coupled with good management practices, it is possible for race teams to remain in form for extended periods. For example, as mentioned earlier, a fancier may find that trichomonads (wet canker) reappear on his crop flushes every third week. Given a constant training regime, this will be predictable and repeated. Rather than wait for the associated loss of form to occur, 2 days on Turbosole can be given. In the same way most problems

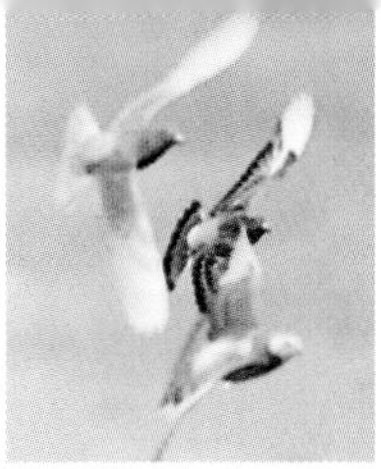

Chapter 16

DISEASE CONTROL IN THE RACE SEASON –

A summary

Diseases active in the loft during racing can be divided into two types:-

1 **Diseases that should be eradicated from the loft and can be treated at any time –** These are:
- Worms,
- Lice, and
- Mites (including airsac mites).

The birds should be free of these at all times and so birds should be treated for them whenever they are identified. It is particularly important that the birds are free of these problems before long tossing starts before racing.

Further exposure in race baskets will occur once competition commences and fanciers need to monitor their birds and treat them if necessary.

2 **Diseases that may be able to be eradicated but are often better controlled through the development of a strong natural immunity**. Treatment is best delayed until just before racing. These are:
- Respiratory infection, including *Mycoplasma* airsac infection,
- Coccidia,
- Wet canker, and
- Viruses – for example, Herpes, Circo viruses.

A strong natural immunity forms in the presence of a good loft environment, good management practices and the correct use of medication. The important thing with these diseases is to avoid medication for them during development until just before racing unless they progress to the stage where they are compromising the youngster's development. Once within 3 – 4 weeks of racing, tests can be done and if any of these diseases is still active then medication is used to get the birds completely healthy before the commencement of racing. In most lofts, there is controlled exposure from a young age to resident diseases – this allows immunity to form. Mild disease exposure during growth acts like a vaccination and is necessary for natural immunity to form. Overuse of medication during this time interferes with this exposure. The natural immunity the birds form is then not as strong, and as a result they are more likely to 'break down' with these diseases during the stress of racing, necessitating further medication. Fanciers can then become locked into an on-going need for medication.

Once racing starts, with its inherent stress, the level of immunity developed by the birds will be put to the test. If it is not high enough, the birds will 'break down' and disease will occur. It should be remembered that once racing starts, drugs only control a disease. It is the birds' natural immunity that protects them in the longer term.

Also, once racing starts, there may be exposure to new diseases and new strains of disease and, as we want absolutely no disease in race birds, medication may be necessary for this reason.

Certain diseases, e.g. wet canker and respiratory infection, cause problems in lofts during racing either through exposure to new strains to which the birds do not have an immunity or alternatively where the stress that the birds are under allows resident strains to flare up. In lofts that have on-going problems with these diseases, programs can be set in place to control them. Other problems are more prevalent in certain lofts but can occur in any loft where management errors occur, e.g. *E. coli*, yeast, fungi.

The correct use of medication, therefore, varies with each part of the pigeon year and also from loft to loft.

As a rough guide, I list below a basic health control program that I recommend for most lofts during racing.

Before racing, ensure that the birds are parasite-free:

- Worm for roundworm and hairworm.
- Worm for tapeworm, if tapeworm segments are observed in the droppings or the loft is situated in a high-risk area.
- Treat for mites (the usual drug used for worming, i.e. Moxidectin, also treats this).
- Dip for lice.
- Treat for Coccidia – leave until last 4 weeks before racing unless the birds are actually unwell.

If wet canker and respiratory infection have been a loft problem in previous years, give anticanker treatment and respiratory treatment finishing 2 or 3 weeks before the first race (see the chapter Health Management Programs for All Stages of the Pigeon Year).

Once racing starts:

- Anticanker medication for 2 days every 2 – 3 weeks unless crop flushes can be done to show that this is unnecessary. Once racing starts, 90% of birds will have wet canker if they have not had treatment for it for more than 3 weeks.
- Respiratory medication for 2 – 3 days every third week unless regular testing shows this to be unnecessary or the flier is 100% confident that he can detect birds with respiratory infection. This can be hard with mycoplasmal airsac infection. Always follow antibiotic use during racing with 1 – 2 days on an avian probiotic.
- Avian probiotic in the water whenever droppings are green and watery or preventively whenever conditions that favour *E. coli* or thrush occur (cold damp weather).
- Regular avian probiotic in lofts prone to *E. coli*/thrush problems, e.g. Wednesday and Sunday, which sets birds up for the coming race and helps them get over the race they have just flown.
- Dropping analysis every 3 weeks or earlier if fancier suspects a problem.

The matters discussed here are dealt with more fully in the chapter Health Management Programs for All Stages of the Pigeon Year.

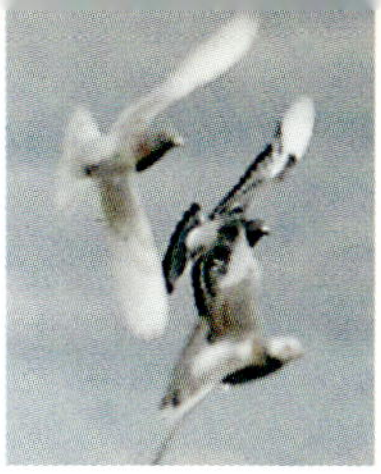

Chapter 17

DEVELOPING RACE FITNESS

As the start of the race season approaches, it is important for the birds to develop their race fitness if they are to achieve good results. For pigeons to win, they must have genetic quality, be motivated, be healthy and also be fit. No matter how keen a pigeon is to return home, he will not be able to do so in winning time unless, like any other athlete, he has become fit. Racing fitness is the result of the interplay of a number of factors, including exercise, feeding, and the overall health of the bird.

An important factor for success in pigeon racing is to understand the principles behind what you are doing. Some fanciers have a good season and then for years afterwards mimic exactly the feeding and tossing routine, etc., of that successful year. But every year is different. Racing can be harder, the weather can be colder, and there can be unforeseen hiccups, such as a bad toss. The skill comes in modifying a basic system so that the birds can again be got into winning form. Unfortunately, there are no strict rules and it comes down to the experience, common sense, skill and observation of the individual fancier and to some extent his ability to think like a pigeon. There are, however, some basic guidelines.

Feeding

For the purposes of management during racing, I find it easiest to divide seeds into two types: energy based (containing a lot of sugars and fats) and protein based. Sugars and fats provide the energy for activity, flight and exertion, while protein units are the building blocks necessary for growth, moulting and the healing of damaged tissue. Peas, beans and vetches are the commonly used protein-based grains, while corn, sorghum, wheat, safflower and also peanuts are the commonly used energy-based grains. In some situations, it can be a trap to buy a premixed race mix because this standardizes the calorie and energy intake of the birds every day no matter whether it is hot or cold or whether they have spent a lot of time on the wing or been locked in the loft. I prefer to buy all my seeds individually and make a mix up each day, altering the proportions of each grain depending on the birds' condition and factors that affect it. I work around a basic mix of 30 – 40% dun peas, 15 – 20% corn, 15 – 20% safflower, 10% milo, 5% wheat, 5% small seeds (e.g. millet, linseed, rice, rape) and 1% peanuts (1 – 3 per bird per day) during racing.

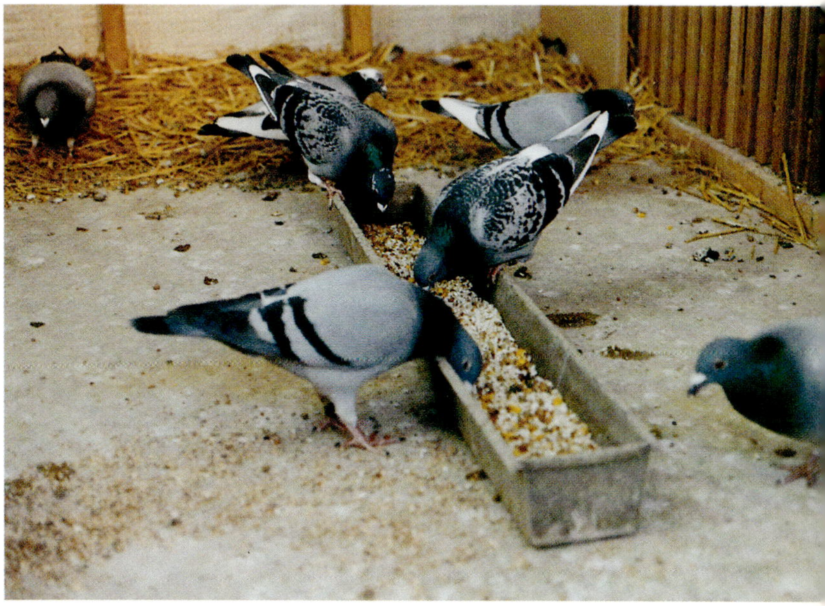

Several of the author's 2-year-old hens feeding.

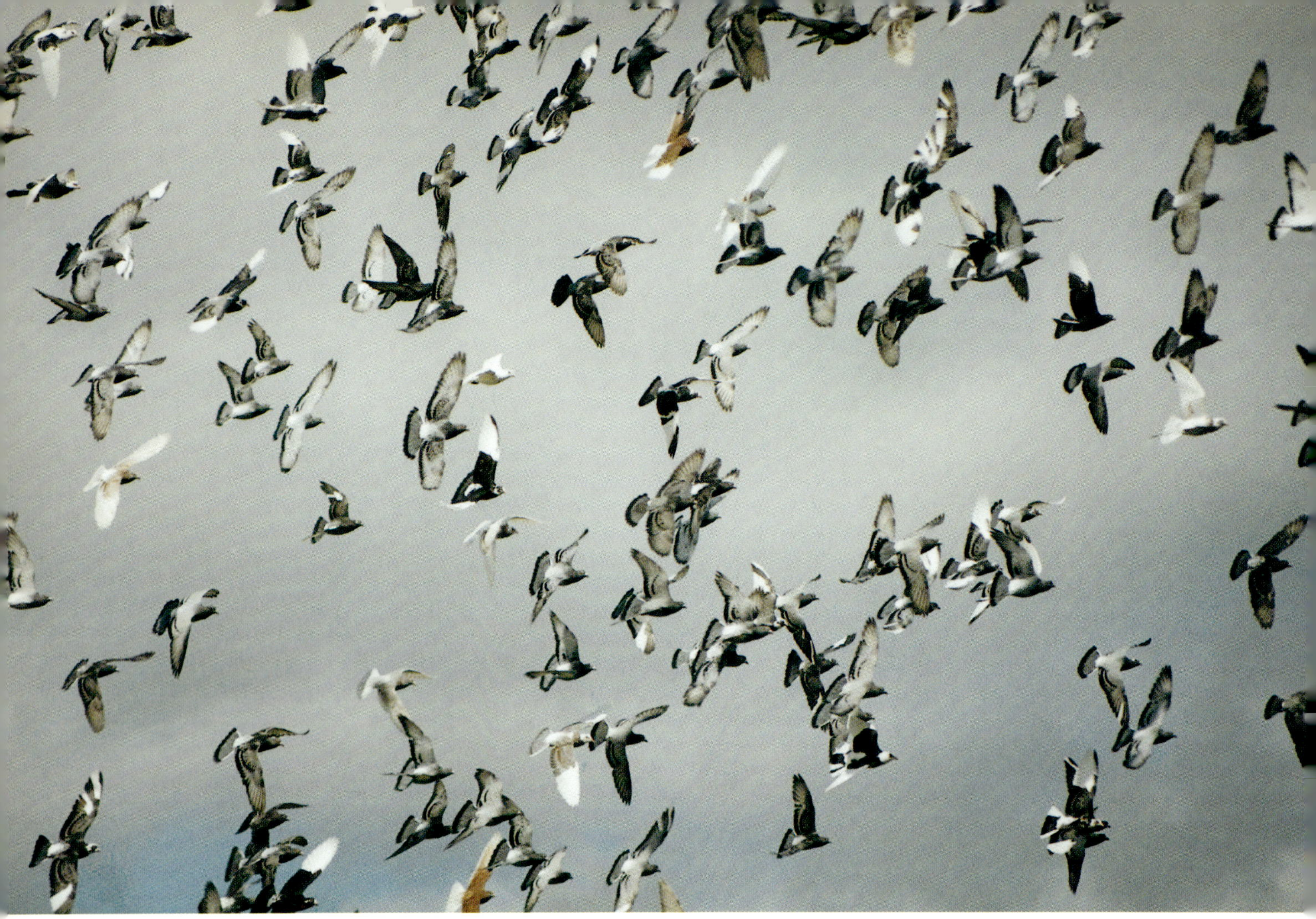

Race birds exercising.

If the weather is cold and raining during morning exercise, or if something has frightened the birds and they have spent several hours on the wing, then, when called in, their blood sugar and other energy levels will be low. It is important that these levels return to normal as quickly as possible because otherwise the pigeons will start mobilizing stored energy reserves such as body fat or even mobilize body protein, in the process losing pectoral muscle bulk and with it fitness, something that may have taken some time to develop. To achieve this, a high percentage of energy-based grains in the seed mix is fed and there may even be an advantage in feeding those seeds of smaller diameter, such as safflower and millet, because they have a larger surface area compared to their volume for the digestive enzymes to act upon. The energy and calorie content of the seed mix can also be increased through the addition of oil-based additives such as wheatgerm oil or Polyseed Oil. Conversely on warm days, pigeons often do not want to fly and are not using up energy reserves to keep themselves warm. When called in, their blood sugar levels may be relatively normal. If fed a high-energy mix under these circumstances, the excess sugars and energy will be stored mostly as fat and the pigeons over a period of time will become overweight. One needs to assess each training session and feed accordingly. The seed ration with its energy and calorie content can then be modified a bit each day, correlated to the amount of work that the birds are taking, always working towards a bird that is fit and in the correct body condition for racing. Several of the birds can be handled every few days to assess their condition and thus monitor their program. Remember that all birds do not handle the same when fit. I find it quite straightforward with birds in my own race team to have a mental image of what they handled like last time and can tell if that individual bird has put on or lost weight and I try to remember what each bird handles like when that bird is showing other signs of fitness (e.g. bright and active in loft, dropping down feathers, with leaders in races, etc., etc.).

I find peanuts an extremely useful feed for two reasons. Firstly, because the birds find them so extremely palatable, they can be used for trapping and to bond the birds to you and, secondly, because they are so nutritious, they are an extremely useful conditioning aid. I do, however, only feed them on days when I feel the pigeons need the extra energy they contain and aim to give most birds no more than three. A small amount is also fed after any toss as an additional incentive. Quite a few fanciers use barley. However, I think it should be used with caution. It is a starch-based grain. I see its main role as being one of satiating hunger in birds that are overweight in order for them to lose weight. It should be avoided when the birds need a more nutritious meal. Its misuse in the early races when it can be cold and some of the younger birds are still growing and moulting and in the later races when the birds are spending a lot of time on the wing, can make it hard to put condition on the birds.

Exercise and tossing

The other half of conditioning birds is the amount of exercise that they take. The amount of time that the birds spend on the wing around the loft needs to be long enough to make them fit for the current races without being too long so that the birds are flattened, lose their natural keenness for flying or fly off any race condition that they may have. Ideally, I feel that birds should spend $\frac{1}{2}$ – $1\frac{1}{2}$ hours per day on the wing around the loft. They do need to have some longish time on the wing to build up the enzyme pathways that release energy to them during the longer races when sustained flight is required. I do not, however, know of any consistently successful fliers whose birds regularly fly for more than $1\frac{1}{2}$ hours per day around the loft. Any longer than this and I think there is the risk that they may fly their race around the loft during the week.

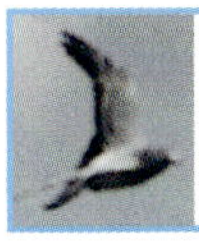

Tossing serves to educate the birds and develop fitness but if overdone can destroy race form.

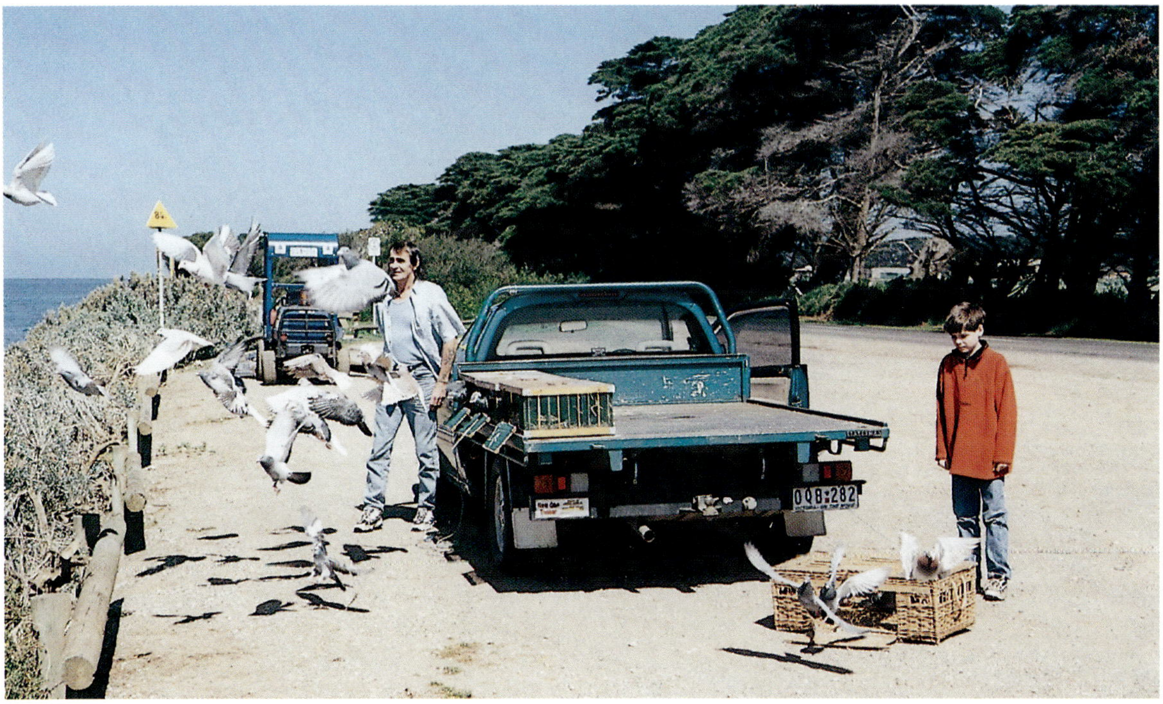

Well-known Australian fancier Keith Saggers and the author's eldest son Christopher tossing their birds 3 days before basketing for the V.H.A.'s first 500-mile race in 1998. Interestingly, both Keith and the author had two birds each in the top 30 in the Federation result with approximately 2500 birds competing.

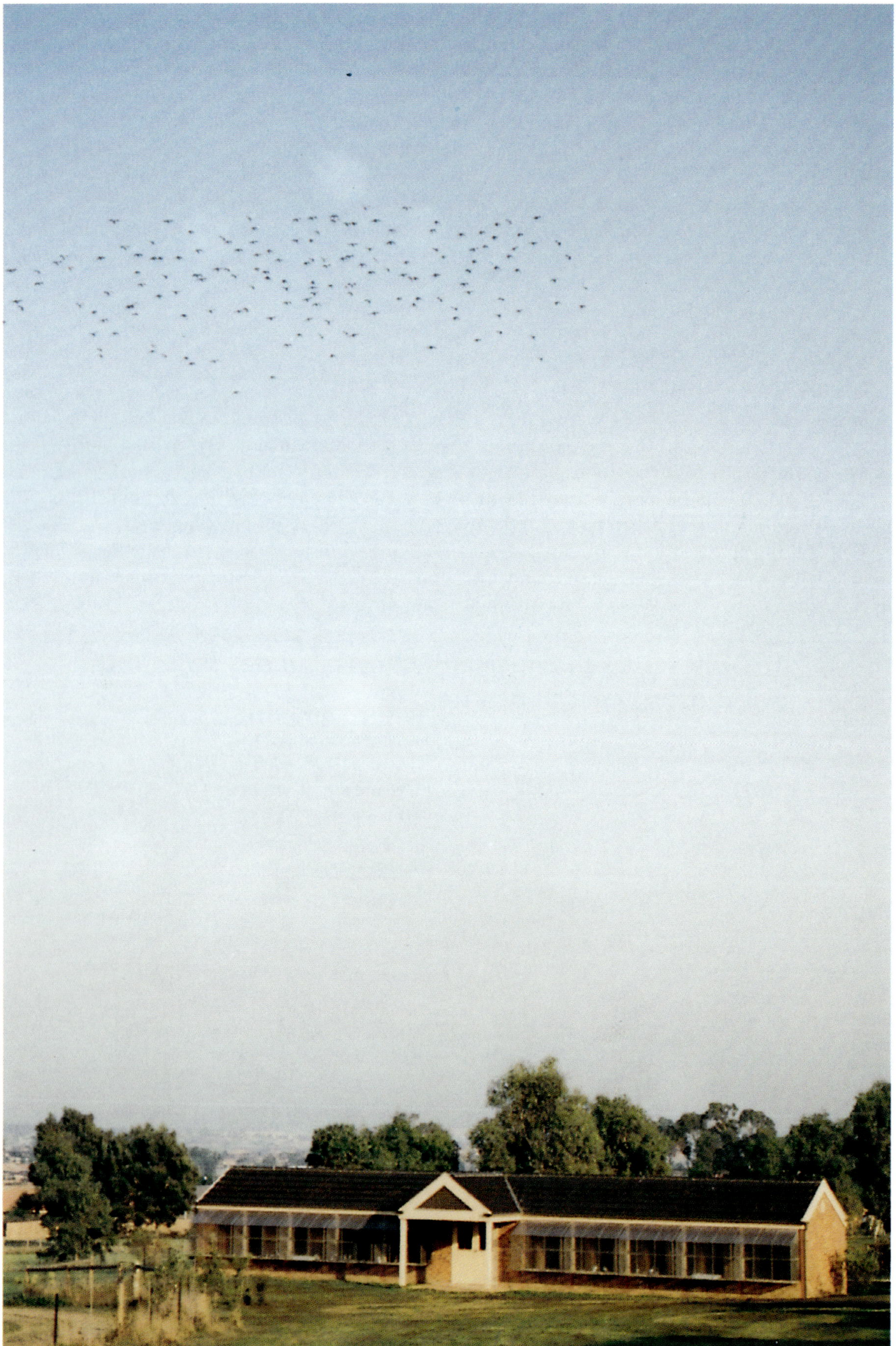

Similarly, the amount of tossing given to the birds must be assessed. Apart from the early educational training tosses, the fancier must assess what level of tossing his birds need to make them race-fit. In tossing his birds, the fancier should be making a conscious decision that his birds will benefit from this. After all, he is deliberately giving the birds work in excess of the amount that they are voluntarily taking around the loft. Some fliers believe that the more you toss, the better it is and the more likely it is that the birds will succeed. I feel that this is not necessarily the case and in fact sometimes tossing can be viewed as simply an attempt to salvage a season that is already going badly. If the birds are not racing competitively, it may be that they are underweight and tired. Tossing will only worsen their performance. If, however, the birds are overweight and reluctant to fly, tossing may be the answer. It seems that when everything is coming together well, and the birds are in form, e.g. feeding, health, loft environment and exercise, the birds through their own vigour will want to fly and winning form will come. Tossing under these circumstances is just not necessary. Once birds are fully educated, if you can open the loft door and a pigeon will fly voluntarily around the loft for an hour, putting it in a basket is probably wrong. The bird may be being unnecessarily exposed to injury and predation and is running the risk of becoming basket-weary and losing the desire to race.

As fliers would appreciate, there are, however, other factors involved. In some country lofts, some birds will simply not leave the loft through fear of falcons, while under some motivation methods birds are also reluctant to exercise. With my own 2-year-olds, which I fly naturally, I find it is the birds that I do not clock that fly well around the loft. The clock birds keep coming down and checking in their boxes to make sure that another bird has not gone in there. With my own birds on eggs, I find that when exercised in the mornings, the hens will not come off their eggs, and in the afternoon the cocks will not come off their eggs. These birds, although motivated to win, simply lose pectoral muscle bulk to the point of being unraceable unless tossed fairly hard. Even postpubertal cocks and hens racing to their perches are more interested in being flirty than working properly if running together. Deliberate tossing of such birds has strong advantages. When tossing, I usually do not toss all of my birds but simply the ones I feel will benefit from that toss. I usually toss the birds 50 miles, looking for 1 hour – 1 hour 20 minutes on the wing. Birds that I feel will exercise around the loft well are let out for a fly before the toss birds get back.

The fancier must therefore decide on what level of tossing to give his birds. This will depend on how many hours they are spending on the wing around the loft and in recent races, their age, the weather, the method they are being raced under and many other factors that will vary from year to year. The skill of the successful flier is in deciding, through handling and observation of the birds, what level of training and feeding is appropriate for that season.

Left: The author's race team exercising in the morning, high in the sky above his stock loft.

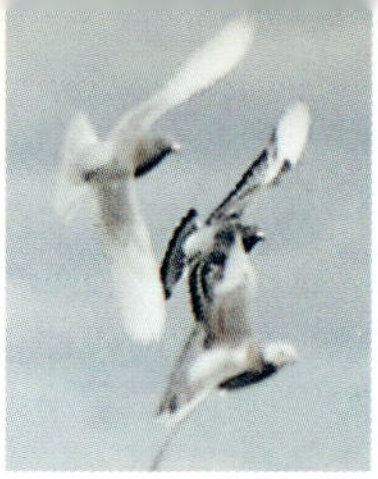

Chapter 18

SELECTION OF BIRDS FOR THE RACE TEAM

How to tell if a bird is fit is one of the important skills that a fancier must develop if he is to achieve continued success. The selection of the race team each week is never easy for, apart from certain races when birds need to go for conditioning, experience or for which they have been nominated, the fancier aims to send the birds that are at their best that week and to avoid sending birds that are not right and might be lost. Simply flying teams rarely achieves the best results as birds that are really fit may be left at home simply because it is not their turn, while unfit birds may be sent and lost. The fancier must get to know his birds as individuals so that the correct decision for each of them can be made during a basketing session. If a fancier has 80 birds to select from, in effect he should try to make 80 correct decisions during each basketing. Essentially, these decisions are based on:

- How the birds handle and look,
- Their behavior, and
- Their droppings.

To help, there are guidelines that can be followed.

Handling

It is not possible to tell if a bird is fit by handling it. Indeed, stock birds that are fed correctly will often handle the same as members of the race team and yet, if forced to fly, their exercise intolerance quickly becomes apparent. It is possible, however, to tell if a bird is well through handling it. Fitness can only be determined through observation of a bird's behaviour around the loft and following exercise.

And so, how do we tell through handling that a bird is healthy with the potential to be fit? Incredibly, there are signs in its muscles, keel, weight, feet, eye, mouth, wattle and feathers that give us the answer.

Muscles

The feel and appearance of the bird's flight (pectoral) muscles gives a good indication of its potential to be fit. Understanding what causes the changes we are assessing makes interpreting them easier. The size, feel and appearance of muscles depend on a variety of factors, including what work requirements are being made of them. As a muscle works, it adapts to its job, increasing in size and strength. A circulation develops to meet the muscle's requirements. As a muscle works, lactic acid forms within it. In a fit muscle, the circulation carries lactic acid away. If the muscle works beyond its fitness capability, the circulation cannot keep up and lactic acid accumulates in the muscle. This essentially chemically bruises the muscle, causing it to become inflamed. This makes the muscle swell, become hard and develop a bluish hue. These muscles are sore and such birds often resent handling.

Size

The muscles of different birds vary in size when each bird is fit. This means that different birds will handle differently when they are ready to race. Some fliers have the idea of a mould into which a pigeon is poured. One opens the mould and all the pigeons handle the same. When they handle like that, they are fit. I believe this not to be the case. Some feel fuller when right, e.g. Janssens tend to 'blow out' more readily, while in other birds their muscles tend to V away from the keel when right. In addition, there is variation of individuals within strains and families. As a general rule, however, the flight muscles do tend to increase in size as fitness comes. Do, however, remember that the muscles of overflown birds will increase in size through inflammation, sometimes giving them the appearance of being superfit. Also, as fat can be deposited within muscles, an increase in size can be associated with overfeeding.

Tone

The muscles of a fit pigeon should be toned, i.e. neither hard nor soft. Unfit muscles, such as those of a stock hen sitting on eggs, tend to have no substance, while the muscles of a bird that is likely to be fit have a resilience within them. An experienced flier once told me that when fit, a pigeon's muscles should feel like a woman's breast. I guess it all depends on which breast you compare it to! Excessively hard muscles are associated with inflammation in birds that have been exercised beyond their fitness capability.

Colour

The muscles of a fit pigeon vary in colour from a rosy pink through a variety of purple shades. However, most birds when well do have pink muscles. This indicates a muscle with a well-developed circulation and well perfused with blood. Such muscles usually have the potential for a lot of work. However, some birds are fit when their muscles appear slightly purple. This is probably due to some melanin pigment (the same pigment that gives the 'blue' to feathers) either scattered through the muscles or the skin. This is why most reds, mealies and white birds almost always have pink muscles. Blue muscles occur in three situations:

1. In birds that have been overworked and have become chemically bruised through lactic acid accumulation.
2. In unhealthy or unfit birds for a short period after exercise until they catch their breath and reoxygenate their blood. This process will take longer in birds with any form of respiratory problem.
3. In birds in generally poor health.

Skin over flight muscles

In fit birds, the skin over the flight muscles often appears thin and transparent with little flake. These changes usually relate to the increase in muscle size that can be associated with fitness. The skin is elastic and tends to stretch in a manner similar to a balloon filling with air, leading to the changes that we notice. In birds that have been fit for a long time, the skin can accommodate the increase and these changes are not so apparent.

Keel

The keel should preferably be white, not pink. The muscle inflammation and bruising that occur with overwork tend to turn the keel generally pink. The clearly defined pink 'blood spot' that contrasts against a white keel indicates health and a stress-free environment but not fitness. You can get this in stock birds as well.

As a general rule, if the muscles are full but toned, remain pink and the keel is white, the birds are exercising within their fitness capability. If they are spending a lot of time on the wing, then this, in turn, means that their stamina and fitness are developing.

Weight

The fit bird's body needs to feel full and toned, yet at the same time not be heavy. It should be light but have a strength to it. It should be buoyant. It is here that the skill of the fancier comes into play. He must be able to not only detect changes in the bird's weight and condition but know how to alter his management and feeding to get the birds right. Birds that are fat become heavy in the hand, while birds that are not working properly tend to become 'leady'. Anything that makes the birds feel unwell, the most common example here being wet canker, will mean that they will still fly around the loft if forced but simply do their laps. They will spend time on the wing but will not push beyond their own comfort zone and actually improve their fitness. These birds tend to float rather than really exercise. This means that they fail to become fit and buoyant, instead developing a heaviness to them, described as being 'leady'. Birds that are fat need to have the energy and calorie content of their seed mix decreased (i.e. fewer oil and starchy seeds). I feel this is a much better approach than simply reducing the volume of grain fed. Conversely, birds that are light need a richer ration, perhaps supplemented with a conditioning agent such as wheatgerm oil or Polyseed Oil.

Feet

Birds are no different from ourselves. When unwell, we get a low peripheral blood pressure, making us pale and sensitive to cold. Pigeons are the same. In birds with a poor peripheral circulation, the feet appear pale and cold, and in birds that are dehydrated, the feet can actually become a bit shrivelled. In well birds, the feet appear full and pink and are usually clean and warm, even in cold or damp conditions.

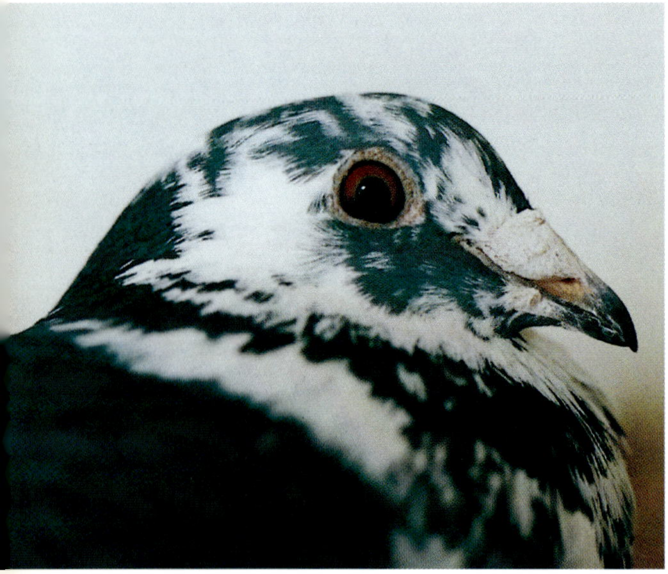

Often good distance birds appear always to be in good health, as shown here. This is 1st V.H.A. Federation, 530 miles, 3000 birds competing, released at 6:00 a.m. and clocked at 6:30 p.m. for B. Willemsen.

Eye

The eye itself should appear wet, glistening and bright. However, there should be no excess moisture. Some fanciers use the term 'glass eye' to describe this appearance. The iris should be full of colour and the pupil should have a quick response to light. The third eyelid should be tucked right back and will sometimes quiver with the beat of the heart in well birds. Increased prominence of 1 the third eyelid is usually associated with respiratory infection. This makes the membrane covering the third eyelid become inflamed and thickened, making it harder to fit under the main upper and lower lids. The blink in the fit bird should be virtually undetectable. However, it is interesting to note that pigeons only blink with their lower eyelid as it is the only eyelid with muscles. The main eyelids should be well retracted but covering the eye to the edge of the iris, making the eyes look round and prominent. Some birds do, however, have an oversized eyelid opening, which is heritable.

Mouth

The lining of the mouth should be rosy pink, not pale (associated with anaemia or general ill health), red (inflammation) or dirty grey (due to long-term inflammation, usually associated with respiratory infection or wet canker). The mouth should be moist but free of excess mucus. Any mucus present should preferably be clear. The tonsils (above the fringe and at the entrance to the windpipe) should lie flat and match the surrounding tissue in colour. The windpipe should be still and elliptical. The slot (choana or palatine slit) should have no discharge and preferably be open. Respiratory infection can cause the edges here to swell, narrowing its opening. The tongue should lie flat on the floor of the mouth and should in most birds be a pale pink colour to its tip, although some birds do naturally have pigmented tongue tips. The beak should be closed when the bird is being handled. Remember not to examine the mouth soon after feeding or exercise as there will be more mucus present and the mouth will appear redder.

Wattle

The cere at the base of the beak should be white, chalky and free of associated discharge. However, sometimes in health, it can be pale pink due to the birds having flown in rain, billing or genetic factors. With respiratory infection, mucus forms in the sinuses, which then drains under the cere and on through the slot into the mouth. The cere acts a bit like a sponge, absorbing this discharge and becoming stained a yellow to brown colour. With mild respiratory infection, a small amount of clear mucus may appear at the nostrils, making the beak here look a bit darker and shiny. The eye cere should be white and covered in bloom, except in birds that have genetically pink eye ceres.

Feathers

The feathers should be covered in bloom and be held close to the body and tight. They should appear shiny and feel silky. The tail should be the width of a single feather. Sometimes, the marking and colours will appear just that bit more distinct. The white feathers of a pied might contrast more. The main or contour feathers are all lost and replaced just once a year in the annual moult. Conversely, powder down feathers can be lost all year round. However, they are only lost when the birds are feeling well. The disintegrating powder down feathers are one of the main components of a bird's bloom. Bloom production and powder down feather drop are therefore a good indication of general health. Bloom gives a silky feel and a lustrous shine to the feathers. When being produced in good quantities, it will accumulate on the outer edges of the flight feathers as a white covering.

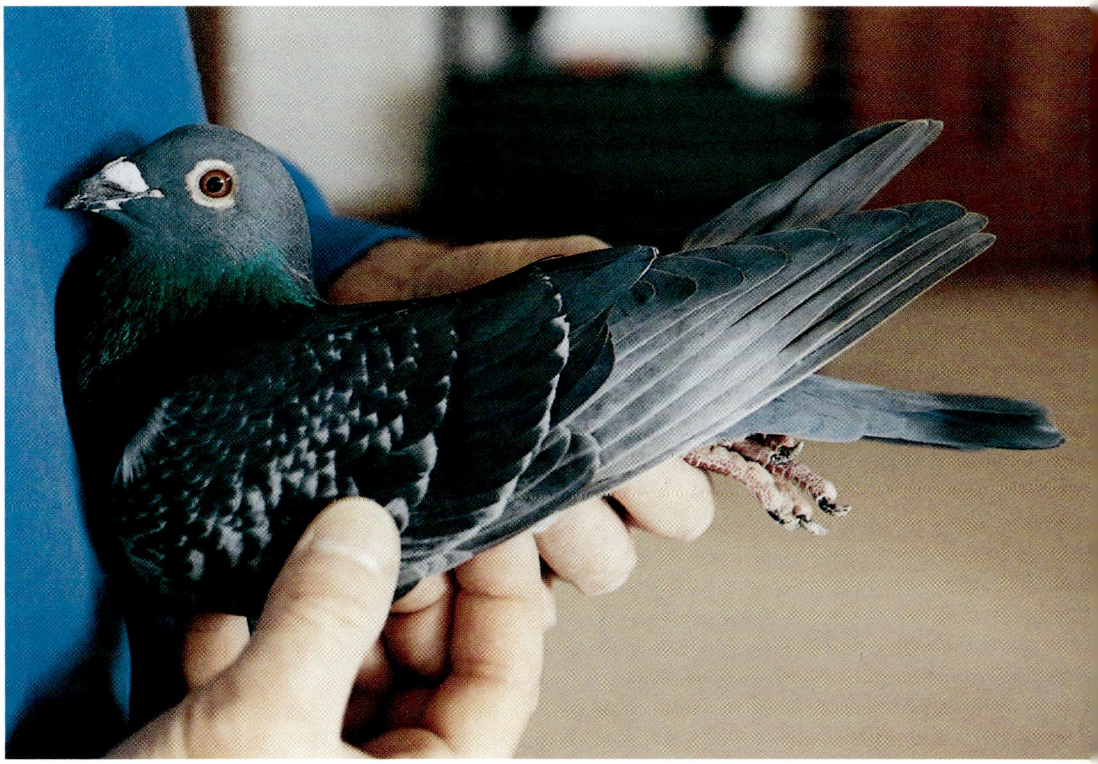

Right and overleaf: Bloom accumulated on the outer edges of the flight feathers as a white covering, indicating good health.

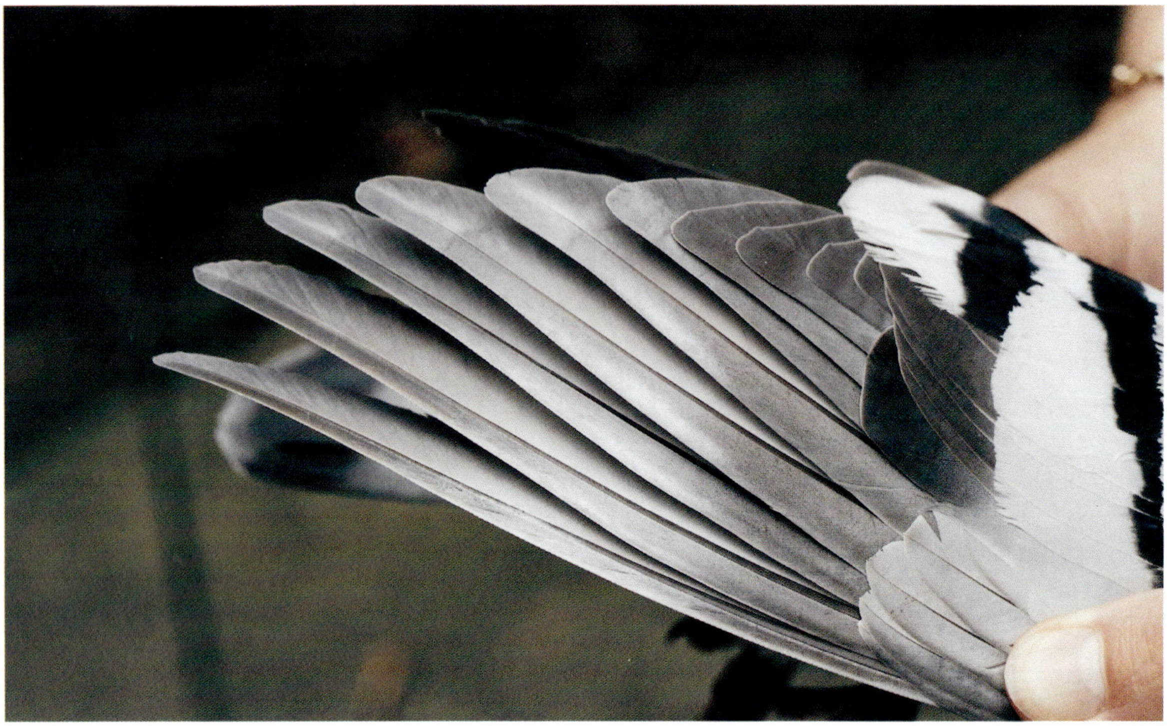

This in turn leads to white marks, called friction rubs, on the vane of the flights being produced when the bird flies. When fit birds are handled, bloom will accumulate on the hands and clothes of the fancier, and Graeme Davison (Davo) states that when his birds are well, his loft actually turns white. More bloom will, however, be produced on hot days and it quickly accumulates in healthy birds if they are not flown or bathed. In some fit birds, the feathers become puffed over their ears, in others not.

Behaviour

As stated earlier, I feel that it is very difficult to pick a race team simply by handling the birds during a basketing session. I feel it is vital to make an assessment of the birds' fitness by observation of their behaviour in and around the loft during the week, the way they exercise around the loft, and, in particular, how they look when they land, both from loft exercise and from a toss. It is only through observation of these behaviours that one gets an idea of how a bird feels in itself and its exercise tolerance. Handling, in addition to ruling out certain things that would prevent a bird from being sent, e.g. a hen that has become eggy, a minor injury or flights at an awkward stage, usually simply reinforces the impression one has already gained of the bird and confirms that there are no indicators of ill health. Jo Herbots of Belgium informed me that his father's main job, and a very important one, around the loft is observation of the birds to ensure that the correct birds are sent to the races and the correct ones pooled.

Loft signs

Fit pigeons should be bright and active and be keen to exercise. When well, some birds will fly alone. Others can exhibit a variety of behavioural changes, e.g. a cock may parade along the top of a door or take over a second nest box or a hen may be reluctant to come into the loft when called. An observant fancier can correlate such behavioural changes in individual birds with their corresponding performance. For a bird to become truly fit, it must be mentally happy. This is why it is not possible to force fitness, no matter what tossing or feeding regime is used. How many times does one see a young cock take over a vacant box or a young hen become flirty and start to really glow.

For true fitness to come, the birds must be happy and content in their loft. Successful Australian fancier, Keith Saggers uses the term 'loft happy' and it is very apt. Fit birds are confident of their position within the loft. This shows itself in a number of ways. They rest and sleep well, sometimes to the point of letting a wing hang from the perch. They are tame and confident with the fancier but are alert and interested in his actions, watching him when in the loft. Fit birds are keen to protect their perch and are prepared to squabble over food. Lofts that house fit birds are therefore noisy and active.

Loft-flying signs

Fit birds are usually keen to leave the loft at their usual exercise time. They fly high and with purpose, are prepared to range, will become strung out in single lines, and duck and weave. As mentioned earlier, they do not float when flying in the way that tired pigeons or pigeons that are scared of their loft will, but rather fly with purpose. Fit teams will usually exercise for $^1/_2$ – $1^1/_2$ hours. Do, however, remember that some birds, e.g. mated birds, particularly cocks, get anxious if away from their perch or box too long and will come back to the loft to make sure that no other bird is there. It is rare for birds that are properly bonded to their loft to fly for more than $1^1/_2$ hours. I hear of fliers saying that their birds fly for 2 – 4 hours but I feel that a bird that is truly bonded to its loft would become anxious being away from it for this long. Similarly, I would start to wonder if there was actually something scaring the birds from the loft. It is always nice to see the birds exercise but it is important that they do not overfly, in the process losing condition that would be better used up in the next race.

Tossing signs

Fit birds look bright in the basket and, when released, group up and exit the toss point quickly. Upon arrival at the loft, they recover quickly. I very much use this sign with my own birds and take particular note of the way particular candidates for that weekend's race look when they land. I feel that if a bird lands from an approximately 1-hour headwind toss, still looking good and keen to re-establish itself on its perch, then it must be well. I also take note of the way the birds come at the loft and like to see them coming hard and pushing. I take an aerobic toss, where the birds arrive panting but recover quickly, as a good sign. Here they are not panting from fatigue but because they feel fit and well enough in themselves to try as hard as they can to reach the loft. Birds from an unfit team arrive at their loft in a strung-out fashion, appear initially confused, and take a long time to recover.

Droppings

The appearance of the droppings on the perch gives an indication of the birds' health. The droppings should preferably be brown, although sometimes greenish droppings (if the birds are fed greens or seed containing chlorophyll, such as dun peas) are all right. Always, however, the droppings should be well formed and tight. An undisturbed dropping on the perch in the morning indicates a restful night, which is conducive to fitness. Down feathers stuck to the droppings indicate an on-going down feather drop and is a good indication of health. The droppings should be uniform throughout the loft, indicating that flock health is good. Problems such as wet canker, which affect different birds within the loft to different extents, result in varied droppings throughout the loft. Some fliers mention that the uric acid (white) should be on the top or bottom of the dropping and that the droppings should be at a distance from the bird, indicating that they are dry, nut-like and have been spat out.

All of these signs may appear a bit disjointed but with experience it becomes almost second nature to monitor them. As stated above, there are no fixed rules when selecting a fit bird and the fancier must use his eyes, hands and common sense. With experience, one can detect that extra glow that a truly fit bird will get about it and indeed finding that a lot of one's birds have become like this by the time of basketing is a truly satisfying experience for the conscientious fancier.

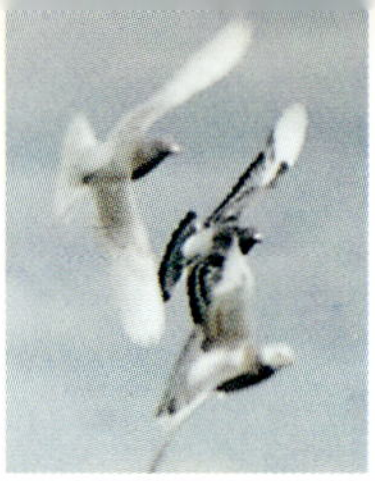

Chapter 19

BASKETING, RACE DAY AND RACE RECOVERY PROTOCOL

Basketing day

As the day of basketing approaches, it becomes increasingly important that everything is done correctly. An error now means that there is little time to correct it or for the pigeons to forget. The fancier should walk into his basketing centre with healthy, fit, motivated pigeons that are calm in themselves and ready for the task at hand. The fancier's efforts during the week culminate on the day of basketing. The result on race day is a direct quantitative assessment of these efforts.

What to drink

Of prime importance is that the birds drink well during the day. Often, clean, plain water is the best. Many medications are bitter and these are best avoided. Anything added to the water should be familiar to the birds and very palatable. Benefit can be obtained in some birds by giving probiotics, multivitamins or half-strength electrolytes. Do be careful, however, as sugar-based or electrolyte preparations put in the water too concentrated can actually dehydrate the birds.

What to feed

Carbohydrates and fats are the energy sources during flight. This does not, however, mean that the birds should be gorged with these types of seed. This only leads to the accumulation of body fat, which is a hindrance. The diet should be based on these grains but should be fed at a level matching the birds' exercise to allow them to become full and buoyant but not heavy in the hand. A grain mix based on corn, safflower, milo, wheat and rice is good. It makes no sense to feed more than approximately 25% legumes (peas and beans) now. Any grits, pick stones or other supplements that contain excessive (more than 2%) salt should be removed 1 – 2 days before basketing but returned to the loft before the birds return.

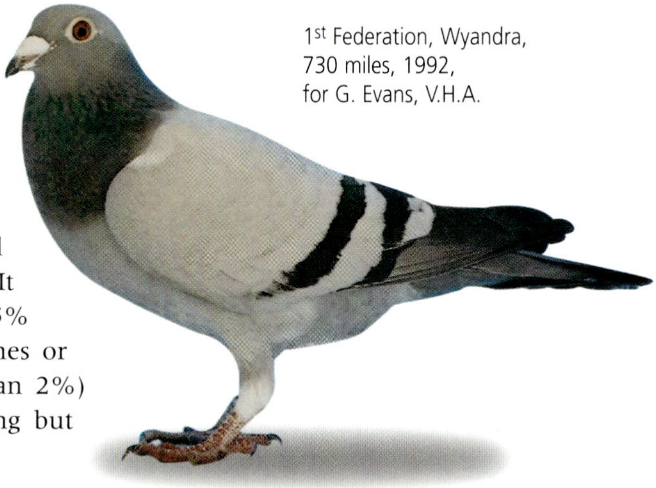

1st Federation, Wyandra, 730 miles, 1992, for G. Evans, V.H.A.

When to exercise

Some fliers prefer to keep the birds in the loft on basketing day. This prevents the risk of the birds overflying due to their race readiness or a loft scare. The last thing anyone wants is for the birds to fly their race around the loft on basketing day. Keeping them in also allows for controlled feeding. With the birds in the loft, there is no chance of the first birds through the trap eating substantially more than the last ones in or getting more of an opportunity to selectively eat more of the tastier grains, e.g. safflower. If kept in the loft, the birds also cannot get wet if it does happen to rain. It is nice to send birds covered in bloom and definitely bad to send birds that are damp.

The decision to keep the birds in or not is more important for sprint racing. The advantage of letting them out is that the birds stay in their loft routine. All pigeons, particularly youngsters, get a feeling of security from a daily routine that is predictable for them. A day that is relatively normal puts them more at ease. If accustomed to a fly and not let out, the birds can often be extremely restless in the loft. If flown normally, they are more likely to drink normally and rest properly in the loft as basketing approaches. A moderate fly also allows them to stretch and tone their muscles.

The act of basketing itself should proceed routinely and calmly. Remember to be kind and quiet with the birds and to conceal any excitement you may be feeling. Any motivation techniques used can be negated by a rough basketing, which in turn can result in a bad trap on race day.

Race day

What happens as the birds arrive from a race very much affects subsequent race results. It is easy to be distracted by the excitement of the moment, with people phoning to compare clocking times, etc., but it is important to remember what is happening from the pigeon's point of view. When a bird returns from a race, it must be given the opportunity to recover physically and also be rewarded for its effort.

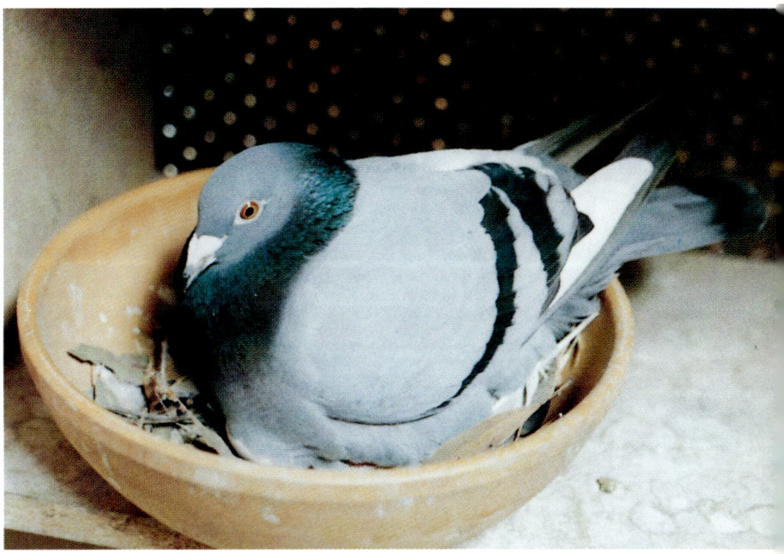

1st Federation, Barringun, 600 miles, 1992, in V.H.A., 2634 birds, clocked by the author, 7:36 p.m. (13 hours 6 minutes on the wing). Photo taken the day after her win.

Physical recovery

When a bird returns, it is hungry and thirsty, its body energy and electrolyte reserves have been depleted, and it is tired. Poorly managed, this means prolonged recovery, decreased opportunity to race the bird and decreased motivation on subsequent races. Correct management means the race can be a positive experience, adding to the bird's fitness capability and also its keenness in subsequent races. For physical recovery to occur, the bird must be provided with several basics: food, water and electrolytes, and rest.

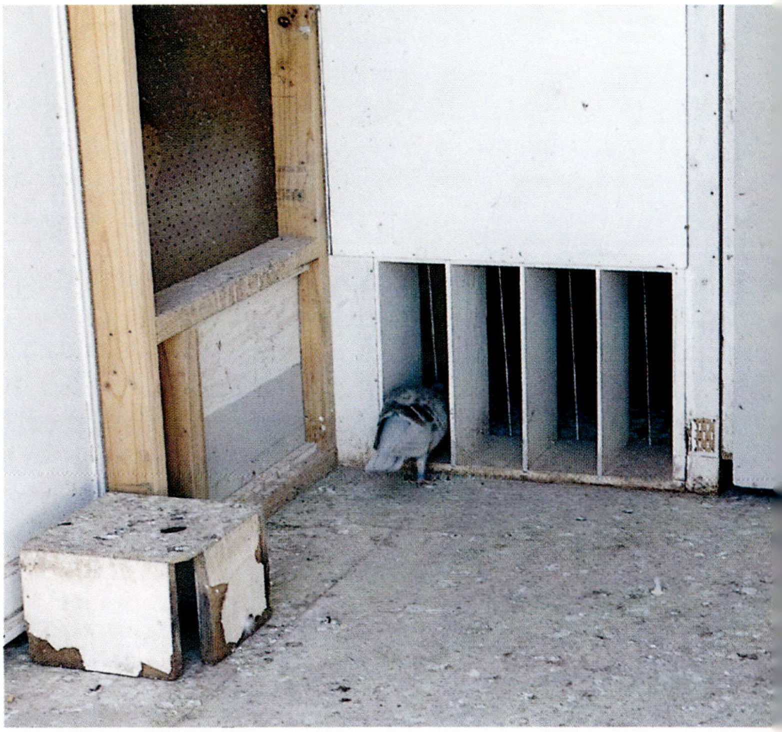

Journey's end for a tired race bird. How the fancier manages this bird now will affect both its physical and psychological recovery.

Food

Obviously food must be available to the returning birds, and all the better if it is the right type. The aim here is to quickly restore blood sugar levels and start to replace organ glycogen reserves. Basically, the birds initially need a mix that is high in energy and calories and low in protein, a mix that is often described as a 'light' mix. The mix needs to contain carbohydrate- and oil-based grains that are readily digestible such as milo, safflower, wheat, rice and corn. In addition, there is advantage if small seeds with similar composition, such as white millet, canary, canola, hulled oats and linseed, are used. These have a larger surface area compared to their volume on which digestive enzymes can act and so their nutrients are released more quickly to the birds. There is also advantage in adding to the seed a small amount of blended conditioning oils, such as Polyseed Oil (e.g. 1/2 – 1 ml/kg). However, several hours after return or the next day after the birds have rested, depending on the type of race, a more substantial mix with peas and beans should be offered. These are protein-based grains. Proteins are the building blocks for healing and tissue repair.

For distance racing, the practice of feeding a high-carbohydrate mix, often called a 'depurative' mix, for several days after the race should be discouraged. A man working hard all day does not want to sit down to a piece of cake but is looking for a steak and pigeons are no different. Essentially, we need a quick replacement of lost calories and energy, followed by access to foods that will rebuild the body's energy reserves.

Water and electrolytes

During exertion, both water and electrolytes are lost from the bird's system. These need to be correctly replaced to restore the bird's sense of well-being and to speed recovery. With short or easy races, plain water and access to grit and a pink miner al (e.g. PVM Powder) will be sufficient. However, with extreme exertion, significant levels of electrolytes will be lost. If the birds are allowed to drink plain water upon return, this further dilutes those remaining electrolytes, leading to a condition called 'water intoxication' and results in a prolonged recovery.Recovery is therefore speeded by the use of electrolytes in the water. At my clinic, I recommend an electrolyte preparation (Electrolyte P180) be placed in the water on long races and in particular on hot days when the birds arrive at the loft distressed. Alternatively, products such as Probactrin can be used. Probactrin contains electrolytes, multivitamins, avian probiotics and simple sugars. These simple sugars do not need to be digested and in pigeons are passively absorbed through the bowel wall. This means a quick replacement of lost energy. Probiotics (beneficial bacteria from the bowel) are necessary for digestion and absorption of nutrients. These organisms are essential for health but yet are the first to be lost with any stress. Quick replacement enables bowel function to return more quickly, meaning the droppings in the postrace bird return to normal more quickly and that feather down drop resumes. Probactrin replenishes body fluids, provides energy and nutrition, helping to re-establish blood sugar levels and replace depleted glycogen reserves, and floods the bowel with beneficial bacteria, replacing those lost during the race. On the Continent, where widowers are often sent to a 200-mile race each weekend, the use of such medications has particular advantages. Quick recovery means a quick return to race form.

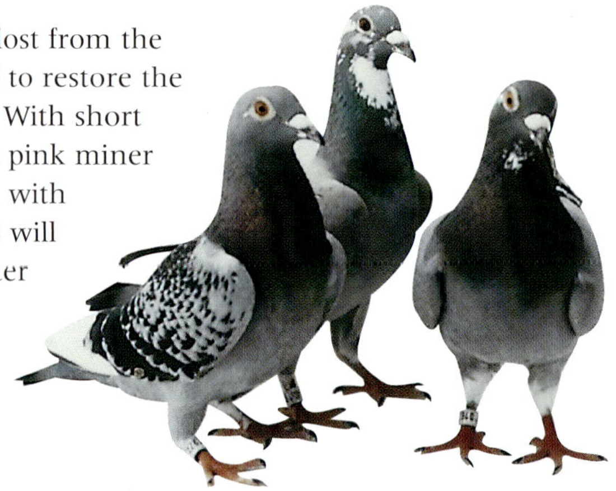

A trio of 500-mile winners. The three young hens that landed together to win 1st and 2nd V.H.A. 500 miles for Godfrey Stevens. The bird on the right is his champion 'Double Dip', which had already won 1st Federation 300 miles. This bird is still the only bird since the Second World War to win two V.H.A. Federation races.

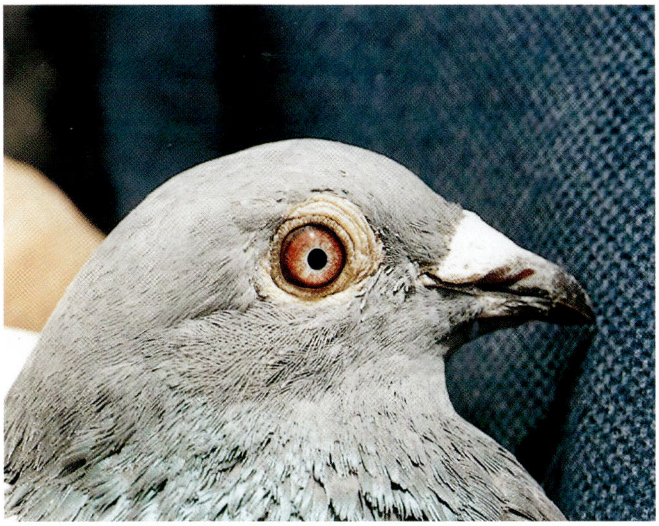

1st Federation 700 miles for K. Fawcett, 1999, clocking at approximately 8:30 p.m. in the dark on the day of liberation.

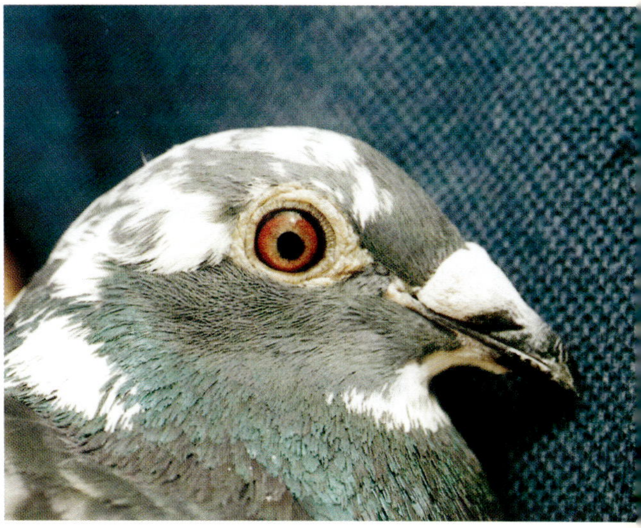

2nd Federation 700 miles for K. Fawcett, 1999, clocking at approximately 10:00 p.m. in the dark on the day of liberation.

Rest

All fanciers are keen to check on their birds as they return and in particular to check that all of their fancied birds are back. But it is important that the birds are given a chance to rest and sleep. Try and avoid unnecessary disruption.

Psychological recovery

It is important to remember the three cardinal requirements of a pigeon to win: it must be fit and healthy, have genetic quality, and be motivated. If the bird is fit, healthy and of quality, then it is relatively straightforward to get it to home. What makes it a winner is its keenness to return. This is why, on the Continent, where fanciers provide each other with the world's toughest competition, that so much effort is put into motivation systems such as widowhood. Too often, this aspect is overlooked by Australian fanciers. In Australia, because the vast majority of birds only compete in their first year of life, our season can be viewed as simply an extended European young bird program, with many fliers relying on food and love of the perch to draw their birds home quickly. The Australian practice of separating the sexes as puberty approaches before or during a season would appear alien and bizarre to most Continental fliers. Behaviouralists tell us that when an animal is doing something for a reward, the benefit of the reward is halved if it occurs more than 5 seconds after the event. It is therefore important that the returning bird has access to its own perch, box, section, hen, eggs, etc. One can imagine the negative effect on a bird when it arrives late to a closed trap or returns and has to wait in a trapping section to be counted, etc. Obviously, other factors like loft security from cats, etc. must be considered here but the fancier must keep in his mind

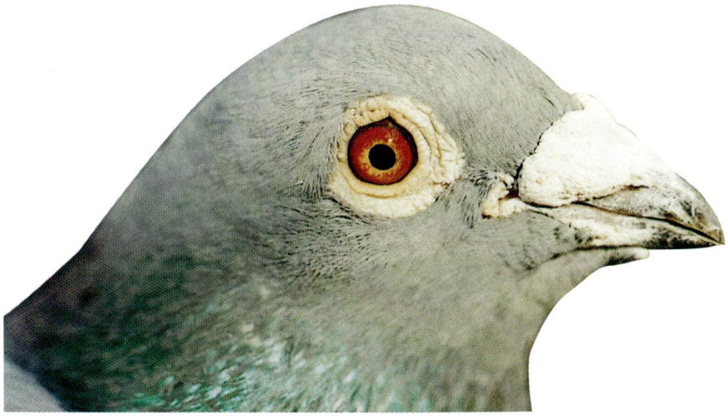

Champion BBC raced by S. Mazurkiewiecz, which was placed 2nd Federation V.H.A. 350 miles 1998 and then 1st Federation V.H.A. and 1st National 400 miles, 1998. Subsequently sold at auction for AUD$7500.

what is going through his bird's mind as it returns from a race. The pigeon must feel welcomed back into the loft, anticipating during the journey a reward, be it simply food and a secure perch for a young bird, eggs for a naturally raced bird, or the hen of a widower.

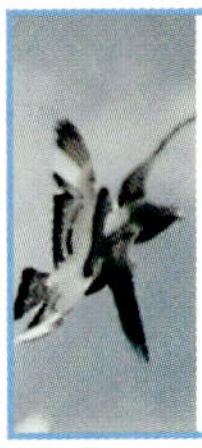

The pigeon must feel welcomed back into the loft, anticipating during the journey a reward, be it simply food and a secure perch for a young bird, eggs for a naturally raced bird, or the hen of a widower.

Interpreting the results of race day

Obviously, a good indicator of how the team and loft are fairing is the position in the race. This can, however, be deceptive in Australia where in many organizations only the first bird is clocked. One competitive bird can make a bad team look good. What one should be looking for, in addition to the time of arrival of the first bird, is a good percentage of the team arriving in competitive time. Essentially, what we want is for large numbers of birds to come at the loft quickly and for them to look neither mentally nor physically distressed. Look for the following four indications of health and fitness.

1 **How quickly droppings return to normal –** As fliers would be aware, pigeon droppings are made up of three basic components: digested food from the bowel (browny green), solid urine (white) and liquid urine (clear liquid). Bile in pigeons is green and is produced by the liver. Bile digests grain, releasing its nutrients. When birds are away, their food intake is reduced or absent. However, urine production in a well-hydrated bird is constant. The droppings of a healthy bird on arrival are therefore made up of just urine and appear as a creamy patch of liquid. In races that birds find particularly taxing, either because of their difficulty or the non-preparedness of the birds, bile is produced because of the bird's hunger and exertion. And so, in these birds, the droppings on return contain urine and bile, appearing as a creamy liquid tinged to a variable extent with fluorescent green. Once the birds are back and eating normal-

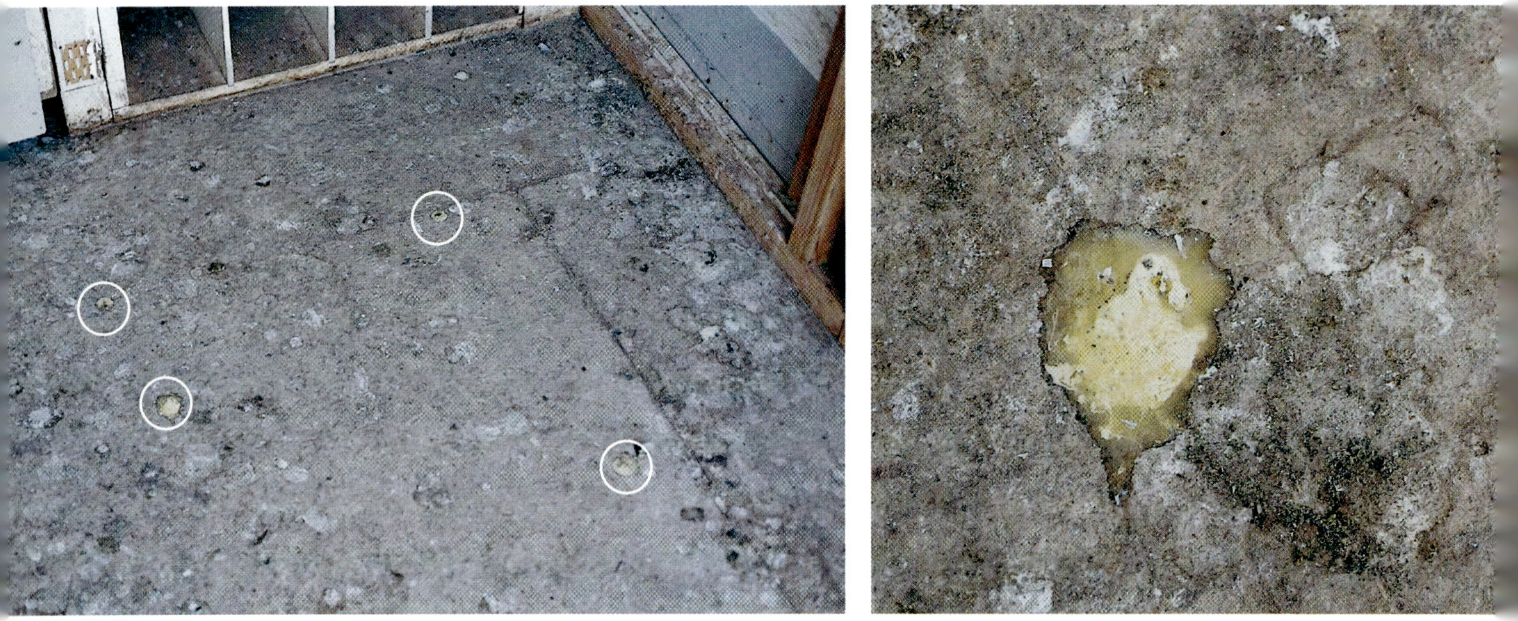

A mistake for beginners. Not the droppings of sick birds but the droppings of healthy, recently returned race birds. The droppings are made up of liquid and solid urine and appear as a creamy patch. With feeding, the droppings quickly return to their normal appearance.

ly, digested food will appear in the droppings and the droppings will start to look the way they did when the birds were sent. In healthy fit birds, this occurs within a couple of hours. Supplementing with normal digestive bacteria (probiotics) and electrolytes hastens this process. It is important that any supplements used are sweet tasting and readily taken by the birds. Returning race birds must drink readily so that any dehydration is quickly reversed. Birds that drink well upon return will produce a good amount of urine, making the first couple of droppings passed very watery. Fanciers should look for these to ensure that the birds have drunk enough.

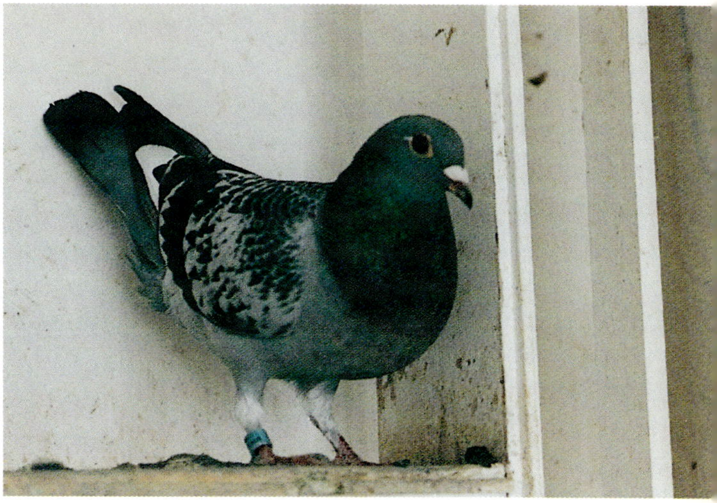

1st V.H.A. Federation 500 miles, 1997, released at 6:00 a.m., clocked approximately 7:30 p.m. on the day of liberation, 2500 birds competing. Raced by G. and N. Mountjoy, bred by the author.

2 **How quickly birds recover after returning, with food and rest –** Within 1 hour on a short race.

3 **Crop emptying –** Birds that recover well will have an empty crop the next morning. Electrolyte imbalance and slow recovery interfere with crop muscle function, leading to delayed crop emptying.

4 **Comparing results and returns with other fliers.**

Some fliers look to whether the birds go to the food or the water first, as an indicator of how taxing the birds have found the race. With exertion and heat, moisture is lost from the surface of the airsacs. With airsac inflammation, this loss can be excessive, leading to birds being more inclined to drink first upon arrival. Healthy birds, however, will drink initially on a hot day, if suffering from transporter dehydration, or simply if the race has been long. Eating first does, however, indicate that the race has not been overly draining and that the bird has been exercising well within its fitness capability.

Postrace recovery

The day after the race is essentially a day of rest and recovery. Just how quickly the birds recover depends on the length and difficulty of the race and the condition that the birds were in when sent. Birds from low velocity, 'long hours on the wing'-type races are obviously going to take longer to recover than birds from sprints, i.e. races of less than 3 hours duration, and the basic postrace management has to vary accordingly. Similarly, birds that are sent healthy and fit recover quicker than those that are healthy but unfit. Fit, healthy birds arrive at the loft and look as if they could keep going. They do not eat or drink excessively. They go to their perch where they may look tired for a short time before appearing normal and relaxed. Healthy but unfit birds are more tired, more distressed and are sometimes disoriented upon arrival, which sometimes results in abnormal behaviour, such as sitting on the loft roof or sitting on the landing board for an extended time. These birds often simply want to drink and sleep on arrival; however, 1/2– 2 hours later they will eat food and often grit. Crop emptying time and the droppings take longer to return to normal. Birds that are sent with a health problem and are therefore unfit, not only need a prolonged recovery but also veterinary intervention. These birds arrive distressed, will often just sit on the loft floor and are not interested in food or water initially. Sick birds still look tired and have green watery droppings 24 hours after the race.

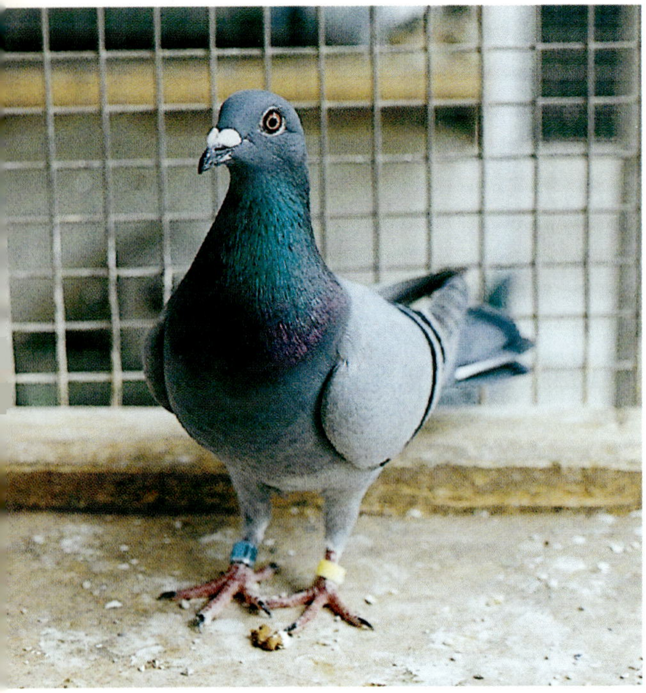

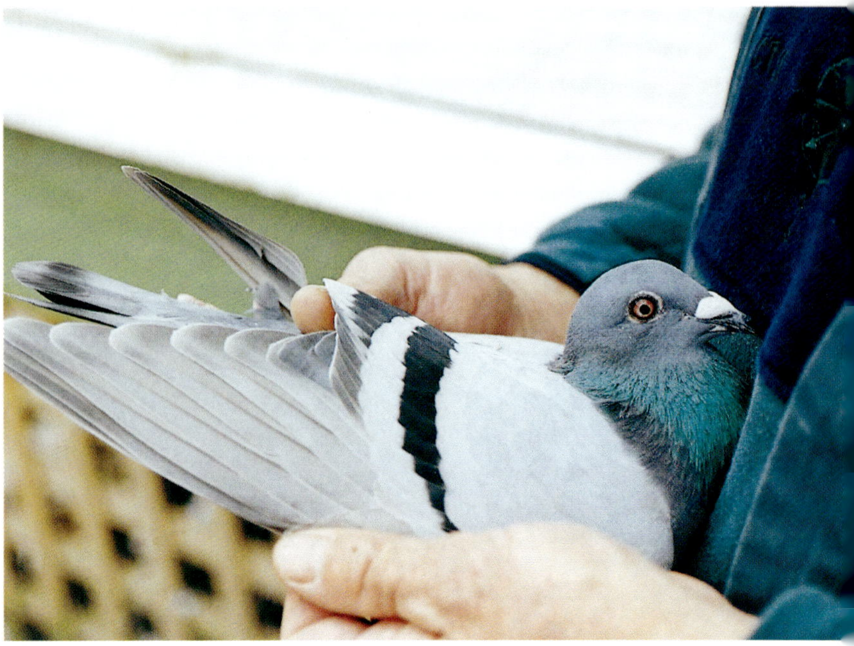

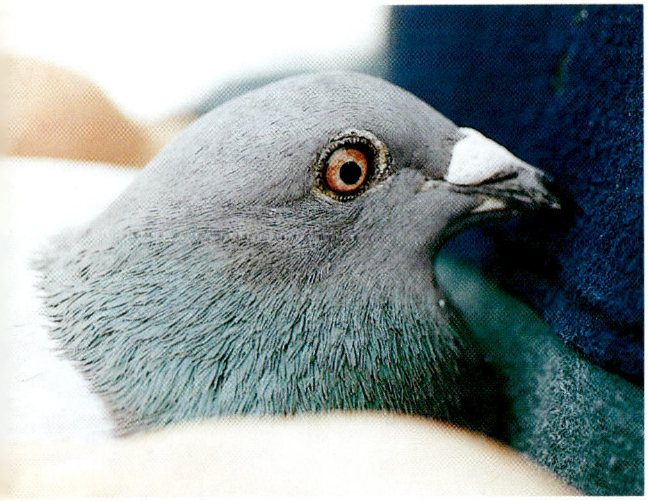

Above: 1st Federation 700 miles for R. and B. Harkom, clocking at 4:30 a.m. in the dark on the morning of the second day, approximately 1500 birds competing. These photos were taken about 3 days after her win and she is still clearly displaying the superhealth that enabled her to achieve this result. This hen was weaned in March and she won on the first weekend of October the same year.

What to drink

Probiotics, electrolytes and multivitamins can be continued for 24 hours depending on the speed of the bird's recovery. If the birds still look tired from the race the following day, there are significant race stragglers or the birds that did not go to the race are tossed, preventive health medication is best left until Monday. It is best to initially focus on the race birds' recovery as prolonged race recovery can, in itself, create a vulnerability to disease.

What to feed

Continue with the light mix for 24 hours after arrival unless birds look completely normal. After this, reintroduce legumes at normal levels for a team in training (i.e. 30 – 40%). Ensure that grit and pink minerals, e.g. PVM Powder, are available.

When to exercise

It is best if birds are given the opportunity to fly the day after the race. They should be let out but not forced to fly. This gives them an opportunity to stretch their wings and to relieve any muscle stiffness. A bath is also a good idea and some fliers like to warm this.

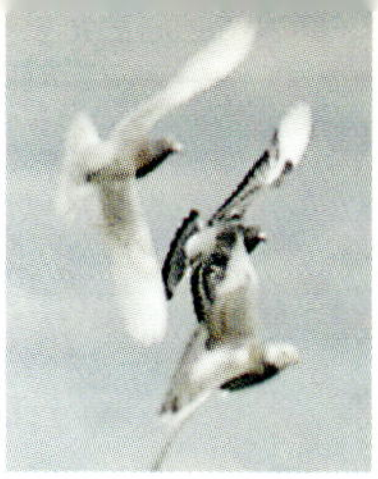

Chapter 20

STRESS*

Most pigeons carry within their systems a wide range of potential disease-causing organisms. Why don't they get sick? An adult pigeon that is well cared for is a fairly robust animal and disease in this situation is relatively uncommon. The reason that some get sick is stress. Often the best thing that the fancier can do as prevention against disease is use good management practices. Drugs can be viewed as the equivalent of a fire fighter, only coming in when problems arise.

It is often stated by pigeon veterinarians that stress is the underlying cause of disease but exactly what does this mean to you, the health-conscious pigeon fancier. Stress is anything that affects the bird's ability to resist disease or develop race fitness. It is a major cause of all illnesses in pigeons in that it weakens the birds, creating a vulnerability to disease. There are four types of stress that every fancier must understand if he is to effectively control the health and fitness of the thoroughbred flock:

1 Loft stress,
2 Feed stress,
3 Flying stress, and
4 Disease stress.

Loft stress

The fancier must understand that the loft is the place where the pigeons rest. In order for the pigeons to rest there, the loft must fulfil two basic criteria: it must promote a feeling of security and provide a healthy environment. Loft stress is therefore anything that prevents the thoroughbred pigeon from resting properly. The causes of loft stress are overcrowding, high humidity, temperature extremes and insecurity.

Overcrowding

Overcrowding is the single most important cause of loft stress. Twenty-five racing birds or six pairs of stock pairs in a loft section with a height, width and depth of 2 m is the maximum recommended number of birds to maintain health.

High humidity and temperature extremes

Humidity greater than 65% during the evening rest period is a major cause of stress. Essentially, the loft must provide a dry atmosphere without being dusty, while at the same time provide sufficient ventilation without exposing the birds to extremes of temperature and humidity. High humidity, apart from being stressful in itself, means that the droppings do not dry out overnight and, unless strict hygiene is applied, this provides an ideal environment for problems such as *E. coli* and Coccidia.

* Portions of this chapter were co-written with Dr Rob Marshall of Sydney, N.S.W. I would like to thank him for his contribution and permission to use this material.

Although cold is a recognized stress in pigeons, it is not so much the low temperature but rather the dampness that can be associated with it that contributes to stress. A rapid change in temperature is also an important factor in loft stress, more so than simply a low temperature.

Ideally the loft temperature should be around 20°C, with a change of not more than 5°C over a 24-hour period. The conditions of the loft at night must favour restful sleep. Therefore, in high-humidity areas or during times of high humidity, it is necessary to review the loft ventilation to control this. In very cold areas (<0°C), the loft must be warmed, even to the extent of providing a heater. A correctly insulated and ventilated loft is necessary to prevent high humidity and maintain a less variable temperature within the loft. All roofs must be ventilated, and especially metal roofs. Condensation beneath the ceiling in the morning must be avoided and is an instant sign of loft stress. Dew on the grass or on the windscreen of the car can alert the flier to periods of high humidity. The correct level of humidity can be detected by the dryness on the surface of a piece of rock salt in the loft. The humidity is too high if the surface of the rock salt becomes wet, and is an indication that procedures should be introduced to decrease the humidity.

Possible changes can include lining the roof, installing louvres on the front of the loft, and adding sliding roof panels and adjustable vents. A high/low thermometer can be used to measure temperature fluctuations within the loft and a hygrometer can be installed to measure humidity levels. The successful race loft is therefore designed to control temperature extremes and to maintain low levels of humidity, which in turn ensure a good night's rest for the pigeon in full training.

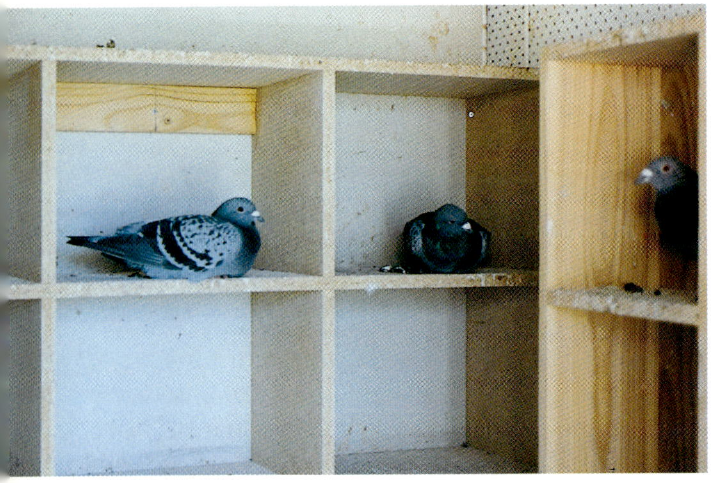

Above: No stress here. Birds lying on their keel or better still with a wing relaxed and hanging from the body indicate that they are relaxed and feel secure in their loft.

Loft security

Basically, the pigeon is looking for a safe little corner within the loft that it knows is its and where it feels safe. This means that there is no cat, snake, goshawk, noise or rodent worry for the birds. The loft manager must also be kind and gentle to the birds within the loft. Signs of loft stress include birds on the ground before sun-up, and watery droppings in the morning, which turn normal in the afternoon. Both urinary and bowel waste accumulate in the cloaca where a significant amount of fluid is resorbed. If disturbed, the pigeon will evacuate his cloaca before this process is completed.

A disturbed or watery dropping that improves through the day indicates a restless night's sleep. A bird whose perch has disturbed droppings in the morning has not had a good night's sleep and will have trouble attaining race form. The cause may be an uncomfortable ('stuffy', cold or draughty) loft, noise, light, rodents, red mite, or alternatively a disease (such as respiratory infection, which causes sneezing, or *E. coli*, which causes a 'gut ache'). Morning droppings are not only a good indication of a bird's general health but indicate how well the bird has slept. The perfect morning dropping should be a tight little nut that is brown in colour and has a down feather stuck to it.

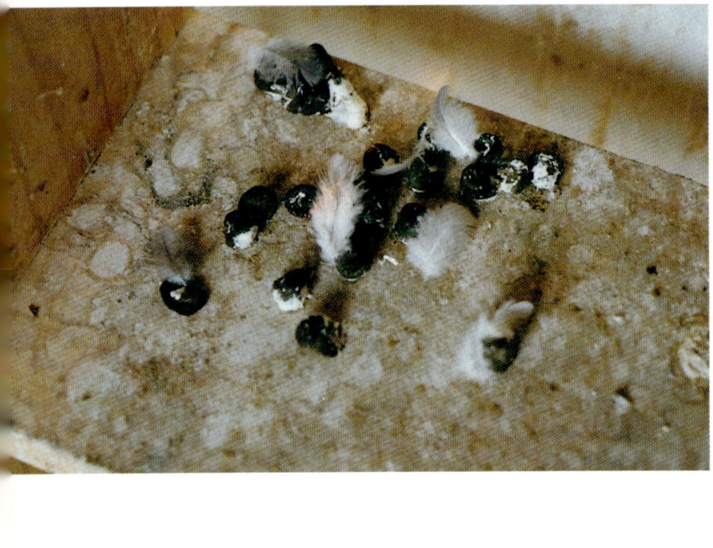

Left: Perfect morning droppings.

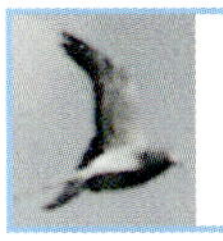

A disturbed or watery dropping that improves through the day indicates a restless night's sleep.

Feed stress

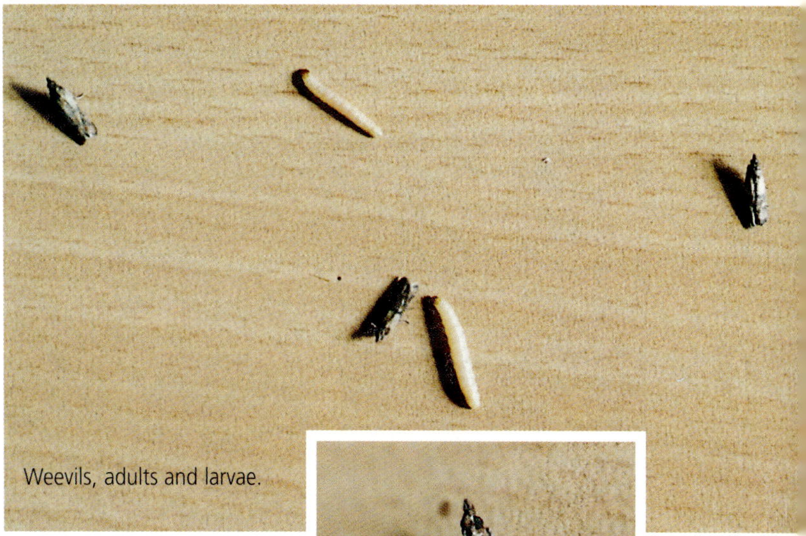

Weevils, adults and larvae.

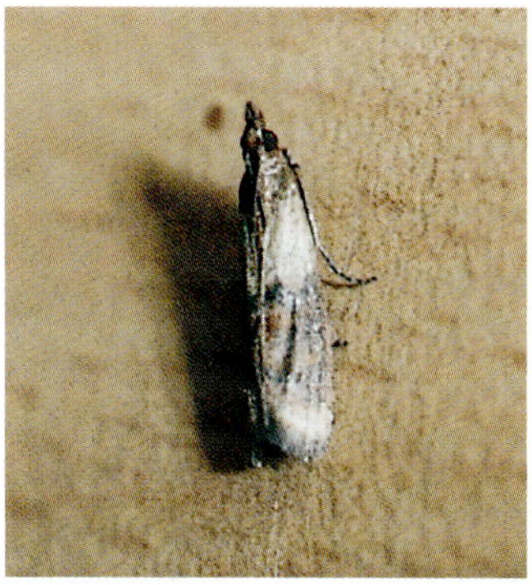

Feed stress relates to poor quality and incorrect quantity of anything fed to the thoroughbred pigeon. The thoroughbred pigeon requires the best-quality feed in the correct amounts. Feed is fresh if 80% of the grain sprouts after 48 hours of growth under sprouting conditions. Feed is clean if it is free of harmful bacteria, fungus and insects. Dust on the feed favours bacterial contamination, whereas high moisture content of the feed predisposes it to fungal contamination. Weevils in the feed indicate old or improperly stored grain and this must not be fed to healthy birds. Weevils are one of the intermediate hosts for the pigeon tapeworm. Bacteria and insects, by damaging the grain, not only decrease its nutritional value but also result in the birds swallowing an amount of infectious debris. The importance of fungal toxins cannot be overstated. They are colourless, odourless and tasteless. They are what we call 'immunosuppressive', which means that they interfere with the body's normal ability to resist disease and also directly damage the liver and kidney. (Refer to the chapter Fungi, Feed and Form.)

Quality feed, therefore, is fresh and clean. Quality feed also contains the correct balance of protein, starch, fat, vitamin and minerals. Vitamins and minerals must be of high quality and if provided regularly, e.g. twice weekly, will help avoid deficiency. Remember also that wet grit can be a source of bacterial infection.

The incorrect level of feeding can also contribute to feed stress. The racing pigeon must not be fed too much or too little. A bird that is too heavy will fail to perform in the race, show and breeding arenas. A bird that is underfed immediately exposes itself to illness. The level of feeding must be related to the training level.

The feeding pattern is also relevant here. Young birds, in particular, do better in a routine and should be fed at about the same time(s) each day.

Flying stress

Flying stress not only refers to the amount of work (training or racing) done by the pigeon in relation to its fitness and feeding level but also to the various stresses associated with the race itself. The amount of time spent on the wing by a racing pigeon must relate to its level of fitness and calorie intake. Forcing a bird that is underfed, underweight or overweight, unfit or already tired to fly is a significant stress. Tired birds must be given a chance to recover, both physically and mentally, before being brought back into work. Overtossing or over-racing early in a pigeon's career not only provide on-going stress but are a sure way of destroying its potential as a distance bird. Flying stress is exacerbated by moulting, particularly in young birds and particularly when involving the flights and tail.

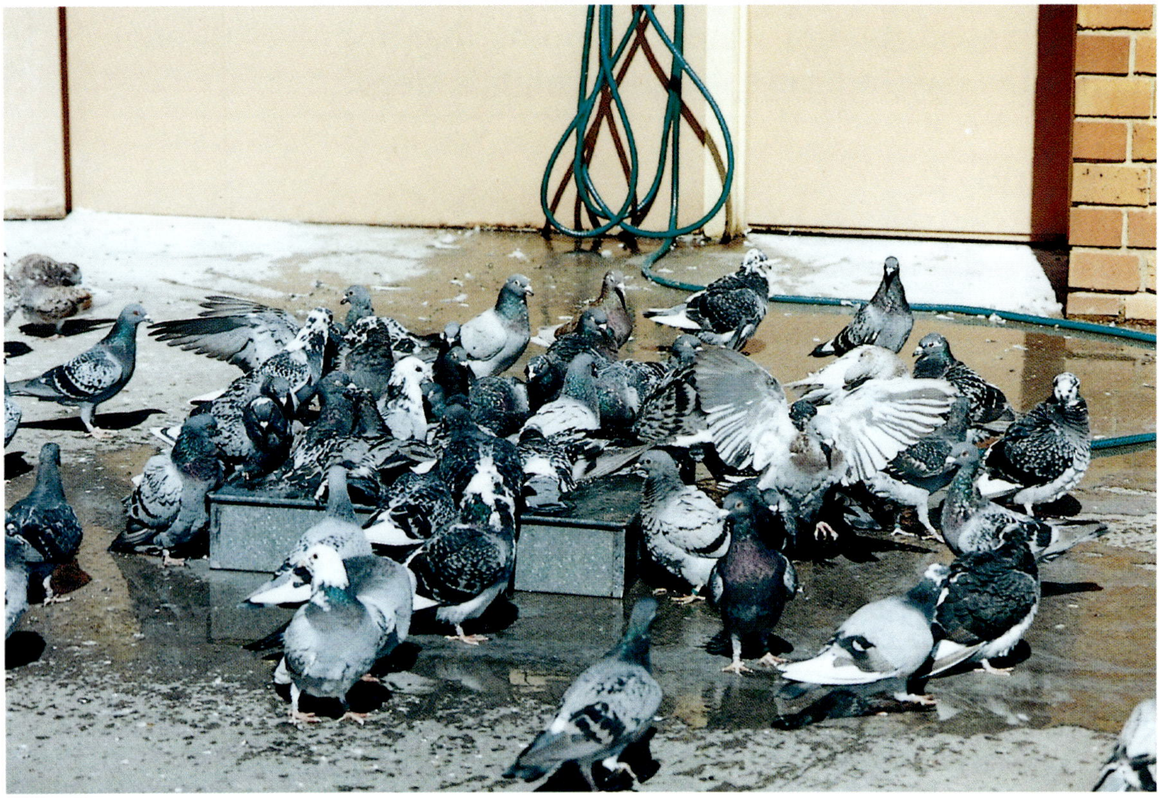

Bathing, although not essential for health, is a good stress reliever.

The very nature of racing provides stresses related to the toss and race basket, including transport, exposure to disease, exertion, and exposure to predation. The correct management of the bird upon return, involving rest, diet and effective disease control, helps to reduce any flying stress.

Interestingly, during the racing season it is often the good fliers whose birds 'break down', associated with flying stress. Less competitive fliers may provide their birds with plenty to eat and keep tossing to a minimum. These birds have no stress-related disease and when checked in a veterinary sense no problems are apparent, but they are not fit or competitive either. The more competitive fliers get their birds fit through monitored exercise and controlled feeding, in the process, stripping out excess body fat, creating buoyancy and superhealth. It is easy, however, to push the birds over their limit and when tested these birds may show evidence of breaking down, having problems with *E. coli*, thrush or wet canker, etc.

Disease stress

Typically in pigeons, there is a disease cascade, with well-recognized connections between the various diseases. For example, elevated yeasts (thrush) often are an early indicator of stress. Unless the stress is identified, the birds become further run down and problems such as wet canker and respiratory infection start appearing.

A very common problem between January and March in Australia is respiratory infection. Typically, this affects young birds and birds that are in a heavy body moult. They show signs of eye colds, dirty ceres and increased sneezing. Pigeons can often tolerate a single stress, but when stresses start overlapping any natural immunity that these young ones have already formed is put to the test. When a crop flush and faecal smear are done on youngsters with respiratory disease, most of them have one of the three primary parasitic diseases, namely worms, Coccidia or wet canker. Indeed, approximately 80% of moulting youngsters with respiratory disease have high trichomonad counts. It is these trichomonads exerting their parasitic effect that provide the further stress

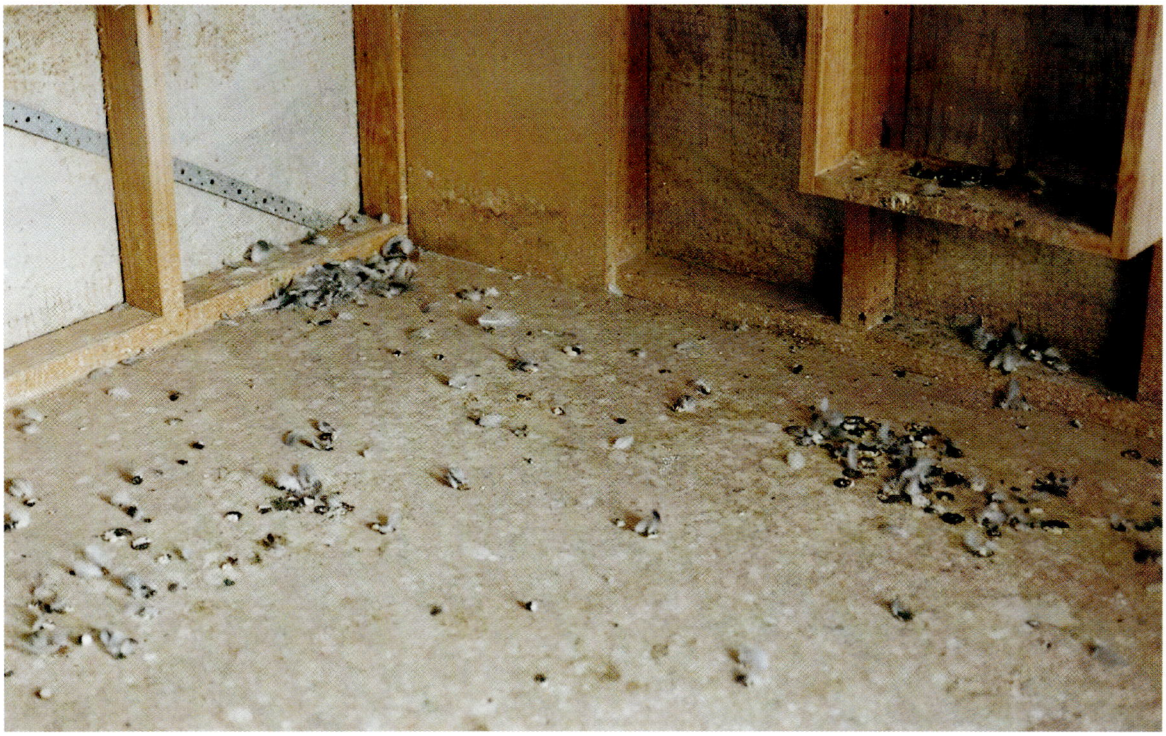

A pleasing sight in the morning to pigeon fanciers, indicating a stress-free night. Tight nut droppings and an abundance of down feathers cover the floor.

necessary for the *Chlamydia*, which is already within the system of the young birds, to flare up and cause disease. Without identification of these concurrent problems, we find that the response to treatment with respiratory antibiotics is poor or alternatively the problem quickly recurs once treatment is withdrawn. Often treatment of the wet canker (i.e. the elevated trichomonad level), for example with 2 days Turbosole, will result in such an increase in vigour of the young ones that they are then able to clear the respiratory infection by themselves. In the same way, other loft, feed or training problems can provide the stresses that enable respiratory infection to flare up.

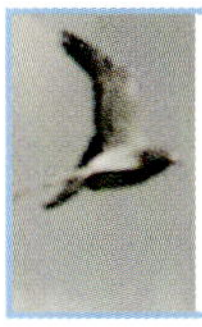

It is possible sometimes to tell what sort of loft a fancier has simply by looking at his birds' droppings under the microscope.

There are also well-recognized connections between various loft design and management practices and certain diseases. For example, birds from cold, damp lofts often register positive on their *Chlamydia* tests and have mildly elevated Coccidia counts. Lofts with high humidity often have problems with *E. coli* and thrush infections. Fliers are often surprised when I can tell what kind of loft they have simply by testing their birds' droppings. The overtraining or underfeeding of young ones often leads to thrush. High Coccidia levels not only indicate major stress but also poor hygiene and dampness. As a pigeon veterinarian, when my own pigeons are just not performing, what I have to try to figure out is what diseases are active and what precipitating stresses are at work. The solution is usually a combination of medication suggestions and a review of recent management practices, e.g. the level of tossing. In the same way, I have to nut out the same problems presented to me by clients.

The appropriate combination of stress minimization through the provision of a good loft environment and good management practices coupled with the correct use of medication is the way of achieving optimal results with the birds.

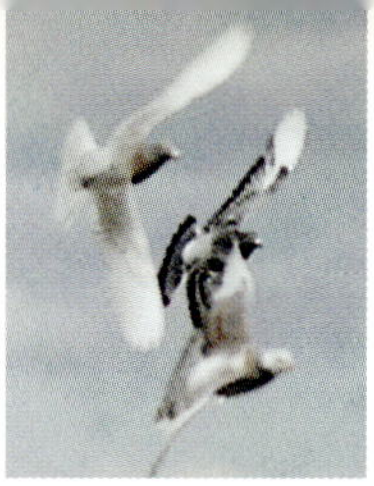

Chapter 21

WINNING

Pigeons have a natural desire to return home. Through selective breeding, they can now do this from great distances and at high speeds. It is the job of the competitive pigeon flier to not only get his birds home but to get his birds home quicker than everybody else. In order to do this, his pigeons must have three characteristics:

1 Quality,
2 Fitness and health, and
3 Motivation (psychologically right).

Quality

To draw any analogy between the pigeon seen pecking in the parks and a racing pigeon would be like considering entering a Shetland pony in the Melbourne Cup. Today's competitive bird is a thoroughbred animal, each bird carrying its own pedigree and bloodlines, with various strains being better for short or long-distance races or for fast or slow days. These strains tend to carry various characteristics that enable identification to an experienced eye.

The trouble with picking good racing pigeons is that when one looks at them, one sees the colour of their feathers, the colour of their eyes, the shape of their head, etc. However, these things have little correlation with the bird's ability to win races. The most important things are the things that one cannot see. These include the bird's determination, intelligence and stamina. Birds on long-distance races, when they do not make the loft on the first day, find themselves alone, having had nothing to eat or drink, and still a long way from home. They must have the presence of mind to orientate and the constitution to continue on.

Things that can be seen and may give an indication that the bird has the potential to do well are:

- **The bird's personality and temperament –** It can be hard to assess this when buying at a sale. It is only when the bird is home in the loft that one can see how quiet and sensible it is, or alternatively, how flighty it is.
- **Outward signs of good health –** Very often, good birds always seem to be well.
- **Balance –** Most good birds give the impression in the hand of being full in the chest but at the same time long. They possess a sternum that is deeper at the front and tapers to a pair of tight vent or pubic bones.

But above all else, the most important thing that one can see is the bird's

- **Pedigree –** The bird, at best, can only realize its full genetic potential and if the winning genes are just not there, it cannot win.

However, as with other competitive animals, just having a good pedigree does not make that individual a champion. As in any competition, some birds will appear as the best. It is the job of the pigeon fancier to obtain as a good a pigeon as he can, to thoroughly test the progeny racing, and, in turn, only breed from the best. As a general rule, it is the winners or their close relatives that tend to breed the winners. This is particularly so in the longer-distance races. If the pigeon does not have the genetic potential to perform, particularly at the distance, it simply cannot do so.

Fitness and health

No matter how well bred or motivated a pigeon might be, if it is not fit and healthy not only will it be unable to win but to simply return to its loft might be an impossible task. The development and maintenance of fitness and the attainment of superhealth are dealt with in the chapters covering these areas.

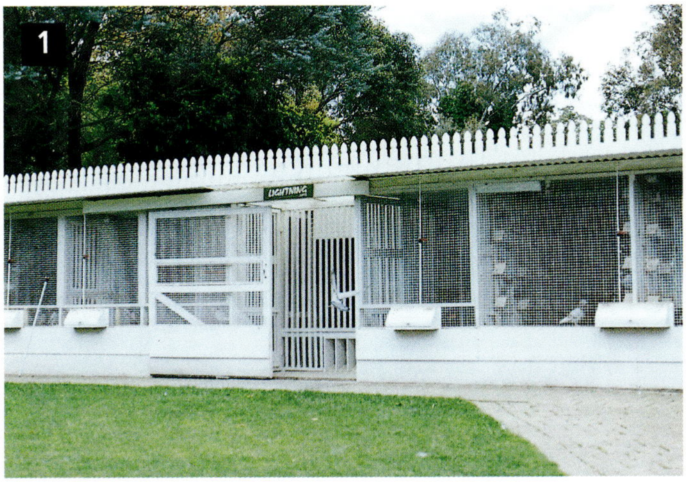

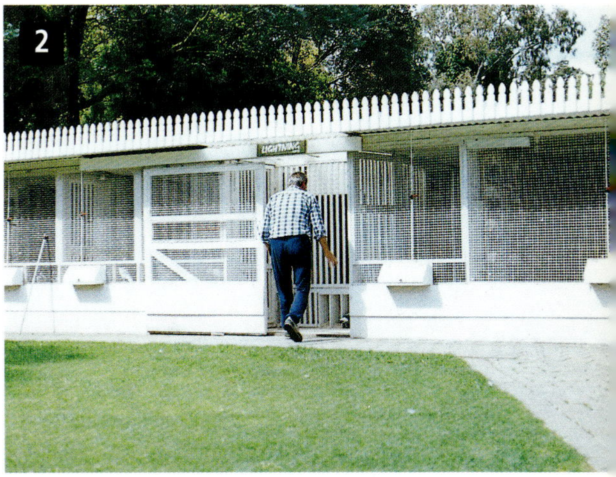

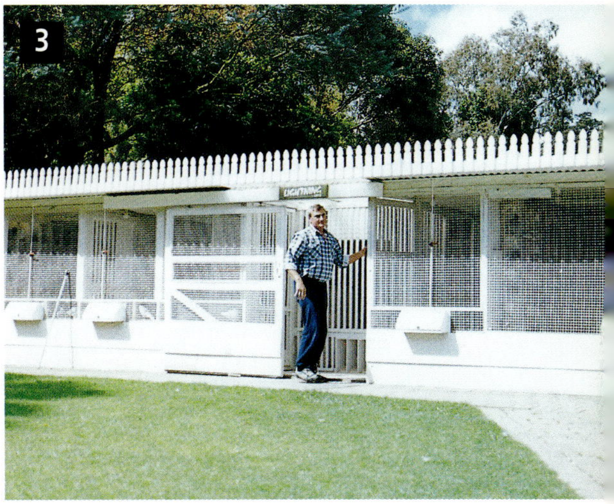

Photos 1 – 3: V.H.A. champion George Vella, clocking in V.H.A. fourth 300-mile race in 1997. He gained 26th overall with approximately 4500 birds competing.
1: The clock bird arrives and flies in to his fly-in.
2: No time is wasted and George quickly follows behind the bird and clocks her in.
3: Clocking completed, a good result is hoped for.

Motivation

Although beyond the scope of this book to discuss motivational techniques in detail, the basic methods and how they aim to motivate the birds will be briefly discussed.

It is important that the loft provides an environment in which the birds feel safe and secure and to which they want to return quickly, as discussed in the chapter Loft Design. Having created such an environment, the fancier has several methods at his disposal to increase their level of incentive to return. In Australia, most pigeons are only raced during their first year of life. For most of this time, they are, in fact, prepubertal (onset of puberty is variable but usually occurs between 7 and 8 months of age). These birds home and home quickly, simply because of the bond they have developed with their perch, loft, and possibly their owner. However, as the year progresses and the old bird season commences (in July), the birds start to go through puberty. For several weeks, the young cocks and hens flirt with each other and at this time their motivation to return increases dramatically. Astute fanciers can capitalize on this and some good races have been won with birds in such condition.

Following puberty, the hens start to ovulate and lay. Care must be taken with the hens to ensure they are not sent to races after ovulation as they can be easily lost. Four days after ovulation, the eggs are laid. After ovulation, the hen's abdomen will start to increase in size and feel puffy. Her pectoral muscle mass may appear smaller. Any pressure on the abdomen will cause 'open beak respiration' due to the volume of the developing egg interfering with distention of the abdominal airsacs during inspiration. Postovulation, the smooth edge of the egg can be felt high on the right-hand side of the abdomen just behind the ribs. This becomes progressively more obvious until laying occurs.

Many Australian fanciers prefer to race their cocks and hens separately. In this situation, the eggs are removed and the hens will then intermittently lay through the rest of the season. This system has the advantage of making management less complicated. For example, the hens may be exercised in the morning and the cocks in the evening. No record needs to be kept of the hens' laying cycle. The hens tend to lay less and so can be raced more frequently. Similarly, some cocks, when with the hens, will be so active sexually as to run themselves ragged, thus proving very difficult to get into race condition. Sometimes, the sexes are allowed together for short periods, just before basketing or upon return from racing.

Other fanciers prefer to leave the cocks and hens together, in particular taking advantage of the flirty hens as puberty approaches, but then providing them with nest bowls and nest boxes once laying commences. This is called the **natural system**. Most birds race best when they are sitting on their eggs for 8 – 12 days, however, it must be remembered that all pigeons are different and the fancier must observe his birds individually and assess at which stage of the reproductive cycle each bird will perform best. Birds that are sitting are often reluctant to exercise around the loft, to the point of losing so much pectoral muscle bulk as to become unraceable. The level of tossing, therefore, has to be increased accordingly.

The main advantage of the natural system is that, in certain birds who race well under this system, a predictable level of motivation can be achieved so that birds can be set for particularly important races. Fanciers using this method usually work around a 20-day cycle. Most hens will lay

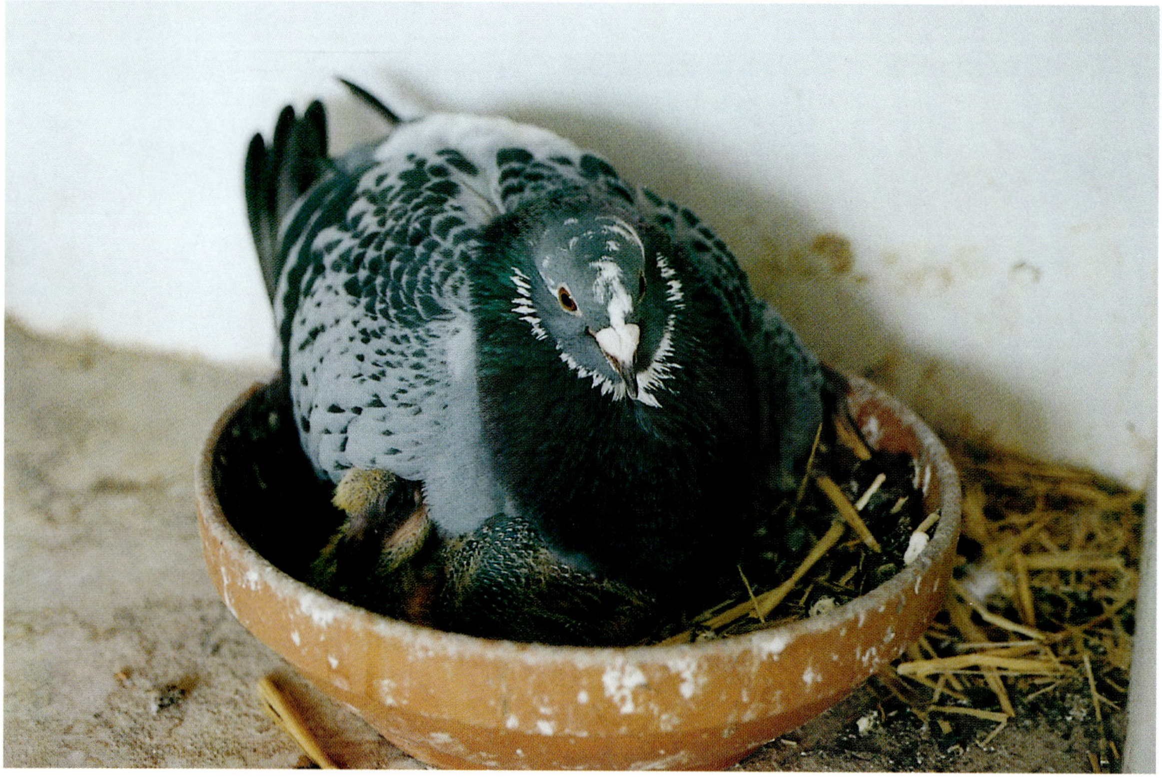

A 2-year-old race hen on a 7-day-old baby illustrates the strong bond that some hens have with their box, which creates an incentive to return quickly on race day.

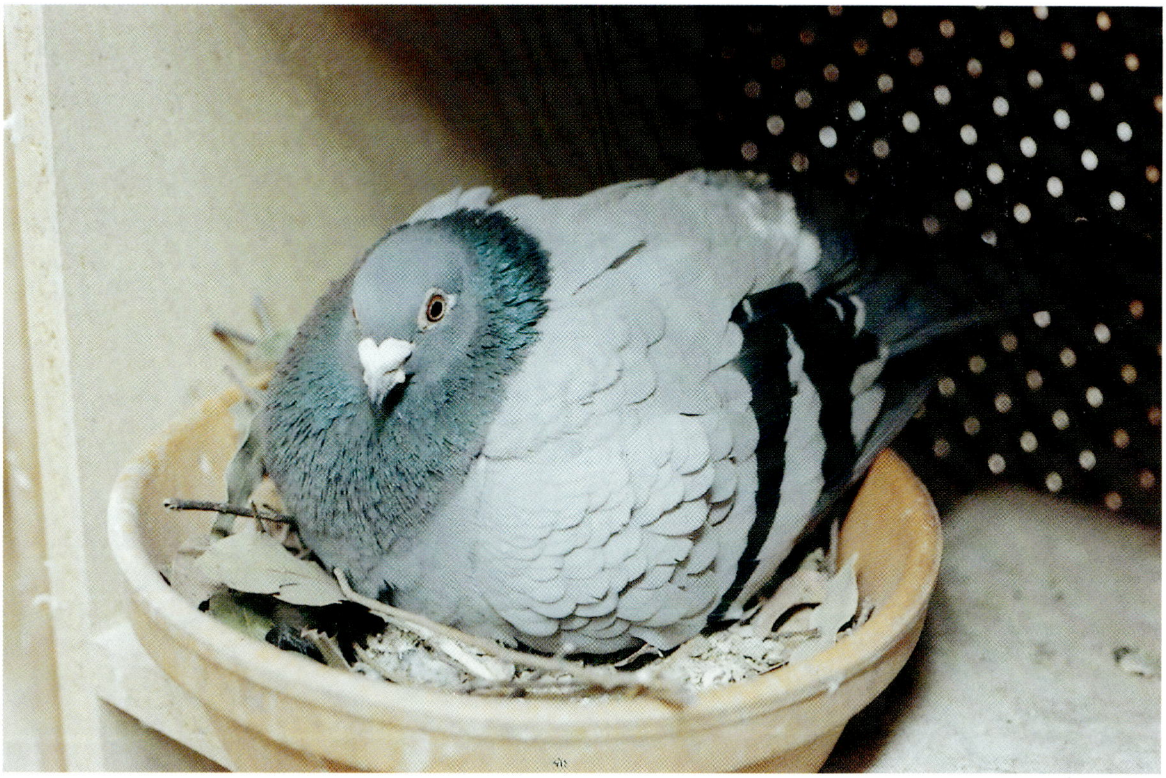

The author's 'Baby' BBH. This hen flew the V.H.A. smash 700-mile race in 1990 at 20 weeks of age when only 20 birds were clocked within 6 days of release. She flew the 700 again in 1991 and was the author's fifth bird on the day in the 1992 600-mile race, arriving at 10:45 p.m.

approximately 10 days after being introduced to a cock or after having eggs that they are incubating removed. Once she has laid, she is allowed to sit and bond herself to her eggs and box for 2 –3 days, just being kept in her normal loft exercise routine. Following this period, she and the cock are deliberately tossed and often quite hard, e.g. three 50-mile tosses in 5 days, and then sent racing at approximately 10 days after laying.

If the racing is short and easy, then according to the condition and capability of the individual bird, she can be sent to a second race between 15 and 17 days. Upon return, she is allowed to sit for a further 2 – 3 days and then the eggs are removed. Most hens will then, fairly predictably, lay again in 10 days and may be sent racing again in approximately 20 days. There are a variety of extensions of this method, with the pairs being allowed to continue sitting, eggs hatching and birds being raced to one or both youngsters. Indeed, some hens will race particularly well to a 12 – 15-day-old youngster.

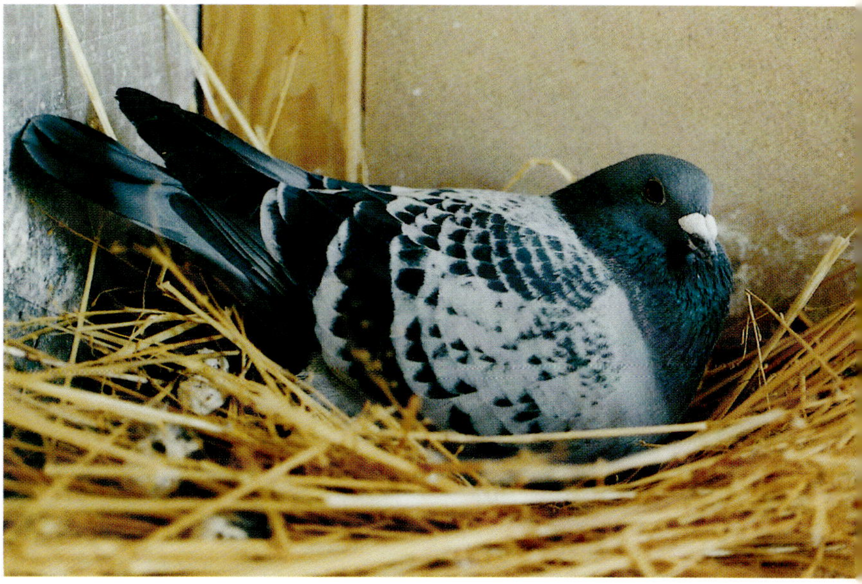

Every pigeon is looking for a special little spot that it regards as its own. This cock has built this huge nest and it will be this that he is thinking of when coming from a long tiring race.

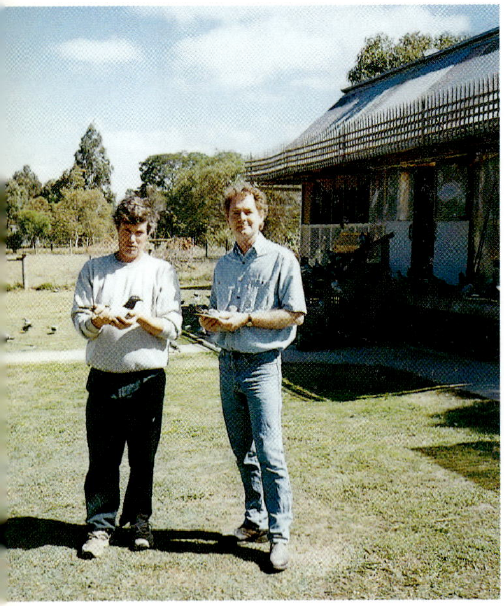

The author with his friend V.H.A. champion Grenville Evans in front of Grenville's racing loft. Grenville was V.H.A. champion in 1997 and 1998 and was third overall in 1999.

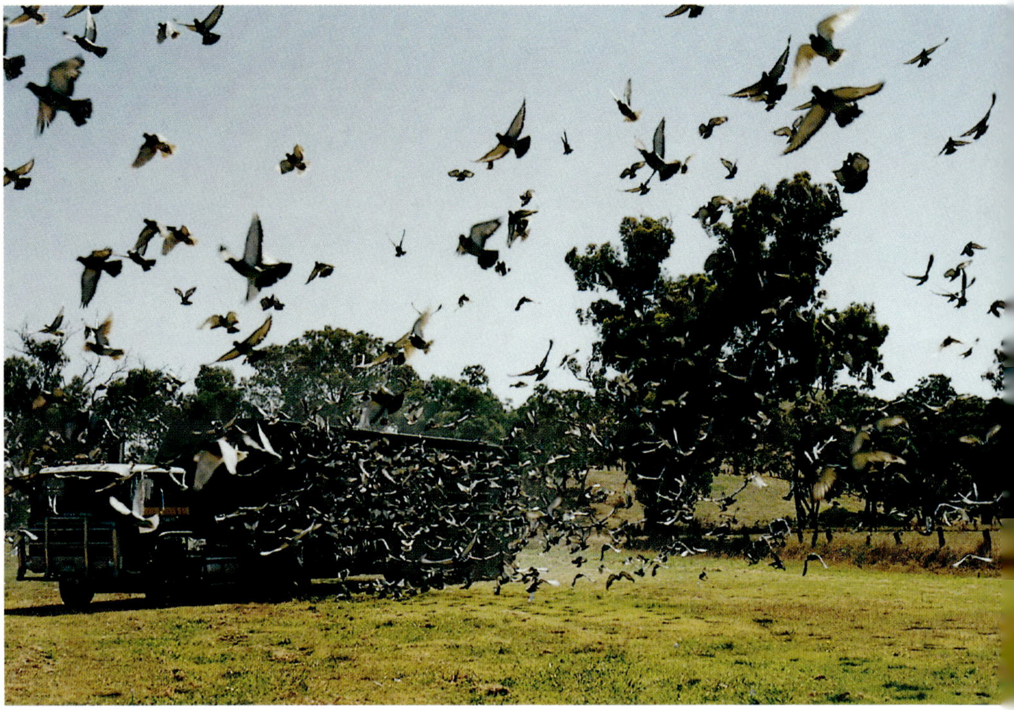

Young birds head for home in the first V.H.A. young bird race for the year from Avenel, 80 miles.

Other more elaborate systems have been developed. These include:

- **Widowhood system –** This is more widely practised on the Continent where pigeons tend to be raced for several years, and, in fact, is the most popular method used there, with many of the big race winners racing under this method. At the completion of their first year of racing, promising young cocks are mated to hens and allowed to raise a pair of youngsters. When the hen lays again, she is removed after a period of time. This can be shortly after laying or, alternatively, after the eggs have hatched, when the cock can be left to finish raising any youngsters by himself. From this time on, the cock will only see the hen upon return from a race or, sometimes, training tosses. The aim is to bond him to his nest box so that he not only breeds but rests and sometimes feeds there.

  When the cocks are away, the hens are placed in the nest boxes. The returning cocks must find their hens waiting and soon correlate quick return with seeing their hens sooner. This method can become quite involved, with details varying from fancier to fancier. Some show the hen for a short time before the cock is basketed, others put a nest bowl in the box or, alternatively, leave a nest bowl in the box all the time but simply turn it the correct way up the day the cocks are sent away. The feeding of widowhood cocks can also become involved. The essential features of this method are, however, the bonding of the cock to his nest box and the cock's anticipation of the hen waiting in that box upon his return.

- **Double widowhood –** Double widowhood is essentially the same method, but both the cocks and hens are raced to the same box, each anticipating the other's presence upon return. A strong disadvantage is that one of the pair may be lost and cocks, in particular, hate to return to an empty box. Some fanciers keep a number of high-libido hens to act as spares, just in case.

- **Roundabout system –** This is a relatively new method that is gaining popularity and allows for both sexes to be raced. The loft used is made of two sections, one containing nest boxes and the other perches. The section with nest boxes has a trap such as a sputnik on the front, while the perch section has a door for the birds to exit. A door joins the two sections. Before racing, the pairs are allowed to bond to the nest boxes by breeding there, but, with the onset of racing, the sexes are separated.

Both sexes are exercised independently, with, for example, the hens being released from the perch section for exercise and, while the hens are flying, the cocks are moved through the adjoining door to this section. The hens, following exercise, return through the trap to the nest-box section, which the cocks have just vacated. When the cocks are exercised, the process is repeated. Following exercise, including tossing and racing, the birds, therefore, always return to their nest boxes, which, in itself, is an incentive but, of course, when racing both sexes are sent so that returning pairs, in addition, find each other in their nest boxes. This greatly adds to their incentive. Sometimes, towards the end of the racing season, when the longer races are on, the pairs can be left together and must race as a sitting pair.

Length of flight feathers in distance birds

Did you know that, as a general rule, distance birds have longer primary and shorter secondary flight feathers than sprint birds? The short cup-shaped wings of sprinters can be moved quickly up and down, resulting in a fast flight. By contrast, the longer wings of distance birds take longer to move up and down but each stroke propels the pigeon a greater distance, in the same way that the step of an animal with longer legs covers more ground. This means that distance birds travel further for a given number of wing beats and, as it is each down stroke that causes most fatigue, can fly further before becoming tired. Because of the extra effort involved in flying on short wings, sprint birds can only maintain their speed for a short period of time.

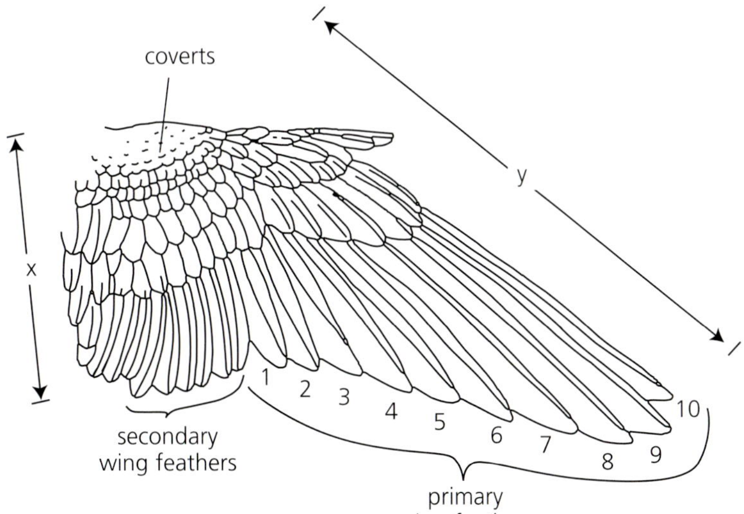

A quick and easy test to check on the extension of the outer primary feather is to, while holding the bird, simply flick the secondary feathers adjacent to the first primary feather out so that it sits on top of the wing coverts. In distance birds, the length from the wing butt to the end of this secondary is usually half or less than half the length from the wing butt to the end of the tenth flight.

Above: The length from the wrist to the tips of the longest flights (y) is a lot longer relative to the length from the wrist to the end of the secondary feathers (x) in distance birds

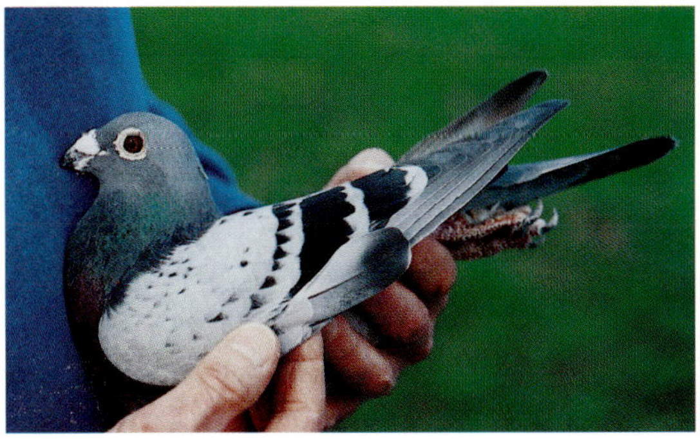

Right: Checking the relative length of the primary and secondary feathers by flicking the outermost secondary feather on top of the wing covert.

Many different but correct answers to the one question

If a new flier asks several fanciers what each does to win, it is likely that he will get several different answers. This is because, although all are being truthful, the answer they give is based on their personal experience. In Australia, there are several large and successful racing studs where birds of different genetic backgrounds are raced. These studs offer a great opportunity to study the effect that genes have on a winning race management system. Most fliers' birds are related to some extent, or are from at least the same background. The methods used by successful fliers have developed over time to suit their birds and situation. As in other lofts, the birds in a stud are all in the same environment, are under the same tossing and feeding regime and are also receiving the same medication. The main variable is that studs often house a variety of strains. In the studs, groups of birds from genetic backgrounds as diverse as, for example, the Janssen's and Goodgers (an established Australian strain that is known for its long-distance ability) are present. Janssen's are a fast strain but many birds do not form a strong natural immunity to common health problems such as wet canker, as do the Goodgers. After a race (particularly a hard one), trichomonad numbers are more likely to flare in Janssens, necessitating either a course of an anticanker drug or a longer spell before the bird is sent racing again. In Goodgers, a steady fly often tends to condition the birds and so sometimes doubling them back the very next week can give a good result.

If a new flier asks the owner of a Janssen-based loft how often an anticanker treatment should be given during racing or how often the bird should be raced, he may be told to give 1 day per week of treatment or alternatively a 2-week spell between each race. A Goodger flier may answer that giving anticanker medication is unnecessary and that sending birds 2 or even 3 weeks running brings the best out in them.

The advice that each fancier is giving is correct for his situation. For a new flier, the information received from a successful flier who races a similar type of pigeon is perhaps the most valuable. In the same way, other individual loft parameters, such as loft location, affect what needs to be done to achieve form and so fliers who are in a similar location can give more applicable advice. However, to some extent it is through health monitoring and trial and error with various management practices that a fancier learns what is best for his situation.

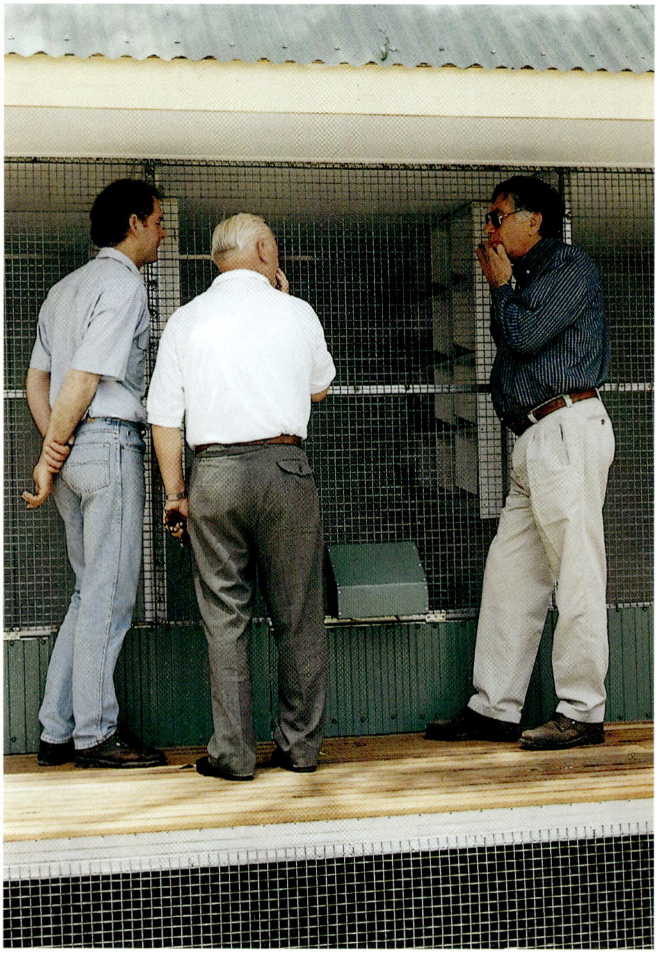

The author, Mr Silvere Toye of Belgium, and Mr George Kypreos talk pigeons in front of the Sydney Futurity loft, 1998.

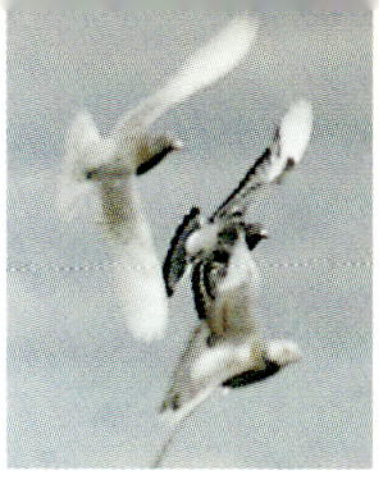

Chapter 22

CORTISONE USE IN PIGEONS

Cortisone is one of the body's natural secretions. It is produced by two small glands called the adrenal glands that sit just in front of the kidneys. Cortisone is one of the body's great regulators in that it is involved in controlling many of the body's metabolic processes. The mechanism of cortisone production in the body is fascinating. As blood flows through a gland in the brain called the pituitary gland, the gland registers the level of cortisone present and then via a hormone tells the adrenal gland to either stop producing cortisone or produce more so that the body's cortisone level is kept within a healthy range.

Cortisone is involved in a whole array of the body's processes, including maintenance of normal fluid and electrolyte levels, sugar metabolism, bone, feather and skin growth, immune and inflammatory responses, appetite and sex drive, to name only a few. Abnormal levels of the substances that control the body's processes lead to an imbalance, which confuses the body's regulatory mechanisms, leading to health problems. Cortisone is no exception.

Effect of cortisone

As most fanciers will be aware, it has become the practice of some flyers, more so in some countries than others, to give their birds cortisone. Why would they do this? The reason is that when we give cortisone and confuse the natural hormonal messages, some of the results can be useful for racing in the short term. These are:

- **Effect on moulting –** Cortisone is one of the hormones involved in controlling the moult. If cortisone levels become high, the moult will stop. This has obvious benefits for young bird racing where the birds can be raced with a full wing of nest flights.
- **Effect on inflammation –** Cortisone has an anti-inflammatory effect. If cortisone levels rise, this inhibits the body's normal inflammatory response and to some extent any soreness associated with it. This means that tiring race birds are more likely to fly on at speed.
- **Effect on frame of mind –** Cortisone is a mood-altering drug. It promotes a general feeling of well-being. Youngsters on cortisone are described as being tireless, being happy to fly for extended periods around the loft and taking well to any motivation system used.

The problem is that in inducing these changes, we also get all the other effects of cortisone overdose, which includes suppression of the immune system leading to an increased vulnerability to disease, interference with the deposition of calcium in bones leading to the formation of a weak skeleton, and interference with growth generally so that birds given cortisone, particularly early in life, cannot grow into normal strong pigeons.

Large amounts of cortisone given suddenly interfere with the normal body's metabolic processes to such an extent that the birds become severely unwell. So when giving cortisone, only small amounts must be given initially, which are then gradually increased. In this way, as the level of artificial cortisone gradually rises, the pituitary gland, trying to keep a normal level, tells the adrenal gland over a period of time to gradually produce less and less of the body's own natural cortisone. Slowly a tolerance is built up to the artificial cortisone and eventually, with continued supplementation, the cortisone level becomes higher and higher, eventually becoming higher than it would be normally. Supplementation is then continued until there is sufficient cortisone in the body for the above effects to be seen.

A veterinarian can give a gradually increasing dose of cortisone to a pigeon by injection or tablet. However, these options are not readily available to fanciers and so cortisone eye drops are used. When drops are placed in the eye, they flow down the tear duct into the back of the throat, where they are swallowed. Using the drop as the unit of measure, both the number of drops and frequency can be increased with time. For example, one drop may be placed in the eye every third day initially before increasing to one drop every second day and then two drops every second day. Once the required threshold is passed and there is sufficient cortisone in the system, this dose is maintained for as long as the fancier wants to exert the effect or the bird starts to become unwell with cortisone overdose (usually about 8 weeks).

If cortisone treatment is suddenly withdrawn, the birds also become severely unwell and can die. This condition is called Addisons disease. Because the adrenal gland has not had to produce cortisone for a period of time during supplementation, it temporarily loses the ability to produce normal levels. This means that if cortisone treatment is suddenly withdrawn, the blood level of cortisone will fall. The pituitary gland will register this and immediately tell the adrenal gland to produce a lot of cortisone. It cannot do this immediately and so the cortisone level plummets, with the bird becoming unwell. This means that, in the same way as cortisone supplementation has to be gradually built up, it must also be gradually withdrawn.

Dangers of cortisone use

And so why is cortisone such a bad thing? It could be argued that it is simply another drug that can be used to advantage in, say, the same way that anticanker drugs are used to lift performance in lofts with a wet canker problem. The reason is that the bird's whole metabolism is generally disrupted, leading to general ill health after a relatively short period of time. It is only a few of the drug's effects that are of benefit to racing. Cortisone compromises growth and predisposes the pigeon to disease. In the longer term, it has serious effects on health and the bird's quality of life. Prescribed medicines, on the other hand, such as wet canker treatments, increase the birds' health and enable them to realize their genetic potential.

Monitoring cortisone use

How is cortisone use monitored? Mature birds that are carrying baby nest flights or are behind in their body moult and are not on the darkness system always make one suspicious. Laboratory tests used in horses and dogs to monitor cortisone levels in blood have been adapted to measure cortisone levels in droppings. Tamper-proof collection bags are supplied and a Federation official collects droppings from perches and the loft floor at random in the owner's presence. Several Australian metropolitan Federations have incorporated in their rules the right to collect droppings from members if they feel it is appropriate.

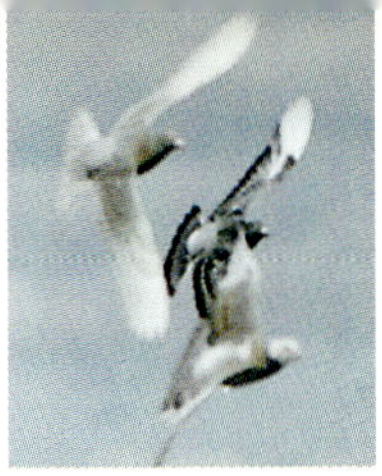

Chapter 23

VISIBLE INDICATORS OF HEALTH IN THE HEAD AND THROAT

Many of the factors that influence the health of our birds are hidden to the naked eye and it is only through veterinary examination that these things are revealed. However, there are external signs that reflect whether or not various internal systems are working well. The informed fancier must learn how to identify and interpret these signs. This chapter deals with indicators of health involving the head and throat.

Tonsils

After opening the bird's beak, an important structure to look at initially are the bird's tonsils. The tonsils are a visible part of the bird's immune system and, as such, can react to potentially harmful organisms. Pigeons have two tonsillar areas in the mouth. One is small (about the size of a match head) and is located on the floor of, and just inside the opening (epiglottis) of, the windpipe (trachea). The second is comparatively large and includes approximately two-thirds of the bird's soft palate. It is divided into two segments with a groove running down the centre. Flyers are familiar with the bird's fringe (spicules) along the base of the soft palate. The tonsils form a triangle within the soft palate with the fringe forming the lower edge of the triangle. In health, the area is just discernible from surrounding tissue, being a slightly redder colour.

When stimulated, the tonsils become inflamed. They become inflamed in response to disease and in pigeons the two usual problems are wet canker or respiratory infection. When inflamed, the tonsils become redder and swollen and so contrast more with the surrounding tissue.

As the tonsils on the palate swell out, if both sides do so uniformly, the central groove becomes deeper. If one side enlarges more than the other, the groove will deviate to one side, with the swollen segment pushing across onto the other side. This swelling may cause the fringe to disappear. If associated with respiratory infection, then, as the swelling subsides, the fringe will reappear. However, if the tonsillitis is due to canker, sections of the fringe and, indeed, the tonsil itself will be lost permanently.

With longer-term tonsil inflammation, small abscesses form, which appear as small yellow dots scattered through the tonsillar tissue. Microscopically, these consist of clumps of white blood cells, called lymphoid aggregates, and other inflammatory changes. Tonsillar abscesses are almost invariably associated with wet canker. When the disease is active, i.e. the trichomonad count is high, these abscesses are yellow and bulge out from the tonsillar tissue, and the immediately surrounding tonsillar tissue forms a red zone of inflammation. At this stage, as a consequence of the wet canker flare-up, the birds cannot perform. As the condition resolves and the tonsil is no longer inflamed, the abscesses gradually lose their colour, changing to white and then becoming a translucent plaque on the tonsil. At this stage the condition is no longer active and cannot affect race form. The spots may, however, take weeks or even months to disappear. Teams containing birds with white spots in their tonsil therefore tell us that they have had a wet canker flare-up in the past and alert us to the possibility of repeat flare-ups with the stress of racing ahead. Where individual birds are developing new yellow spots in the tonsil, the fancier should, if racing, organize an immediate crop flush or, alternatively, instigate treatment with an effective anticanker medication and seek veterinary advice.

Similar changes can be observed in the tonsil on the floor of the windpipe. However, they are indicators of respiratory disease.

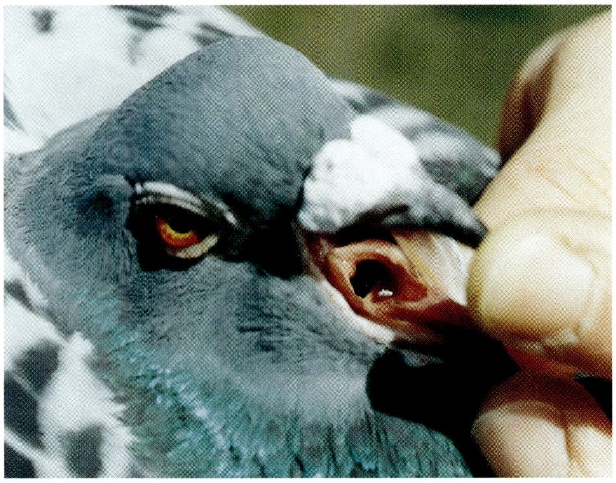

Bird with an abscess in the tonsil that sits on the floor of the windpipe. The abscess is the small raised white line at the entrance of the windpipe.

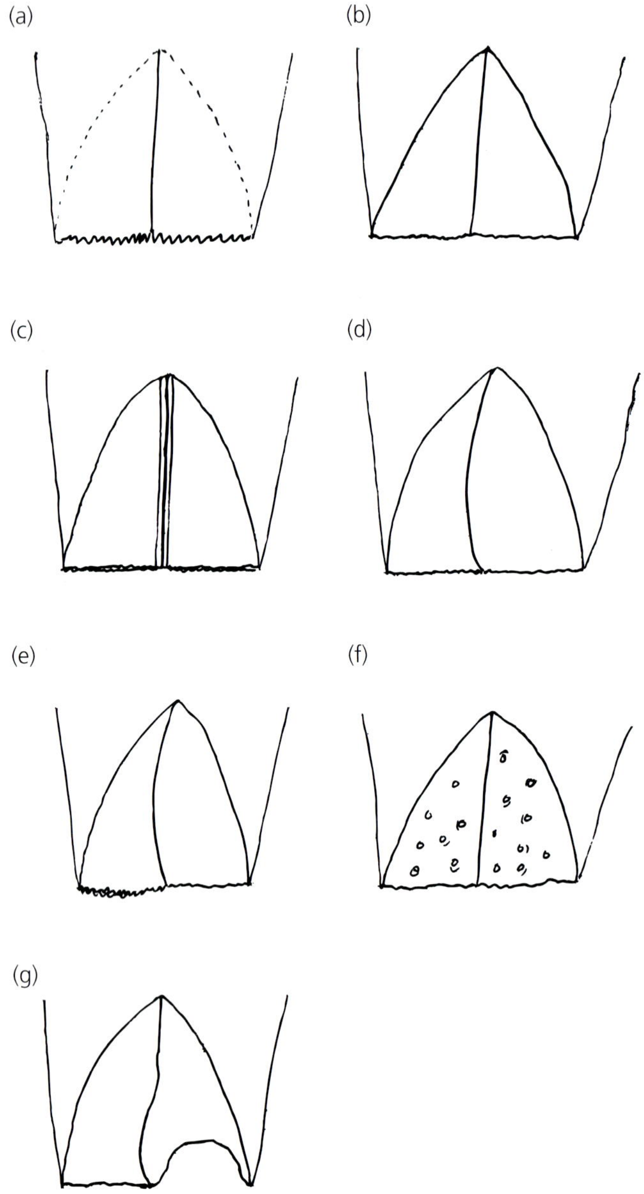

Interpreting tonsil changes.

(a) A healthy tonsil, spicules (the fringe) intact, a straight shallow central groove, tonsil edge barely discernible from surrounding tissue.

(b) Loss of spicules. This may be temporary with inflammatory conditions causing tonsil swelling, such as respiratory infection, or permanent, if associated with canker.

(c) Uniform swelling of both tonsils: central groove deeper and spicules less obvious.

(d) Tonsils with chronic degenerative changes. This bird has a history of wet canker or respiratory infection when young and may or may not be vulnerable to further problems during racing, depending on its genetic make-up, the natural immunity it has now formed, and how well it is managed. Without proper management, problems will continue and it will not race well. With correct management, it may be a champion.

(e) As the central groove is formed by the inner edges of each tonsil, when one tonsil swells and increases in size, it causes the central groove to curve. At the same time, the spicules on that tonsil become less prominent.

(f) Microabscesses dotted through both tonsils, indicating longer-term inflammation.

(g) Large section of tonsil lost, indicating earlier canker nodule formation.

Mucus

The level and appearance of mucus in the throat can also give an indication of the bird's health. In health, the throat should appear wet but with no accumulation of mucus apparent. The level of clear mucus can marginally increase in birds that are 'just not right' and is more often than not associated with stress-producing circumstances, such as problems with the loft environment or a recent flaw in the birds' management. Rather than reach for medication, correction of the underlying problem is the more appropriate course of action. When bubbly clear mucus starts accumulating at the back of the throat, particularly if the throat appears red and inflamed, this is indicative of inflammation in the area. This is almost invariably associated with wet canker. The fancier should monitor the birds for other signs associated with wet canker, as discussed in earlier chapters, and seek veterinary advice. The mucus becoming white, coloured or turbid often indicates secondary bacterial infection and is usually due to *E. coli*.

Nostril discharge. A respiratory infection?

Not all discharges from the nostrils are associated with respiratory infection. It is not unusual to find dried discharge or clear fluid at the opening of the cere in short-faced breeds, such as Turbits, Owls and Oriental Frills. The sinuses that drain under the cere release fluid from their lining, which evaporates as the birds breathe. In short-faced breeds, the sinuses are compressed and there is not the same opportunity for this fluid to evaporate away, with the result that some trickles from the nostrils. The same occurs in short-faced breeds of dogs, such as the Boxer and Pug, and in Persian cats. A similar mechanism occurs in race birds that are exercised on cold mornings. The moisture in the warm, expired air condenses on the cold surface of the beak, leaving a wet ring at the opening of the cere.

With respiratory infection, thick, white slime can accumulate in the throat. This slime, however, does not form in the throat but rather moves into the throat from neighbouring respiratory structures, namely the sinuses and trachea. Pigeons have several hollow cavities in the bones of their skulls, called sinuses. These are lined by a sensory membrane, which produces mucus in response to irritation. They open into the slit in the roof of the mouth called the choana. With inflammation of these sinuses, i.e. sinusitis, as in a human with a cold, mucus forms but then drains through the slit into the mouth. Mucus that forms in the trachea is coughed up into the throat. Sometimes these birds can be heard to cough or may have a mucus component to their 'grunt'. Such mucus will sometimes run in a thread from the top of the trachea, which may appear red and inflamed, to the roof of the mouth. Dutch veterinarians believe this mucus to be associated with *Mycoplasma* and state that it is very common, affecting 90% of lofts there.

Mycoplasma is a difficult disease to diagnose in the live bird. Only certain labs culture *Mycoplasma*, and it is an expensive procedure. Blood tests are used to diagnose the conditions in chickens. In Australia, the condition is usually diagnosed by suggestive changes found either grossly (white mucus lining the upper 20 – 30% of the trachea) or microscopically (lymphoid aggregates scattered in increased numbers throughout the respiratory system and increased level of mucus-producing glands in the upper trachea, following autopsy). A tentative diagnosis can also be based not only on the signs shown by the birds, but also by response to treatment. Some European veterinarians state that the problem is so common that a loft is assumed to be infected unless it has been treated before racing or recently during racing, and feel that, although it does not clinically affect the birds' health, it has a big affect on race form. With severe respiratory infections, mucus will accumulate at the beak margins where it becomes air dried and yellow.

When assessing the level of mucus, the birds should not be examined after feeding or exercise as some mucus found normally in the upper crop can, during this time, move into the throat. Similarly, this mucus can be massaged into the throat.

Colour

The lining (mucus membrane) of the throat should be rosy pink in health. It becomes pale with anaemia (low red-blood-cell count) and low blood pressure, which occurs with poor health. With a normal red-blood-cell count and blood pressure, the blood vessel at the back of the throat should be turgid and pulsate with the beat of the heart. With respiratory problems, the lining will become pale blue due to the blood not containing enough oxygen. The tongue in health should also be rosy pink. A purple tip can indicate respiratory problems. Some birds, however, do have a naturally pigmented tongue tip and so it is a matter of knowing your birds so as not to become confused.

Defects in the tongue outline usually indicate an earlier pigeon pox infection. Yellow plaques on the tongue or throat are either a pox vesicle or trichomonad ulcer. As a general rule, if a line is drawn through the base of the beak, a yellow plaque in front of this will be pox and behind it will be canker. Trichomonads are fragile organisms and the environment from the base of the beak forward is too hostile for them.

Windpipe shape

A bird that is breathing with ease can relax the muscles of the windpipe and its opening will appear narrow and elongated. If the bird is having trouble getting its breath, several mechanisms are available to it to provide more oxygen. It can contract the muscles of the windpipe, which dilate it and gives the opening a rounded shape. The healthy pigeon has an epiglottis (windpipe opening), that is narrow, elongated with sharp edges and with small spicules along the side. The more rounded the epiglottis, the more distressed the bird. To provide more oxygen, the bird can also breathe faster and deeper. This will cause the epiglottis to move, in the process elevating the tongue tip. In health, the tongue will lie flat on the floor of the mouth and the epiglottis will appear still but I am cautious to attach too much significance to a tongue that is elevated in profile with the beak open, placing more significance on other signs. Obesity and egg laying can cause these signs, but also space-occupying abdominal lesions and respiratory infections, particularly of the airsac. The shape of the epiglottis also varies between families and, as a general rule, cocks have a slightly more slit-like opening.

The slot in the roof of the mouth should be free of debris and slightly open. Birds that are breathing with ease should, when in the hand, have their beaks tightly closed. If it is difficult to see whether there is a slight space, the beak can be held closed while monitoring the birds for signs of distress.

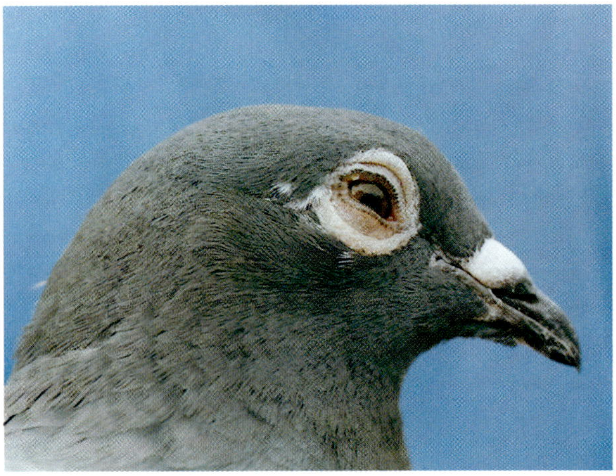

Sinuses

As mentioned earlier, within the skull of the pigeon are several small cavities called sinuses. One of these encircles the eye in the shape of a doughnut. The sinuses interconnect through narrow channels, which means they are poorly drained. With respiratory infection, fluid can accumulate in the sinuses, causing them to bulge, leading to swellings around the eye. These swellings can physically **1a** squash the tear duct (which carries tears from the eye to

Bird with a sinus infection. Birds have a doughnut-shaped sinus that runs around the eye. When inflamed, fluid forms in it, which, with gravity, accumulates at its base, causing the section of face below the eye to bulge. This bird also has a concurrent conjunctivitis (inflammation of the membrane that lines the eyelid). Over the next few days, as the inflammatory fluid drains away, the cere will start to become stained.

the inside of the choana), causing tears to overflow the eyelid margin and wet the face. When checking for bulges, the head should be looked at not only from the side but also from the front and top.

Eyelids

Pigeons have, in addition to the two eyelids that we have, a third eyelid (nictitating membrane). All eyelids are lined by a membrane called the conjunctiva. When inflamed, this becomes red and swollen. This is usually associated with respiratory infection. When infection is mild, the third eyelid can have trouble fitting behind the main eyelids because of the thickened membrane covering it. Severe infection is the classic 'one eye cold'. However, not all red watery eyes are associated with respiratory infection. Some older birds, particularly if heavily wattled, develop loose-fitting eyelids, leading to air drying of the conjunctiva and irritation. This is compounded by the bird attempting to relieve the irritation by rubbing the eye on its wing butt.

The eyelids, particularly in pieds, are a site for U.V.-induced tumours. Goblet cell cysts also occur. Goblet cells produce a mucus that enables the tears to stick to the eyeball surface, in the process preventing the eye drying out as the bird flies through wind. A mammal's eyeball with air passing over it at the speed a pigeon flies would dry out.

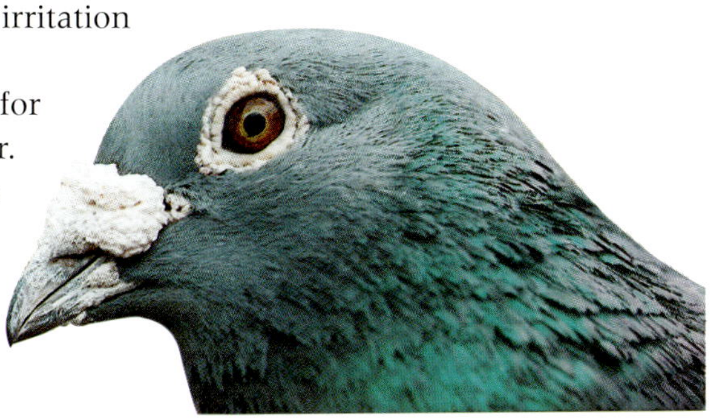

Richly coloured eye and shiny feathers of a healthy stock cock.

Ceres

Birds produce a white powder, which covers the eye and nose ceres. They fail to produce this when sick and so the ceres become dull. In addition, with respiratory infection, they become stained with discharge. Inflammatory material that forms in the sinuses drains underneath the nose cere and then through the slot in the roof of the mouth into the back of the throat. As this material flows under the nose cere, the cere acts like a sponge, absorbing this material, which stains it various shades of brown depending on the volume of material present. Not all 'less than white' ceres, however, indicate a problem. Rain can wash off the white powder covering the cere, exposing the red blood below to give the cere a pink hue. Also, young hens can lose this white powder through excessive billing.

Eye

In health, the eye should have a quick blink, a responsive pupil and a rich iris. A bird in which one eye becomes pale usually has a uveitis (inflammation of the uvea). The uvea is the iris and its support structures. It floats like a web within the fluid bag that is the eyeball. It loses colour in one of two situations:

1. **A physical knock to the eye –** This causes the uvea to flap within the eyeball, in the process damaging itself.
2. **A blood-borne generalized disease, which inflames it –** The only diseases in which this occurs with any frequency in pigeons are pigeon pox (including vaccination) and some forms of respiratory infection.

A loss of colour in both eyes usually indicates severe illness. Anaemia or the drop in blood pressure associated with severe disease means that there is less blood flowing through the eye, giving it a washed-out appearance. Also with disease, fat is resorbed from the iris, which makes it look dull.

It is surprising, perhaps, just how much information can be gained by a look at the head followed by opening the beak and looking down the throat. Many fanciers seem to do this almost routinely when first handed a bird and it is important for this not to simply become a habit where important signs are overlooked.

Eye cere problems

With age, the eye cere of some birds, particularly cocks, becomes so developed that the eyelids become heavy. This leads to the eyelid, particularly the lower one, falling away from the eyeball surface. This not only interferes with normal tear drainage from the eye but exposes the delicate membrane lining the eyelids, called the conjunctiva, to both the air and sun. Both of these cause irritation to the bird, who often attempts to relieve this irritation by either scratching at the eye or swinging its head around to rub the eye on the top of the wing butt. This self-trauma leads to further inflammation and sometimes secondary infection. With long-term exposure to the sun, the conjunctiva can also become cancerous. The birds presented to my clinic with this problem are usually quite old, because the eye cere does tend to slowly increase in size with age, and are usually cocks, because the eye cere is bigger in cocks. Heavily cered strains of racing pigeons are predisposed to this problem, as are the heavily cered breeds of fancy pigeons, such as carriers.

Treatment involves surgical resection under general anaesthetic of all excessive eye cere tissue and sometimes removal of the eyelid margin. Removal of the eyelid margin is not a practical procedure in mammals but birds have a third eyelid, called the nictitating membrane, which can protect the eyeball if one or both of the two main eyelids are removed.

Aged cock with heavy cere.

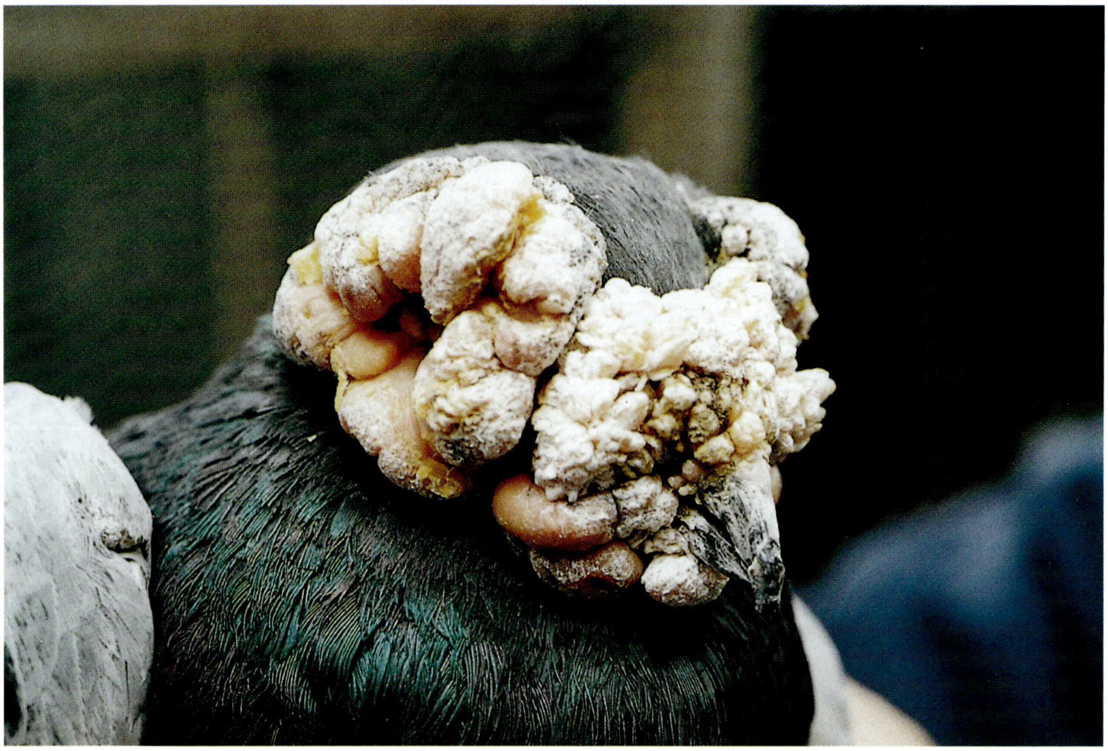

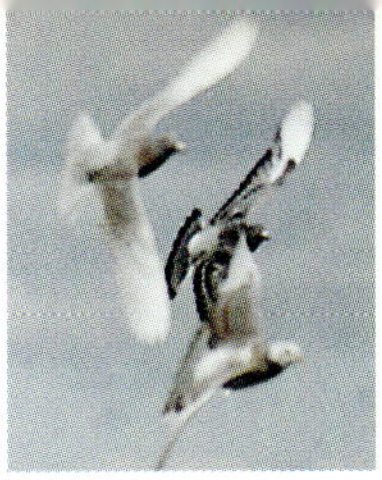

Chapter 24

MANAGEMENT OF PIGEON HEALTH BY SUCCESSFUL FLIERS DURING THE RACE SEASON

Just how do winning fliers manage the health of their birds? At times, this seems a bit abstract and so to make it a bit more real, at the start of 1998 I rang the top twelve place-getters in the V.H.A. Old Bird Aggregate in 1997 and asked them that question. The V.H.A., with 360 members, is Victoria's largest Federation and last year they were its most successful fliers. This is how they answered.

Although most said they would not mind their names being mentioned, I thought it would be more objective if their comments remained anonymous. Their summarized answers, below, are in no particular order.

1 Antibiotic combination for respiratory infection and anticanker medication mixed together to all birds Saturday and Sunday every week of the race season. Avian probiotic Wednesday and Thursday, water-soluble multivitamin once a fortnight. Microscope test weekly.

2 Antibiotic combination for respiratory infection and anticanker medication mixed together to all birds Saturday and Sunday every week of the race season. Late pigeons receive respiratory antibiotic tablet and anticanker tablet. Avian probiotic Wednesday and Thursday. Worming before racing and half-way through season (Ivomec). Microscope test every 1 – 3 weeks. Treatment for Coccidia only if detected in these tests.

3 Worming before racing (Ivomec) and again during the season only if felt to be necessary. No testing done. No routine preventive medication given.

4 Antibiotic combination for respiratory infection and anticanker medication mixed with multivitamin and given to returning race birds on Saturday. Natural herbal extract given in the water on Monday. Apple cider vinegar (acetic acid) given on Tuesday.

5 Anticanker and anticoccidia medication given Saturday and Sunday to all birds every 2 weeks. Respiratory antibiotic combination given on Monday every third week. Water-soluble multivitamin given 1 day every 2 weeks. Avian probiotic given when droppings poor. Microscopic testing as needed (on average every 2 – 3 weeks). Pink mineral available.

6 Before racing, anticoccidia drug for 2 days, sulfur antibiotic for 5 days, finishing 2 weeks before first race. Once racing starts, anticanker medication for 3 days every 2 – 3 weeks, anti-biotic combination for respiratory infection for 2 days every 2 weeks, microscopic testing on Sunday or Monday every week, and further treatment as indicated. Electrolytes/vitamins given Sunday, water-soluble vitamins on Wednesday, pink mineral available but removed the day before basketing.

7 Before racing, all birds wormed (Levamisole), given 6-day course of anticanker medication and then 6-day course of sulfur antibiotic. Once racing starts, 2 days anticanker medication given Friday and Saturday every 4 – 6 weeks. If the birds are going well, no further medication given.

8 Anticanker medication given for 2 days every 3 weeks. Two different anticanker drugs used in rotation. Antibiotic combination for respiratory infection given for 2 days every 3 weeks. Anticoccidia drug given for 2 days every 3 weeks. Sunday and Monday are treatment days. Birds are not provided with grit during race season.

9 Birds wormed before season and half-way through season (Ivomec). 2 days anticanker medication and 2 days anticoccidia medication given on alternate Saturday and Sunday. Microscope testing every 3 – 4 weeks. Pink mineral always available.

10 Anticanker medication given on Saturday and Sunday every fourth week. Two different antibiotic combinations for respiratory infections given on Saturday and Sunday every third or fourth week in rotation. Probiotics and multivitamins provided for returning race birds. Pink mineral always available.

11 Before racing, all birds wormed (piperazine). Once racing starts, anticanker medication (sometimes mixed with vitamins) given Saturday night and Sunday every week. Antibiotic for respiratory infection given on Monday and Tuesday, depending on how birds are going. Following this, dilute hydrochloric acid placed in the water for 24 hours. Clear water given on Thursday. On Friday, either vitamins or probiotics given. If droppings deteriorate, 1 – 2-day course of sulfur-based antibiotic given. Race birds are not provided with grit.

12 Before racing, all birds wormed (Levamisole). Anticanker medication given on Sunday and Monday to returning race birds (most birds race every third or fourth week). Every 4 weeks, all birds given 2 days of anticanker medication and on one of these days, antibiotic combination for respiratory infection added. Grit removed on Tuesday and replaced on Friday for Thursday night basketing. Garlic given most days either on feed or in water and yeast supplement sometimes used.

As can be seen, there are differences in the health control protocol used from one loft to another. They are all, however, successful programs in that, in all cases, the loft that used them was successful. What conclusions can we draw?

- The two diseases of most concern were far and away wet canker and respiratory infection, with 11 of the 12 fliers regularly using anticanker medication and 10 regularly using medication to control respiratory infection, with most lofts allocating Saturday and Sunday as their treatment days.
- Following this was concern about the droppings as an indication of digestive tract health, with 5 of the 12 lofts regularly using probiotics (which acidify the bowel amongst other things; see chapter The Use of Probiotics in Racing Pigeons). And a further two using apple cider vinegar (acetic acid) and hydrochloric acid to acidify the bowel, in the process making it harder for bowel infections to establish.
- Four lofts regularly treated for Coccidia, while another two only treated if Coccidia was detected under the microscope. In the other six lofts, coccidiosis was not a concern.
- Six lofts regularly wormed the birds either before or during the season. The others either felt it was not a problem or treated only if worms were detected under the microscope.
- Six lofts used multivitamin supplements regularly, with four using this in the form of a pink mineral.
- Five lofts had samples regularly tested or had their own microscope. Seven treated as a matter of routine.
- Two lofts did not provide grit or any other calcium supplement during the entire season.
- One loft used no medication apart from worming before the season.

Veterinary comments

The concern regarding the control of wet canker and respiratory infection is a valid one. These are the two main diseases that will put a good team off form. They affect good lofts and the best managers because of race unit exposure and the unavoidable stress associated with racing. When I have birds in my clinic for testing, if they have not been treated for wet canker for more than 3 weeks during the season, at least some birds in 80% of teams will have this problem. All but one of the fliers interviewed did, however, rely on only a single anticanker product to control this disease, which can be a bit risky. Using the one product year after year opens the door for resistance to develop and I usually recommend using one drug as the main controlling agent but every fourth or fifth treatment using an alternative. Similarly, only one loft used more than one antibiotic mixture to manage respiratory infection.

The use of probiotics (to acidify the bowel) and other acidifying agents is pleasing as it shows an understanding of the need to maintain a normal bowel bacterial population and an understanding of how this can be disrupted by stress.

It was a bit disappointing to note that diagnostic microscopes were not used more. However, I gained the impression that these winning lofts had used their health management protocols for some time and as they were winning they felt little need to change them. However, without testing it is impossible to know whether the frequency of drug use is really necessary or whether a new problem has entered the loft. For some fliers, the time involved in testing did seem a relevant factor.

I was surprised that two lofts did not supply grit as I feel that this should be available to the race team. If there is concern about any salt it may contain, leading to a thirst in the race units, it would be best to remove it on Tuesday afternoon and replace it on Friday (the day after basketing).

The mixing of two drugs together seemed common practice. This can make the birds less likely to drink and there is some evidence that this may slightly decrease medication effectiveness, but there are only so many days in the week and sometimes it is necessary to combine drugs for the birds to get the necessary medication.

Some of the ways in which drugs are used are a bit questionable and it is likely that some birds do well despite a particular practice of the flier. Some older drugs were still being used, e.g. Tricon, a chlortetracycline, which is more likely to have side-effects and is less effective than the more recent doxycycline, and piperazine (a wormer that kills only roundworm) whereas more effective wormers that kill hairworm, roundworm and mites are available. To me, some drug use seemed inappropriate, e.g. a lengthy course of a sulfur antibiotic before racing.

Overall, however, I felt that these winning fanciers had a good understanding of the diseases likely to affect their birds' health during racing and the way to control them.

It is pleasing that the 12 fliers involved were so generous with their information.

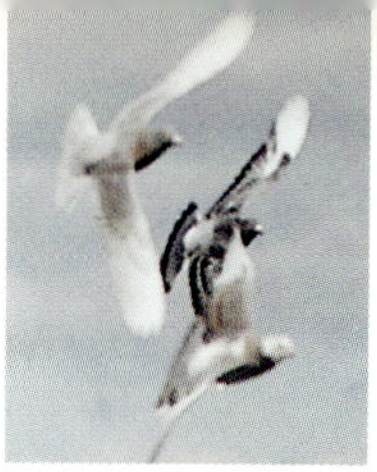

Chapter 25

EXERCISE, DIET AND ELECTROLYTES – Their effect on race form

A common request at my clinic from fanciers is for me to comment on their birds' condition and suggest modifications to a tossing or feeding regime based on this. As fanciers would be aware, many factors affect whether or not a team is in form. One thing is for certain, and that is that birds that are unhealthy cannot be in form. As a veterinarian, I see the assessment of the birds' health as my primary role. Getting the birds healthy sets the stage for fanciers to then realize the genetic potential of their birds. If every year was the same, then once a fancier had achieved success it would simply be a matter of reapplying the same tossing and feeding regime and, depending to some extent on the individual ability of the birds in the team that particular year, results hopefully could be duplicated. But of course, each year is different. Racing may be harder or the weather may be colder, etc., and so it is a matter of modifying a basic system so that form, and with it success, can again be found. It is the skill of the successful fancier in modifying a basic system, using as his guidelines the birds' behaviour in the loft, their willingness to fly, how they handle, and a realistic assessment of their race results, that enables him to decide what his birds need regarding tossing and feeding to again bring them into form. It is important that the fancier has a basic knowledge of just how these things affect his birds so that an informed decision can be made. One must be careful not to fall into the trap of simply repeating what has been done in earlier years as this often leads to failure, given the number of variables involved. For example, what does one do if the birds are heavy in the hand or become light and are reluctant to fly? The following information will help fanciers make an informed decision as to what to do with their birds if they are out of form. The answer as to what to do if the birds are heavy or light is at the end of the chapter, but I hope that you will already know the answer before then.

Energy requirements of exercise

During exercise, the processes of muscle contraction require the provision of large amounts of energy. Various sources of this energy are available within the body. All are broken down into a substance called ATP, which in turn is broken down to ADP, and it is this process that releases that energy. The contribution of these sources and their ultimate efficiency (i.e. how much ATP is produced) will depend on the speed and duration of exercise. Energy can be released either in the presence or absence of oxygen.

Aerobic (with oxygen) processes

ATP can be produced from the oxidation of two substances:

1 **Glucose** – Glucose, stored in the muscles and liver of the body as glycogen, is metabolized to pyruvate in the presence of oxygen via the Krebs cycle, and then to ATP. One mole of glucose metabolized in this way produces 36 molecules of ATP.

2 **Fat –** Fat is broken down to free fatty acids and in the process produces carbon dioxide, water, heat and energy. The free fatty acids are transported via the blood stream and diffuse into the muscle. This takes approximately 20 minutes. This is of little importance in horses and greyhounds but is important in pigeons because of the longer duration of races. One mole of fatty acids produces 129 molecules of ATP. Thus, oxidation of fatty acids provides more efficient energy production than does glucose oxidation.

Anaerobic (without oxygen) processes

Aerobic processes provide the main mechanism for energy production initially. However, once the pigeon is working hard, insufficient oxygen is delivered to muscles for all energy needs to be met, and therefore anaerobic processes play a major part in the supply of energy. The energy in ATP can be released anaerobically. There are two sources of this ATP:

1 **ATP already present in the circulation and from other processes, including breakdown of creatine phosphate to ATP –** This lasts less than 10 seconds, and then

2 **Glycogen, which is broken down to pyruvate in the absence of oxygen –** This process is less efficient, producing only three molecules of ATP from each mole of glucose. Also, in the absence of oxygen, the pyruvate accumulates and is then metabolized to lactic acid. This lactic acid accumulates in the muscle (see Blue Muscle Syndrome), decreasing the pH of the muscle, and then diffuses out into the blood stream to be metabolized in the liver. How quickly blood lactate levels rise is an indication of fitness.

When exercising comfortably, energy requirements are met aerobically through breakdown of glucose and breakdown of fat. If exercise becomes harder, oxygen uptake increases through various mechanisms such as panting, and reaches a peak. If exercise continues, there is an oxygen requirement that cannot be met. This is called the 'oxygen deficit' and energy then has to be provided from anaerobic energy sources, principally ATP and creatine phosphate and then after 6 – 8 seconds glycogen breakdown in muscle to lactic acid.

When a pigeon lifts into the sky, it is initially relying on its stores of ATP and energy produced from sources such as creatine phosphate. After this initial burst of muscle activity, energy comes from glucose in the blood stream. After 20 minutes, provided it is exercising within its fitness capability, so that it is able to adequately supply oxygen, it starts to break down and use glycogen. This is broken down and continues to supply sugars. The glycogen lasts for 300 – 400 km, half a day at the most. When the glycogen runs out, provided the pigeon is flying easily, it starts to use its body fat as a source of energy. This is why pigeons in races up to 400 km, particularly easy ones, can be sent in quite light condition and succeed. In longer races in which they need to draw on the body's reserve of fat they must be sent in heavier condition otherwise they simply 'run out of petrol'. This is why the best preparation, and the way the birds handle when sent, is different for sprint and long-distance racing. If during the race short periods of intense activity are required, or through sheer fatigue, the pigeon becomes short of breath so that the oxygen threshold is passed, glycogen will be broken down in the absence of oxygen, leading to lactic acid production, which in turn can cause myositis (muscle inflammation) and cramping.

Training

Through regular tossing and training, the bird's respiratory system develops, so that the oxygen threshold becomes higher. Similarly, the muscles become fitter, so that any lactic acid produced can be more efficiently removed by the circulation, with the result that the pigeon can exercise for longer periods without developing cramp or muscle inflammation through lactic acid accumulation. Endurance training results in decreased muscle glycogen utilization and increased reliance on fats

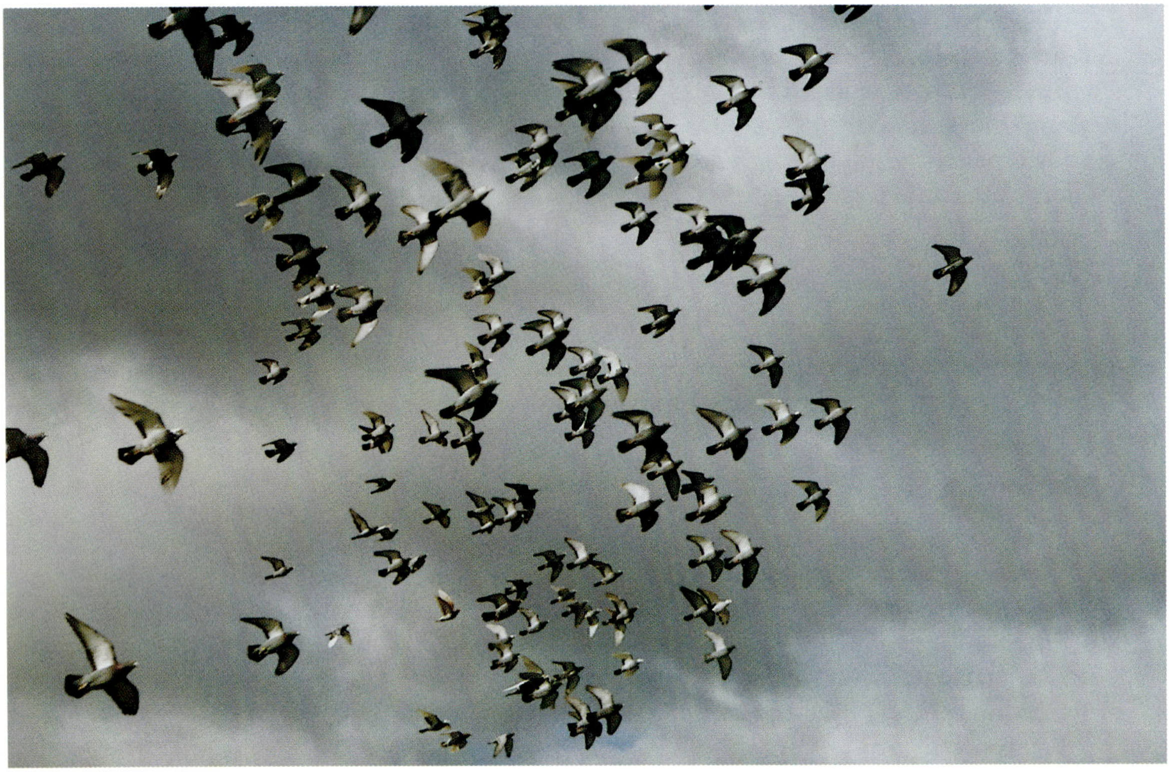

A team of race birds show their control and agility in a strong wind on a stormy day.

as energy sources. This is shown by increased levels of enzymes involved in fat metabolism. It therefore becomes obvious that to be competitive in the longer races, birds need periods of sustained exercise. Young birds will usually fly well around the loft because of their youth, vigour and perhaps the novelty of flying. However, postpubertal birds, particularly once they have flown a few races, often will not fly for extended periods. Therefore, they need to be made to exercise. This can be done either through tossing or forced flying (flagging) around the loft. Both have their disadvantages. Flagging has the potential to decrease the birds' bond to the loft, through scaring the birds away from the thing to which you want them to race, and can also lead to bad traps. Tossing can lead to loss of and injury to birds. Obviously, birds that are sick or fatigued should be rested and then, when well, gradually brought back into work.

It is important to match the level of tossing given a team with the current fitness of that team. Ideally at the start of the season, there should be a gradual increase in the amount of time spent in the air around the loft and on tosses, and later in the season, once the birds are fit, tosses should be of sufficient length to benefit the birds. At the same time, diets should contain appropriate levels of carbohydrates and fats to accommodate the work done.

Care should be taken not to confuse birds with muscle inflammation (myositis) with fit birds. The pectoral muscles of birds that exercise well beyond their fitness level will, because of the inflammation, swell and feel firm several days later. Because these birds will have used up their body fat, they will also be buoyant and they can be mistaken for birds that are superfit. However, these birds will be reluctant to fly and will resent handling because of the pain within the muscles. Sometimes, also, the muscles will take on a bluish tinge and the keel will take on a generalized pinkish colour. These birds should be rested while the muscles heal before gradually being brought back into work.

Electrolytes

As the various energy sources within the body are utilized, the body's reserves of water and electrolytes (or salts), in particular sodium and potassium, are also used. After moderate, aerobic exercise, when the bird's breathing can continue to supply adequate oxygen, if the pigeon can drink, it will quickly recover as long as its sodium levels have not been reduced. In more strenuous, anaerobic exercise, when the bird's breathing cannot supply sufficient oxygen and lactic acid is produced, this sodium bonds to the lactic acid before passing from the muscle cell and is eventually lost to the system in the urine component of the dropping. In addition to sodium and potassium, to a lesser extent calcium and magnesium are also lost. As the total body potassium level falls, this leads to muscle weakness and fatigue. After a long race, the pigeon is therefore deficient in these electrolytes, and if the pigeon drinks water alone, this further dilutes what electrolytes remain, leading to 'water intoxication' and a more prolonged recovery. If electrolytes are added to the water, obviously normal levels are more quickly re-established and recovery is more rapid. This has particular application to the Continental style of racing, where widowhood is common. Here, all cocks in a given section are often sent to the race. Many races are about 500 km and, being experienced birds, this means that the time from first to last arrival is often less than half an hour. Some fanciers aim to send these birds each week. In such a situation, the electrolyte requirements of all birds are similar and it is an advantage to hasten recovery so that the birds can be that bit more competitive the following weekend. In Australia, returning race birds enter loft sections and share drinkers with birds that have not raced and the time during which race birds return may be extended over several hours. Also, the need to get individual birds quickly back into condition is not as pressing. All the same, it is obviously good to offer the birds as quick recovery as possible. If birds that have not raced or other birds that do not need electrolytes drink them, it does them no harm. Their system simply retains what they need and harmlessly excretes the rest, and so there are situations where electrolytes are of definite benefit. If a flier wants to use an electrolyte mixture, even if only after long or hot flights, there are several good ones on the market now specifically made for birds.

Grits and pick stones also contain mineral salts and if electrolytes are not provided, the birds will eat these, and their electrolyte levels will gradually return to normal. Birds that become tired and come late from races, probably pick at natural sources, such as clay, during the journey.

Food

On return to the loft, in addition to replacing its electrolytes and fluids, the bird also needs to replace its lost energy reserves. After the race, blood sugar levels are low. It is the aim of the fancier to get the pigeon's blood sugar levels within normal range as quickly as possible so that the bird's energy reserves are not further depleted, and then to start to replace the energy reserves used up before the next race. For this reason, initial seed mixtures should be fed that contain seeds with readily digestible forms of carbohydrate, such as starches and sugars, e.g. maize, milo, wheat and safflower. It may also be a good idea to use seeds of a small diameter as these offer the birds' digestive enzymes a relatively larger surface area so that digestion can occur more quickly and the seeds' nutrients can become available to the birds more quickly.

Once the birds are rested and fed, after 24 hours a mixture higher in protein-based grains, e.g. peas and beans, should be offered each day through the week, so that the birds' energy stores can be replaced. The actual levels will vary somewhat on a daily basis, depending on what work the birds are taking and the temperature. For example, if the birds have flown a lot on a cold day, when called in their blood sugar levels will be low. It is important to re-establish this and so the seed mix that day should contain higher levels of carbohydrate-based grains. Conversely, if the day is warm and the birds have not flown much, when called in their blood sugar levels will probably be normal. If fed such a high carbohydrate mix, this extra energy will be converted to fat and the birds may become overweight. It is here that the skill of the individual fancier comes into play, where, by observation and handling of the birds, a basic system can be modified to suit the current situation. This should continue until the day of basketing for the next race, when again a mixture with high levels of readily digestible carbohydrates should be fed. It can also be a good idea to put half-strength electrolytes in the water on the day of basketing.

It can be seen, therefore, that if the birds are heavy in the hand it is probably because their mixture is too high in carbohydrate relative to the work they are doing and they have become fat. One would therefore decrease the amount of carbohydrate and fat-based grains in the diet and increase the amount of work they are taking. This would make them use fat as an energy source and they would lose weight and become more buoyant. If, conversely, they were light, one would increase the amount of carbohydrate and fats in the diet and decrease their work. The excess energy content of the diet would replace lost energy reserves, such as glycogen and fats. As this occurred, the birds would feel better, regain some of their vigour and become keener to fly. Once this had occurred, they could gradually be brought back into work and hopefully regain form, As to what to use as a basic diet, there are most definitely no strict rules, but as an example the following is a good basic mixture: 35% peas, 18% safflower, 18% corn, 15% milo, 5% wheat, 5% rice and 4% mixed small seeds.

Blue Muscle Syndrome

If a pigeon racer is assessing his birds for race readiness, one of the things that he will almost invariably do is roll the birds over and, amongst other things, assess their muscle colour. Here the desired colour is a rosy pink. However, many times the muscles are found to have a bluish discolouration. Much has been said and written about this condition and I am sure that there is still much to learn as to its cause but it seems to be associated with one of three situations:

1. **When birds have difficulty oxygenating their blood or breathing –** Blood with a low oxygen content develops a bluish colour. As this blood perfuses the muscle, it in turn gives the muscles themselves a bluish hue. Possible causes include respiratory infection, in which the blood is not given the opportunity to oxygenate, or anything that interferes with breathing, such as an abdominal space-occupying mass that interferes with distension of the airsacs or obesity. The muscle remains bluish for only a short time until the birds catch their breath.

2. **Healthy birds that are exercised beyond their fitness capability –** These birds develop myositis (muscle inflammation) or 'cramping'. In a fit working muscle, energy reserves are broken down during exercise. By-products of this metabolism are carried away by the muscle circulation. As a muscle becomes fit, it develops both the ability to store energy and a circulation to cope with the removal of the various by-products of exertion. If a muscle is exercised beyond its fitness level, the circulation cannot cope with the amount of by-products (mostly lactic acid) formed. As a result, these accumulate in the muscle and damage it. In minor cases, this causes the muscle to become a bluish colour, a bit similar to a bruise, and in more severe cases the muscles will also swell and become painful. In this situation, the discolouration is persistent until the muscles have healed (usually 4 – 5 days).

3. **Poor health or mismanagement practices, which inhibit the development of fitness –** From a disease point of view, wet canker and respiratory infection, in particular, prevent birds from coping with even moderate exercise. From a management point of view, it is important to match dietary components such as fats and proteins with the energy requirements of the birds and the amount of time that they are spending on the wing. Overcrowding or excessively humid lofts can also be an underlying cause.

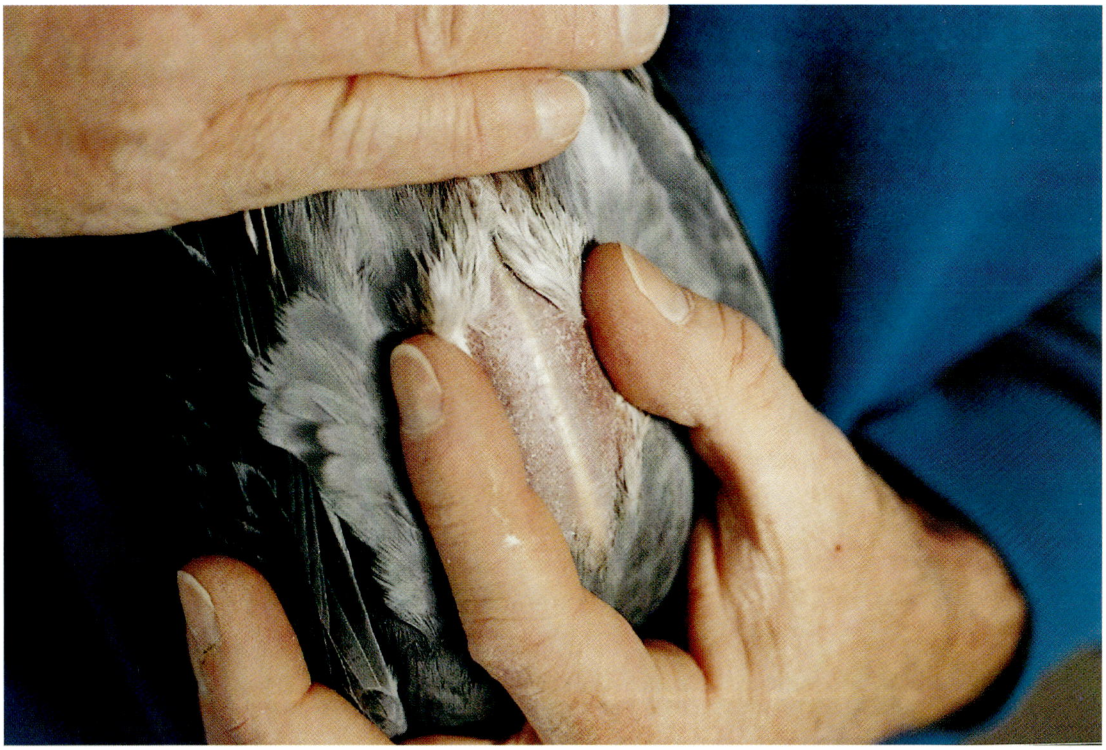

The desirable rosy pink muscle colour and white keel of the healthy bird that is not being overworked.

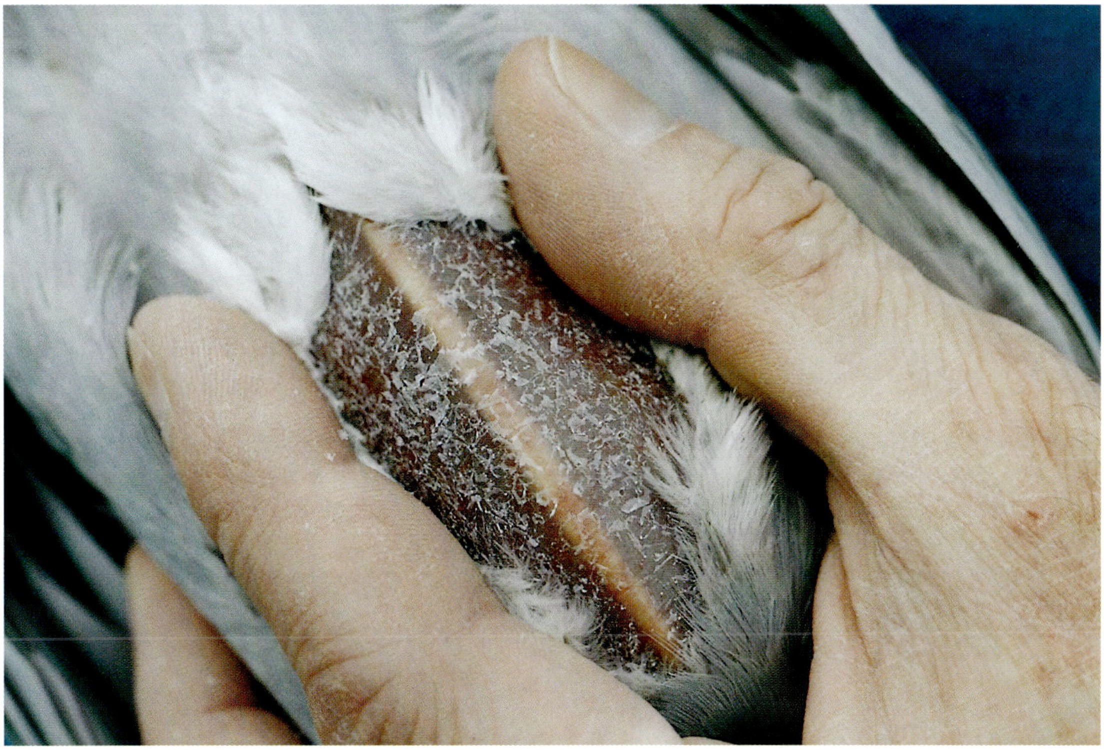

A bird with myositis (muscle inflammation) that has been exercised beyond its fitness capability. Note the deep purple discolouration of the muscles and the red blush across the keel.

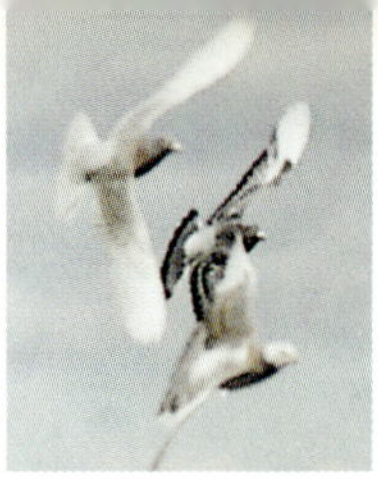

Chapter 26

JUST HAD A BAD SEASON? POSSIBLE ANSWERS

The completion of the race program is a time of reflection for most fliers. Many will have achieved success, but for some the season will have been disappointing. It is hoped that the following notes may help explain poor results and aid in avoiding a recurrence next year.

Poor bird quality

The first thing to look at is bird quality. Even with poor management, if the birds are good, occasionally an individual bird will get itself right and achieve a good result almost by accident or despite its owner. If the birds are good, I feel that probably just an open loft with hoppers would achieve some good results. Tossing and all the other things we do just maximize any potential that the birds may have. As the well-known Australian fancier John Brislin says: "Good birds make good fanciers". Think to yourself this year as you slide the ring over a baby's foot – were the results from this pair disappointing last year. If so and nothing else has changed, prepare to be disappointed again. One thing that is very common at my clinic, when we are investigating possible causes of a disappointing race season, is that fliers are reluctant to question the quality of their own birds. Most fliers think that they have good birds. Interestingly, it is often the better fliers, who presumably do have the best birds, that are the most critical of their birds.

As part of the overall assessment of the birds, it is important to make a realistic assessment of the team's results. Beware of placing too much emphasis on wind-biased races or races where loft location is a significant factor. Look at the races that are long enough or hard enough to give birds a chance to show how good and fit they are. Fanciers who quote that they had five birds, for example, that could have been placed in the first 20 in the competition in fact cast doubt on the quality of their competitors. As an example, for the first time the V.H.A. in Melbourne this year transported a second smaller Federation's birds. In races over 400 miles, the birds were released together and the loft locations of both Federations overlap. In some of these races, some of the better V.H.A. fliers had ten of their own birds in time to win the other Federation. If these lofts were in the other Federation, they could be achieving significantly below their best and yet still be deemed as flying well. Fliers should not be frightened to test their birds against the best opposition available and in the more telling races. Where possible, a realistic interpretation of results must be made. This helps in selecting the current race birds to retire to the stock loft, in the process leading to a stronger stock loft and better youngsters being bred each year.

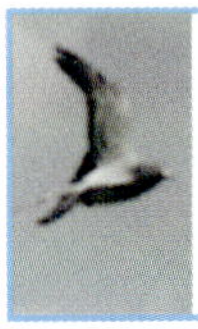

Aim to improve your birds by 1% per year. That doesn't sound like much but after 10 years that's 10% and that is significant.

When selecting a bird for stock, try not to be distracted by the bird's appearance. The ones with the pretty eyes, big white eye ticks, etc., always look nice but a winner after clocking always looks nicer. The ones to go for are the birds that are consistently early to the loft, and I personally have found that the ones that are early on the harder days, when the hours on the wing are up and velocities are down, have a higher strike rate in the stock loft.

Lack of motivation

Fanciers should think that perhaps managing the birds differently may improve results. Pigeons want a secure little spot that is theirs in their loft, where they know they will find food and water and be safe. The natural desire to return to this can be maximized by a number of methods well known to fliers, including the natural method and widowhood, etc. For years in Australia, some fliers have achieved success by simply managing the whole year's racing as an extended young bird program. Hens becoming 'rank' or flirty have been viewed as a problem, and when considered necessary the two sexes are separated. And yet, the natural instincts of the pigeon when harnessed can tremendously enhance the individual bird's desire to return home with the associated lift in loft results. However, cocks not given the opportunity to have a box with a hen will continually drive and fight, eventually running themselves ragged, to the point of being unraceable. Many quality cocks that have the potential to do well at the distance are ruined this way in Australia. Hens will lay anyway, and will be deprived of the opportunity to incubate if not provided with boxes. They have therefore had a big drain on their system without any incentive enhancement. Unmated, postpubertal hens when fit are prone to fly-aways and will just disappear from the loft. In the past, much of the success of Australian fliers who keep postpubertal sexes apart is due to the fact that their competitors did the same. Australia is following the way of the Europeans with successful fliers placing more and more emphasis on motivation.

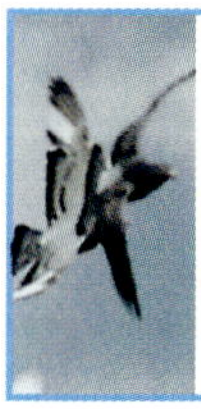

Health problems are not as obvious in older birds because, through a longer exposure, they have a higher natural immunity, which modifies their disease response.

Inadequate disease control and poor use of medication

In younger pigeons, disease is often obvious. However, older race-age birds, simply because of their age and therefore their longer exposure to disease-causing organisms, have had a chance to develop some natural immunity, thereby modifying their response to disease. With the stress of racing, this immunity is put to the test. With the continual exposure to disease in race units, in which many birds from many different lofts are in intimate contact, disease is a common cause of poor race performance. However, the effect of disease in the race bird is very subtle with often little outward sign other than disappointing race results and perhaps a reluctance to fly. All birds are exposed to worm eggs, Coccidia, ectoparasites and new strains of canker in the race units. All the race birds are under stress, so that the trichomonads, *Chlamydia* (a principal cause of respiratory infection), thrush, and bacteria such as *E. coli* that they carry have the potential to flare up. Although obviously important, it is wrong for a fancier to think that good care at home makes his birds immune.

These days, testing of the saliva (a crop flush) and droppings (a faecal smear) can be done quickly, routinely and cheaply. At my clinic, fliers drop off or mail in droppings. Results are available within hours. Saliva tests require a live bird to be presented. The fancier usually holds the bird while a sample of saliva is taken; results are viewed on a video connected to the microscope and the test is completed in minutes. Regular tests, usually every 2 weeks during racing, are recommended so that the common problems (wet canker, respiratory, *E. coli*, Coccidia, worms, thrush) can be detected and treated before they have a chance to affect the team's form. For some problems, however, a 'live bird' test is not available. If there are severe on-going problems, autopsy and pathology can be done. This applies to a common yet serious respiratory infection called mycoplasmosis. With *Mycoplasma*, there is often a history of the birds doing well in the early races and tossing well, but as soon as the races get longer and harder, race performance drops and losses increase. Definitive diagnosis of this and other less common conditions is made through microscopic examination of tissue samples. Results take up to 7 days.

Where routine testing is not possible, preventive programs are recommended; these are covered in other chapters. The indiscriminate use of medication is to be discouraged. All medication should only be used on the advice of a veterinarian. Most medications, if used inappropriately, have the potential to make the birds worse. However, to steer away from all medications across the board is simply 'sticking one's head in the sand' and the correct use of modern medication has the potential to enhance most teams' performance.

Other factors

Other factors such as loft design, training and feeding regimes, feed and water quality, time of mating and resultant age of youngster, etc., are all relevant and warrant review if the results are below expectations.

Keep a record of when all youngsters are weaned. Most pigeons in Australia only race in their first year of life, and in particular times of the year certain age groups of pigeons are more likely to do well. For example, in Victoria, the later-bred pigeons often score in the distance races, while youngsters too young or conversely too old are less likely to do well in the Victorian young bird program. Be prepared to carry over more 2-year-olds. If not over-raced as yearlings and have not become hawk-shy, they are disproportionately over-represented in some long hard races. They are more easily motivated. A motivated, experienced 2 year old can be very handy on a hard day. Perhaps consider racing them to a separate section or better still a separate loft to their eggs, etc. Fliers not practising specific motivation systems such as widowhood should consider them.

Feed and water must be provided in an hygienic way. Ingestion of excessive bacteria with these is a recognized stress on the birds. Once stresses start overlapping, the birds' natural resistance to disease and vigour break down. Water should come directly from the tap, preferably without plastic fittings, and not from a hose. Birds should always be fed from trays and never on the floor. Feed can also be contaminated by fungi before purchase or during storage. Something as simple as this can have a profound effect on racing. If in doubt, the testing of batches of grain prior to feeding is a straightforward matter.

If the birds are difficult to bring into form, consider changes to the loft design, in particular, ventilation and temperature control mechanisms. If the loft performs better in the warmer times of year, this may mean that the loft is too open and closing it in will bring success also in the colder months. At my clinic, many more Tasmanian dropping samples tested, when compared with those from the mainland, have significant levels of Coccidia and are *Chlamydia*-positive. Both of these are more likely to occur with on-going stress. Tasmania, being further south than the mainland, has a generally cooler and wetter climate. Cold is a well-recognized stress for pigeons and in particular Coccidia is more likely to be a problem in damp conditions. At my clinic, we describe this as the 'Tasmanian syndrome'. These results suggest that in Tasmania the tendency should be toward lofts that are more Continental in design.

Don't fall into the trap of simply repeating feeding and tossing regimes used in earlier years. A particular system used with success one year will not necessarily work other years. Weather and racing conditions change from one year to the next and one must modify feeding and tossing regimes to suit the current season so that form can again be found. If one year three 50-mile tosses per week brought success, the next year the racing may be harder and this degree of tossing will only flatten the birds. Harder racing and colder conditions require giving seed mixes containing higher levels of energy and carbohydrate. With easy racing, this just makes the birds fat.

When good results are coming, they can seem easy. However, when they are not, they seem impossible. When things aren't going well, everybody is an expert. Ask the same question of five fliers and you will sometimes get five different answers. If you are frustrated, seek the advice of successful local fliers, look to the fliers that achieve consistent success, particularly from the distance, or, if available, veterinarians experienced with pigeons.

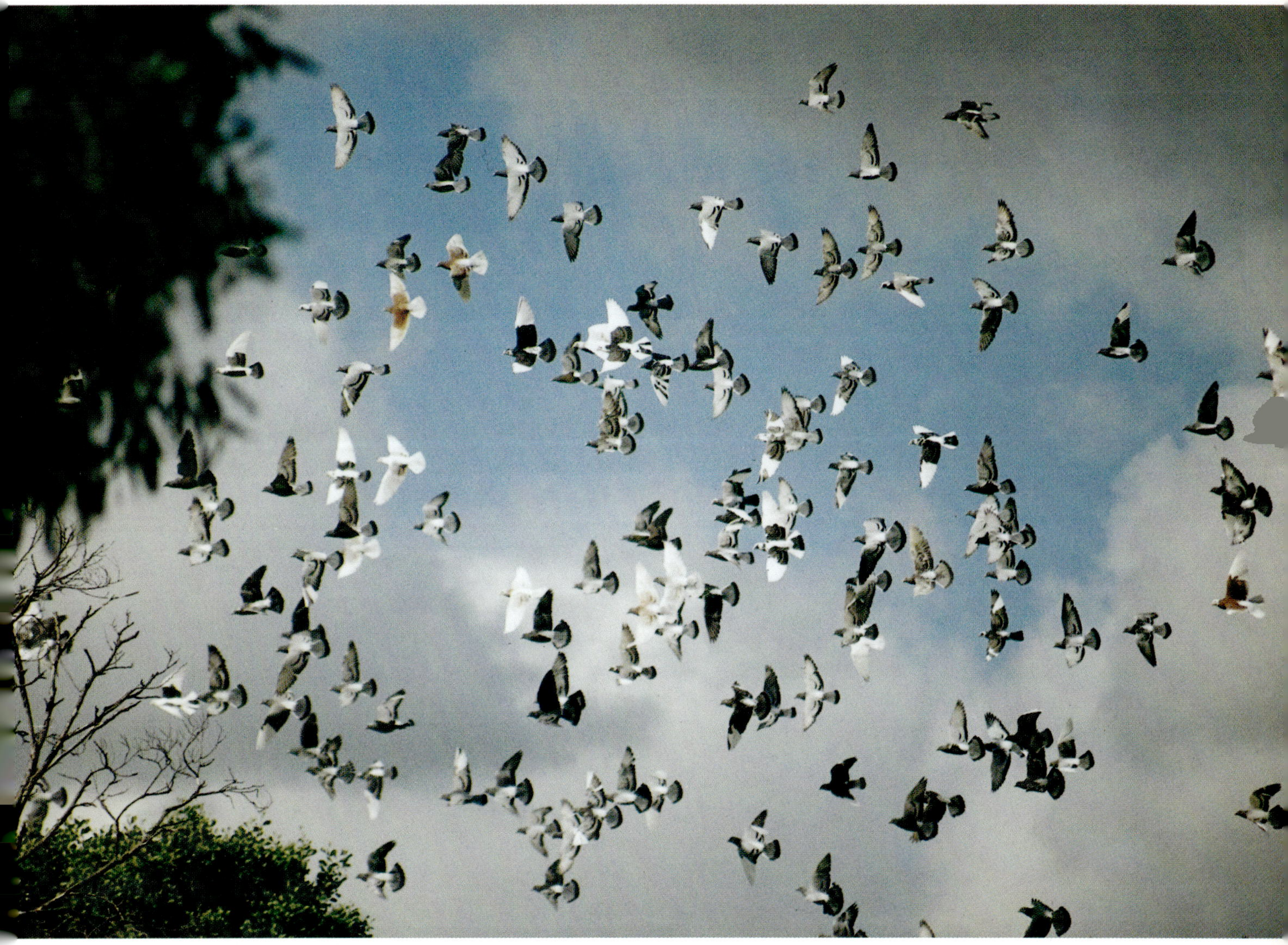

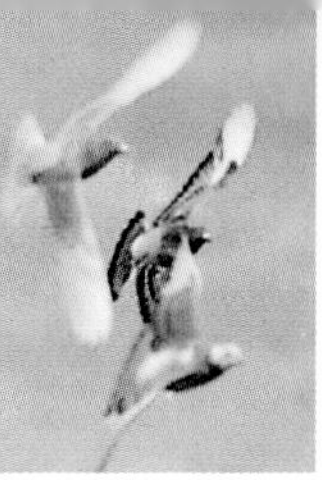

Chapter 27

PIGEON RACING IN AUSTRALIA

Young bird racing in Australia

On the Continent, when people discuss young bird racing, they discuss a variety of modifications around a basic system. In Australia, by necessity, a much wider variety of systems are used. Partially, this is because Australia is such a large country. Young birds are raced in to Hobart in the southern part of Tasmania, where the winters are cold and the summers mild, while birds of a similar age are raced 2000 miles to the north in Townsville, Queensland. In these warmer areas, it is the summer heat and humidity that need to be avoided and so stock birds are mated in July and August, with some fliers finishing breeding by Christmas. These young birds then commence racing in April and May, with the season extending through to October. In the south, it is the cold winters that must be avoided and so for many fliers breeding occurs later and two seasons are flown. Fliers pair their birds in late August – early September (or later) and breed through into March. A first series strictly for young birds commences in early March and runs for 8 weeks. There is no racing through the winter months of May, June and early July, with a second series starting in mid-July and being completed in November.

As overseas, it is difficult for fliers in Australia to be successful for an entire season and so different fliers adopt different methods aiming for success, often in different parts of the season. For example, in Victoria, rings are issued on 1 July and some (only a few) fliers have 7-day-old winter youngsters ready for ringing immediately. These birds, although considered to be early-breds, in fact moult more as if they were late-breds from the previous breeding season. When maintained on normal light, they undergo a complete body moult but often hold their flight feathers or perhaps drop one or two. They go through puberty, pair and develop all the incentives associated with this. Some of the young hens will lay as early as January and these birds can then be raced on the natural system. There is even the potential to race young bird widowhood. The disadvantage here is that these birds often start moulting again in March, not only completing their flight moult but actually completing a second flight moult. During this time, they are in full training. Fliers who practice this method often keep the work up to the birds and at the same time keep them a bit hungry, both of which tend to slow the flight moult. The combination of hard training while young, early puberty, and for some birds a double moult seems to put a big strain on these birds and few go on to race well as 2- or 3-year-olds or even in the later races in the same year.

Conversely, other fliers (the majority) breed later, weaning birds through November. These birds undergo a single moult and often do not go through puberty until the race season has already commenced, which means that some incentive aids are just not present. Also, the immaturity of some of these younger birds means that racing is simply beyond them. The distances are too great for their young age. It does, however, appear that most birds, provided they are weaned by the beginning of November, will be able to handle tossing by early February and short races of 70 – 100 miles by early March. This is not the case with all birds and some individuals seem to really struggle. Often, if withdrawn from the race team and retrained for racing in the second season, these birds can in fact do quite well when older. Some fliers attempt to fly birds much younger than this in the first season and indeed a few manage to win major prizes. However, if fanciers attempt to race birds weaned through December and even January, the percentage lost becomes progressively higher. Those young birds weaned through November and raced in the first series undergo a single moult and, provided they are not raced too hard and are fed correctly, tend to mature into very useful race birds for the second series. In fact, the experience gained in the first series is usually beneficial for them.

Very few fliers in Australia manage their young birds on the darkness system.

Old bird racing in Australia

The term 'old bird racing' in Australia is somewhat confusing because most of the birds that compete are, in fact, not old birds at all. In most races, 90% of entries are still 1 year old or younger. Most are birds that flew the early young bird races or birds that were bred later and were too young to fly in the first series. For many Australian fanciers, old bird racing is simply an extension of young bird racing, with similar techniques being used. Some fliers race their pigeons on the natural method and a small percentage race widowhood. Most fliers use the basic system of providing a clean loft, good-quality feed and a regular training routine around the loft, coupled with tosses as deemed necessary. Many Australian fliers toss a lot by European standards, with it not being unusual for birds to receive two, three or four 50-mile tosses per week towards the end of the season when the longer races are on. The birds' sex drive is regarded as a nuisance by many fliers, with the sexes being separated once most of the birds have gone through puberty. Many fanciers regard postpubertal cocks as a nuisance and cull them heavily. These methods would seem alien and bizarre to most European fanciers and yet the returns and velocities of these birds are often remarkable. Many of the birds weaned in January, February and March and sometimes even April are sent to 500-, 600- and 700-mile races in October and November and not only fly these races but win and in good time. It is not unusual for them to fly 600 miles on the day and 10% of 700-mile races are also flown on the day.

Importation of pigeons into Australia has only been legal since 1989 after an import ban for quarantine reasons was imposed in 1956. To some extent, it may be that Australian pigeons have been under different selection criteria than European birds because of the different racing system. Characteristics associated with many Australian strains are quickness to mature physically with the hens going through a late puberty, winning ability being passed along the hen line, ability to orientate a long way from home at a young age and the ability to fly all day. The availability of European pigeons in Australia has had a big impact. However, for the most part, these new Australians have been more successful in the shorter races, although European birds have now won at all distances.

A NEW ZEALAND CHAMPION:

John and Dwayne MacNeil of Auckland, New Zealand, their champion loft and ace pigeon '1090'

There are approximately 180 fliers in Auckland with about 800 in New Zealand. John and Dwayne race in the Manukau club in Auckland. Both John and Dwayne share equally in the success of this loft and although John has raced for many years, Dwayne at 25 years of age has a very modern approach to the way pigeons should be raced. Youngsters are raced to a two-section loft, which is part of their house, while the main old bird racing loft is a widowhood loft. The results of the usual team of approximately 20 widowhood cocks are excellent with sometimes the first six positions in the club being taken. In particular, they have one exceptional cock , slate cock MA 94 1090. He is arguably the best-performed race bird in all Australasia, being placed in the top 10 positions no fewer than 17 times in races containing between 700 and 1500 birds, with nine of these being outright Auckland Federation wins. As Dwayne explained, 1090 is a leader. Even though he was clocked many times, he always trapped well, flying straight into his widowhood box and waiting for Dwayne to come and get him. He appears to like being handled. Already at stock, 1090 has bred three outright Auckland Federation winners. 1090 is a Janssen. His father is bred from a son of 'James Bond' when mated to a grand-daughter of 'James Bond', while his mother is bred off a daughter of 'Stamvater'.

1090 race results

Position	Race point	Distance (km)	Number of birds
1st	Raetihi	284	1199
1st	Ashurst	395	854
1st	Raetihi	284	1051
1st	Palmerston	390	394
1st	Waiouru	295	804
1st	Raetihi	284	1313
1st	Johnsonville	484	566
1st	Palmerston	390	466
1st	Ashurst	395	908
2nd	Kuratau Junction	220	1412
2nd	Palmerston	390	531
3rd	Raetihi	284	477
5th	Levin	420	875
7th	Taupo	210	1236
7th	Johnsonville	484	768
8th	Taupo	210	1210
10th	Palmerston	390	790

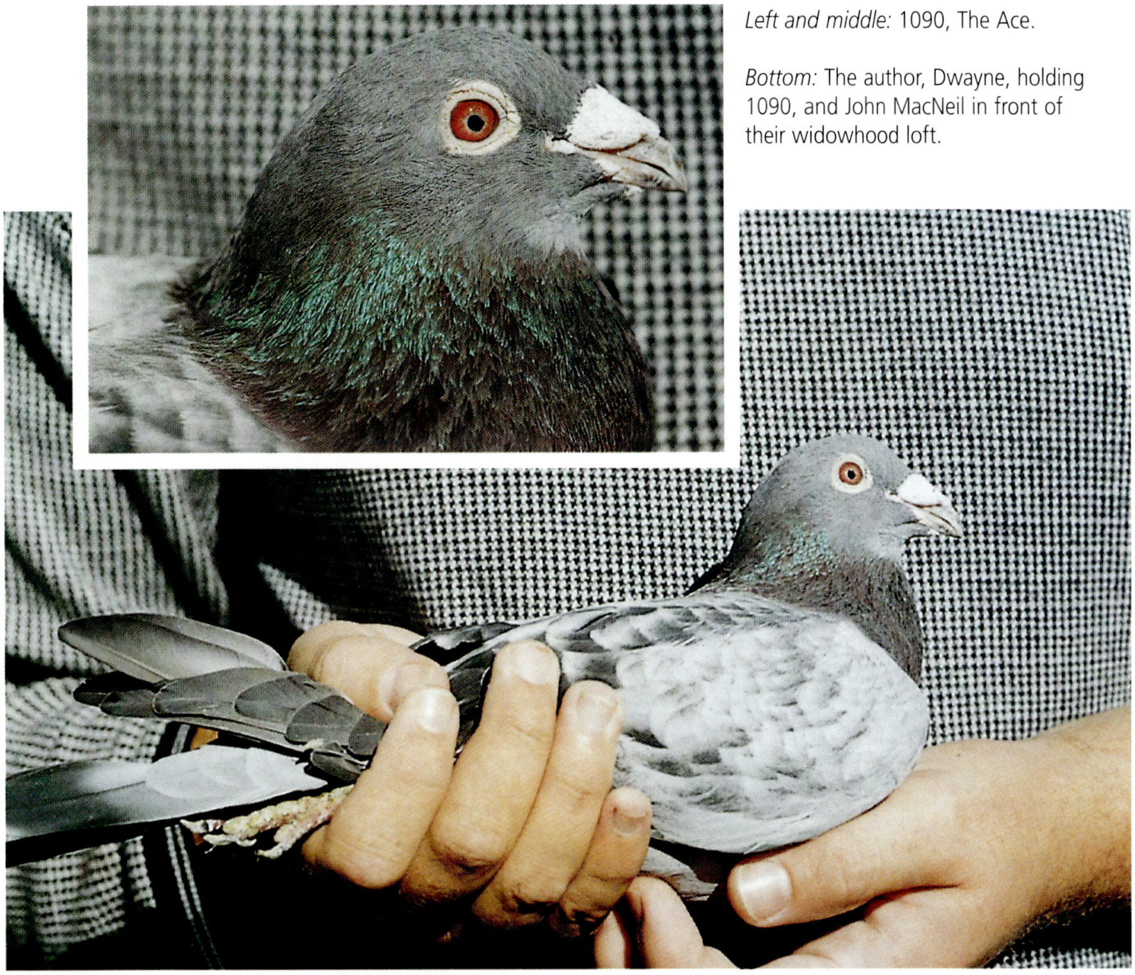

Left and middle: 1090, The Ace.

Bottom: The author, Dwayne, holding 1090, and John MacNeil in front of their widowhood loft.

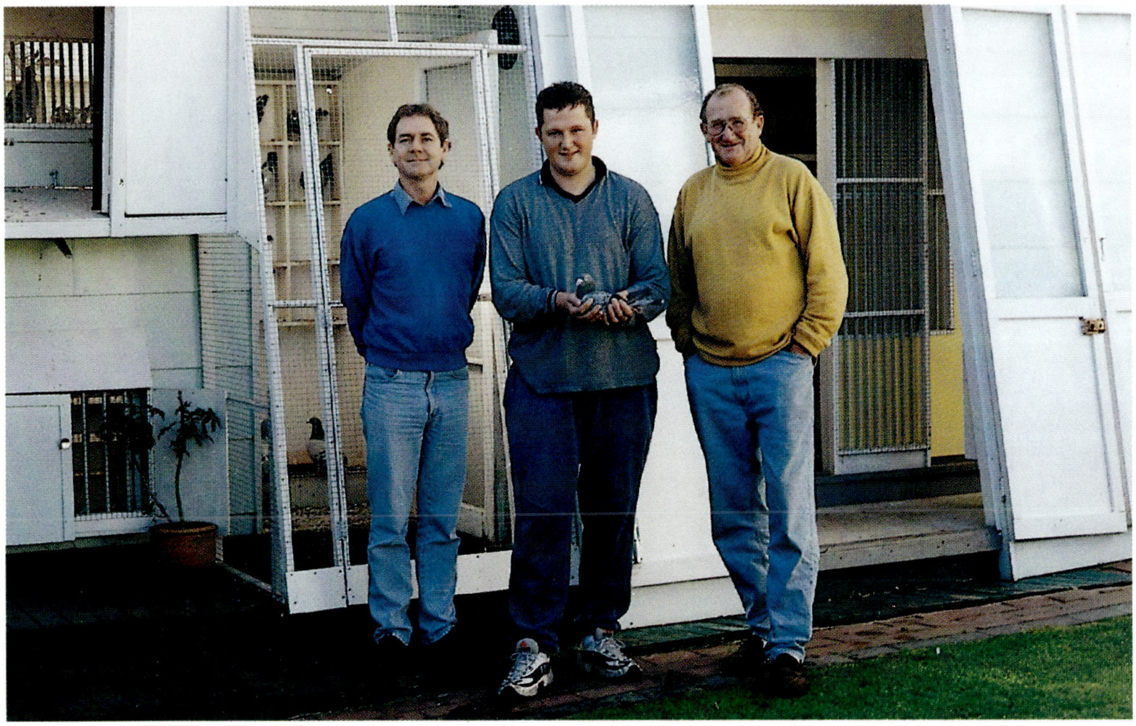

Photos 1 – 21: Basketing protocol in Australia.

These photos illustrate the technique used to send birds to a race at V.H.A. headquarters in Melbourne, Australia.

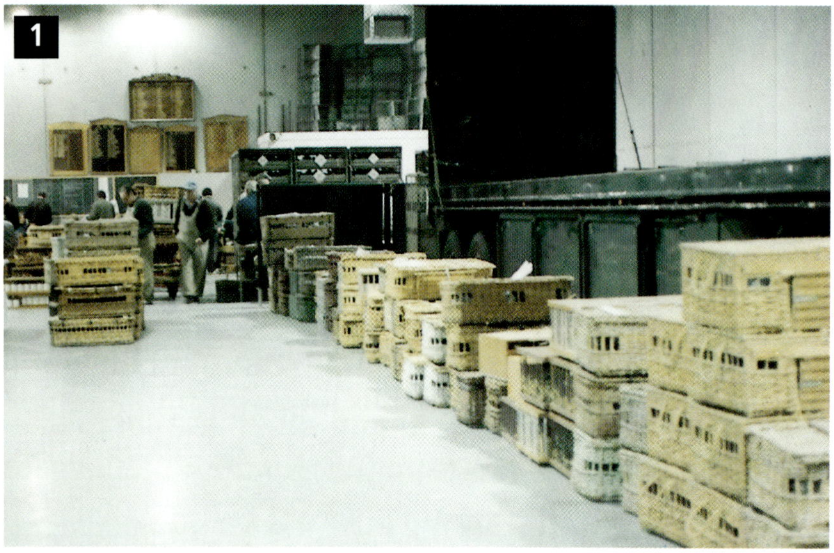

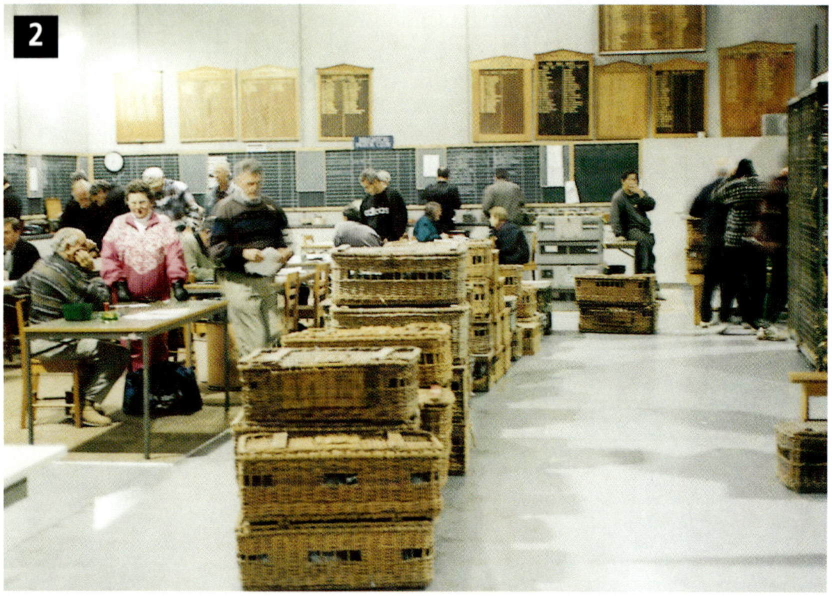

1 and 2: Thursday evening, members arrive and place their baskets containing their entries in a queue, waiting to be processed.

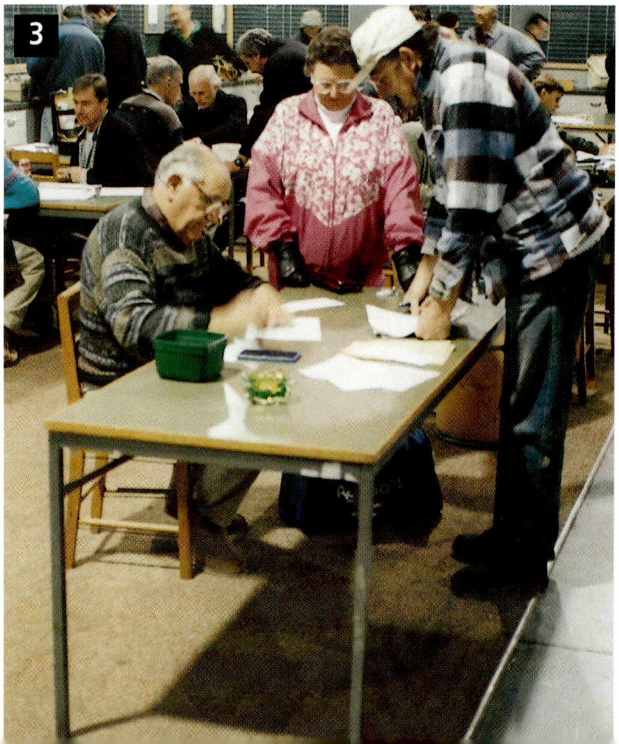

3: Members go to their club secretary, who checks their entry forms, attends to other paperwork and accepts payment.

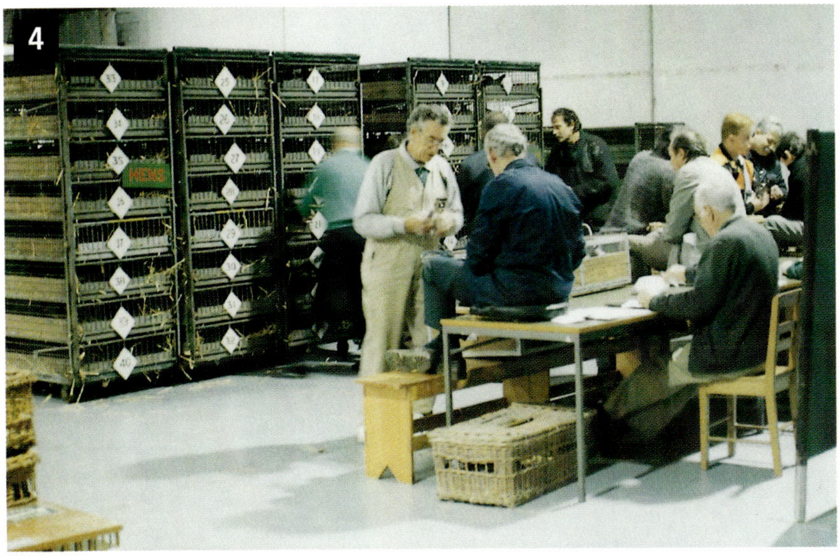

4: Fanciers work in teams of three to process the birds. The 'handler' removes the bird from the basket and reads its life ring number.

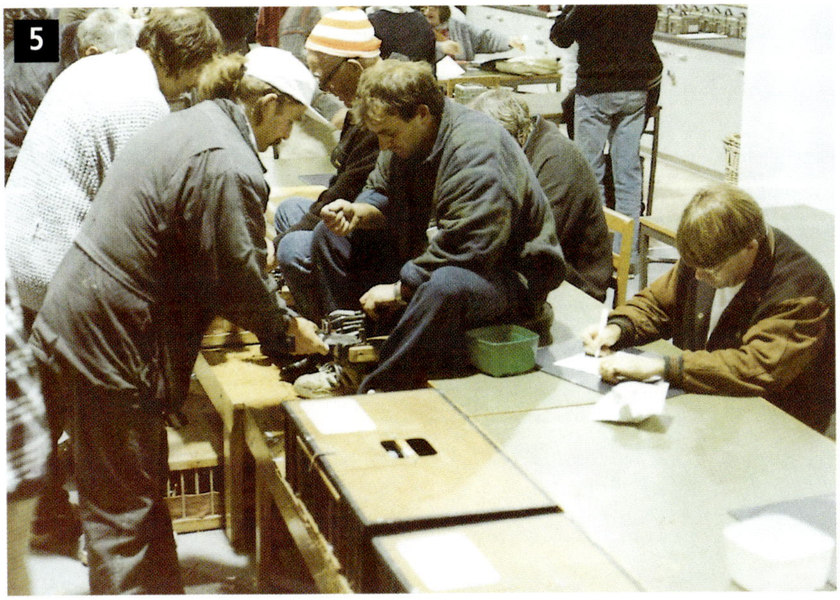

5: The handler then places the pigeon's leg in a machine operated by the 'ringer', who places a race rubber ring on the bird's leg. The 'penciller' records the number on the race rubber beside the bird's life ring number on the member's entry form.

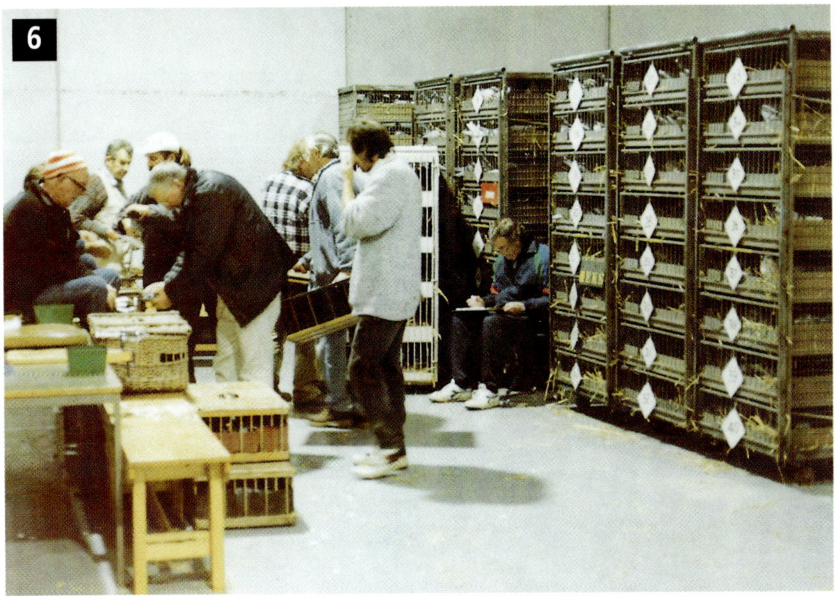

6: Once the race rubber has been placed on the bird's leg, the handler is then directed (in this case by the man in blue sitting by the race baskets) as to which race basket the bird should be placed in. An even number of birds are placed in each basket and cocks and hens are separated.

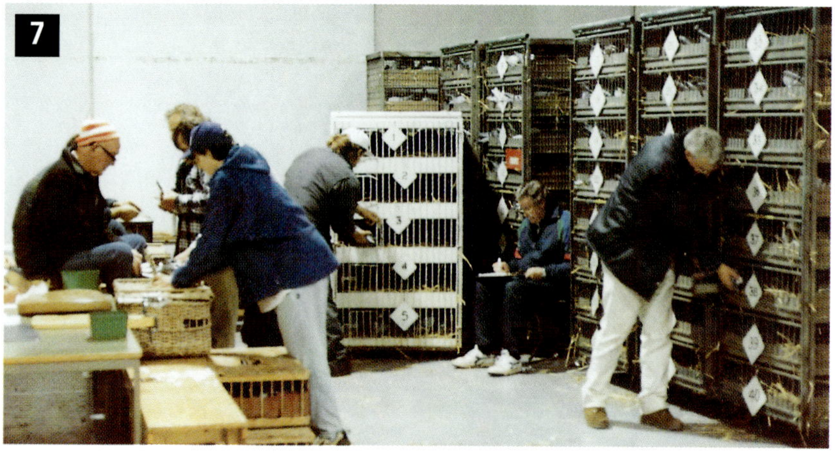

7: The handler then gently places the bird in this basket. The bird is now in the race.

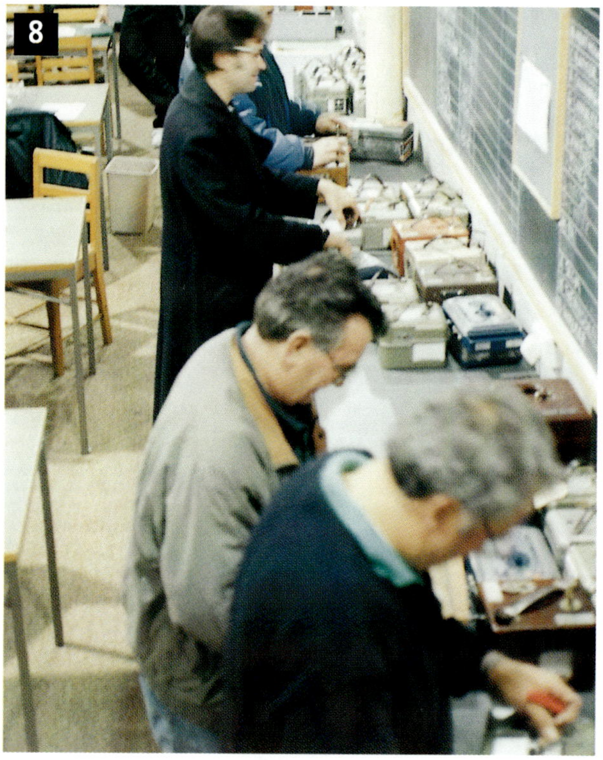

8: Competitors' clocks are set and sealed in readiness to record bird arrivals.

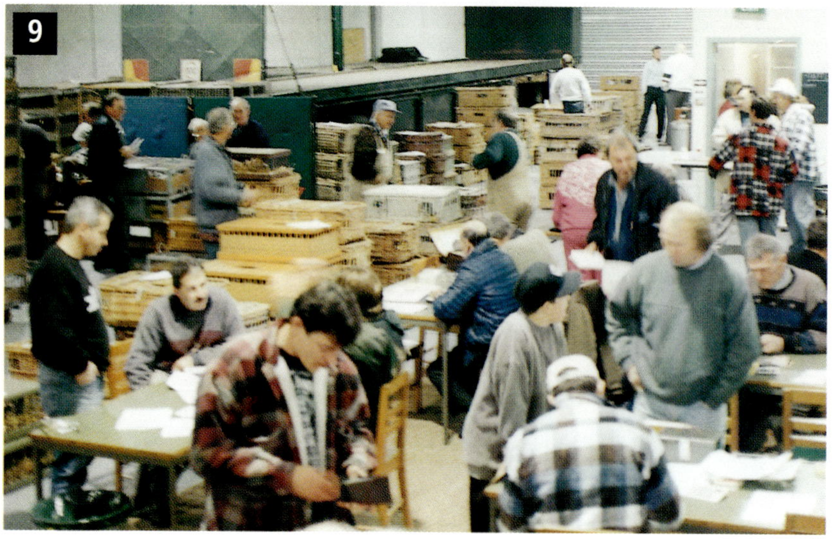

9: At the completion of basketing, race baskets are loaded on to the semitrailer tray in the background. Local carriers bring birds in from other basketing centres. Loading is completed late Thursday evening and the truck carrying the birds leaves immediately for the race point.

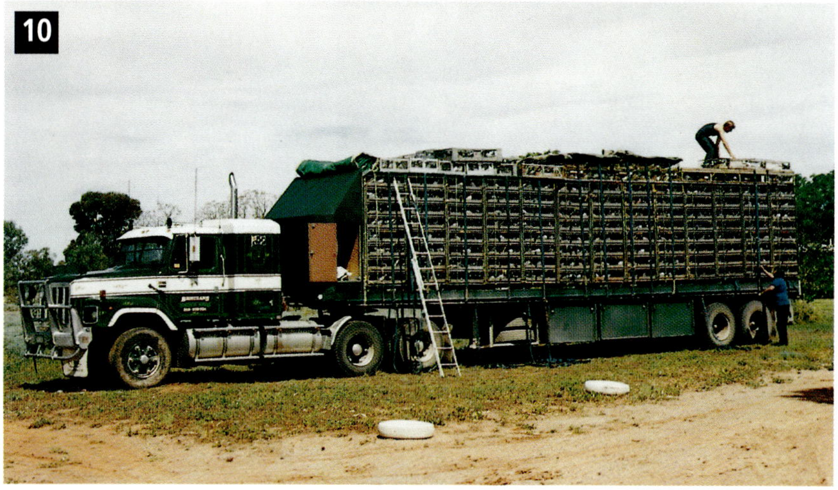

10: Arrival of the transporter at the race point early Friday afternoon, in this case in the V.H.A. 530-mile race from Bourke, N.S.W., on Saturday 23 October 1993, 4923 birds competing.

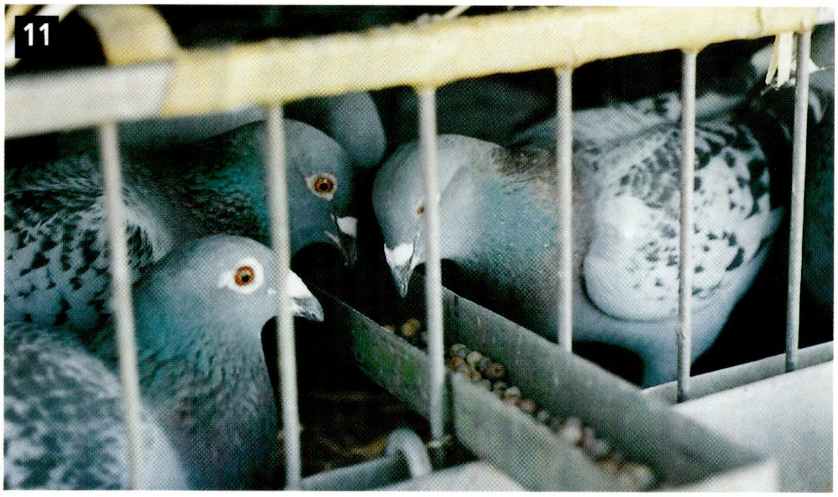

11: Birds are fed immediately on arrival at the race point from trays, filled with grain, that are slid into the baskets.

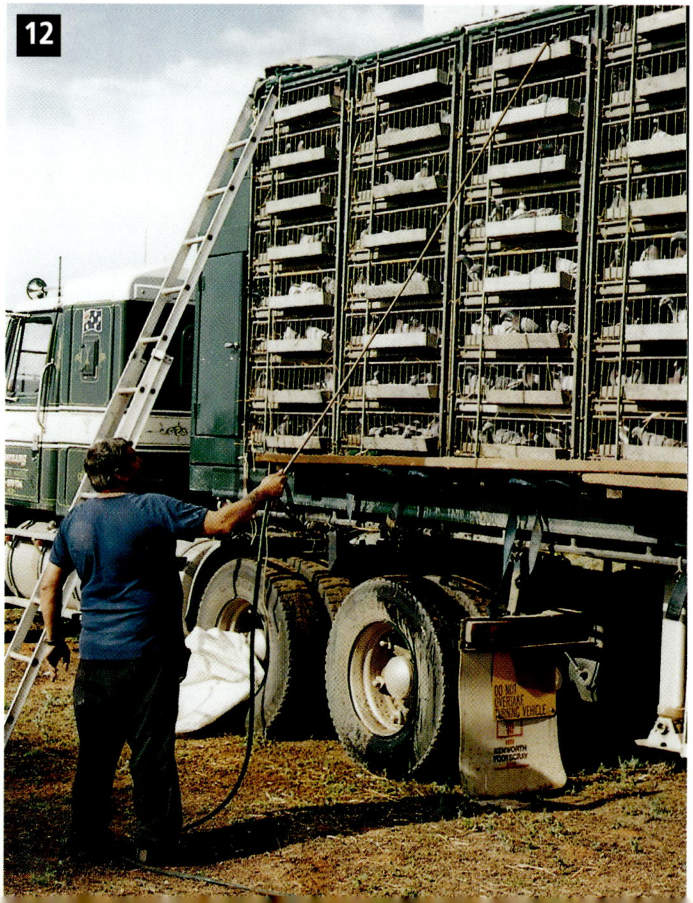

12: Drinkers are attached to the outside of each basket so that the birds can drink.

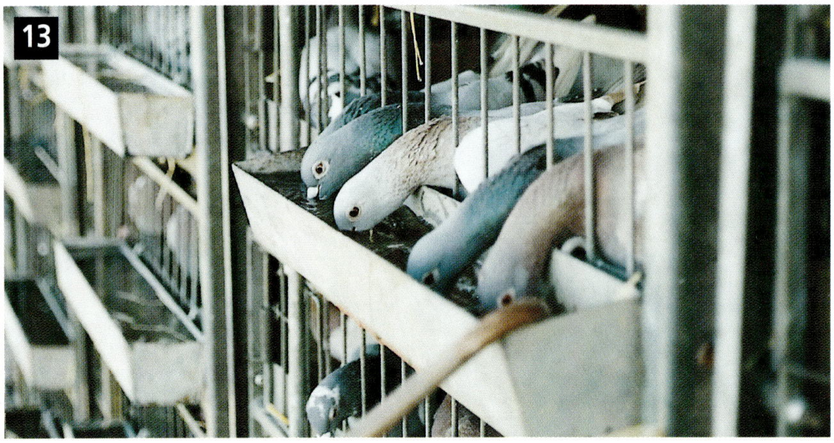

13: Birds come to the front in turn and drink.

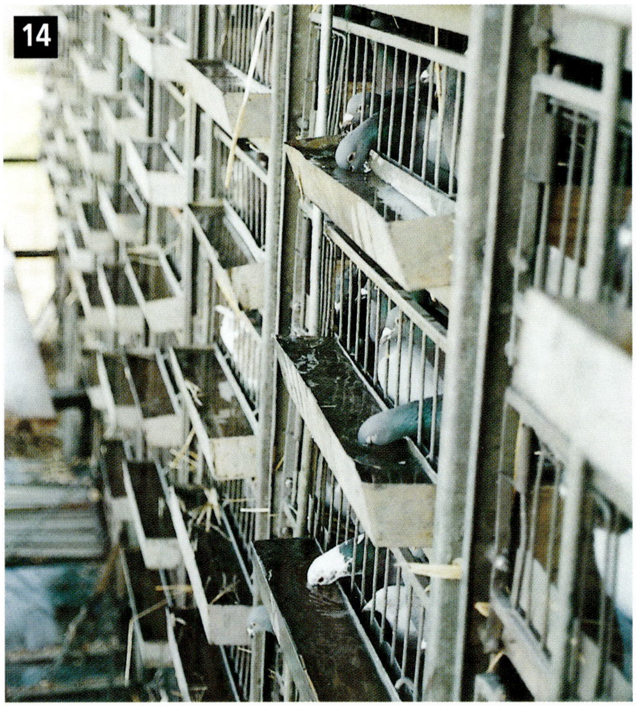

14: View along the front of the transporter, all birds having been fed and watered within approximately 2 hours of arrival at the race point.

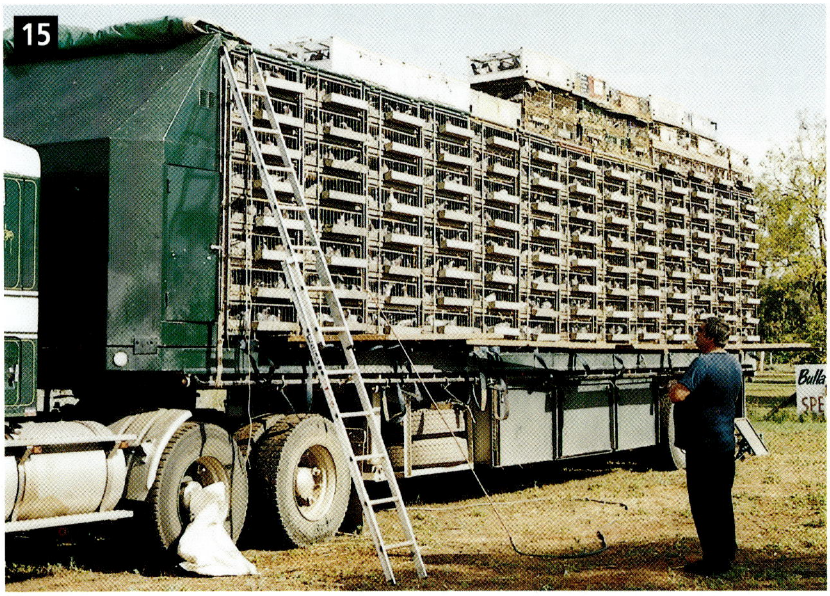

15: Head convoyer, Mr G. Camillieri, supervises the birds.

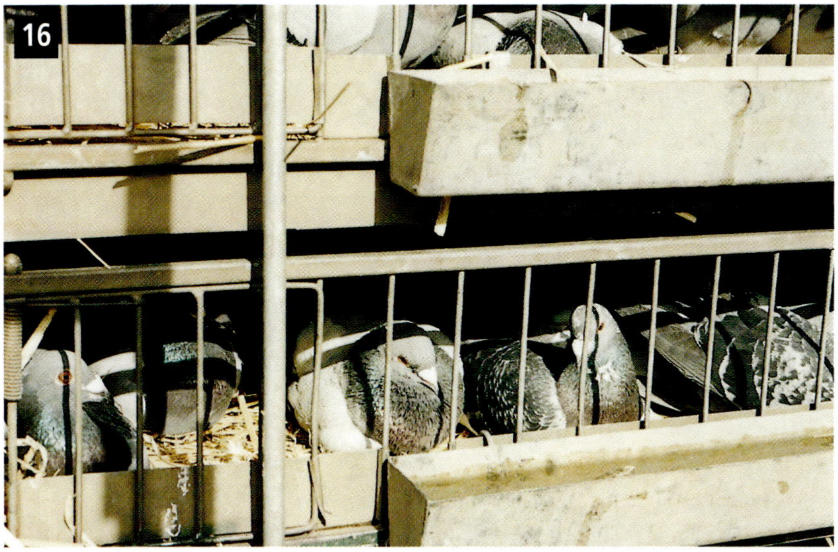

16: At dusk, the birds settle down, ready to spend their second night in the baskets.

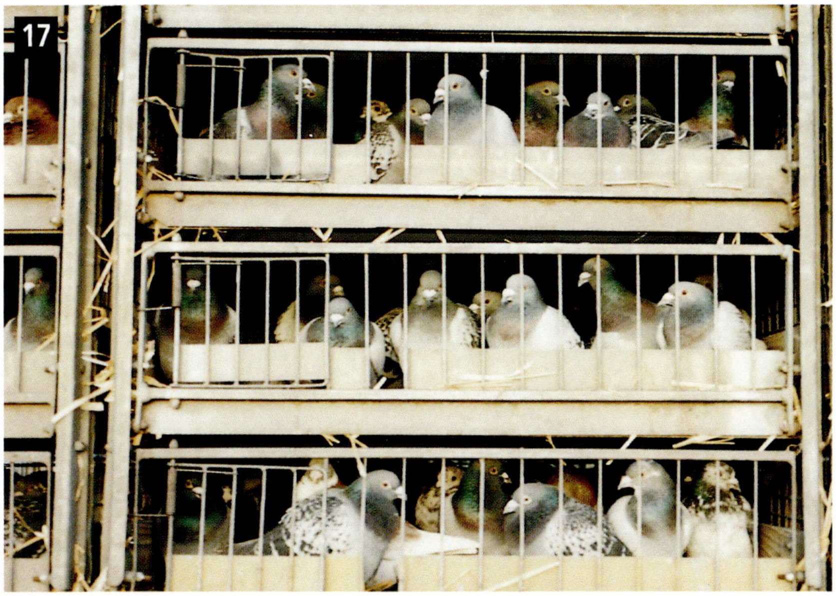

17: 5:30 a.m. Saturday morning, half an hour before release. The drinkers have just been removed.

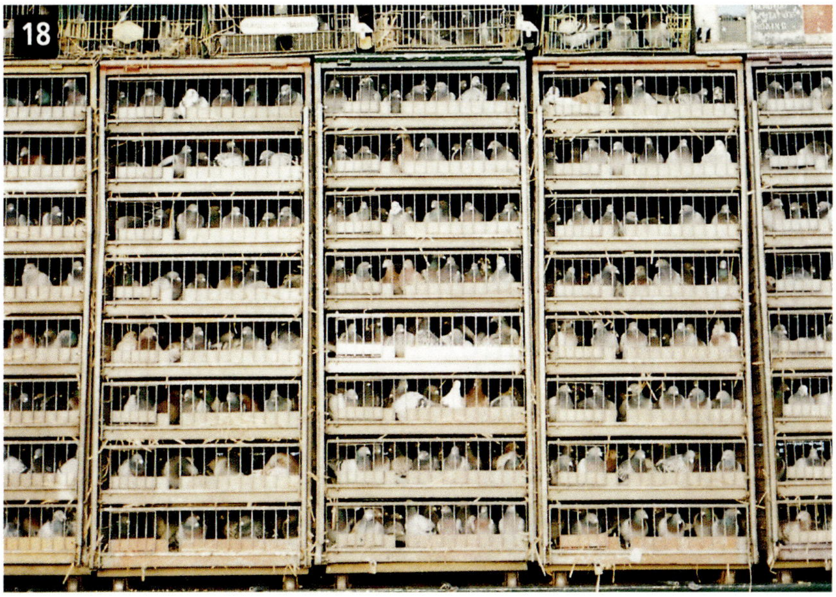

18: 5:59 a.m. The opening mechanisms have been unlocked and the birds sense their impending release.

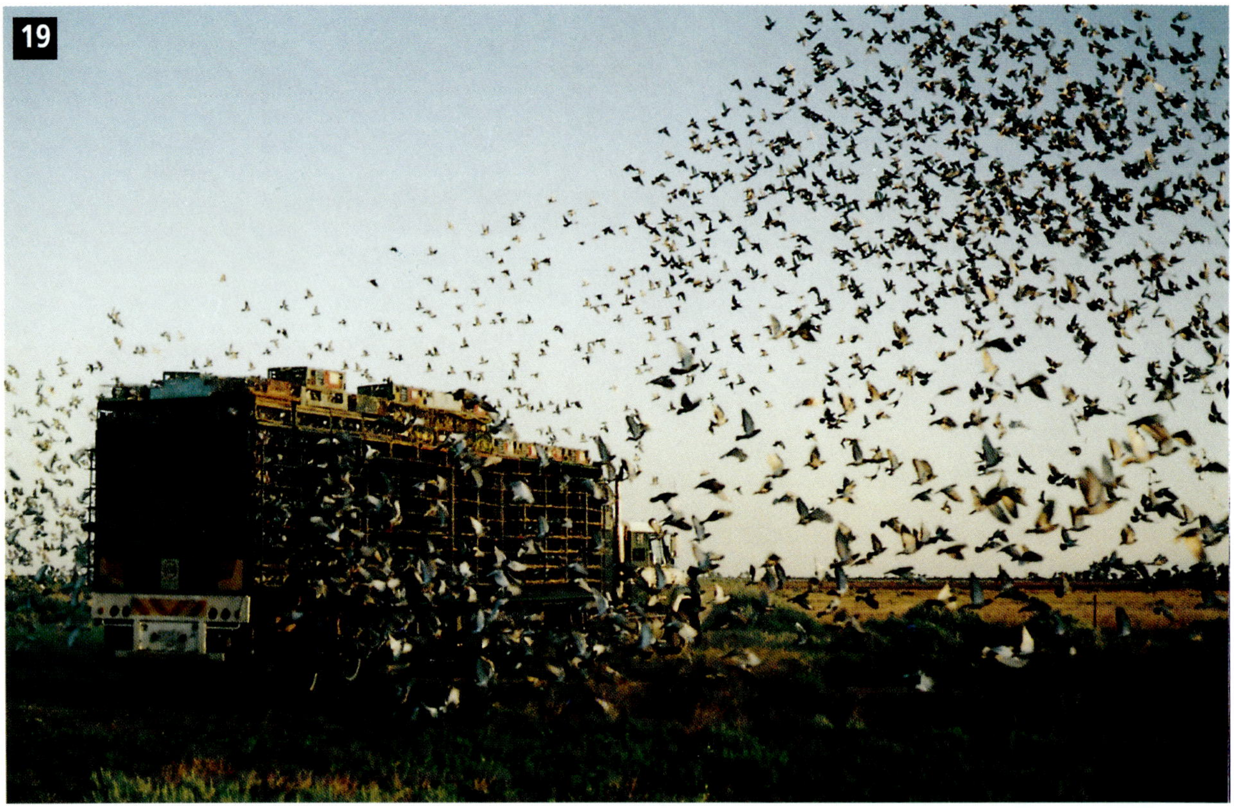

19: 6:00 a.m. Away they go. In this particular 530-mile race, the leading birds had returned to Melbourne by 4:30 p.m., at an average speed of 50 miles per hour.

20: Race birds, high in the sky, streak across the countryside on their way home.

21: Journey's end. A bird having completed the 530-mile race arrives and swoops into the fly-in of competitor Bernie Willemsen, Melbourne.

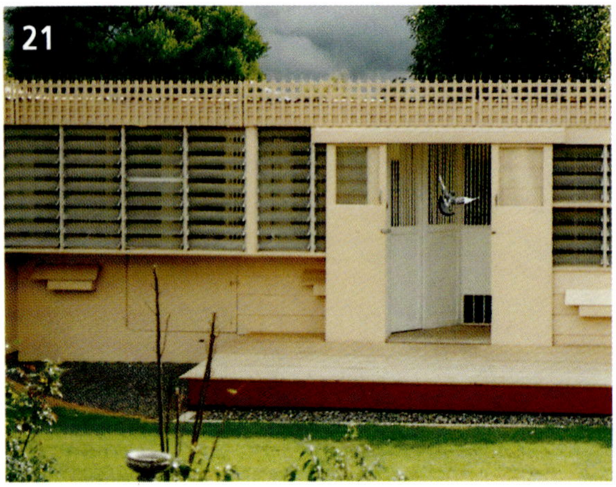

Birds of prey

Falcons and hawks are a significant threat to pigeons. In Australia, there are six species of falcon, all of which are native, and the main one that bothers pigeons is the Peregrine falcon. Falcons have adapted to hunt birds at speed in the sky. Peregrines, although they will occasionally snatch a bird from a loft roof, essentially hunt the birds on the wing. In level flight, a fit well pigeon can outfly a falcon (just). However, the bird's usual mode of hunting is to circle high, waiting for appropriate prey, such as a pigeon, to appear below. It then dives down at great speed after selecting a potential victim. The pigeons' response usually depends on their number, age and experience. A flock of pigeons greater than 300 in number will often group together and attempt to outfly the falcon, particularly if fit. Small numbers of birds, particularly if tired towards the end of a race or younger inexperienced birds, will often scatter and seek shelter in trees or anything else available. Unfortunately, the loss of pigeons is greater than the one the falcon actually gets, as many more pigeons injure themselves in the panic to avoid the falcon.

Hawks have adapted to hunt small birds in the cover of trees and so are more of a danger to the pigeons around the loft, particularly youngsters. Only a limited number of options are available to the pigeon fancier to protect his birds from birds of prey. Keeping a tree-free zone around the loft and always being in attendance when the birds are out make it harder for hawks to stalk the birds. To discourage falcons from attacking a flock, a variety of bells and patterns have been placed on birds in an attempt to frighten the falcons away. These strategies seem, at best, only moderately successful.

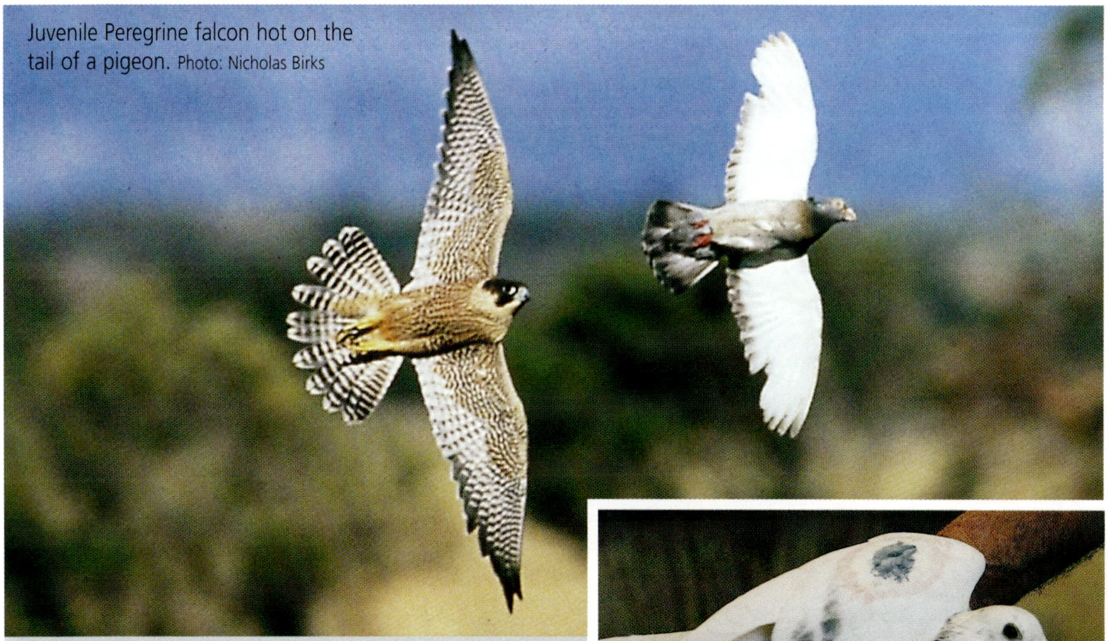

Juvenile Peregrine falcon hot on the tail of a pigeon. Photo: Nicholas Birks

This falcon (on the left) has lost his altitude advantage and the team of pigeons is attempting to outfly him.

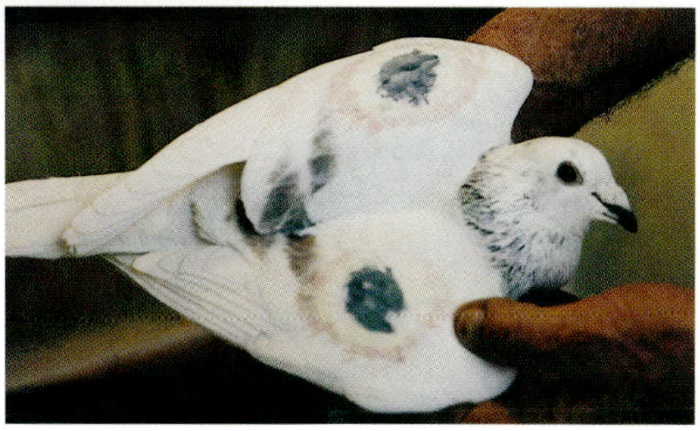

One ploy adopted by fanciers is to paint a 'terror eye' pattern onto several of the lighter-coloured birds. This pattern is intended to represent a large eye in an attempt to scare an attacking falcon.

Section 5

BREEDING

28 Problems Of the Breeding Season

18th Fed 730 miles (approx. 650 birds competing) for the author in October 1999.
This hen also flew the V.H.A. 600-mile event in November 1998 and 1999.

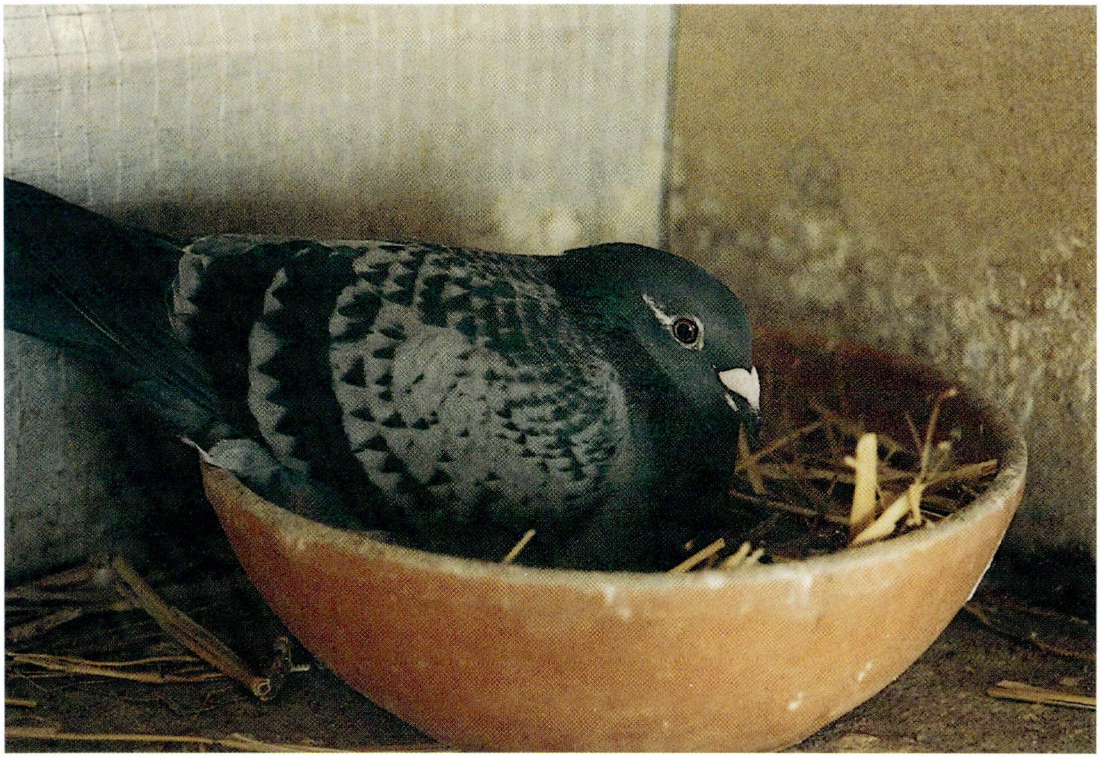

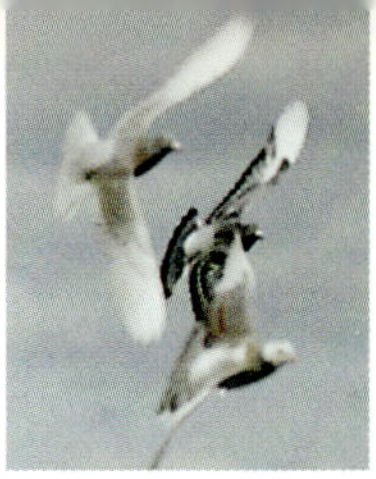

Chapter 28

PROBLEMS OF THE BREEDING SEASON

The main ingredients of a good breeding season are healthy stock birds and good loft management. Prebreeding health checks and preventive programs as outlined in other chapters should ensure that the birds are healthy. Good loft management essentially means good food, an hygienic loft, no overcrowding, and disease control. However, there are several problems that are seen commonly once the stock birds have been paired.

Canker

By far, the most common disease affecting youngsters during breeding is canker, and indeed most ill health in stock birds at this time also relates to this problem. Control is outlined extensively in the chapter Canker. Any stock bird that appears unwell during breeding should immediately be suspected of having canker, even if no sign is visible on examination of the throat. Most canker that affects feeding stock birds occurs internally around the outlet of the crop or lining of the proventriculus (the first compartment of the stomach). Feeding stock birds almost invariably have some trichomonads in these areas and anything that creates a small abrasion in the lining here gives an opportunity for canker organisms to invade and form a canker nodule. Sometimes the birds develop a 'sour crop' through occlusion of the crop outlet by the canker nodule, or breathlessness due to squashing of the windpipe by a canker nodule, but more often than not just adopt the sick bird pose of being quiet, fluffed up and a bit underweight. As the condition quickly passes the stage where it will respond to treatment and as anticanker drugs, if given to an individual bird in this situation, do no harm, I feel that a fancier finding an unwell breeding stock bird should immediately start treatment for canker (such as 1/4 Flagyl tablet) and seek veterinary advice. Grains with a large diameter, such as maize, abrasive grains such as unhulled barley, or poor-quality grit containing larger segments, although not directly giving the birds canker, can predispose vulnerable birds to the problem through the increased likelihood of damage to the lining of the crop and stomach. It is good practice to avoid these during breeding, particularly in lofts experiencing problems.

Some fanciers may notice 2 – 3-week-old youngsters with what appears excessive mucus in the throat or making a clicking sound when they breathe and mistakenly diagnose this as a respiratory infection. Respiratory infection is very uncommon in nestlings because of the immunity passed to them passively in the egg and in the parents' milk. These birds usually have canker. The number of trichomonads present here has either not crossed the threshold where sufficient are present for visible yellow material to form, or the trichomonads may be one of the non-yellow-producing strains.

The canker organism has evolved to increase in number in breeding stock birds around the time their eggs are hatching and levels remain high until the youngsters are 10 days of age, so that most cases of canker are seen in youngsters under 10 days old. Fanciers need to be particularly vigilant during this time. Youngsters should be checked daily, with individual treatments and flock treatments being given as is appropriate for that loft's situation as outlined in the chapter Canker.

Wet nests

Once the birds are paired and youngsters have appeared in the nest bowls, every fancier has experienced the odd pair of stock birds that are wet feeders. This results in a nest bowl, surrounded by smelly wet droppings, in which the youngsters are not 100%.

Hormones and wet nests

Recent veterinary research has shown that the wet nests observed with certain feeding pairs when their youngsters are about 10 days old are associated with changing hormone levels in the parents. A hormone called prolactin is produced and triggers the production of the parents' crop milk. After 10 – 14 days of feeding youngsters, prolactin levels fall. Falling prolactin levels lead to a number of physiological changes, with the result that some birds feed a very watery meal to their youngsters. This fluid is in turn passed by the youngsters in their droppings, leading to a wet nest. The significance for us as fanciers is that these youngsters fail to thrive on these dilute watery meals. As a result, they may not grow properly and become vulnerable to secondary infections, in particular wet canker and *E. coli*. Problems can be decreased by supplementing the parents with probiotics (Probac) and water-soluble sugar-free multivitamins (Multivite Plus) so that the water they then feed to their youngsters, in turn, contains these. Youngsters from such nests should be regularly checked for canker and, if canker is observed, dosed daily with an anticanker medication (Spartrix tablet or Turbosole paste) until well.

Any condition that makes the parents thirsty will also predispose pairs to wet nests. This will make them drink more water, with the result that they feed more water to the babies, which, in turn, causes the youngsters to pass wet droppings. Things that will make stock birds thirsty include:

- **Incorrect use of grits or medication –** Because of the minerals, in particular calcium, that grit contains, it is important that feeding stock birds have grit in front of them all of the time. Poor-quality grits will contain an excessive level of salt. Because the birds eat the grit to gain access to the minerals it contains, they are forced to take in the salt and therefore develop a thirst. Many medications, e.g. multivitamins and antibiotics, contain high levels of sugar, which, if inappropriately used, can also create a thirst. Also, some medications, in particular antibiotics, if used incorrectly, can cause diarrhoea, which also can create a thirst.

- **Diseases –** Any inflammatory condition of the crop, stomach or bowel causes fluid to be lost and will create thirst. In feeding stock birds, the usual problems here are wet canker, coccidiosis or bacterial infections, in particular *E. coli*. If wet nests are a problem, it is best to have a dropping analysed. In the absence of testing, treat affected pairs for canker. If there is no response, a probiotic in the water or on the feed may help.

- **The pigeon fly –** The small flies with prominent wings and legs that pigeon fanciers see in nest boxes are a specific pigeon pathogen called *Pseudolynchia canariensis*. Their lifecycle is fascinating in that the maggots grow and pupate in the droppings around the nest bowl. The adults are blood-suckers, feeding on the youngsters in the nest, with their saliva giving the youngsters diarrhoea to facilitate the development of the flies' maggots. It is best to steer away from the older, more toxic insecticides, such as the organophosphates and hydrocarbons. I suggest using Permethrin, which is a synthetic pyrethroid. This comes in a variety of forms including water-soluble powders and solutions. I find the solutions easier to use. It is a good practice to spray the nest boxes out with a Permethrin Solution before mating. However, if necessary, after normal cleaning and temporarily removing the birds, boxes can be sprayed during breeding.

Lack of vigour in youngsters

Failure of the youngsters to thrive is usually associated with a poor diet, dietary deficiency or disease.

Diet

It is obvious that the breeding bird requires better nutrition than a bird that is not breeding. The seed must be clean and fresh. Dirty seed may carry bacteria, which may harm the youngster and retard its development. Old seed may be of lower nutritional value than fresh seed. A good test of food value is to sprout the seed. Good-quality seed will be sweet-smelling and 90 – 100% will sprout after 2 – 4 days. The growing baby requires considerably more energy and protein than the adult and, for this reason, a high-protein seed mix, which is also high in energy, is necessary to produce robust babies. Seeds high in protein include peas and beans, and these seeds should make up at least 40% of the breeding mix. Corn is a very high-energy food but is not recommended if canker is a problem in the loft. Corn does not directly give the birds canker but can damage the throat and the canker organism finds it easier to establish in damaged tissue.

Dietary deficiency

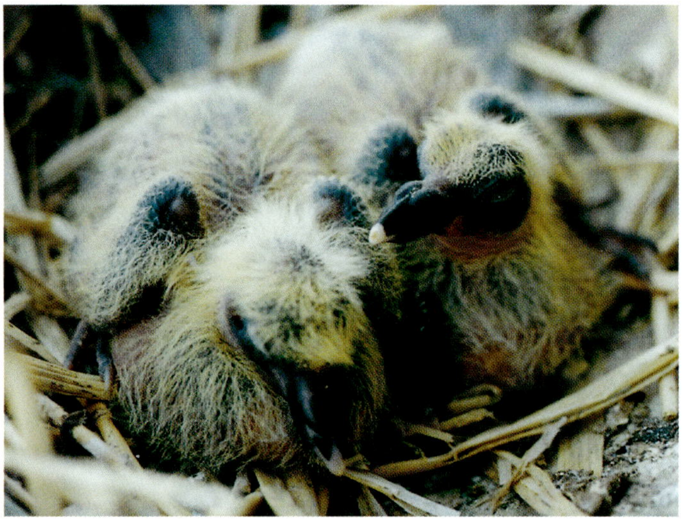

Healthy pair of recently hatched youngsters.

Breeding is one of the times of year when supplementation with vitamins and minerals can give definite benefits. Feeding youngsters places a big nutritional drain on the stock birds and, when dietary levels are marginal, deficiency can develop, leading to disease problems. Most commonly during breeding, this involves the mineral calcium. No matter how much shell grit the birds eat once paired, they cannot assimilate sufficient to compensate for the amount lost in pigeon milk production and in the hens' egg shell formation. The difference is made up from calcium stored in the skeleton before pairing. This is why it is so important that birds have access to grit for the entire year. The amount that can be mobilized from skeletal stores is self-limiting, and when this threshold is passed, a number of problems appear. Calcium is necessary for normal nerve and muscle activity, and so the birds may appear reluctant to walk, floppy, and weak or just quiet. The oviduct is a muscle and should act as a muscular tube pushing the egg down. With a fall in calcium levels, it loses this ability, leading to egg binding. Similarly, if there is insufficient calcium to supply the shell gland within the oviduct wall, rough or soft-shelled eggs may be produced. The quality of crop milk may deteriorate with reduced levels of calcium, leading to soft bones in the youngsters. This is often best assessed where the beak attaches to the head. Similarly, the youngsters are predisposed to 'splay leg', although nest-bowl size and genetic factors are involved here. I feel it is of benefit to not only provide a continuous source of calcium in the form of grit and pink minerals but also to supplement with calcium syrup in the water, particularly in the latter part of the breeding season as the stock birds' calcium reserves are being depleted (e.g. the Australian Pigeon Company's Calcium / Vitamin D_3 Syrup, 5 – 10 ml per litre of water, 1 or 2 days per week). Using an avian water-soluble multivitamin several days per week is also a good idea.

Disease control

The best way to control disease during the breeding season is to pretreat the stock birds against the diseases known to be present before pairing. The main problems of the breeding season, which should be controlled before the season, are worms, external parasites, coccidiosis, canker, respiratory infection and *Salmonella*, in that order, although it will not be necessary to treat for all problems in each loft. The need for treatment depends on problems experienced in the loft in earlier years and how long the loft has been established. These matters are discussed in the chapter Health Management Programs for All Stages of the Pigeon Year.

The main reason for treating before pairing is that all birds in the loft must be treated to control disease. During breeding, this obviously includes youngsters in the nest and there are problems associated with accurate medication of these youngsters. Any medication placed in the drinking water is absorbed by the stock birds to a variable extent. When feeding young youngsters, i.e. less than 10 days old, by the time the parents have produced milk, any medication ingested by them has long since been absorbed and metabolized. This is why, for example, if canker appears in youngsters in this age group, they must be individually dosed with tablets. With older youngsters, i.e. older than 20 days, where the parents are essentially eating and drinking and then pumping the wet grain into the youngsters, the medication will be received by the youngsters. In fact, because the amount of food taken by large, rapidly growing youngsters is much more on a weight basis than adults, there is the potential for gross overdose. Ten-day-old youngsters eat four times as much as an adult, although only a quarter their weight. Therefore, there is the potential for them to receive sixteen times the recommended dose. This becomes progressively less marked as the pigeon matures, but the fancier must be careful. It is important that doses are accurately measured and drugs with wide safety margins are used.

Some problems can only be 'band-aided' until the end of the season, when a control program can be instituted. This is usually only possible when all youngsters are over 6 weeks of age and drinking for themselves. An example here is hairworm infection. Before the stress of breeding, stock birds will often carry these asymptomatically. However, by the third round, particularly in the hens, they can cause severe weight loss, anaemia, diarrhoea and sometimes death. Because of the heavy environmental contamination, and youngsters reinfecting treated adults, usually only the worst

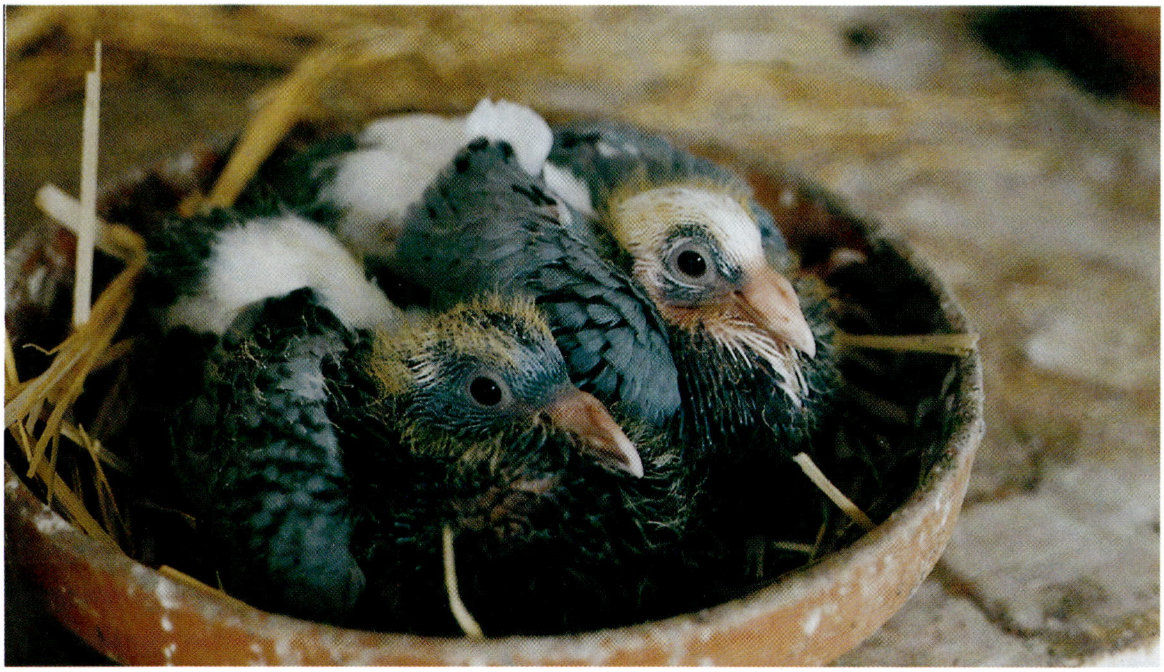

Robust pair of 2½ -week-old nestlings.

affected individuals are treated until the pairs are split up. Once all birds are old enough to eat and drink for themselves, and there are no youngsters in the nest boxes making thorough cleaning possible, it is feasible to eradicate the parasite.

One would expect the odd youngster to be less vigorous than the others for a variety of reasons, including congenital deformities. However, if there is a problem, it should be investigated, even if it only means that once identified the problem can be prevented in the following breeding season. It is good for the fancier to be familiar with, and recognize, the common problems. It is also important for him to know when he needs to seek veterinary advice. Most problems can be identified through straightforward testing involving a throat swab and faecal tests or, occasionally, an autopsy.

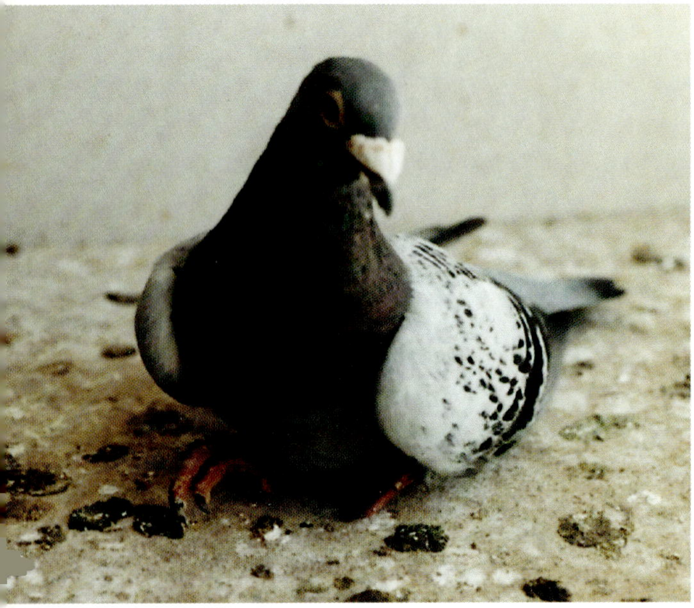

Hen affected with post-egg-laying paralysis.

Post-egg-laying paralysis

Sometimes, a hen will have difficulty walking after laying an egg. This can range from a simple inability to straighten her toes so that she walks on her knuckles, through to a total flaccid paralysis of both legs, forcing her to get about by lifting herself by her wing butts. The main nerve that supplies each leg is called the sciatic nerve. After each sciatic nerve exits the spine, it passes through a kidney before tracking its way around the inside of the pelvis and running into the leg. Sometimes during laying, this nerve can be pinched between the inside of the pelvis and the egg shell. This causes the nerve to become inflamed and means that any nerve impulse passed along its length is garbled. This inflammation is reversible and most hens will get better in 3 days to 3 weeks, depending on the severity of the inflammation. It is usually a matter of separating the bird so that other loft mates do not peck and harass her, often placing her in a spare nest box or basket lined with straw to prevent any pressure sores forming, together with food, water and calcium source within easy reach.

Anything that makes eggs more difficult to lay can predispose the hen to this problem. For example, calcium deficiency can either decrease the strength of oviduct contraction or interfere with shell formation, both of which lead to prolonged egg laying. In the same way, hens that are overweight or lay big eggs are also vulnerable.

Parents abandoning the nest

As all fanciers will know, pigeons have an amazing bond to their young and nest box. Youngster and egg desertion is a problem of loft management rather than disease. External loft stimuli, in particular cats, may be relevant here. Fanciers should, however, also consider the possibility of red mite. Adult mites live in nooks and crannies within the loft, particularly under the nest bowl. They become active at night and will crawl freely over both the youngsters and the incubating parents, biting and sucking blood in the process. Occasionally during the day, individual mites may be found hiding under the wings of the youngsters. Alternatively, only the small scabby attachment sites may be seen, or the youngsters may be pale because of lost blood or have swollen feet because of the associated protein loss. If red mite are suspected, investigate the incubating birds with a torch at night or run a knife down a crack in the loft, which may be covered in blood if mites are present. The measures discussed to control pigeon fly are also effective in controlling red mite.

Egg-bound hen

When a hen is unable to lay an egg, she is said to be 'egg bound'. This is a serious condition, which is almost always fatal. Calcium is necessary for strong coordinated contractions of the oviduct and if the hen has been egg bound for less than 24 – 48 hours, it is worth giving her some calcium in case she is deficient. Usually 20 mg of calcium is given every 24 hours. Calcium tablets can be obtained from a pharmacist or veterinarian and a proportion of these given, e.g. 1/5 of a 100-mg tablet. Alternatively, calcium syrup (1/2 ml of Australian Pigeon Company Calcium Syrup) can be given neat direct to the beak, or failing that, several big pinches of PVM Powder can be placed in the back of the throat. If this does not work in 24 – 48 hours, or if the hen starts to become distressed, she should be taken to a veterinarian. Injections are sometimes given to stimulate the oviduct to contract. Alternatively, a hypodermic needle is passed through the wall of the cloaca (the sac inside the bottom, into which the oviduct enters) into the egg and its contents aspirated. Once empty, the egg shell is then collapsed inside the oviduct. With on-going calcium supplementation, most hens are able to pass this collapsed shell. It is important to empty the egg before collapse, otherwise the egg shell can lacerate the wall of the oviduct, causing egg content to leak into the abdominal cavity, which can be fatal. If these measures fail, then the abdomen and oviduct can be opened under anaesthetic and the egg shell surgically removed.

An older technique is to put paraffin oil into the cloaca in an attempt to lubricate the egg and make its passing easier. This practice is not encouraged. Oil can safely be put into the cloaca only. However, this is not an advantage because if the egg has been able to reach here, it will be passed. If the oil is inserted too deeply and enters the oviduct, it runs the risk of introducing infection, which in itself could be fatal or damage the oviduct, affecting subsequent fertility.

Fortunately, in hens that are in good condition, egg binding is not very common, but do ensure that palatable calcium supplements are always available before and during breeding to minimize problems. If individual hens do develop problems, it is worth trying direct calcium supplementation for a short time, but if this does fail, your veterinarian can help.

Abnormal egg shell surface

Occasionally, eggs with abnormal egg shells are produced. These can range from ones that have an irregular rough texture on the surface through to eggs that have virtually no shell at all. There are a number of possible causes, and indeed occasionally a quite normal healthy hen will lay an egg like this. If it is becoming a common problem through the loft or one hen does it persistently, it is usually due to one of two reasons.

1 **Calcium deficiency –** The shell gland sits in the wall of the oviduct (the tube that carries the egg to the exterior) and secretes the egg shell onto the expanding egg. A healthy functional shell gland cannot produce a normal shell if the pigeon is deficient in calcium. It is important that palatable sources of calcium, such as mineral blocks, pink minerals and shell grit, are always available before and during breeding. As the developing egg passes along the oviduct, it rotates along its longitudinal axis. In early calcium deficiency ,this movement can be seen as translucent lines, where the egg shell is thin, forming a spiral in the shell.

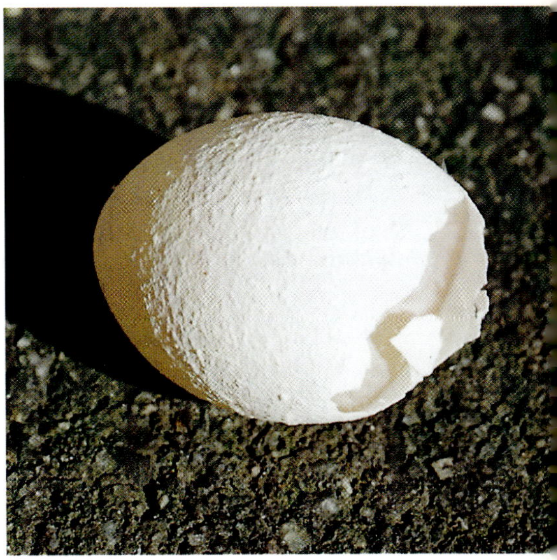

Egg produced either as a result of oviduct disease or calcium deficiency. Note the irregular roughened surface and thinner-than-normal shell.

2 **Diseased shell gland –** If problems persist despite adequate calcium supplementation, it is likely that the shell gland is diseased. If it is diseased, the most likely problem is an infection. The usual bacteria that cause these infections are ones that live in the bowel and backtrack from the cloaca into the oviduct. If the infection has been there for a long time (several weeks),

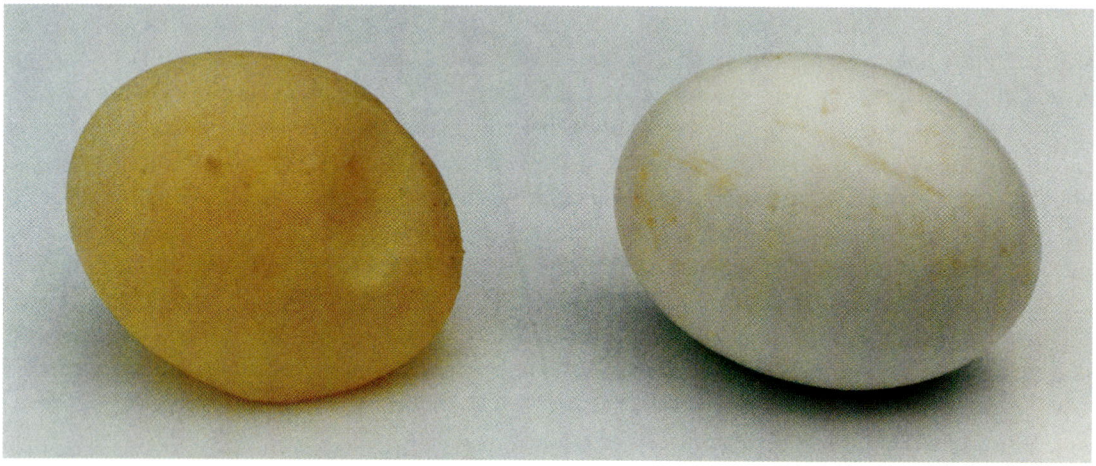

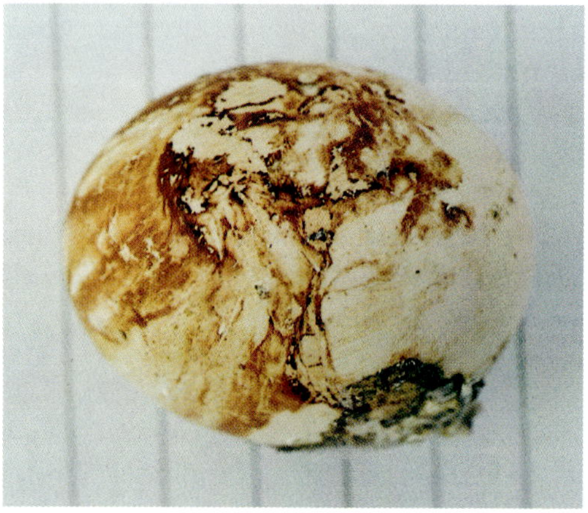

Above: Soft-shelled compared with a normal egg.

Left: This egg has been laid with difficulty, which may be associated with calcium deficiency or oviduct disease.

they respond poorly to treatment. However, if caught early, they can respond quite well. The usual antibiotic we use is Baytril. I usually recommend separating the problem hen, treating her with Baytril (three drops twice daily for 10 days) and then waiting a further 2 weeks before reintroducing her to the cock, while all the time making calcium supplements available.

Confined hens unable to fly or walk after laying

A common query at my clinic regards hens in good health that have been placed in individual nest boxes to pair and lay but when let out into the rest of the loft, either limp or cannot fly properly. This problem is primarily due to calcium deficiency. Once pigeons are breeding, a lot of calcium is lost from both the cock's and hen's system through the production of crop milk but, in addition, in the hen in the production of the eggs. It is therefore important that the birds are provided with an on-going supply of calcium to compensate for this loss. If calcium access is denied through a critical time, such as egg shell production, calcium stored in the bird's bones will be mobilized to meet this demand. This loss of calcium from the bones makes the bones sore, making the birds reluctant to fly or to walk so that after taking a few steps they prefer to rest on their keel. Alternatively, the loss can lead to microfractures, which will make the birds limp or fly with a wobble. If movement is restricted, e.g. being in an individual run that is too small, this exacerbates the problem because it leads to muscle stiffness and can compromise blood supply to the bone itself. The answer is to ensure that, even if birds are confined for a short period of time during breeding, a palatable calcium source such as grit or PVM Powder is in front of the birds. A sugar-free calcium syrup can also be added to the water. If practical, rotating pairs out into the main loft until the pair bond has established will also help.

Hardware disease

Pigeons, being natural foragers, will often find and swallow any bits of wire or nails that are left around the loft. Once swallowed, these usually pass into the gizzard where the grinding action of this organ usually leads to them perforating or sometimes completely penetrating the stomach wall. Although this could happen at any time of year, almost invariably these birds present at the start of the breeding season when they are building their nests. It is vital that a meticulous clean up occurs following any loft renovation. Birds with this condition are lethargic, underweight, have green diarrhoea and delayed crop emptying. The diagnosis is confirmed by x-ray, where the swallowed metal is immediately obvious. Most of these birds respond well to surgery, which involves opening the abdominal cavity and then the gizzard itself to remove the swallowed objects. Antibiotics and another drug called Calcium EDTA are given after surgery. The Calcium EDTA chelates out any metals that have been absorbed into the system before surgery.

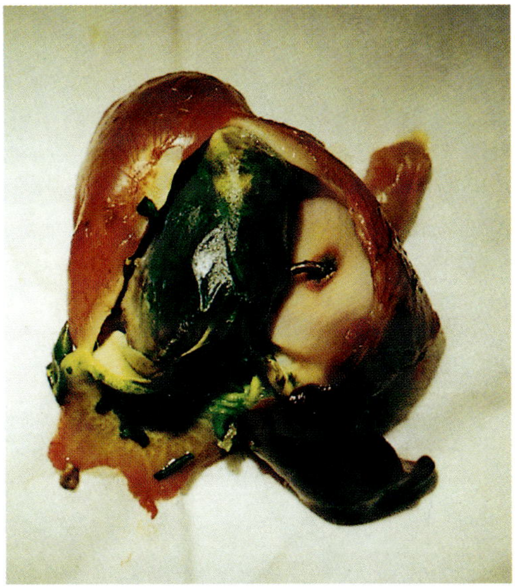

Autopsy specimen of a bird's gizzard with hardware disease. Note the piece of wire extending through the inner layer of the gizzard (green) into the muscle of the gizzard wall on the right-hand-side of the photo.

Angel wing

We have all seen the single-nest youngster with its lower wings turned out. This condition occurs in a number of different types of bird, including geese and chickens as well as pigeons, and is called 'angel wing'. During growth, the shafts of the primary feathers (as with all feathers) are full of blood. This makes them heavy. Also, initially during growth, bones are made of cartilage, which, unlike mature bone, can be shaped and bent. As the bird matures, calcium is deposited into this cartilage matrix, which, as a result, gradually becomes harder and harder, in the end forming the hard bone of the adult. Until they become mineralized with calcium, the bones of the wrist (carpus) are not strong enough to support the weight of the blood-filled feathers, which cause an outward rotation of the lower wing at the wrist. Fortunately, in most cases, the condition is self-correcting. With time, calcium is deposited in the cartilage and the bones gradually increase in strength. As the feathers stop growing, blood is withdrawn from the shaft and they become lighter. As a result, the wing gradually moves into a normal position.

This condition usually does not occur when two youngsters are in the nest as each youngster tends to offer support for the other while they pass through this growth phase. Interestingly, in some other heavy birds, such as geese, the deformity can be permanent unless the wing is strapped into a normal position until growth is complete.

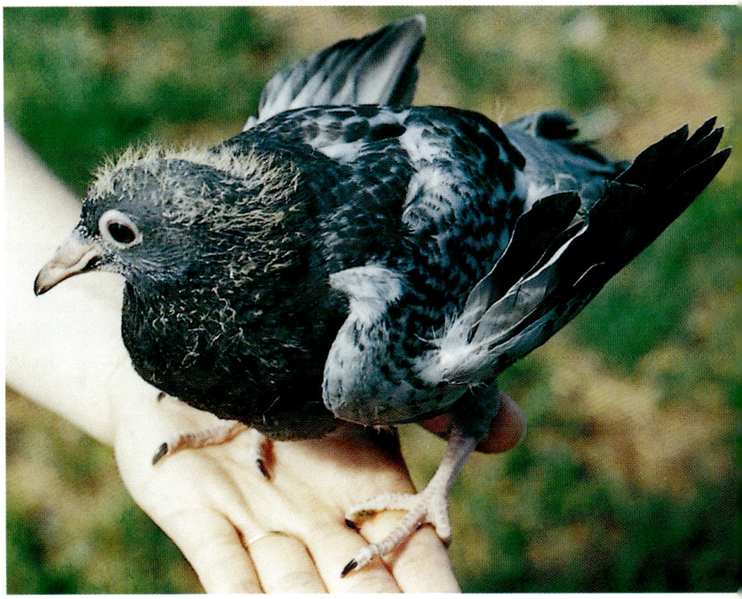

Youngster with angel wing.

Splay leg

'Splay leg' refers to a condition where one or both legs of a nestling project from the side of the body so that, as the bird matures, the leg cannot be brought underneath it for normal standing or walking. The actual deformity is an outward deviation of the long bones of the leg, so that they are bent rather than being straight. There may be genetic and nutritional factors involved here. However, the usual cause is a combination of particularly tight-sitting parents and inadequate nest material. Certain birds brood particularly tightly to the point of almost squashing their youngsters. If the youngsters have inadequate nesting material against which to brace themselves or are in an oversized nest bowl, the legs tend to push out to the side. The condition is more common in single-nest youngsters because they lack a nestmate against which to brace. If caught early, providing a smaller nest bowl, packing the nest bowl with nesting material or fostering two single-nest youngsters of the same age together will help. In bigger youngsters, hobbles can be tried. However, usually the prognosis is hopeless in these cases.

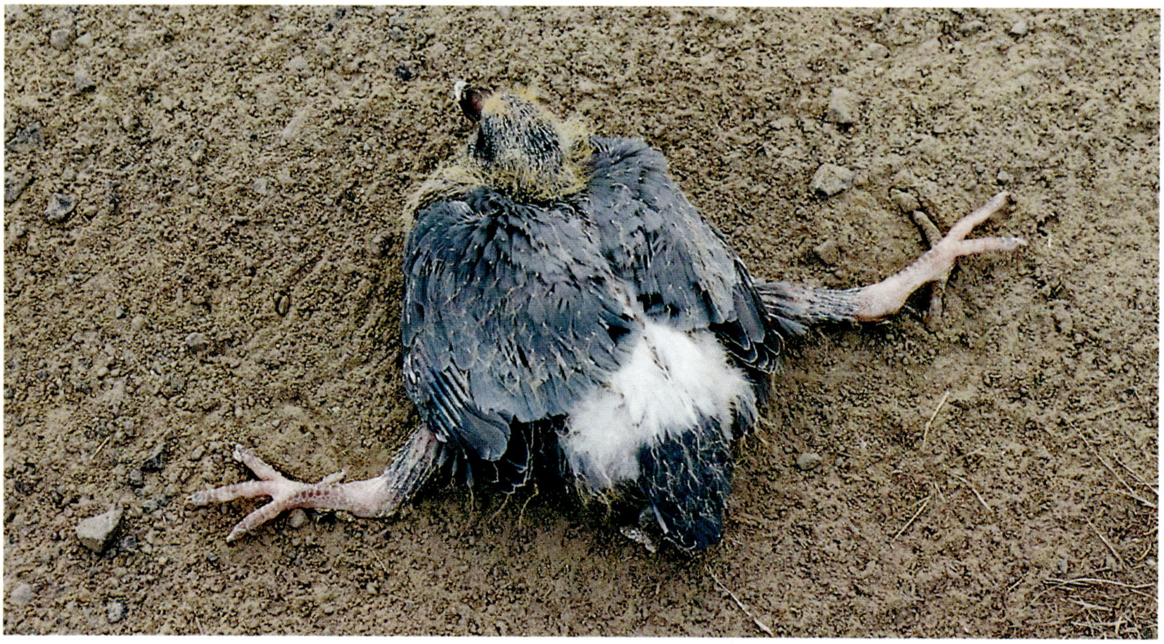

Youngster affected with bilateral splay leg.

Bent keel

As some youngsters mature in the nest, it becomes apparent that the keel deviates to a variable extent from the midline rather than being straight. There does seem to be a genetic component to this condition in that some birds are more likely to breed such youngsters even when their eggs are fostered to other birds. Birds with calcium deficiency are more likely to develop this condition. Stock birds that sit too tightly on their youngsters or fail to provide adequate nesting material can predispose youngsters to this condition.

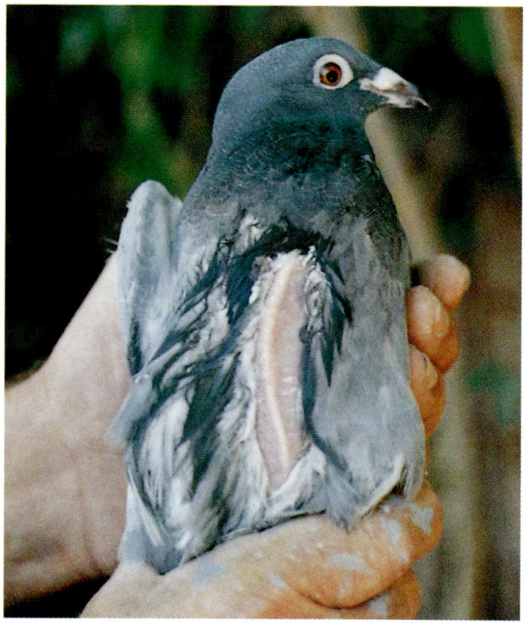

Weaned youngster with a bent keel.

Cloacal prolapse

Persistent straining can lead to either stretching or tearing of the support structures of the cloaca. When this happens, the cloaca is everted and pushed through the cloacal opening so that it becomes visible. Fanciers usually notice that an affected bird looks unwell and on examination a red fleshy mass is visible at the cloacal opening. Anything that leads to straining can cause this condition and so it is sometimes seen in birds with chronic diarrhoea. However, it is most often seen in hens that have had difficulty laying an egg. Sometimes egg laying is difficult for no apparent reason. However, hens that are calcium deficient are much more likely to have difficulty laying eggs because calcium is necessary for strong coordinated contractions of the oviduct. Often the egg that causes the prolapse, if passed, will be soft-shelled or streaked with blood or mucus.

Provided the condition is noticed soon after it occurs so that the internal structures have not been damaged, the prognosis for these birds is quite good. Under general anaesthetic, the cloaca is cleaned and replaced, and sutures are placed at the cloacal opening to prevent reprolapse. These stitches are usually left in position for 10 – 14 days. These birds must be

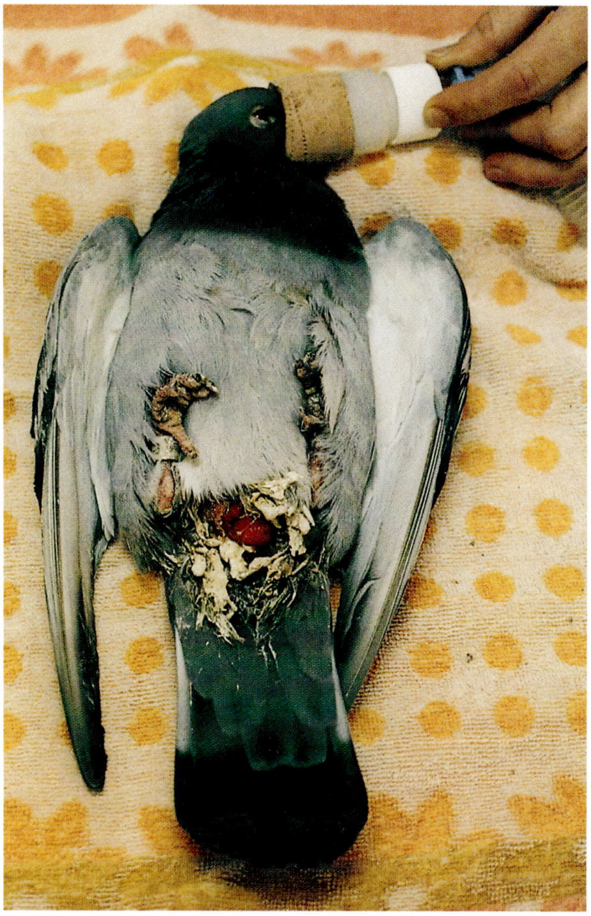

Above: Anaesthetized bird being prepared for surgery to repair its cloacal prolapse.

Below: Close-up of the above bird's prolapsed cloaca.

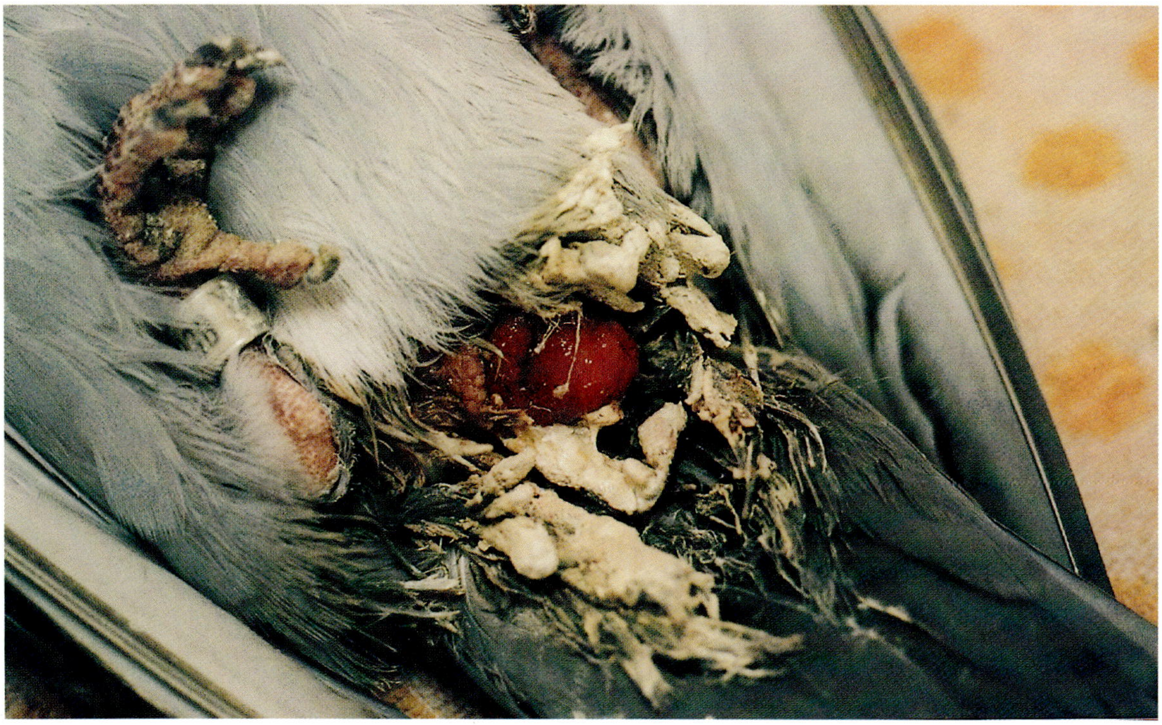

monitored to ensure that they can defaecate normally and that no further eggs appear. Calcium and antibiotics are routinely given. Droppings should be examined microscopically to ensure that diarrhoea is not the cause of the straining.

Internal ovulation

When a hen ovulates, a cone-shaped structure called the infundibulum at the top of the oviduct (the tube that carries the egg to the exterior) initiates a gentle waving action that sucks and guides the immature egg into the oviduct. As the egg passes down the oviduct, it swells and a gland inside the oviduct wall called the shell gland secretes the shell onto it. In some hens, for one reason or another, the infundibulum fails to suck the young egg into the oviduct and it floats free into the abdomen. It does not carry infection with it but it does, however, initiate an inflammatory response. What happens next depends on how severe this inflammation is. Sometimes the hen can actually die, being found dead sitting in her nest bowl. At other times, she may be transiently unwell and it will simply be noted that she is late to lay or only lays one egg, etc. However, usually, she fails to lay, looks unwell and inflammatory fluid starts to accumulate in her abdomen, so that it becomes swollen. Other conditions such as problems with the liver or heart or cancer can also cause fluid to accumulate in the abdomen. However, when the abdomen of a hen that was healthy at pairing fills with fluid and her egg laying is erratic, an internal ovulation should be suspected. Treatment involves rest and time and sometimes antibiotics to guard against secondary infection. As the damage caused by the internal ovulation heals, the fluid is resorbed and the hen becomes well. However, as internal ovulations occur as a result of a defect in normal ovulation, they tend to recur in these hens. Also, as damage from an earlier internal ovulation heals, scars can form around the ovary, which can predispose the bird to further ovulation problems. This can lead to the hen, perhaps, laying later than other hens paired at the same time or producing a clutch of only one egg, etc.

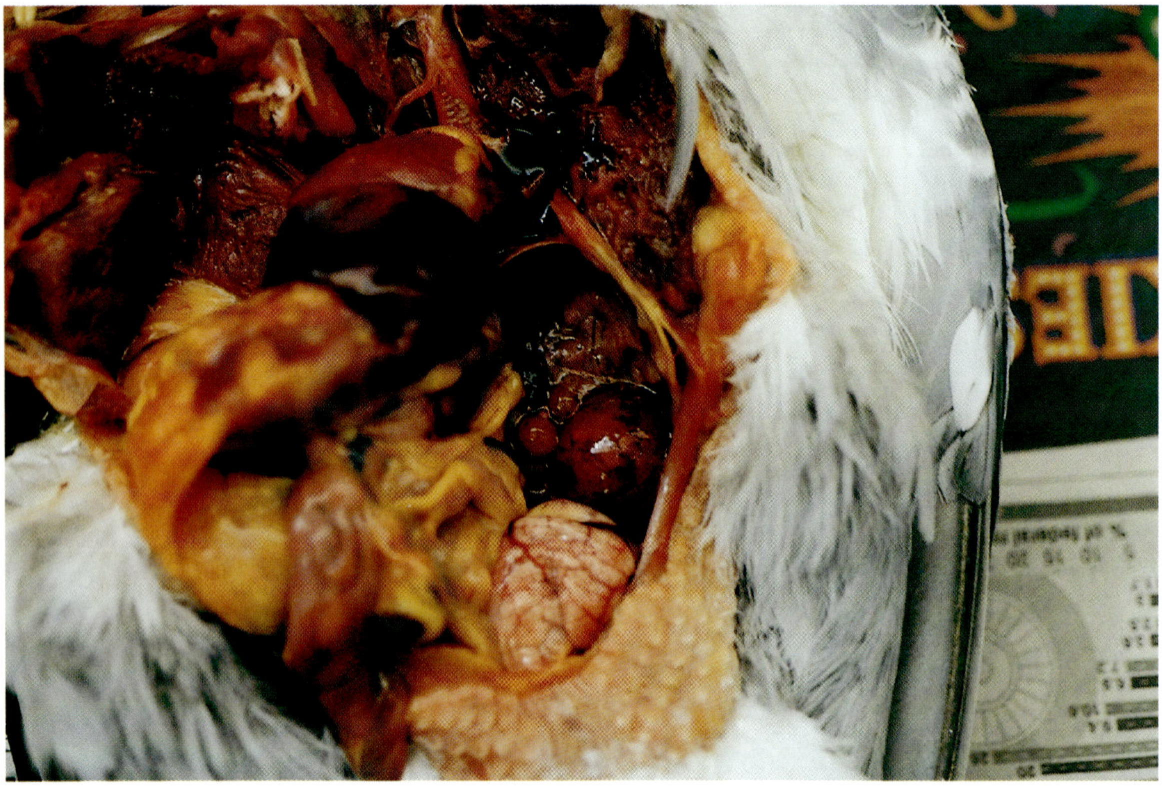

Autopsy specimen of a hen with internal ovulation. The bowel and liver have been retracted to the left. The abdominal fat is visibly stained yellow, indicating an earlier ovulation. More inflamed blood-filled follicles of various sizes can be seen on the surface of the ovary. The pink fleshy object at the base of the abdomen is the bird's oviduct.

Breeding stock birds and race winners, from a genetic point of view

The aim of breeding is to stabilize the winning genes. Winners are often the result of cross-breeding and, as such, contain a wide variety of genes. This means that the youngsters they produce will range considerably in quality. Some will be good but just as many will not. To stabilize the winner's genes, one needs to mate it to close relatives, e.g. if the winner is a cock, to its mother, sister or daughter. Some of the resultant youngsters will have the genes required. The only way of telling which for sure is to breed off these and, in turn, race their youngsters. However, it is likely, but not necessarily so, to be the ones that look like the winning bird that are carrying the winning genes. Physical appearance is the external indicator that genes might be shared with the winner. Once a good bird here is identified, because it is the result of inbreeding, it has little genetic variation and is likely to breed birds as good as itself and with less variation.

In this way, inbred lines carrying the winning genes can be established in the stock birds. Through a phenomenon of genetics called 'hybrid vigour', where the youngsters produced from crossing two inbred lines are especially vital, these inbred lines can be used to produce race birds.

Racing identifies the birds that are carrying the required genes. Inbreeding to these birds stabilizes these genes so that they are concentrated and preserved in a proportion of the progeny. These individual birds, once identified, are of enormous value in the stock loft. Inbred birds of different lines are then crossed to breed the winners!

A new champion in the making? A stock cock feeds his youngster.

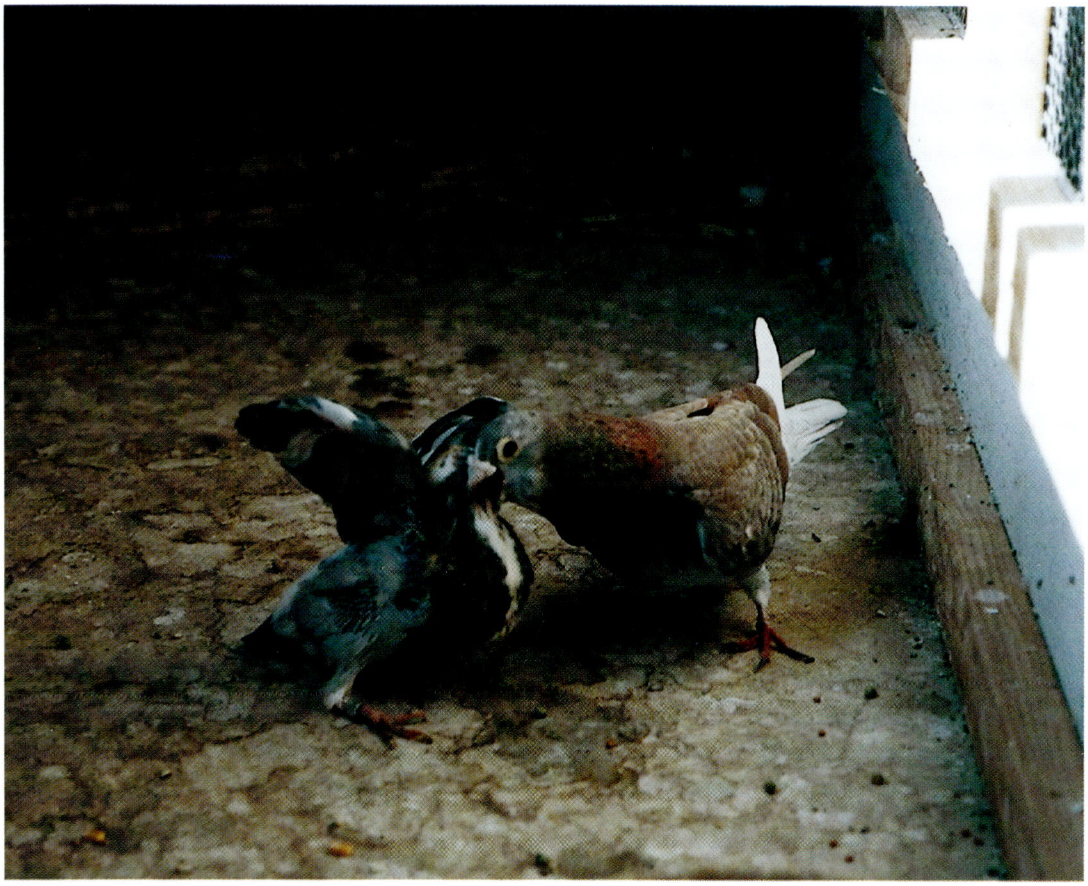

Non-hatching eggs

A big factor that affects the success of the current racing season is the success of the previous breeding season; remember, any success gained in the current racing season began in the nest bowl last breeding season. It is important that good-quality youngsters are produced. Similarly, as most of us only carry a certain number of stock pairs, based on the number of birds we wish to breed and race, it is important that each stock pair makes its contribution to the potential race team. Each season, we only have so long to fill each ring with a good-quality youngster. It is therefore very frustrating to have eggs that do not hatch. Eggs do not hatch for one of two reasons: either they are infertile or the egg is fertile but the embryo dies before hatching.

In the normal situation, ova are released from the ovary and swell as they pass down the oviduct. As they swell, they start to rotate along their longitudinal axis. The shell gland, which is a diffuse gland in the wall of the oviduct, secretes the shell onto the outer skin of the ova during this passage. The egg shell is a mineral matrix with pores through it. Through these pores, water, other substances and micro-organisms can pass.

INFERTILITY

Infertility in the flock

Infertility in most birds indicates a flock out of breeding condition. This may indicate an underlying disease, such as parasitism, or a management flaw, possibly associated with inadequate vitamin or mineral intake.

Infertility in the hen

On an individual basis, hens that are healthy but fail to lay may benefit from being paired later in the season, as the natural stimuli for ovulation are increasing daylength and increasing environmental temperature. If egg laying fails to occur, fostering a pair of 1-day-old fertile eggs under the non-laying hen when she is broody is a good idea. Sometimes after raising a fostered pair of eggs at the time the second pair of eggs would be laid, the barren hen will lay. If laying still does not occur, checks should be run to ensure that no disease is being carried latently. Depending on the value of the hen, blood tests, abdominal x-rays or laparotomy to inspect the ovary may be helpful.

Infertility in the cock

For the individual cock who is producing all or some clear eggs, a health check is indicated to ensure no disease is present. Cancer of the testicle is not uncommon in middle-aged to old cocks and can be detected with an abdominal x-ray or alternatively a laparotomy.

Current advice to increase the number of eggs filled by poorly fertile cocks is:

- **Multivitamin supplementation before pairing –** Supplements, particularly those containing vitamin E, e.g. wheatgerm oil or Turbovite Oil, can be beneficial.
- **Pair later in the season –** The natural stimuli of increasing daylength and environmental temperature can stimulate sperm production.
- **Pair in an individual run –** Older cocks are often clumsy when mating and therefore require longer, uninterrupted time to mate. They are easily intimidated by the younger, more virile cocks. Also, with reduced sperm count, more mating attempts may be required for fertilization to occur. Skittish hens are more likely to crouch correctly in an individual run.
- **Use a proven, keen hen**.

Some fanciers will trim the feathers around the cock's or hen's cloaca short, to enhance sperm transfer. This is of dubious value and it is known that some feathers, called 'feeler feathers', are used as a guide by the cock to locate the hen's cloaca.

Fertility injections

Hormone injections are now available to stimulate fertility in both old cocks and hens. A small gland at the base of the brain, called the pituitary, produces, amongst other things, a hormone called gonadotrophin. This stimulates ovulation (which leads to egg laying) in hens and sperm production in cocks. In birds, the pituitary produces this hormone in response to increasing daylength and increasing environmental temperature, which is one of the reasons why birds start to breed in Spring. With age, gonadotrophin production falls. Synthetic gonadotrophin is now available by injection to boost falling natural levels and once a particular threshold is passed, fertility can be restored. The injections work best in older cocks, which may have filled all eggs 3 years ago, perhaps four of six 2 years ago, and only one last year. These birds usually still have some testicular tissue capable of responding to gonadotrophins. The longer birds have been sterile, the less likely they are to respond, and birds that have primary disease of the gonads, e.g. testicular cancer or an ovarian cyst, cannot respond. One injection is given weekly for 3 weeks. These are best given at the beginning of Spring so that they can act together with the birds' naturally produced gonadotrophin. Hens having injections are best left with their cock so that he is there to fill any eggs if and when ovulation occurs. However, cocks are usually best kept away from the hens while having injections because, being a sex hormone, the injections tend to give the cocks a high libido, leading to repeated mating and sometimes wasted poor-quality ejaculates. It is usually best to put treated cocks with their hen as they have their last injection.

Fertile eggs that do not hatch

All fertile eggs that fail to hatch should be examined to see if they were fertile or not. If eggs are not properly opened, it is easy to confuse infertility with early embryonic death. If the egg is infertile, attention obviously focuses on problems that affect this, while if the eggs are fertile, these matters can be investigated.

Egg autopsy

Initially, examine the surface of the egg. Eggs that are mis-shapen, have a roughened surface or appear thin may indicate oviduct disease in the hen. Such eggs may have increased porosity, making the entry of infection easier. Ensure that the surface of the egg is not cracked or broken. If it is, the entry of infection is made easy (I find that small defects can be satisfactorily repaired using Liquid Paper, provided no infection has entered before application). Similarly, check that the egg is not dirty or has heavy faecal contamination.

Next, the internal contents of the egg can be examined. The entry point is ascertained by candling. The egg shell is wiped with alcohol to sterilize it and then a small window is gently teased open. If the egg is infertile, a small, solid, white blastodisc can be seen on the surface of the yolk. Once fertilization has occurred, an embryo will start to develop. In the early stages this may appear as only a 'halo' formation with an indistinct ring formed around the central 'target cell'. If infection is suspected, swabs are taken from the inner surface of the shell membrane and yolk, and if the egg is fertile, also from the embryo and by aspiration from the chick's proventriculus (stomach). If the chick is sufficiently developed, it can be autopsied and tissue samples collected for microscopic examination.

Growing bacteria from egg contents is not uncommon as embryonic death has usually occurred several days before egg autopsy. Contamination through the shell membrane can easily occur, and the bacteria will easily grow if the parents continue to incubate. If autopsies are performed immediately after embryonic death, positive culture could result from a bacteraemia (bacteria in the blood) in the hen or from an oviduct infection. The principal sources of bacterial infection are, however, the cloacal surface and the nest. It is, therefore, very important that the environment within the nest box is hygienic. If the eggs are thin, cracked, poorly formed or with a roughened surface, the potential for bacterial contamination is much greater.

If a potential pathogen is isolated, and particularly if microscopic changes suggest a bacterial infection as the cause of death, measures can be instigated to prevent further problems. Potential infectious agents causing embryonic death include:

- ***Salmonella*** – This bacterium is excreted by carrier stock birds and can contaminate the nest site. In addition, it can infect the ovary and oviduct and can contaminate the egg before it is passed. It is controlled through identification and eradication of carriers, strict hygiene and the use of appropriate medication (e.g. Baytril).
- ***Chlamydia*** – This can also infect the hen and can be passed in the droppings, thereby contaminating the nest site. In certain stock loft situations, where *Chlamydia* has been accounting for a large number of embryonic deaths and respiratory infection in weaned youngsters, it may be appropriate to treat this organism through a 7 – 30-day course of doxycycline, the length of treatment being determined by the severity of the problem. However, as the introduction of further birds would run the risk of re-entry of the organism, it is then necessary to maintain the stock loft as a mini-quarantine station. This is not often possible. Also, developing youngsters do need some exposure to *Chlamydia* to develop a natural immunity to it. The problem can usually be satisfactorily managed through hygiene and good care of the stock birds so that chlamydial shedding is minimal.
- **Other organisms**, such as the bacteria *Staphylococcus* and *E. coli*, and viruses, e.g. Circo virus, and fungi, e.g. *Aspergillus* – Control of these problems can be difficult if they are identified after breeding has commenced. In lofts with a history of failed eggs, testing and appropriate preventive measures should be carried out before subsequent breeding seasons.

Possible causes of embryonic death

A small percentage (less than 5%) of all eggs resulting in dead-in-shell youngsters is normal. Possible causes of embryonic death vary, depending on the length of incubation:

- **During the first 12 days of incubation:**
  - **Improper conditions in the nest box** – Too hot, too cold, poor ventilation.
  - **Excessive jarring or shaking of eggs** – This is of particular relevance when the eggs are being transferred for fostering. The effect of thunderstorms is a total myth.
  - **Improper incubation** – Due to poor parenting, competition with other birds within the loft, older arthritic birds, poor nest-box design, improper nesting material, over-interference by the fancier, inadequate control of nest-bowl parasites, such as red mite and pigeon fly, failure to provide second nest bowl for next pair of eggs, too many birds in a section, disturbance outside loft, etc.
  - **Poor-quality eggs** – As mentioned earlier, cracked, thin, mis-shapened, rough eggs allow easier entry of infection and are more subject to trauma. This can indicate disease of the oviduct, which may be due to infection by such agents as *Salmonella* or *Chlamydia*, or, alternatively, a nutritional deficiency, in particular, calcium deficiency. As mentioned earlier, some fanciers will have noticed eggs with translucent, clear lines running around the outside of the egg, showing the egg's rotations as it was passing down the oviduct. These thin areas can be an early sign of calcium deficiency.
  - **Infection** – It must be emphasized that, even though infection in the egg can be due to an infection in the hen, most infection comes from the nest site itself, and so the maintenance of hygienic nest-box conditions will do much to decrease embryonic death.
  - **Poor parental nutrition** – Vitamin E, A, B and D_3 deficiency, also manganese and zinc deficiency, have all been linked to poor reproductive performance. Provision of a variety of

nutritious grains, one or more types of grit, a pick stone and pink minerals is often adequate to meet the pigeons' nutritional needs. However, if there is any doubt, a number of excellent additives are now available.

- **Genetic factors.**

Embryonic death after 12 – 18 days of incubation:

- **Improper incubation and nest-box environment –** In the last 6 days of incubation, the microenvironment within the nest box comes more into play. In particular, high temperatures or low humidity can cause the shell to become hard and dry, leading to chick exhaustion during hatching. Similarly, this can cause egg and chick dehydration, which can lead to the chick sticking to the shell, unabsorbed yolk sacs and residual albumin. Providing the stock birds with access to rain or a bath around the time of hatching helps to ensure the egg shell is not overdry or excessively hard. It's interesting reading some of the older bird magazine articles, which mention fliers licking eggs at hatching, presumably to achieve the same result. Poor incubation can also lead to differential rates of chick development, with the more developed chick interfering with the hatch and subsequent parenting of the second.
- **Malpositioned embryos –** As a result of poor incubation, abnormal egg size or shape, or other genetic factors.

Some factors that are a problem in early incubation continue to play a role, including:

- **Poor parental nutrition.**
- **Infection.**

In summary, embryo death is caused in most cases either by factors that adversely affect the temperature or humidity at which the egg is kept or alternatively by infection. That infection usually comes from either a dirty nest-bowl site or disease that the hen is carrying.

There are many advantages to examination of non-hatching eggs. The problem may be one of either infertility or of embryonic death. Investigation of this may identify problems with incubation associated with poor parenting, poor nest-box environment, inadequate nutrition, or infection. As some of the infections that affect hatching can also affect race performance, their identification and control are important.

Four-legged pigeons and other oddities

Occasionally pigeons are presented with a variety of congenital or developmental abnormalities. In 1997, a client rang to say that she had bred a pigeon with four legs! The pigeon was duly brought to the clinic. It was bright and well in itself and not only had four legs but also two cloacas. The extra pair of legs had limited function. However, the bird was able to pass normal droppings from each cloaca. For approximately 6 months the four-legged pigeon lived a relatively normal life but then after a short illness died. An autopsy revealed duplication of several internal organs. Such abnormalities are extremely rare and in this case was probably due to incomplete separation of identical twins.

Over the years, pigeons with no wings, extra toes, no rump, two beaks, extra tails and a variety of other abnormalities have been presented. Some are illustrated below.

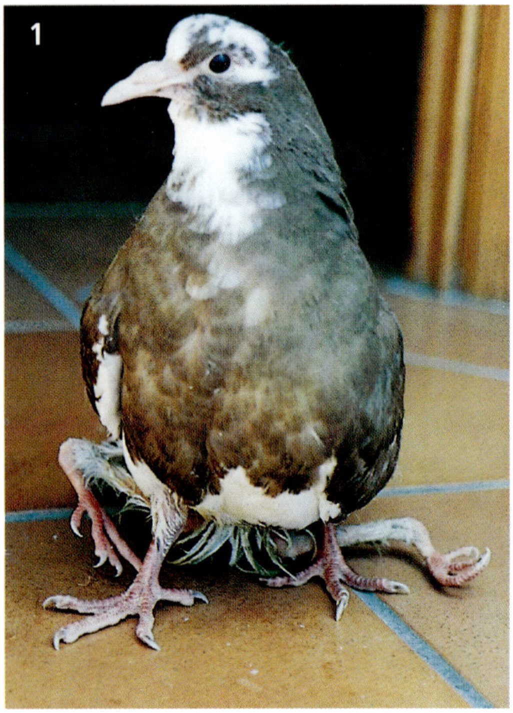

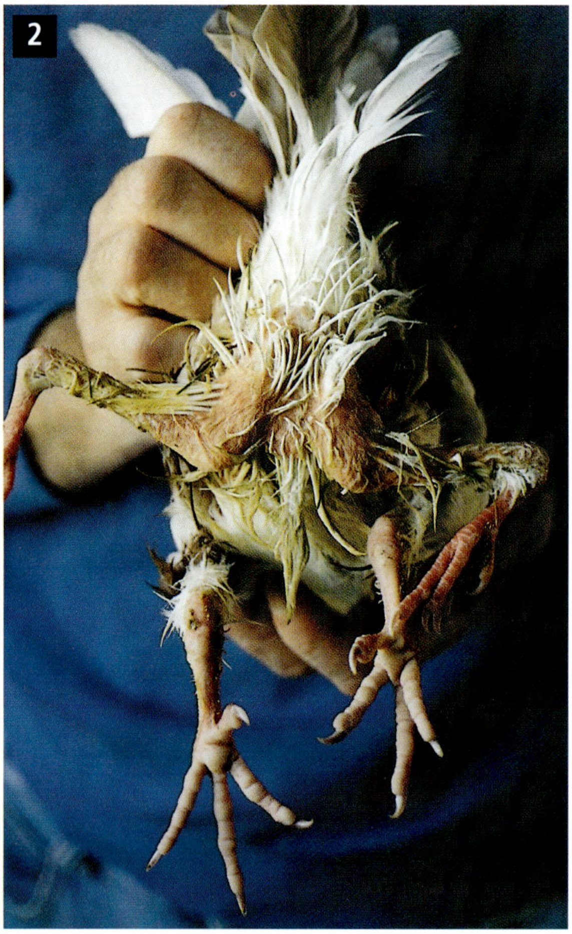

Photos 1 and 2: Four-legged pigeon.

Photos 3 and 4: Two genetic mosaics. Such birds are thought to be the result of two fertilized eggs fusing early in development.

Photos 5 and 6: Porcupine abnormality. A genetic failure of the feather sheaths to disintegrate and release each feather.

Photos 7 and 7a: Split keel. With an incomplete breast bone, this bird's heart was protected only by a thin layer of skin in the middle of the V formed by the shortened keel. The continual movement of the heart, beating against the terracotta nest bowl when it was a nestling, had partially eroded the skin covering it.

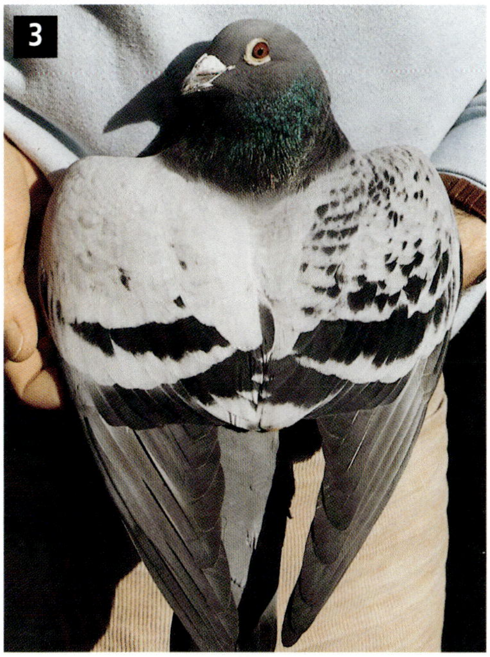
3

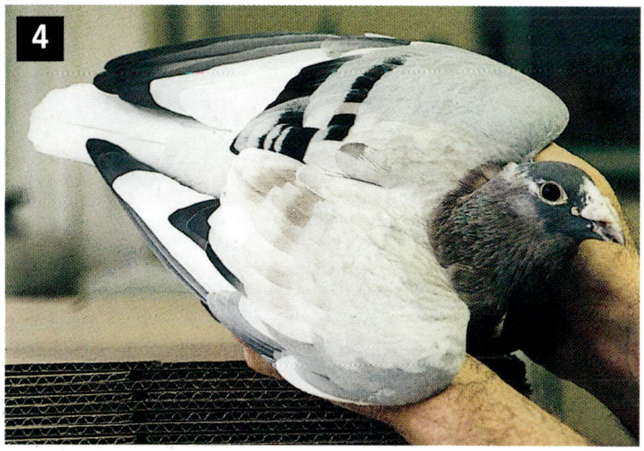
4

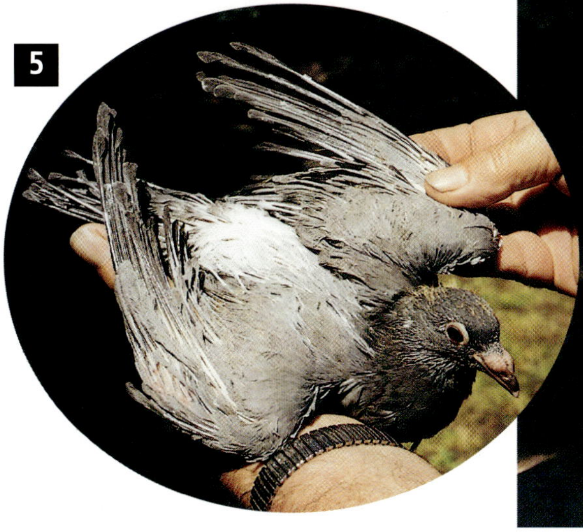
5

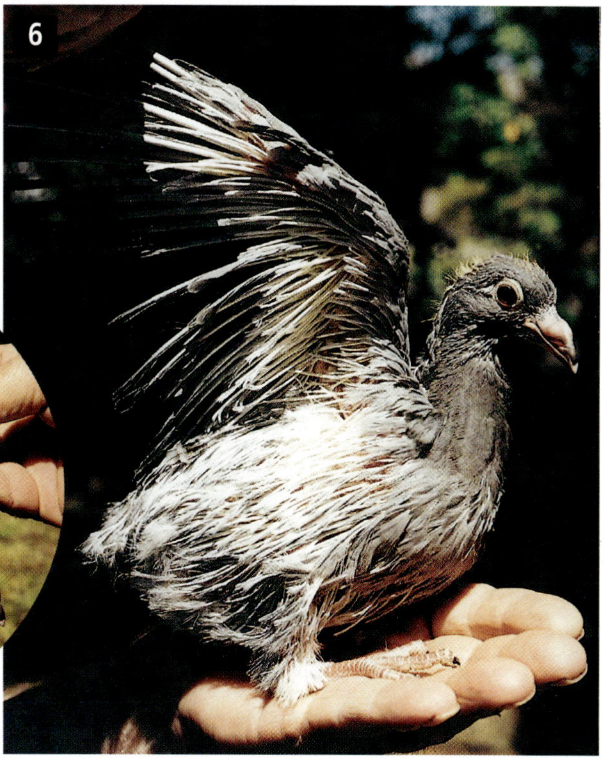
6

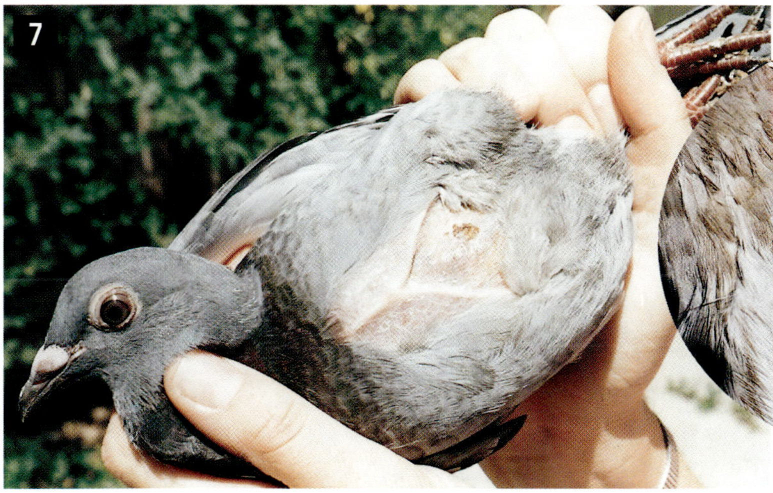
7

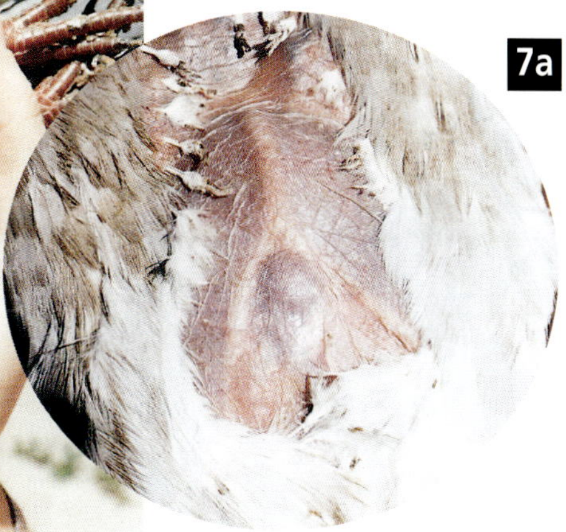
7a

Section 6

HEALTH PROGRAMS

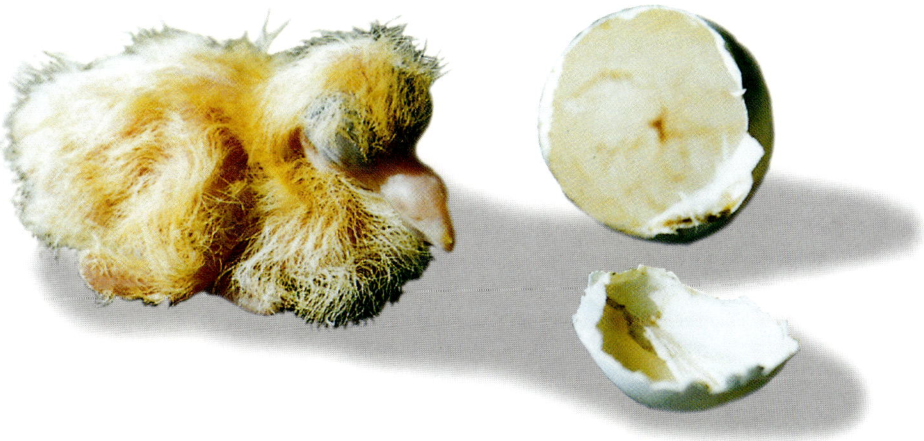

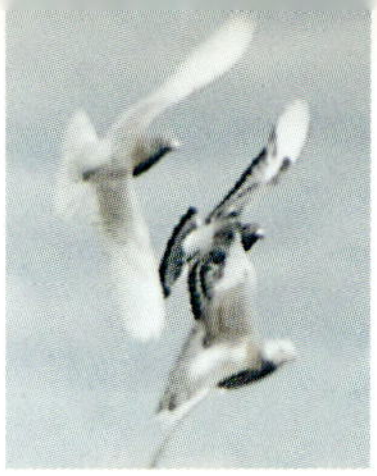

Chapter 29

PROGRAM DEVELOPMENT IN THE RACE LOFT

We have dealt with the diseases that are most likely to affect race birds, and their diagnosis and management during the season. We will now deal with how these diseases are prevented in a coordinated way and explain how programs can be established in various lofts. Veterinarians can always advise fanciers what they should and shouldn't do as regards health management but it is better if the fancier understands how and why these recommendations are made. In this chapter, I will discuss how a program for health management during the race season can be developed. The following chapter discusses health management programs for all parts of the pigeon year.

I think we all prefer to avoid medication during racing if possible, but at the same time don't want our birds' performance to be compromised by health problems. So let's go through how avian veterinarians develop programs to prevent disease. The critical diseases to control initially are the primary parasitic diseases, and in pigeons there are essentially three: worms, Coccidia and wet canker. They all weaken the bird and open the door for secondary problems. With control of these, many other problems will automatically come into line.

Worms

Worms are common and the number present in your race team before racing should be zero. Therefore, it is suggested that a dropping test be done on the birds to see if they are present. For fliers for whom access to an avian veterinarian may be difficult, it is best to assume that worms are present and to worm the birds. We can now develop the beginning of our program as set out below.

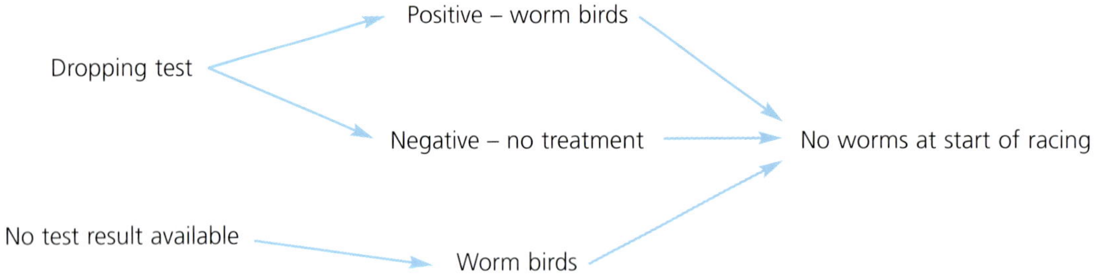

The four 'Ps' – planning prevents poor performance – effectively summarizes the aim of a health progam. Going into the race season free of worms, the birds should remain worm-free until the start of Thursday night basketing when the birds are fed and watered in the units. As the lifecycle of roundworms is 21 days, a test to check for this should ideally be done at least every 21 days after the start of Thursday night basketing. If no testing is available, again it is better to assume they are there rather than wait for the loss of form; treat to clear any that may be there every 21 days. Tapeworms, because of the need for an intermediate host, are not transferred in the race unit.

However, the birds should be monitored for these (segments are passed in the droppings if present) and treated if necessary.

Therefore, once the season starts,

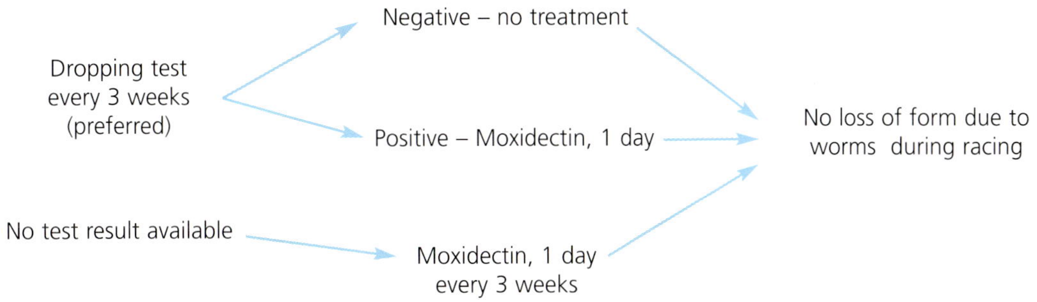

Coccidia

The trap with pigeon disease during racing is that if a bird looks sick then it is sick, but if it looks well it can still be sick. So much disease is hidden and it is only with the exertion of racing that problems become apparent. Our next primary parasite is Coccidia. Remember that birds that are stressed or run down for any reason are more likely to be bothered by Coccidia and it is more likely to be a problem in dirty, damp conditions. In lofts with a Coccidia problem, 2 days on Baycox as a rule will keep the birds' level of Coccidia low for about 4 weeks. To control Coccidia, we can draw up the following plan before racing.

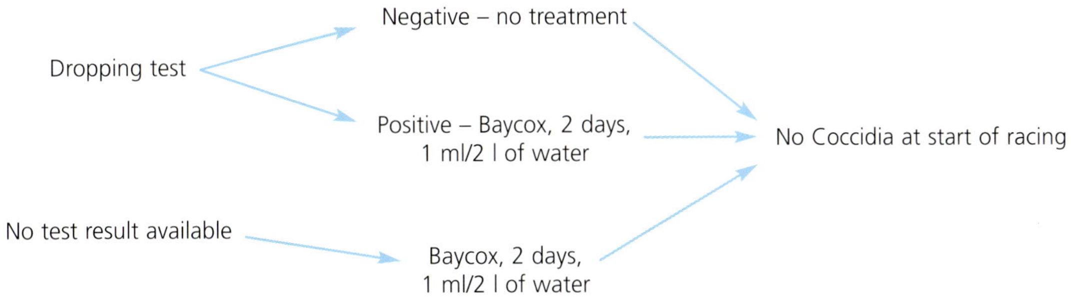

and during racing,

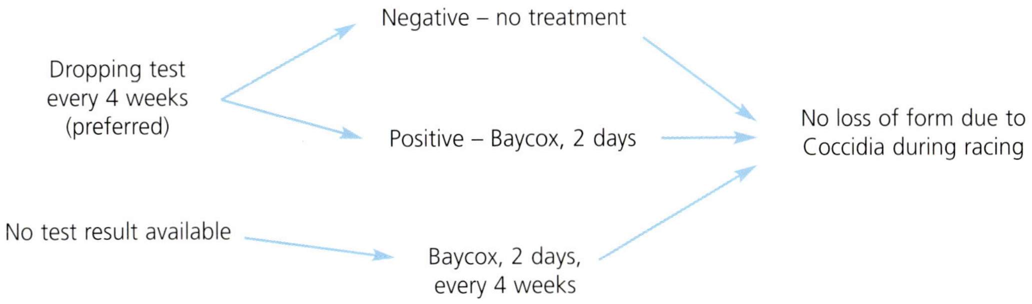

Canker

Dutch researchers now tell us that there are more than 25 strains of canker identified. Of these, only approximately six cause the formation of cheesy material that we as fanciers are familiar with. The others cause the non-visible but more insidious wet form of the disease. As the race season approaches, crop flushing of several members of the race team (it is usually best to test the saddest looking birds) will tell us whether some members of the race team have high trichomonad counts. If so, this means that the level of natural immunity formed by the birds is not yet solid and that with the stress of racing ahead they have the potential to break down and experience trichomonad flare-ups. As trichomonad numbers rise, race performance falls. Ideally, trichomonad numbers should be low at the start of the season. This can only be detected specifically by crop flushing. However, the dropping picture of lots of *E. coli* and yeasts, together with a *Chlamydia*-positive result is very suggestive. In the loft, these droppings are often olivey green and very watery. If testing is not available, and certainly if the birds are showing signs consistent with wet canker (red inflamed throat, exaggerated swallowing, penguin posture, dry feather, etc.), it is better to assume that trichomonads are there. In most lofts with a wet canker problem, it will take about 3 weeks for trichomonads to re-establish in any number after a 2-day course of anticanker medication. As time goes by, and the birds mature and their natural immunity becomes more solid, the treatment interval can be increased.

Before racing:

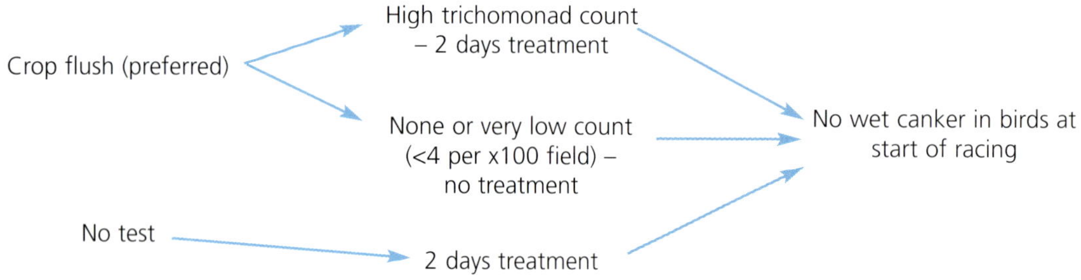

Once racing starts, the canker count needs to be kept low so as not to affect race form.

During racing

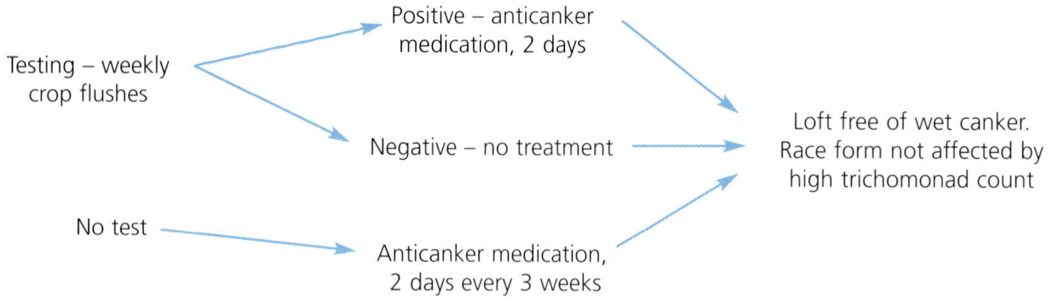

In lofts with a wet canker problem, regular crop flushing can usually establish how long after a 2-day course of an anticanker drug that the trichomonads re-establish. Once that interval is established for that particular loft (with its strain of birds, environment and management system), further testing often becomes unnecessary and medication can just be repeated at that interval.

Respiratory infection

With control of worms, Coccidia and wet canker, many other problems, notably respiratory infection, are less likely to arise. Treatment for respiratory infection is delayed before racing for as long as possible to allow the birds to develop as strong a natural immunity as possible. However, if, as racing approaches, the birds are showing signs of respiratory infection or if tests reveal evidence of an infection or if there has been a problem with respiratory infection once racing has commenced in previous years, medication is given. The aim of any treatment is to reduce the *Chlamydia* level in the birds so that more stress is required to cause it to flare up. In lofts that do not fit into these categories, medication is best avoided.

Before racing:

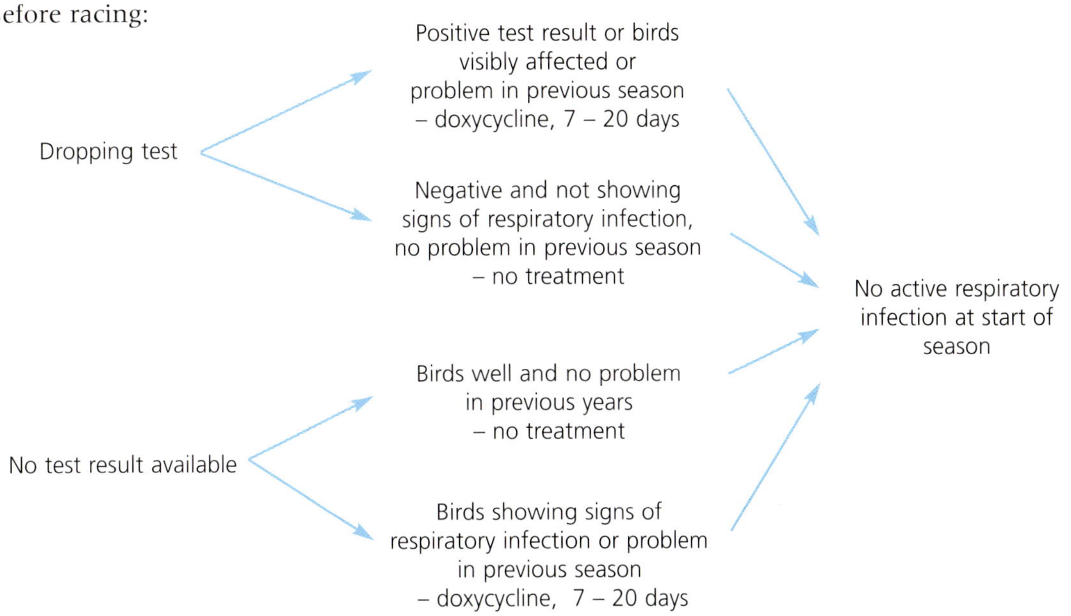

However, during the stress of racing and because of the exposure to potential pathogens in the race unit, respiratory problems are common, particularly in certain lofts and certain strains of birds. It is vital that the fancier vigilantly monitor his birds for respiratory infection, as birds with respiratory infection simply cannot perform optimally. There is no single best way to manage respiratory infection once racing starts. In lofts without a history of respiratory infection and with no clinical signs and where tests show no problem, it is appropriate simply to closely monitor the birds. However, if the birds do develop signs of respiratory infection or veterinary testing indicates the presence of an infection, treatment is given. The usual treatment is a 2 – 5-day course of Doxy-T. If there has been a problem in previous years, then it is likely to recur unless loft parameters have changed. Here, 2 days Doxy-T can be given every second or third Monday and Tuesday. Treatment intervals can be decreased or treatment time increased, depending on the severity of the problem and the control achieved. The basic aim at all times is to avoid antibiotics if possible but at the same time to ensure respiratory infection is controlled.

E. coli and yeasts

A change in the birds' droppings is often the first sign alerting the fancier to health problems in his birds. In race-age birds, olive-green and watery droppings are usually associated with *E. coli* or thrush. If these problems are present in birds before racing, they represent an on-going management or environment flaw. The fancier must evaluate these because both the increased rate of passage and the inflammation that these problems cause within the bowel wall offer the bird a decreased chance of getting the full nutritional benefit from its food. In birds with mild *E. coli* or thrush, the droppings will become olive-green but remain formed. With on-going stress and the advancement of the condition, the droppings become sticky so that the white urates appear smeared over the rest of the dropping. If problems progress further, the dropping becomes olive-green and watery. It is important for the fancier to try and identify any predisposing stress factors and if possible to correct these. If the predisposing factors cannot be avoided, e.g. a south-facing cold loft, then to ensure that the birds are able to get the full nutritional benefit from their food and be at their best at the commencement of racing it may be necessary to periodically use Probac when changes in the dropping are observed. More severe *E. coli* flare-ups may require a short course of an antibiotic, such as Sulfa AVS. If the fancier notices that his birds' droppings are deviating from the desired brown and nut-like quality, the exact cause can often only be evaluated through testing. The following plan can be adopted to control *E. coli* and yeasts (thrush).

Before racing:

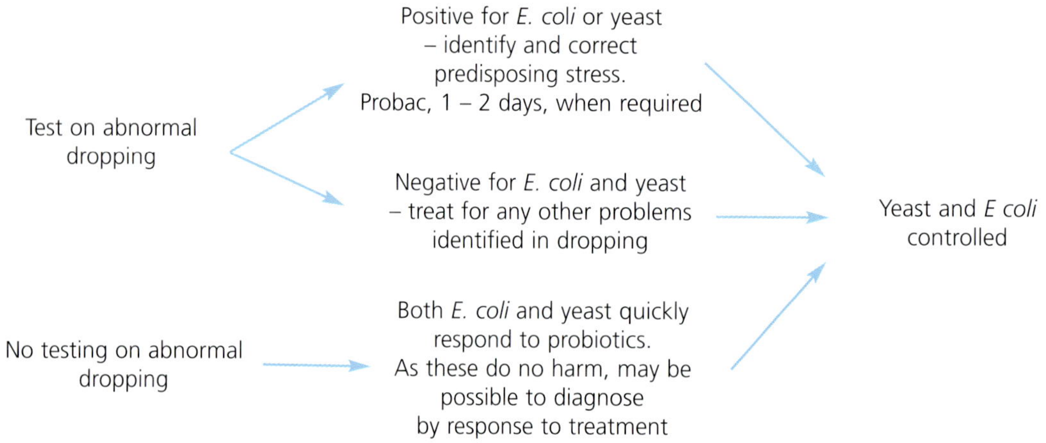

With the on-going stress of racing, *E. coli* and yeast flare-ups are common, particularly in lofts that experience this problem out of the race season, for the superimposed stress of racing exacerbates the problem. The team should be monitored and treated as the need dictates.

During racing:

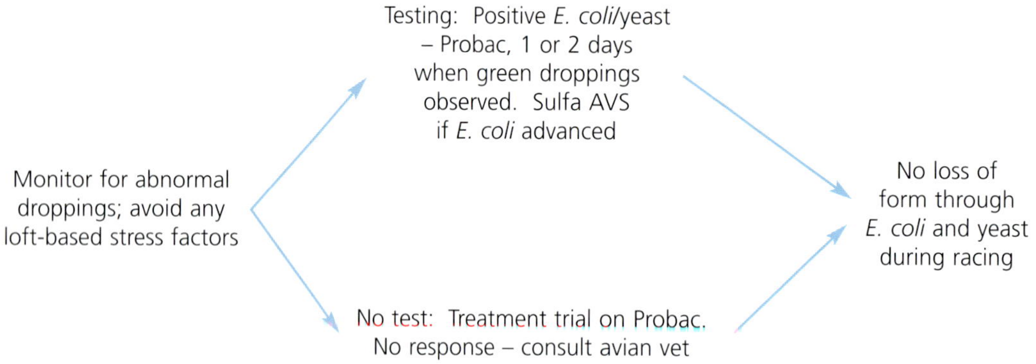

Combined protocols

In many parts of the world, fanciers do not have access to veterinarians with pigeon experience. The following is an attempt to assist both these fliers and fanciers that do have access to an avian veterinarian with their birds' health, both before and during the competitive season. Combining the above protocols, fanciers can see how the following recommendations have been developed.

Before racing

Where testing is available

- Faecal smear to check for worms, Coccidia, *E. coli*, thrush (and others).
- *Chlamydia* antigen test to check for respiratory infection.
- Crop flush to check for wet canker (and others).
- Treat as indicated.

Where testing is unavailable

The basic aim is to eradicate any pathogen that may be present, starting with the primary parasites.

- Moxidectin, 1 day (5 ml to 1 litre of water, 2 mg/ml) for roundworms and hairworms
- Prazivet, 1 day (5 ml to 1 litre of water) for tapeworm in susceptible areas.
- Baycox, 2 days, for Coccidia (1 ml per 2 litres of water).
- Anticanker medication, 2 days.
- If respiratory infection apparent or problem in previous season, doxycycline, 7 – 20 days.
- Monitor for green mushy droppings and use probiotics on the days observed.

During racing

Where testing is available

- Monitor health through dropping and crop flush analysis and treat as necessary.

Where testing is unavailable

- Moxidectin, 1 day every 3 weeks.
- Baycox, 2 days every 4 weeks.
- Anticanker medication, 2 days every 2 – 3 weeks in lofts with a wet canker problem.
- Monitor for green mushy droppings and use Probac for 1 – 2 days when required.
- Monitor for respiratory signs and give Resfite or Doxy-T for 1 – 5 days when observed, or, in a loft with a history of problems, give Resfite or Doxy-T for 2 days every second or third Monday and Tuesday.

A more thorough discussion of these protocols is covered in the following chapter.

Out of the race season, it is unlikely that pigeons in a good loft under a good manager, if fed a balanced diet with access to a good grit, will be lacking anything in their diet. However, pigeons in this regard are no different from us and as the 'Pluravit' (an Australian multivitamin capsule) ad says:

> *If you are working hard* (as pigeons are when tossing and racing) *or*
> *eating irregular meals* (as pigeons are when away in the unit),
> *vitamin and mineral supplements will help.*

Even subtle deficiencies will have dramatic effects on race form. It is important that the correct supplements are used because inappropriate ones, in fact, have the potential to decrease form. I feel that it is therefore a good idea once racing commences to incorporate the regular use of a vitamin/mineral supplement in a health program. Sunday is often a good day for supplementation.

It is best to avoid any unnecessary medication, and so always the preferred way to go is to test regularly through the season and treat as the need dictates. For fliers for whom testing is not available, it is a matter of using preventive medications strategically so that a problem caught in the race basket (bearing in mind that many birds from many different levels of care are in contact in the race unit) is not given a chance to establish and affect form for the rest of the season.

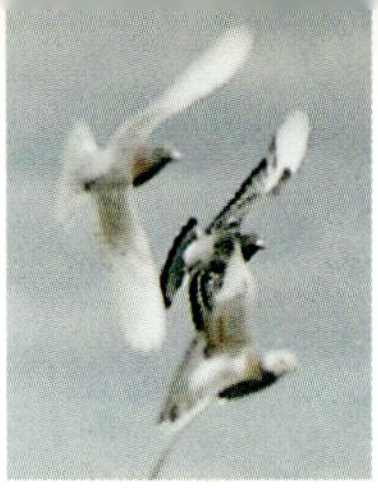

Chapter 30

HEALTH MANAGEMENT PROGRAMS FOR ALL STAGES OF THE PIGEON YEAR

The aim of any health program is simply to keep the birds healthy. Most fanciers don't want to waste time or money on unnecessary or incorrect treatments yet at the same time don't want to compromise the health of their birds by overlooking any beneficial treatment. Programs need not be unnecessarily complex. Mistakes in health management in the long term cause teams not to achieve their full potential and so for a program to be successful it is important that the fancier understands not only what he is doing but also why he is doing it.

For practical purposes, the pigeon year is divided into various stages, and so what should we as fanciers be doing at these various times to manage our birds' health?

Postweaning program 4 – 8 weeks of age

Principal aim: *To allow a controlled exposure to disease organisms so that the youngsters can develop a strong natural immunity to them. This is achieved by providing a stress-free environment and by avoiding the use of medication if possible.*

The routine use of medication during this time should be avoided. During the first few weeks after weaning, the birds are being exposed to a whole range of potentially harmful organisms. A youngster in a well-managed loft, however, does not become sick but rather through this exposure develops an immunity to the organism. Provided the youngsters are well in themselves, a low level of diseases such as wet canker, respiratory infection or Coccidia at this time can be regarded as beneficial in that it reinforces the growing youngsters' developing natural immunity. The use of medications at this time simply interrupts this exposure, with the result that the birds' level of natural immunity is not as high. For this reason, a youngster is only treated if a health problem progresses to the point where the bird is sick in itself and individual bird treatments rather than flock treatments should be given. Flock treatments are only given if there is evidence of a spreading infectious disease or more than 5% of youngsters are affected. Health problems that appear during this time are categorized into one of four types. These are outlined in the chapter Medical Problems in Young Pigeons.

For a youngster to mount a good immune response and, in the process, form a strong natural immunity following exposure to disease organisms, it must be stress-free. Stress compromises the function of the immune system. The avoidance of stress in the postweaning time is also covered in the chapter but essentially it involves weaning batches of youngsters together as groups, being hygienic, avoiding overcrowding and dampness and ensuring that the birds' full nutritional needs are met.

Supplementation

During this time, pink minerals, grit and preferably a pick stone should always be available. A water-soluble multivitamin, e.g. Multivite Plus, can be placed in the water for 1 – 2 days per week, while a probiotic, e.g. Probac, in the water for 1 – 2 days per week helps maintain a full beneficial population of bowel organisms, ensuring full digestion and assimilation of nutrients. Seed oil additives, e.g. Polyseed Oil, can be used to advantage and increase the energy and calorie content of the seed mix. They can be used either by themselves or with a yeast. Garlic Oil is of particular benefit during this time because it is not only nutritious but contains the compound allicin, which is a natural immune stimulant.

Moulting programs

Principal aim: *To have a good moult, resulting in the production of a lustrous set of feathers, and to allow on-going development of a strong natural immunity. This is achieved through the maintenance of a stress-free environment, drug avoidance, parasite elimination and a complete diet.*

Approximately 3 weeks after weaning, the youngsters will start to moult. The process is accelerated in all birds, irrespective of age, in February in Australia with the shortening daylength. As this total replacement of feathers only occurs once a year, a new set of feathers must last the bird for its entire first year of competition. Poor feather quality compromises performance and so it is vital that everything is done to ensure that the new feathers are good.

Healthy stress-free youngsters moult quickly and the feathers they grow are of good quality. Conversely, birds that are sick for any reason take longer to complete their moult and the feathers they produce are not as lustrous. It is therefore important that the basic principles of on-going good care already established in the postweaning time and discussed in the chapter Weaning continue. During this time, medications are still best avoided if possible, the aim being to further strengthen the birds' developing natural immunity through low-grade on-going exposure to various organisms. The parasites, however, must be eliminated now.

Parasites

Internal parasites rob the birds of nutrition that would otherwise be available to them and compromise the moult. It is therefore vital that the birds are free of roundworm, hairworm and tapeworms and either have a low level of Coccidia or none. A low level of Coccidia is still permissible at this time because the youngsters' natural immunity is still developing. Hairworm, roundworm and Coccidia are all detected in a microscopic dropping analysis and this is often the best time for the fancier to send in his first dropping sample for examination for the season. Tapeworms are not a microscopic diagnosis because they can be seen with the naked eye. The different types of tapeworm vary in size. The small ones look like white pieces of cotton trailing through the dropping, larger ones look like pieces of rice stuck on the surface of the dropping, while the largest ones appear as whitish squares up to 0.5 x 0.5 cm either singly or stuck together as ribbons in or on the droppings. What we are actually seeing here are the tapeworm egg packets and, though not continually, they are regularly intermittently passed by infected birds.

Many fliers prefer to routinely treat preventively for worms and Coccidia at this time of year and, unless testing is done to confirm that the birds are free of these parasites, this is a good idea. As some wormers can affect feather quality (e.g. Panacur, Synanthic), it is vital that the correct wormers are used. I recommend for roundworm and hairworm Moxidectin 2 mg/ml (5 ml to 1 litre of water for 24 hours) and for tapeworms Prazivet Liquid (5 ml to 1 litre of water for 24 hours). If Coccidia levels are too high (i.e. more than one every second x100 microscope field), then they are best treated. I recommend Baycox (1 ml to 2 litres of water for 48 hours). Remember after worming for hairworm and roundworm that the loft must be thoroughly cleaned as any droppings passed before treatment may contain worm eggs and therefore have the potential to reinfect the birds. Hygiene is not as vital for tapeworm infection because they do not transfer directly from pigeon to pigeon through the droppings but are instead carried by insects, particularly slaters. (I think this is because slaters, when disturbed, roll themselves into balls, which the birds then mistake for peas.) To prevent reinfection it is therefore best to spray out the loft with Permethrin Solution (see section on parasitic diseases in The Common Diseases for correct use) the following day.

External parasites must be eliminated before the commencement of the moult, otherwise irreparable damage to the feathers is done. Moxidectin, as well as eliminating roundworm and hairworm, also eliminates all external parasites that suck blood. It therefore clears all mites (including airsac mites) but has only limited action against lice. To eliminate lice totally, the birds need to be dipped. The preferred product here is Permethrin Solution. As all lice live on the bird, a single treatment will eliminate all lice from the loft until they are reintroduced with strays, deliberately introduced birds and late returning race birds. However, only a percentage of mites infecting the birds are actually found on the bird at any one time. Many live in the cracks and crevices within the loft. To prevent reinfection, it is therefore important that the loft is sprayed with Permethrin.

MEDICATION

Many of the common drugs used during this time, including, as mentioned earlier, some of the wormers, affect feather quality. Antibiotics (particularly Baytril and Sulfa AVS, and to a lesser extent doxycycline, Resfite and Doxy-T) if used during this time not only interfere with the development of natural immunity by interrupting the on-going exposure to organisms but also compromise feather quality and so their use is best avoided. They compromise feather quality by killing many of the beneficial bacteria in the bowel. These are necessary for digestion and the assimilation of nutrients. Their disruption by antibiotics interrupts the on-going delivery of nutrients to the growing feather within the feather follicle. Turbosole and other anticanker drugs do not disrupt the bowel bacteria and so can be safely used.

SUPPLEMENTATION

Any nutritional deficiency during this time also results in poor-quality feathers and so suggestions made under Supplementation in the Postweaning Program hold true here. In particular, the birds need to have good levels of iodine (found in some pink minerals, e.g. PVM Powder, and some vitamin/mineral supplements, e.g. Multivite Plus) in their diet for the moult to proceed quickly. Supplementation with unsaturated fatty acids (found in seed oils) aid in the production of lustrous silky feathers in birds (and interestingly also a glossy coat in mammals) and so their use is particularly recommended during this time.

If disease appears during this time, the same basic principles are followed as in the Postweaning Program. Flock treatments are avoided unless at least 5% of birds become affected. Unwell birds are treated individually. Those that do not respond within 4 days are usually best eliminated.

Prerace program

Principal aim: *Having allowed as much time as possible for the birds to form their natural immunity, it is now a matter of assessing what health problems are persistent and then using drugs if necessary to get the birds completely healthy before the first race.*

The veterinary attitude toward health management changes 6 – 8 weeks before the first race. Up until this time, apart from parasite control, medication is avoided unless the birds in themselves become unwell. Low levels of various potential health problems, in particular wet canker and respiratory infection, are tolerated so that the birds, through exposure to low-grade disease, can develop as strong a natural immunity as possible to them.

In many well-managed lofts, the birds' natural immunity will be such that, when screened for disease in the last weeks before racing, none is apparent. However, as racing approaches, it is important that any identified health problem be eliminated. I recommend that before fanciers embark on their final long tosses before the first race, and preferably several weeks earlier, droppings and birds be brought to the clinic for a health profile. Any persistent health problem is then cleared with medication so that the birds can be completely healthy at the first race.

For fanciers who are at a distance from the clinic and not able to bring birds to the clinic, droppings can be mailed in. Dropping analysis enables a check for worms (hairworm and roundworm and sometimes tapeworm), Coccidia, *E. coli*, thrush and fungi. Dropping analysis also gives an indication as to the general health of the birds, in particular whether they are likely to have wet canker or respiratory infection. Presentation of a live bird enables a more accurate assessment of not only wet canker and respiratory infection but also of less common problems such as *Hexamita* (a canker-like organism that lives in the bowel).

Parasites

Before the start of racing it is essential that the birds are parasite-free. To this end, if parasites are detected in the droppings, or a dropping analysis is not possible, the following protocol is adopted:

- For hairworm and roundworm, external mites and airsac mites: Moxidectin, 5 ml to 1 litre for 24 hours.
- For tapeworms: Prazivet Liquid, 5 ml to 1 litre for 24 hours.
- For Coccidia: Baycox, 1 ml to 2 litres of water for 48 hours.
- For lice: dipping in Permethrin Solution.

Wet canker

If wet canker is detected on testing, has been a loft problem in earlier years or a test is not possible, all birds are given a 2 – 3-day course of Turbosole. If this is extended to a 7-day course, it will kill any *Hexamita* that may be present.

Respiratory infection

If respiratory infection (including mycoplasmal airsac infection) has been a problem in earlier years, then a 7 – 20-day course of Doxy-T is given. If respiratory infection purely due to *Chlamydia* has been a problem, Doxy-T can be replaced by doxycycline 12%. The course of Doxy-T or doxycycline 12% should be completed 2 – 3 weeks before the first race and should be followed by a 2 – 3 -day course of Probac. It is best, though not essential, to remove the grit, sand or other minerals during Doxy-T treatment.

Supplementation

In addition to actual medication, other preparations can be used to not only maintain health (which is really just the bottom line) but actually promote fitness. Multivitamins, mineral supplements and conditioning oils can be used to build fitness as race day approaches.

Race programs

Principal aim: *To maintain winning form through the entire season by good management and the maintenance of health.*

During competition, medication is used to maintain health. It is vital that the birds are completely free of any health problems to give their best. Winning birds are always not only fit but also healthy. If the natural immunity they have formed is not strong enough to keep them healthy during the inherent stress of racing, then medication is used to ensure that health is maintained, so that success can be on-going and unnecessary losses avoided.

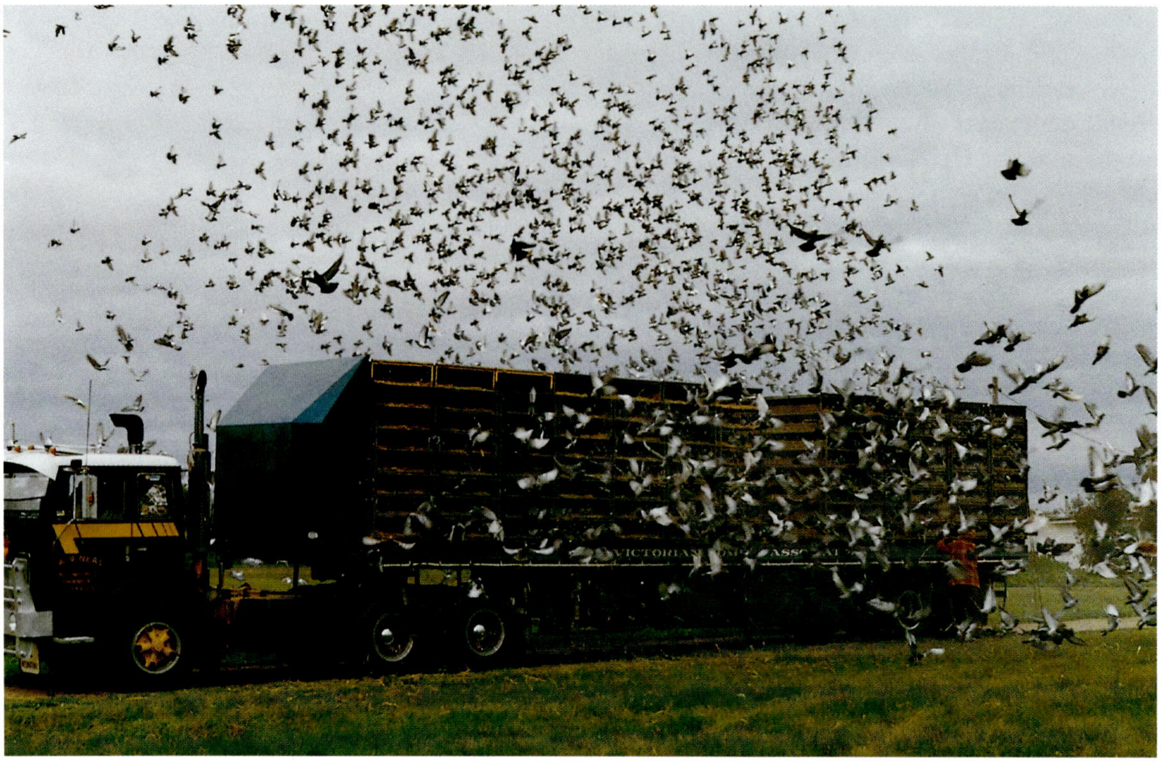

The 15,000 entrants in the first V.H.A. old bird race for 1989, from Wycheproof to Melbourne (150 miles), head for home.

Unless the genetic base of the birds kept has changed, or the way they are managed has altered, then it is very likely that any health problems that occurred in previous years will predictably reappear in a particular loft. This is why successful preventive programs can be reapplied to particular lofts year after year. Some health problems are more likely to occur in particular types of loft and in lofts in particular locations. This explains why a program that works well in one loft is inappropriate in another.

Medication serves another purpose. Out of the race season, exposure of loft members to birds from other lofts is minimal, while once racing starts there is sudden and immediate high exposure to many birds from many different lofts. In this way, birds become exposed to different strains of disease-causing organisms, in particular strains of wet canker and respiratory infection. Because these strains may not be resident in their own loft, they cannot possibly have developed an immunity to them. For this reason, disease can flare up, even in well-managed lofts, with resultant sudden loss of form and variable losses. Medication is used to minimize the impact of this exposure.

When to treat

Veterinary attitude has changed since 1990 as to how to treat birds on race return. Before 1990, many lofts did not contain the wet canker and respiratory strains that are common today. Treatment was aimed at preventing or delaying the entry of these organisms into lofts that were still free of them. To this end, it was recommended that medications such as Turbosole and Resfite were placed in the water of returning race birds usually at slightly higher doses. The medication that the birds took in with the single big drink that they had upon return, although not enough to treat an active infection, was often adequate to prevent infection establishing following a recent exposure. Since this time, through sales, transfers of birds, etc., wet canker and mycoplasmal airsac infection have become steadily more and more common so that now most lofts do in fact contain some strain(s) of these organisms. Treatment protocols have moved away from treating returning race birds (although this is still worthwhile in some lofts) to periodic short courses of medication to keep resident wet canker and respiratory strains in check during the stress of racing. These short courses also serve to lessen the impact of exposure to a new strain on loft health. Regular short courses keep a new strain under control while the birds establish a natural immunity to it.

There are other practical considerations. To be effective in preventing the entry of disease, medication for returning race birds must be given after their return but before these birds mix with other birds in the loft. This usually means treating them as soon as they return. This makes it impossible to use other useful postrace treatments such as electrolytes and probiotics. If returning race birds are treated the next day, i.e. Sunday, this means they must be kept apart from other birds in the loft until this time. If returning race birds have mixed with other non-race birds, there is no point in treating just them on Sunday. Under most management systems, it is important from the birds' motivation point of view that they be allowed access to their perch, box or mate as soon as possible after return. This can be difficult if medication is delayed until Sunday. In addition, some postrace drugs are bitter, which can deter returning race birds from drinking fully, while in fact it is very important that returning birds drink well in order to rehydrate.

These days, the usual recommendation is to focus on recovery from the race on Saturday and then to use either Sunday and Monday or Monday and Tuesday as the days to give any medication that may be necessary. Usually all birds in the loft, i.e. those that have raced that weekend and those that haven't, are treated. If a fancier tosses non-race birds on Sunday or there are stragglers from Saturday's race, then usually Monday and Tuesday are used.

To speed race recovery on Saturday, I recommend either electrolytes, multivitamins or probiotics be given. If the race has been hot, or especially hard, or if the birds look distressed upon return, I think it is best to give electrolytes. Alternatively, if the race has not been especially taxing, multivitamins or probiotics are preferred. I find that the droppings from returned race birds the following morning are more likely to be brown and tight and that the birds will maintain a feather down drop if probiotics are given as they return

Health monitoring

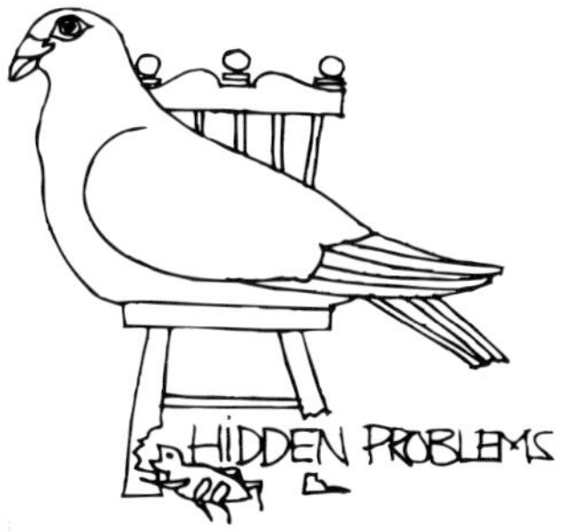

All disease problems that can affect form, except wet canker and respiratory infection, can be detected from the droppings. Birds that have wet canker or respiratory infection because they are sick are not able to mount a good immune response and so opportunists in the bowel, particularly *E. coli* and thrush, sometimes take advantage of the birds' run-down condition and multiply. The presence of elevated numbers of these organisms alerts the fancier to the possibility of these problems. However, their presence is by no means specific, and also, to confuse things, not all birds with wet canker or respiratory infection will have these changes. I recommend that droppings be regularly examined microscopically during racing, usually every 1 – 3 weeks. This detects all other problems and not only enables effective treatment for them but also avoids treatments that may be unnecessary.

Wet canker and respiratory infection are the two most serious and common causes of poor race performance and yet are the two most difficult to detect by the fancier in the loft. Both problems are now so common that I feel that it is not possible to achieve consistent success without vigilant monitoring or regular treatment for them. Wet canker and respiratory infection sooner or later will catch up with the lax fancier. Wet canker can be definitively diagnosed and accurately monitored with crop flushing because the causative agent, the living trichomonad, is seen. Respiratory infection can sometimes be diagnosed with a crop flush. In a respiratory infection, inflammatory material drains from the sinuses through the slot in the roof of the mouth into the throat or alternatively is coughed up from the inflamed windpipe lining into the throat. A crop flush gathers this material, which can be detected microscopically.

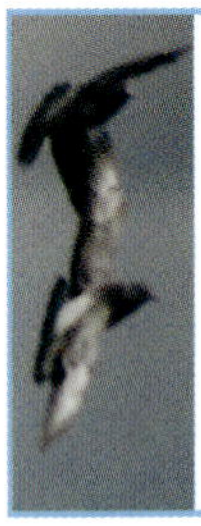

Wet canker and respiratory infection are very common problems during racing. The fancier who does not control these well, and sometimes this will mean the use of medication, can expect to lose more birds and not clock as many prizewinners as the fancier who does.

Medication

It is important to remember that antibiotics should not be given closer than 2 days before basketing. All cause some disruption to the normal bowel bacteria (more so with Baytril and Sulfa AVS, less so with Doxy-T, Resfite and doxycycline), which then take several days to re-establish. An antibiotic course even of only 1 – 2 days during racing should always be followed by 1 day on Probac in order to replace the normal bacteria as quickly as possible. Turbosole is not an antibiotic, only killing canker organisms, and so therefore can be given any day of the week. However, when wet canker is a problem, Turbosole is best given early in the week so that the birds have a chance to 'lift' after having the trichomonads cleared.

E. coli and thrush during racing are usually treated with Probac. This can be given any day of the week and indeed more and more successful lofts are not only using it for this purpose but are also using it to advantage to maintain a healthy beneficial population of bowel bacteria at all times during racing. I usually recommend Wednesday and Sunday (for Thursday night basketing) as the best treatment days for Probac because the first dose sets the birds up for the race and the second helps them recover. However, Probac should always be the first line treatment when the droppings become green or mushy during racing.

It is worth mentioning here the mixing of drugs. The two most commonly mixed drugs are anti-canker drugs such as Turbosole and antibiotics such as Doxy-T. Many fliers do this with success, however, recent evidence shows that mixing any antibiotic with Turbosole does slightly decrease the potency of both. Also, I am concerned that putting several things in the water makes the water less palatable for the birds. This means the birds drink less and may not receive an adequate dose of either medication. However, there are some instances when these disadvantages have to be weighed against the number of days available. With a limited number of days, we sometimes need to mix medications so that the birds receive all medications that they need.

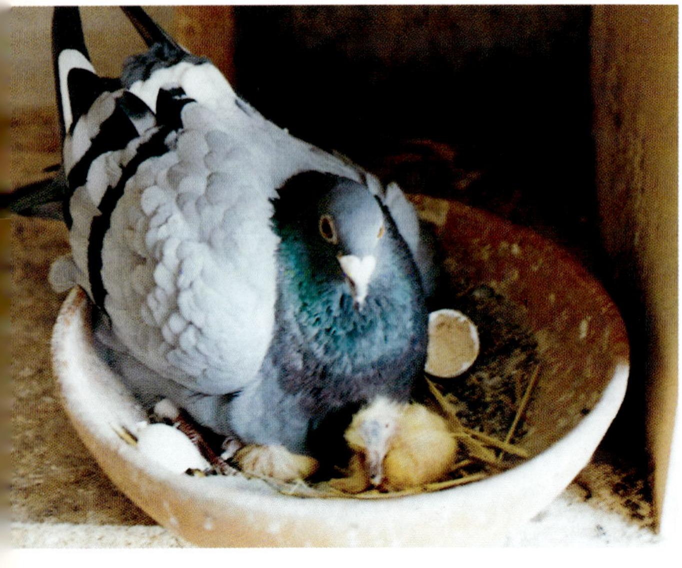

Stock hen with her recently hatched youngsters.

Supplementation

A range of conditioning agents and multivitamins can be used during the season and, although not directly treating disease, do help the birds resist disease by promoting their health generally. I feel that it is good to incorporate a good-quality multivitamin, such as Multivite Plus, in the loft health protocol once or twice weekly. During racing, birds can miss meals through being late and sometimes eat irregularly through being away from the loft racing. The use of a multivitamin helps ensure that they are not lacking something in their diet. Seed oils together with yeasts when added to the grain increase the energy and calorie content of the seed mix and are a way of making an especially nutritious meal for the birds. Some fliers use such agents always on a particular day of the week; however, I feel this to be a mistake. Such products put condition or weight on the birds, which obviously at particular times is advantageous but at other times is not. An astute fancier can use such products as needed to bring his birds into race condition. Just how often they are used should be based on the birds' condition (assessed by handling and observation of loft flying). As a general rule, however, they are of benefit during cold weather, following hard tossing or hard racing, if the birds are underweight and during disease recovery.

I recommend the following base plan for control of wet canker and respiratory infection during racing.

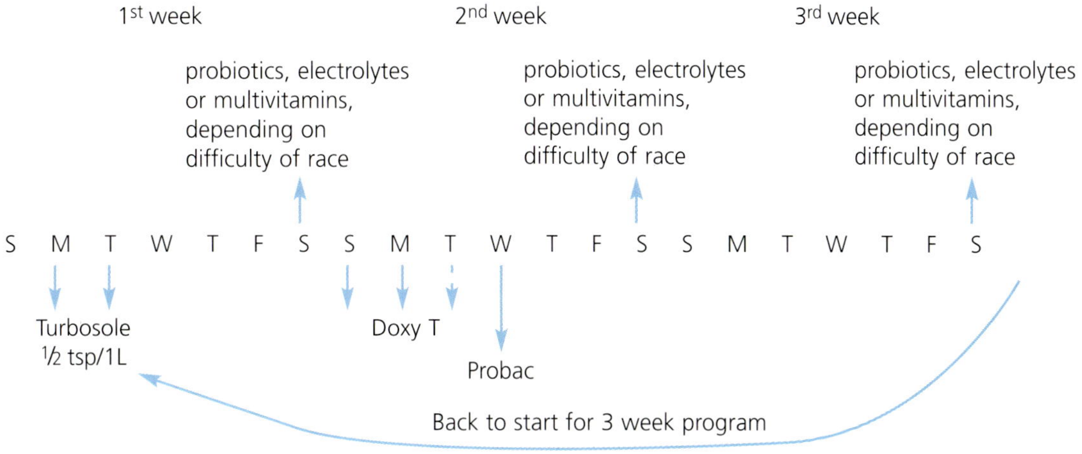

In most lofts, 2 days on Turbosole every 3 weeks will keep wet canker under control while 2 or sometimes 3 days on Doxy-T every 3 weeks will keep respiratory (including airsac) disease under control. If necessary, the week without treatment is eliminated, changing the program from a 3-week rotation into a 2-week one. This means that Turbosole and Doxy-T are given on alternate Mondays and Tuesdays.

With severe flare-ups of respiratory infection, a longer course of Doxy-T needs to be given, usually 4 – 5 days before reverting to 2-day courses every 2 – 3 weeks until the problem is fully resolved. These shorter follow-up courses keep the problem under control while the birds' natural immunity rises and race fitness re-establishes. The onset, however, of respiratory infection during the race season is always a blow because not only do the birds need to throw off infection and become fully healthy, but they then must re-establish their race fitness. Meanwhile, the races are getting longer and longer, which can make it very hard to catch up. Often a loss of form lasting 4 – 6 weeks is experienced.

Drug resistance is always a possibility. I have not seen this with Doxy-T, as yet, probably because Doxy-T already contains two very effective drugs and so an organism would need to develop a multiple resistance for it not to work. If a flyer feels that Turbosole is not giving quick clearance of trichomonads he has three options:

1. **Use Turbosole for longer, i.e. 3 – 4 days –** This is quite reasonable because Turbosole can be given right up to the day of basketing; birds can safely be sent to the race with it in their crop.
2. **Substitute every third or fourth treatment with another anticanker drug –** All birds can be picked up for 2 days in a row and given 1 Spartrix or 1/4 Flagyl tablet each day, or alternatively a 2-day course of Emtryl can be given in the water. Extreme care, however, must be taken using Emtryl during racing because of its narrow safety margin, particularly in hot weather.
3. **Turbosole can be combined with other drugs –** Turbosole can be placed in the water and at the same time all birds are given a 1/4 Flagyl or 1 Spartix each daily for 2 days in a row.

Of the three alternatives, I usually recommend option 2.

Summary

- Turbosole for 2 days every 2 – 3 weeks, usually Monday and Tuesday.
- Doxy-T for 2 – 3 days every 3 weeks, usually Sunday, Monday and sometimes Tuesday.
- Probac –
  - for 24 hours after Doxy-T;
  - when droppings become green or watery; if there is no response, droppings will need microscopic analysis; and
  - considered for use on Wednesday and Sunday as a conditioning agent.
- Seed oils and yeasts added to food on any day of week, based on birds' condition.
- Water-soluble multivitamin in water is best given by itself and can be given 1 day per week on spare days, e.g. Friday.
- Dropping analysis every 1 – 3 weeks. Other treatments, if needed, e.g. for Coccidia and worms, can be given on the third blank week.

This is a good basic program and in most lofts will keep the birds healthy and competitive through the entire season. It must be appreciated, however, that there are many variables affecting health through the season and so modifications to this are sometimes necessary depending on events arising. It is a long season and health varies with time and the change of weather that occurs from the start to the end of the season. Problems that may be present early in the season often disappear as the birds get older, their immunity rises and the weather gets warmer so that the need for certain medications falls away. This occurs with such problems as *E. coli*. At other times, there can be a sudden drastic change in the loft's health status necessitating a change in health management, e.g. the introduction of a new *Mycoplasma* strain.

Prebreeding health program

Principal aim: *To start the breeding season with healthy stock birds.*

Health control in the stock loft is very different from in the racing loft. This is because there is not the continuous potential exposure to disease through strays and returning race birds in the stock loft as there is in the race loft. It should be possible to eradicate many problems, in particular parasites, from the stock loft and then by treating any new birds before introduction to maintain the stock loft as a mini-quarantine station. This is not possible, however, if there is exposure to the droppings of wild birds and so, for this reason, any flights should have suspended or grid floors.

Worms

The level of worms in the stock loft should be absolutely zero. Hairworms and roundworms are cleared by giving a 24-hour course of Moxidectin.

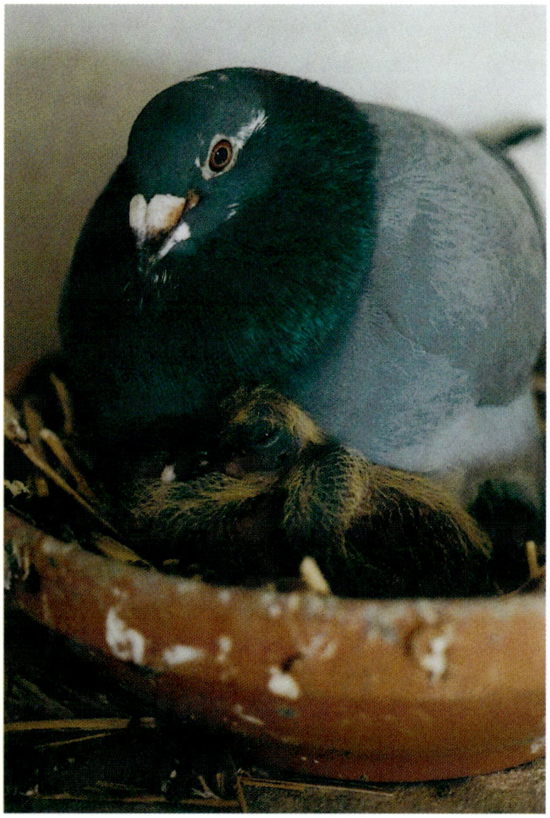

Young stock cock with his week-old baby.

It is vital that the loft is thoroughly cleaned afterwards to ensure that the birds are not reinfected from droppings containing worm eggs passed before medication. If in doubt, it is best to repeat the worming 3 weeks later and again thoroughly clean the loft. The eggs of these parasites can survive for up to 6 months in the environment, If there are aviaries with dirt floors that cannot be thoroughly cleaned, then to achieve control, Moxidectin can be given for 1 day every 3 – 4 weeks spanning this time. The longer-term answer, however, is to insert a suspended or grid floor or a floor that can be thoroughly cleaned.

Tapeworms are treated with Prazivet for 24 hours and reinfection prevented by spraying simultaneously with Permethrin Solution.

Coccidia

In lofts with a Coccidia problem, the Coccidia level can be decreased by giving a 2-day course of Baycox in the 2 weeks before pairing. Repeat 2-day courses in these lofts would need to be given approximately every 4 weeks once the birds are paired to ensure on-going control of this problem. However, on-going coccidial problems are usually associated with environmental or management flaws and often the longer-term answer to controlling this disease is to review these loft factors.

External parasites

Moxidectin will kill all mites on the birds and most lice. To eliminate all lice completely, the birds are dipped in Permethrin Solution. This is a good idea anyway as it has a 4-month residual effect and provides good long-term protection against the insects causing problems during breeding. It is also a good idea to spray out the nest boxes with Permethrin before pairing. Mosquitoes carry pigeon pox, pigeon flies cause irritation, anaemia and are associated with wet nests, mites breed in the warm conditions of the nest box and all other insects, particularly slaters, carry tapeworm. Therefore, before pairing I always spray with Permethrin.

Respiratory infections

Various *Chlamydia* strains are carried latently in some lofts. This means that they are found within the birds' system and flare up, causing problems when the birds come under stress. The outbreaks usually occur during breeding (when the stock birds are under stress) and during racing (when the race birds are under stress). In the stock loft, signs range from infertility, weakened youngsters that die during incubation, during hatching or in the nest, poor babies and excessively run-down parents. In the race loft, we see variable signs of respiratory infection (e.g. eye colds, dirty ceres), poor performance, occasional sneezing, mushy green droppings and failure to come into condition. In lofts that have experienced problems with *Chlamydia* in previous breeding seasons, the birds are treated with doxycycline 12%, not to clear the *Chlamydia* but rather to reduce it to a level at which it is less likely to cause problems. The usual treatment course is 7 – 30 days. The actual length of treatment for a loft is dependent on problems experienced in earlier years. In lofts without these problems, it is best not to treat. Because of the long treatment required in some lofts, ensure that preventive programs are started in sufficient time. Doxycycline does interfere with calcium and vitamin metabolism and does disrupt the normal beneficial population of bowel bacteria. For this reason, treatment courses should cease at least 2 – 3 weeks before pairing and courses should always be followed with multivitamins, calcium and probiotic supplements. If you are unsure about the need for medication, please seek veterinary advice before breeding as the problem is difficult to control once the birds are paired. Once the birds are paired, the best we can do is 'band-aid' the problem, i.e. patch up the problem after it has arisen through strategic short courses of medication to minimize the effect of the disease.

Canker

Control of this problem before breeding has been dealt with extensively in the chapter Canker. In lofts with a canker problem in last year's breeding season, it is usual to decrease the trichomonad burden of the stock birds by giving a 5 – 7-day course of Turbosole 4 weeks before pairing. This means that it will take more stress before the birds shed sufficient numbers of the organism to give their nestlings the disease. In lofts without a canker problem, it is best to give no medication.

Special note on calcium supplementation

Feeding stock birds have high requirements for calcium. It is therefore vital that they are supplemented with calcium once paired. No matter how much they take in (particularly the hens) once paired, they cannot assimilate as much as they are losing from their system in the production of crop milk and egg shells. The difference is made up by mobilizing calcium stored in the skeleton before pairing. It is important that stock birds have access to calcium all year and particularly once mated. Low levels of calcium lead to soft-shelled eggs, egg binding, post-egg-laying paralysis in hens, poor-quality crop milk, slow-growing babies and babies with undermineralized soft bones (the best way to assess this is by gently pushing the lower beak to the side). I recommend that stock birds have pink minerals, shell grit and a mineral block in front of them all year and that, once paired, in addition have calcium solution in the water 1 – 2 days per week.

Summary

- Hairworm and round worm: Moxidectin 24 hours.
- Tape worm: Prazivet 24 hours.
- Coccidia: Baycox 48 hours.
- Dip all birds and spray loft (in particular nest boxes) with Permethrin Solution.
- Doxycycline 12% for 7 – 20 days in lofts with *Chlamydia* problem.
- Turbosole for 5 – 7 days in lofts that had canker last breeding season.
- Finish program 1 – 2 weeks before pairing.
- Upgrade calcium intake once paired.

Breeding season program

Principal aim: *To produce healthy, robust young ready for weaning at 28 days and to maintain the health and condition of the stock birds*

During breeding, it is best to focus on good management (no overcrowding and good hygiene), good feeding and providing the correct supplements. If health problems appear during breeding, it usually reflects a flaw in the prebreeding management of the stock birds. Water-based medications are hard to administer accurately during breeding because of the variable water intake of stock birds feeding youngsters of different ages. Drugs, in particular antibiotics, should be avoided now as many have adverse effects on the youngsters or parents. For example, Baytril has been associated with embryonic deaths and abnormal joints in growing babies.

Most health problems in breeding relate to canker. In lofts where this is a problem it is managed as discussed in the chapter Canker. In summary, decrease the number of babies that develop canker by decreasing the number of trichomonads shed by the parents with periodic 2-day courses of Turbosole given every 1 – 3 weeks as the need dictates. Monitor the youngsters daily and treat those with canker with a daily dose of Spartrix until well. Feeding stock birds that suddenly become unwell and lose weight almost invariably have an internal canker nodule. Separate these and give 4 drops Baytril, twice daily and 1/4 Flagyl or 1 Spartrix daily. Disappointingly, many of these, by the time we realize they are unwell, have passed the stage where they will respond to treatment.

Stock birds that desert nests and pale slow-growing youngsters are often associated with red mite. These move on to the birds during the night to drink blood. Look for the tell-tale crusty 'pin pricks' under the babies' wings where the mites were attached and feeding during the night. This problem can be avoided by dipping the birds and spraying the boxes with Permethrin Solution before breeding. These measures can still be implemented, although not as easily, if mites appear after the birds are paired. Further problems are discussed in the chapter Problems of the Breeding Season.

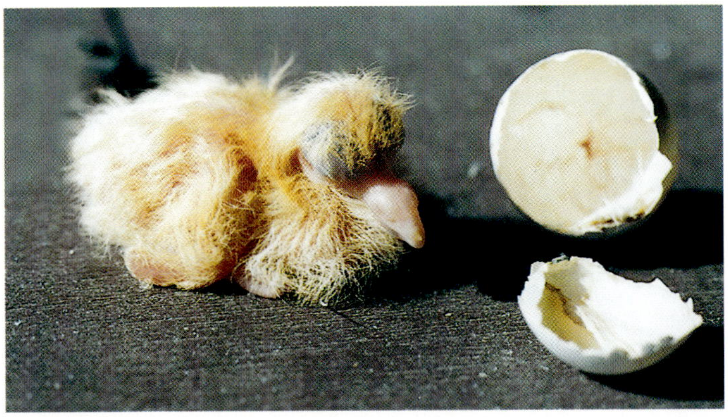

Once stock birds are feeding, the physical and nutritional demands drastically increase. Supplementing with seed oils and yeasts will help them maintain their condition and help them produce robust babies. Pink minerals, grits and pick stones should always be available.

Left: A healthy youngster – the same bird at hatching, and at 7 and 21 days of age.

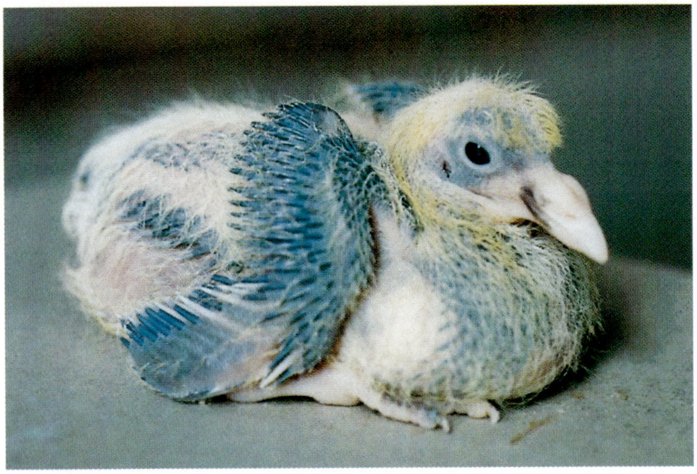

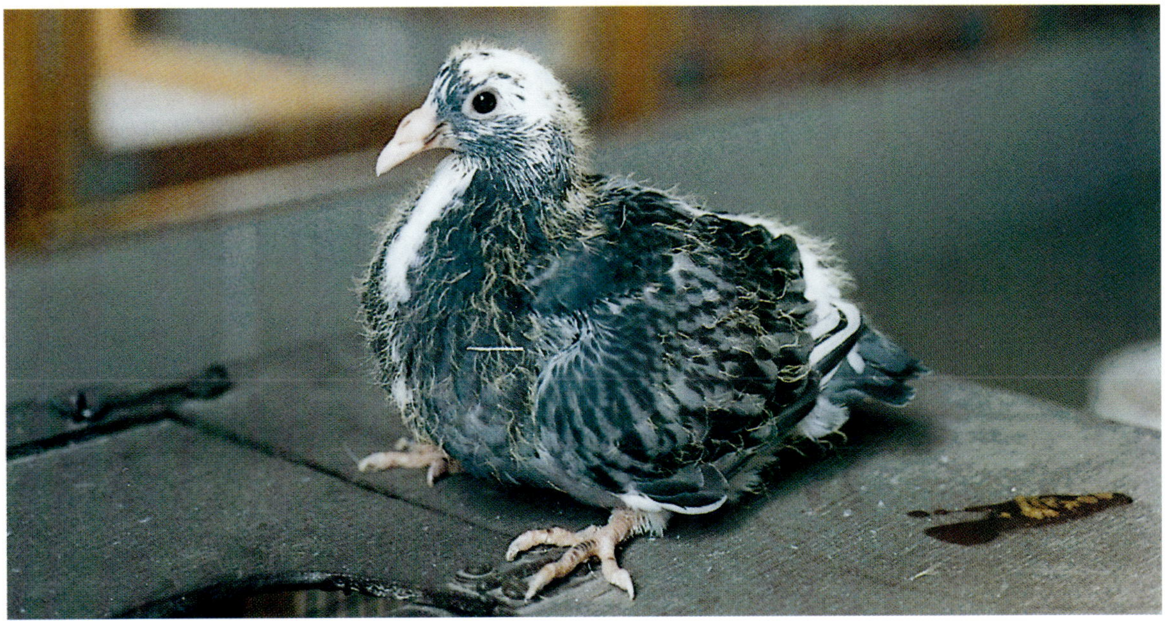

Section 7

MANAGEMENT KEYS TO AID PERFORMANCE AND IMPROVE CLOCKING TIME

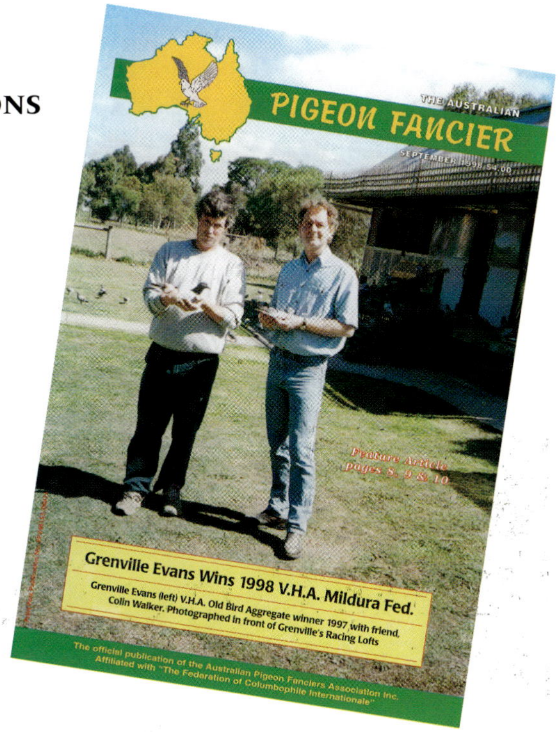

The author with V.H.A. champion for 1998 and 1999, Grenville Evans, in front of Grenville's racing loft.

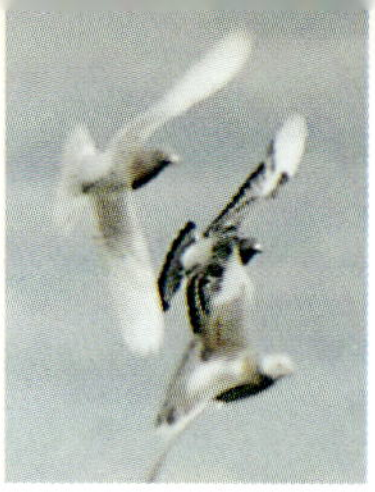

Chapter 31

LOFT DESIGN

There are two things that use a pigeon loft – the fancier and the birds – and a loft should be designed with the needs of both in mind. The importance of a good loft cannot be overstated. Without a well-thought-out loft, it may not only be impossible to get the birds into winning form, but make the fancier's job of managing the birds more difficult.

From the pigeons' point of view, the loft must basically be a place that they like and want to return to quickly. It must be a place where they feel safe and secure, where they know they will find food and water, where they can be healthy, and also where they can breed, if appropriate.

From the fancier's point of view, the loft should make it easy for him to manage and enjoy his birds. It should be easy to catch the birds, both for casual inspection and on a larger scale for tossing and racing. It should be easy to feed and water the birds, easy to clean and provide for easy management of the racing system used, be it natural, widowhood, etc. In addition to these things, for a loft to be competitive, it must create an environment where the birds can come into form. To come into form, the birds must be healthy and motivated. Once healthy and motivated, it is the birds with genetic quality that will win.

Designing a loft to maintain health

For a team to be competitive, the birds must be healthy. To be healthy, they must live in a good loft. A good loft must satisfy the basic criteria of being dry, without being dusty, whilst at the same time provide sufficient ventilation without exposing the birds to extremes of temperature or humidity. If these basic criteria are met, the loft will be successful; however, there are further advantages in being able to control the environment within the loft. Pigeons have a temperature and humidity

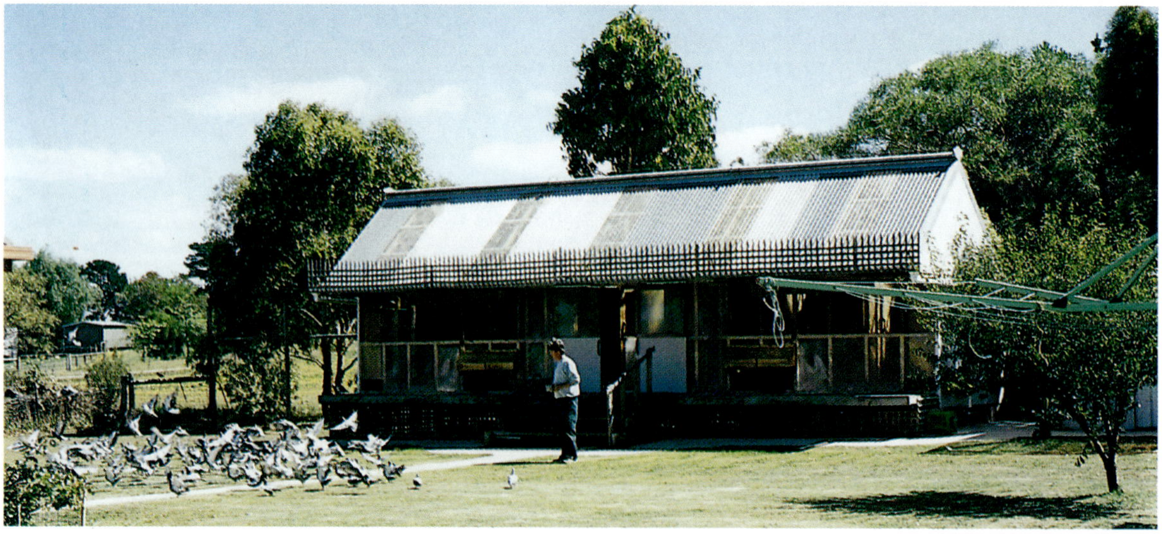

Racing loft of Grenville Evans, Melbourne. This loft contains many features that assist in temperature and humidity control. The loft has a high gable with a capping vent. Panels that clip under the front eave can be lowered to cover the front open sections, depending on the weather.

range that is ideal for them, and within which they are most likely to be in form. The better the loft is at controlling temperature and humidity so that the pigeons are kept close to this optimal, then, logically, the longer the team will spend in form. Designs that achieve this will vary from area to area, so that in cold areas, like Tasmania, in southern Australia, a successful loft will need to be considerably more enclosed than one in Queensland in Australia's warmer north. Obviously, though, in any area, the weather varies, and so the answer is a loft whose ventilation can be adjusted

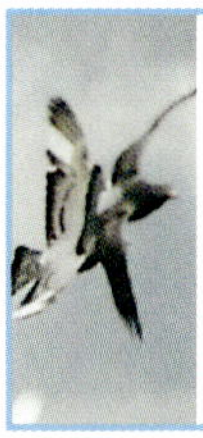

A good loft must satisfy the basic criteria of being dry, without being dusty, whilst at the same time provide sufficient ventilation without exposing the birds to extremes of temperature or humidity.

depending on the weather, so that the environment in the loft remains optimal for the birds. I believe the days of the loft solid on three sides and open at the front, as was common in Australia 20 years ago, are gone. In such lofts, there can be no environmental control, so that when it is cold, the birds are cold, and when it is hot, the birds are hot. Birds in such lofts can be put off form by something as simple as a change in weather, e.g. a cold snap. Obviously, as this is beyond the fancier's control, it is very frustrating if he wishes to be consistently successful. Many successful fliers have realized this for a long time, and this is why such emphasis is placed on systems that control temperature and humidity, such as sliding roof panels, adjustable louvres, loft heating and ventilation systems.

Different sources vary about the optimal temperature for a loft. Some say that the ideal temperature in the loft is 15 – 20°C, others say 20 – 25°C, but all agree that a more critical variable is the temperature fluctuation over a 24-hour period. If the temperature varies more than 5°C over a 24-hour period, it seems harder to achieve consistent form. Fanciers can use a maximum – minimum thermometer to check their own loft's variation. Pigeons can appear healthy at much colder temperatures. However, it has been my experience that birds in cold, open lofts seem to have trouble

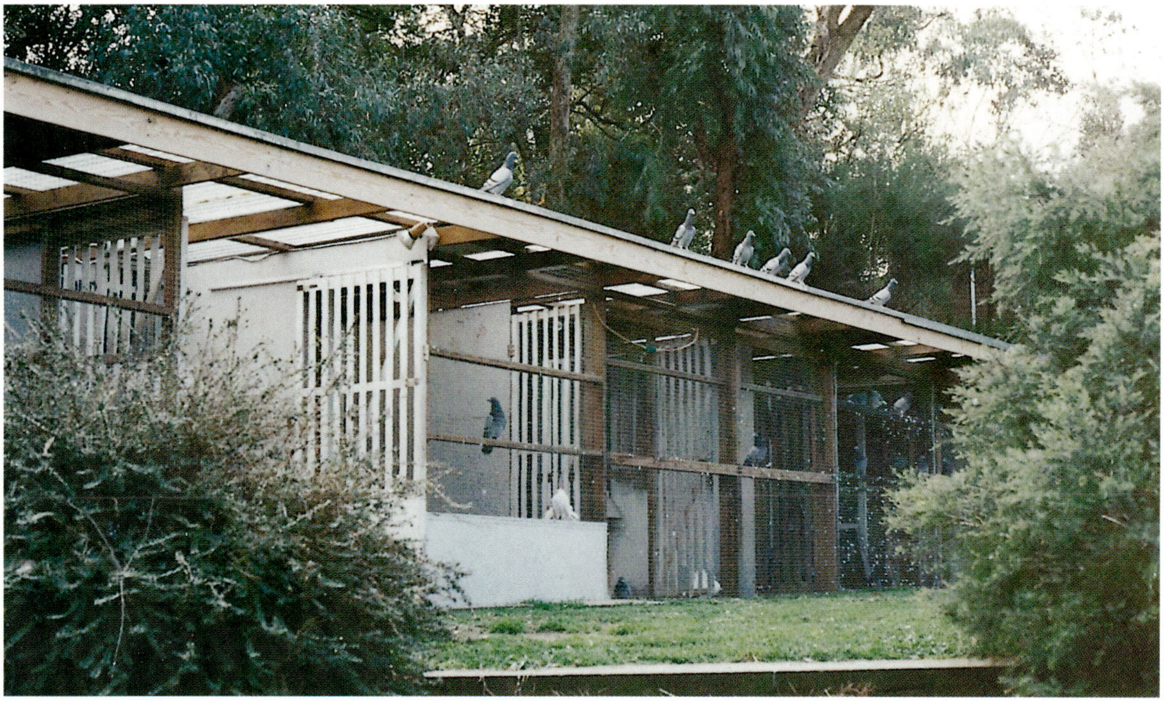

Australian garden loft, the race loft of Geoff Wardle, Melbourne.

with high Coccidia levels. Pigeons are able to tolerate single stresses, such as a cold loft, however, when stresses start to overlap we see a breakdown of the pigeons' defences and a vulnerability to secondary, opportunistic diseases such as Coccidia and subsequent poor race performance. A normal racing pigeon is subject to much stress as part of its normal life in the form of time away from the loft, irregular feeding regimes, and exposure to disease in race units and to predation by birds of prey, quite apart from the exertion of competition. It is therefore important that any controllable stress, such as loft environment, does not compound this. Some lofts work with the birds coming into form easily and others just don't, and the outward appearance and cost of construction may have little bearing on this. However, all lofts that do work satisfy the basic criteria mentioned earlier.

As well as temperature, the humidity will alter daily in the loft. An English fancier told me that if a block of salt, left on the loft floor for the birds, became damp, then the ventilation system in the loft was inadequate. This can serve as a simple loft test to indicate humidity levels. On warm days, the birds cool themselves by evaporation of moisture from their throat and airsacs, and the droppings will dry quickly, all increasing humidity. In cold weather, droppings will remain damp in the loft and moisture will condense on the walls and ceiling. Unless the loft is sufficiently ventilated, a stuffy, humid or damp environment can result; however, if the loft is too open, temperature control then becomes difficult. In this situation, it is important that these droppings, together with their moisture, are removed every morning. But how does one design a loft with these factors in mind?

I think one should begin by assuming that air movement should be basically upward as it is warmed by the birds. This air can carry dust, moisture and gases with it, and must be given an opportunity to escape. Ideally, this is achieved by a gabled roof with tiles with a false ceiling below, alternatively a gabled roof with air vents, or finally a flat roof with vents at the top of the walls. Once we know that stale air is escaping, we can then decide how much air we need to enter. The amount of air entering is controlled by how open the walls are, bearing in mind that too open a design makes temperature and draught control difficult. The amount of air required is dependent on the number of birds within the loft and environmental temperature and humidity, and so, as mentioned, appropriate designs will vary from area to area. The weather changes throughout the year, as does the number of birds, particularly in the race loft. To my way of thinking, the answer here is a wall through which air movement can be controlled, so that on cold windy days the loft can be

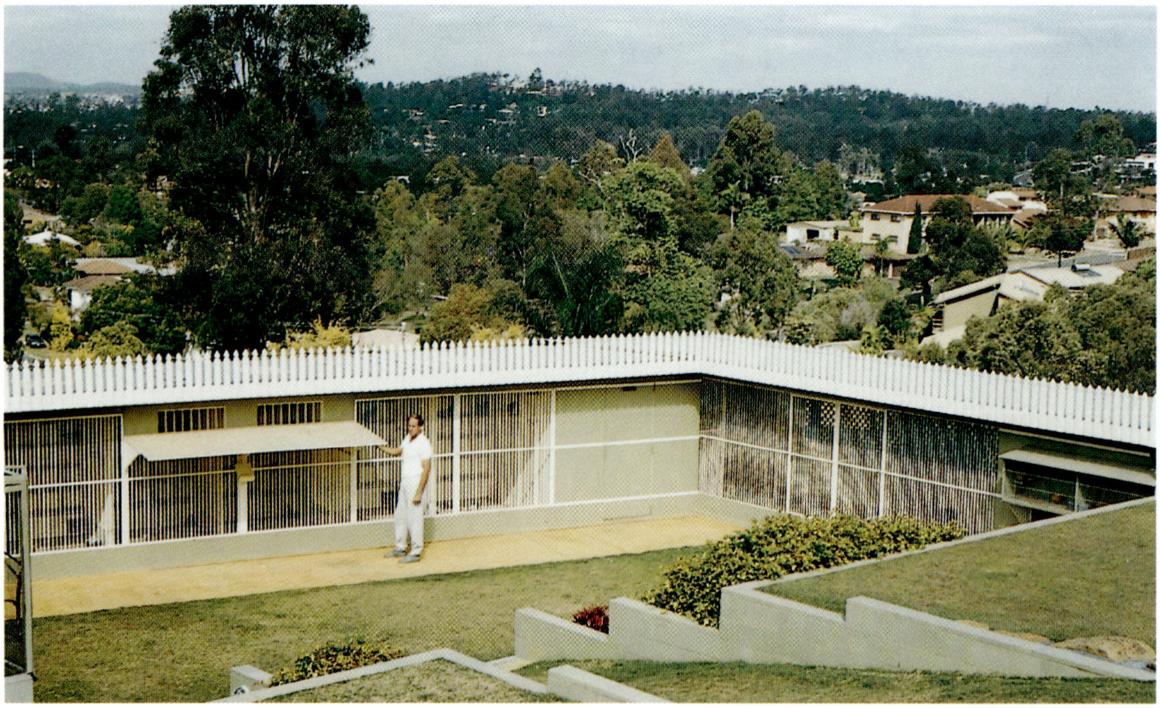

Race loft of Robert North, Brisbane.

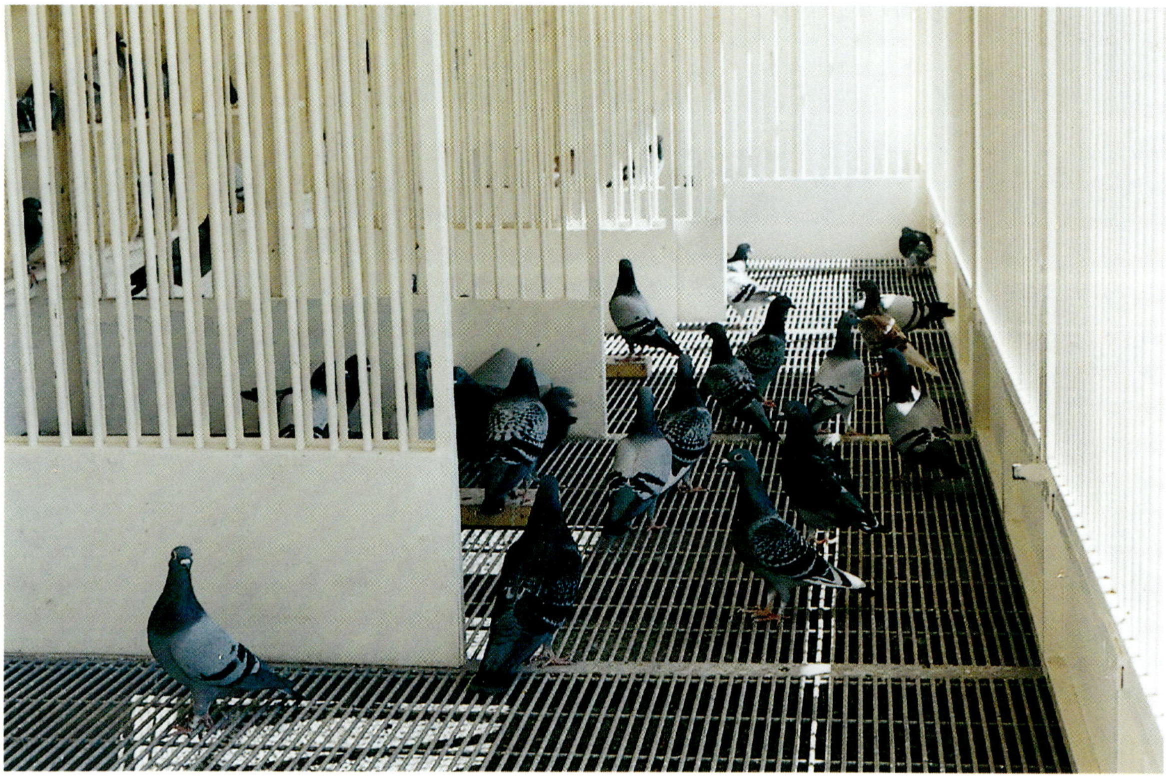

View inside the race loft of Robert North, Brisbane. Note the grid floors.

closed up and on warm sunny days it can be opened. This can be achieved by louvres, which can be opened or closed, or a variety of vents and adjustable windows. If necessary, the false ceiling can be fitted with adjustable panels to control the upward rise of air, and in very warm areas, insulation in the walls may be necessary.

If louvres or windows are used, I feel it is good to have these frosted as there are strong advantages in the birds, once in the loft, not being able to see out. An important part of every exercise program is rest. And when not at liberty, noise and movement outside the loft only disrupt the birds while they are resting. This has particular advantages in Australia where birds of prey are so prevalent. Not only can the pigeons not see them, but goshawks, in particular, cannot see the pigeons and do not aggregate around the loft or hang off the loft wire.

The floor in the ideal loft should be heated. This enables the floor to be quickly dried on cold days and the loft to be warmed if necessary. This can be achieved by heating coils in a concrete slab or, alternatively, by using heating pads. However, I feel the main criterion for flooring is hygiene. In a garden situation, the floor can be made of several materials, including concrete, wooden planks or metal grids. If concrete is used, it should be made as smooth as possible. It has the advantage of being hygienic and easily cleaned. It can, however, become quite cold and sometimes damp and is often best covered by a floor dressing such as a sprinkling of sand or straw. Interestingly a study done in America has shown that the most dustless floor is one covered with a light sprinkling of fresh sand. This apparently traps the dust particles. The pigeons appear to appreciate this as part of their natural behaviour is to scratch and peck. Care must be taken with any floor covering not to allow it to become dusty and it must be changed as necessary. If necessary, a vacuum cleaner can be used. Dusty lofts can predispose birds to respiratory infection. A wooden floor has the advantage of offering a more absorbent surface but, at the same time, is harder to clean because of its irregular texture. It is also virtually impossible to sterilize if an outbreak of disease occurs where the organism survives in the environment, such as paratyphoid. Wood, however, is a surface that pigeons like walking and lying on.

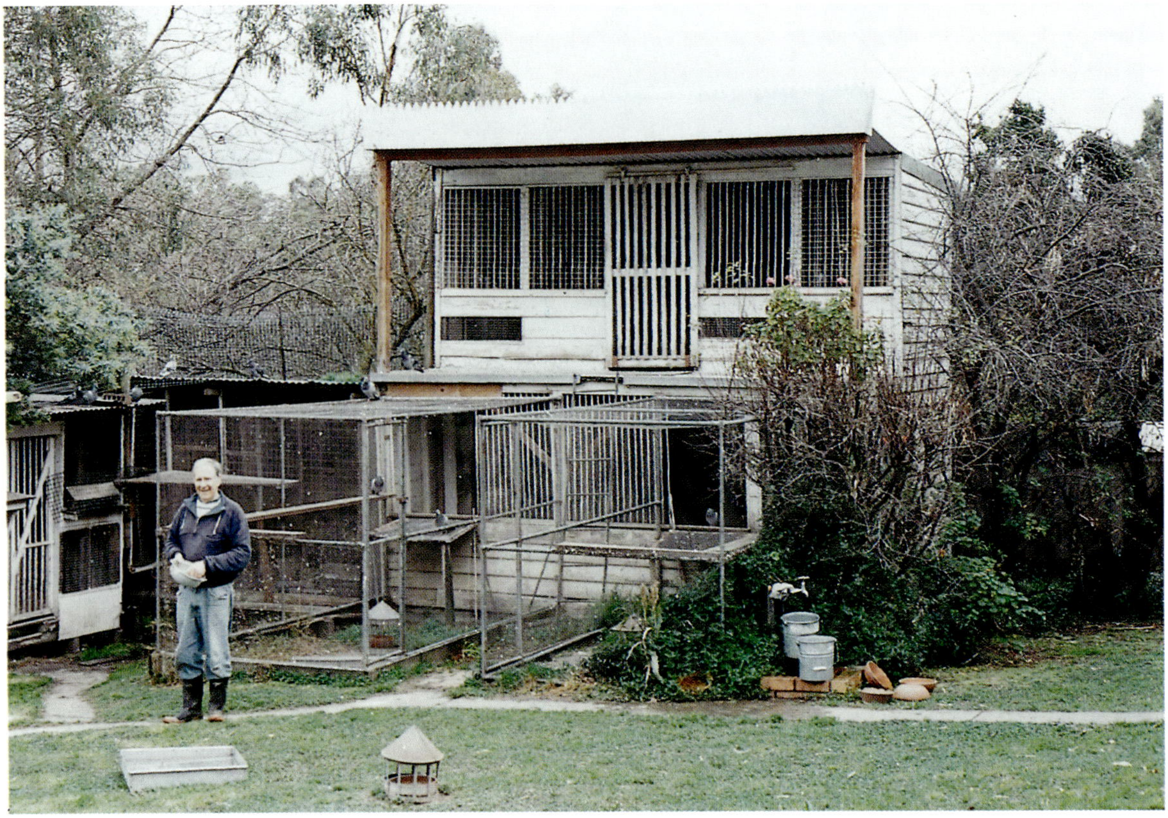

Doug Ince, ouside one of his race lofts in Melbourne.

On a grid floor, the diameter of the mesh should be such that the birds can walk on it but the droppings fall through, sometimes to an underlying pit. This means that the birds' wastes are constantly removed and dust from their droppings cannot become a problem. For the fancier, in particular, with time constraints, this may be the quickest way of maintaining an hygienic environment. However, there may be problems controlling loft temperature and air movement and some birds appear just not to like it and if they do not like it, they may not race as well. Droppings beneath a grid floor must be removed regularly to prevent them from becoming mouldy.

The classic old Continental loft, built within the gable of a heated inhabited house, is a design that has many advantages. The loft floor is warm from the house below, which means that the floor is dry and the warmed air slowly rises, carrying with it dust, moisture and gases from the droppings and exhaled by the birds. This then escapes through the spaces between the tiles. Construction is usually of brick, which is a natural insulator and protects against temperature extremes. The elevated position enhances the pigeons' feeling of security.

The loft as a haven

The pigeon racer must create an environment in his race loft that the pigeons want to return to. Basically, the pigeon must like being there, and want to get back to it quickly. In order to do this, it must :

- **Be a safe place –** Home for a pigeon must be just that, a sanctuary where it is secure and safe. If you watch a wild pigeon living in the roof of a building, perhaps entering through a broken tile, it will dive from some distance, fold its wings and slip straight in without hesitating. It does this because it knows that nothing has ever been there to do it harm. If, however, a cat gets into that roof, the pigeon will fly around trying to look through that hole before landing. It will land hesitantly and will enter cautiously until it is satisfied that no harm awaits it. This is common sense and natural and for the wild pigeon may be a matter of survival.

- **Provide a place to rest –** Pigeons like to go about their daily activities, feeding, preening, sleeping without disturbance. Indeed, as mentioned, the rest period following a training session and meal is just as important in attaining fitness. The loft environment may contain many disturbances, including children, backyard dogs, washing on the clothesline and incinerators. It seems that pigeons become accustomed to anything, particularly if they are exposed to it often or from a young age. However, just because they become accustomed to it does not mean they like it. People living on a busy road get use to the traffic zooming past all the time, but it does not mean they like it.

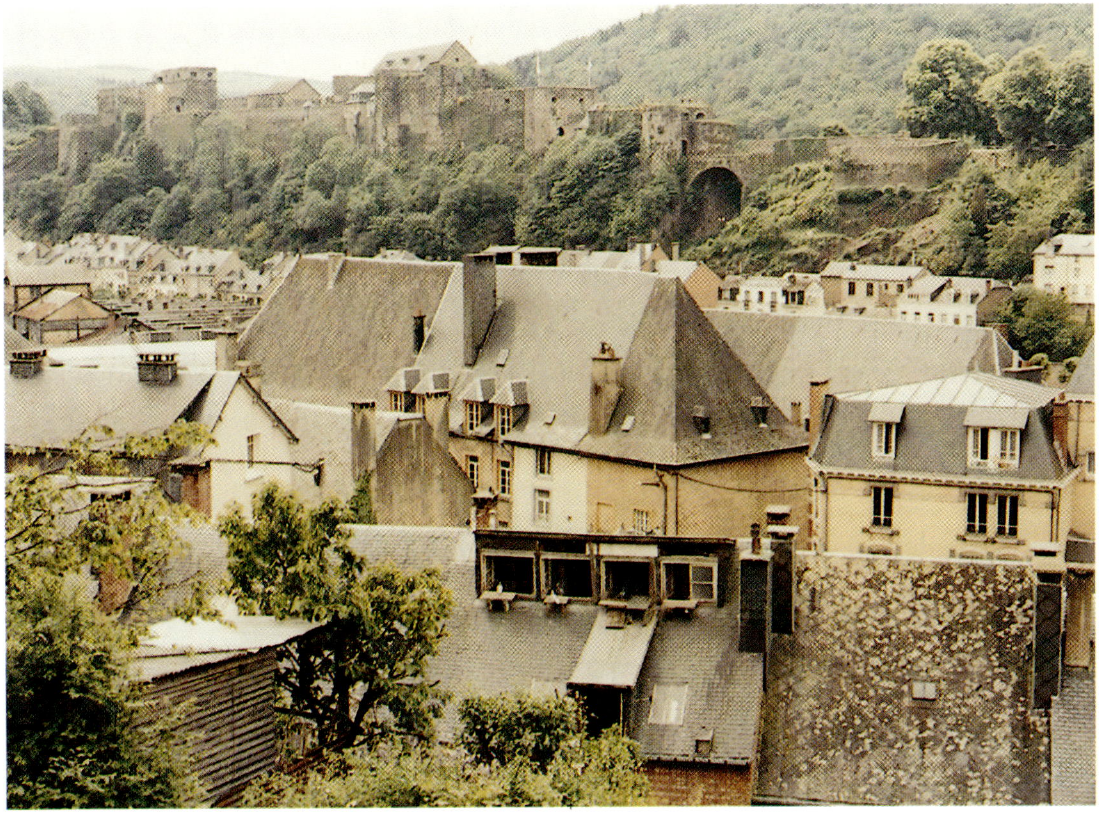

View over the Belgian town of Bouillon. Note the loft set in the roof of the house in the foreground. Such lofts often provide the ideal environment to achieve race form.

- **Provide food and water –** Overseas studies have shown that if the pigeons' reward upon return is delayed by more than five seconds, then the benefit of it is halved. For old birds, this is obviously their box, mate, eggs, etc., but for all birds, in particular young birds, they need to know that food and water are waiting.
- **Provide a place to breed –** In a racing loft this will depend on the method used by the fancier.

Other considerations

Apart from the obvious need to provide a good loft from the pigeons' point of view, so that performance can be optimal, other factors such as the method of racing used, the type of trapping used, basketing of the birds, etc., are all considerations. Working around a basic section size of 2 m x 2 m keeps the birds within reach and tame. Corridors enabling access to all sections also make for easier management. It is easier to care for 200 birds in a good loft than it is to look after 50 in a poorly designed loft.

The maintenance of hygiene within the loft is also an important consideration in any loft design. Few fanciers when speaking honestly would say they enjoy cleaning their lofts and, although not necessarily a chore, it is important that it does not become an onerous task. It is therefore important that the way the loft is going to be cleaned is thought of during its design.

In a loft with an efficient design, cleaning can be done thoroughly and quickly, thus freeing more of the fancier's time to not only enjoy his birds but also to engage in activities that may more directly affect race performance. Similarly, cleaning, if protracted or noisy, may cause undue disturbance to the birds. In particular, attention should be paid to the hoppers and drinkers as some diseases, e.g. canker, are spread through these. Regular cleaning removes germs and, although pigeons will win to lofts that appear dirty, teams cannot be kept consistently in form without reasonable hygiene. In my own loft, I have a hinged door 15 cm x 60 cm at the base of the rear wall of each section. I scrape the perches onto the floor and then, using a wide scraper, scrape all the material from the floor through this door into a collecting bin outside the loft. This helps me clean the loft quickly and minimizes disturbance of the birds.

The final and best assessment of any loft design is the results that the birds achieve racing to it. Some unusual lofts have been the home of champions, while some expensive and attractive lofts house birds whose results are never more than average. Remember that the pigeon is looking for a cosy little spot that he regards as his, where he feels safe and knows he can find food and water. To maximize his ability to return to this spot quickly, he must be fit and healthy when leaving to compete. Loft features have an important role to play in this. If these features can be incorporated into a design that also suits the fancier, the loft should succeed.

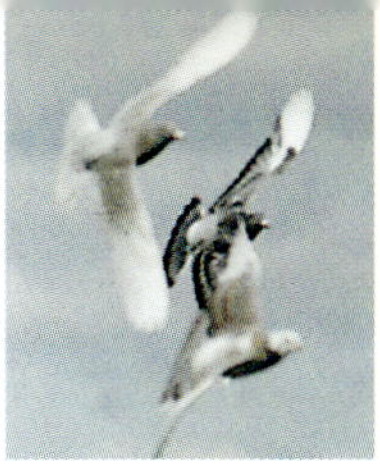

Chapter 32

LOFT HUMIDITY AND TEMPERATURE AND THEIR EFFECT ON HEALTH

It is not possible to design a single loft that is going to be suitable for all areas. Australia, in particular, is such a big country that birds race under an extremely diverse range of conditions, from the cold rainy areas of southern Tasmania to the humid hot areas of northern Queensland, even including islands of the Great Barrier Reef. Other birds race into the dry central deserts, with one of the better-known races – the Silver City Classic – being raced into Broken Hill, in the outback of New South Wales. Fliers in Victoria and New South Wales contend with warm days but very cold nights for much of the year. In the same way, conditions vary throughout Europe and indeed wherever pigeons are raced.

Because of the different conditions, loft designs must vary. Open lofts in warm areas may be conducive to good race form, while similar lofts in colder areas would be a disaster. Many pigeon books, for the most part, discuss a single loft design, which may work well for a particular latitude, and indeed it is important that basic principles are followed. These principles must, however, be adapted to suit a site's unique conditions.

Many things are important when considering what type of loft to build. Quite apart from the loft's geographical location, there are other factors that are site-specific, for example, the way the loft faces, the prevailing wind direction, whether it is in shade from trees, etc. Other factors that will also influence the style of the loft include the type of racing that is to be conducted, i.e. natural or to the perch, the trapping method, the method of basketing, the mode of cleaning, loft security, protection from predators, etc.

The good loft
is one that provides an environment that is conducive to health.

The successful loft
is one that is dry without being dusty, and provides sufficient air exchange without exposing the inmates to extremes of temperature and humidity.

The winning loft
is one that, in addition to this, keeps the temperature and humidity as close to ideal as possible.

The ideal temperature is approximately 20°C. The ideal humidity is 50 – 60%. The installation of a thermometer/hygrometer with a maximum – minimum facility is an excellent way of assessing how good the loft is.

Temperature and ventilation

It is relatively straightforward to build a loft. By definition, it just has to be a cage to confine the birds, and in its simplest form just needs to be a roof and four walls. However, it can be very

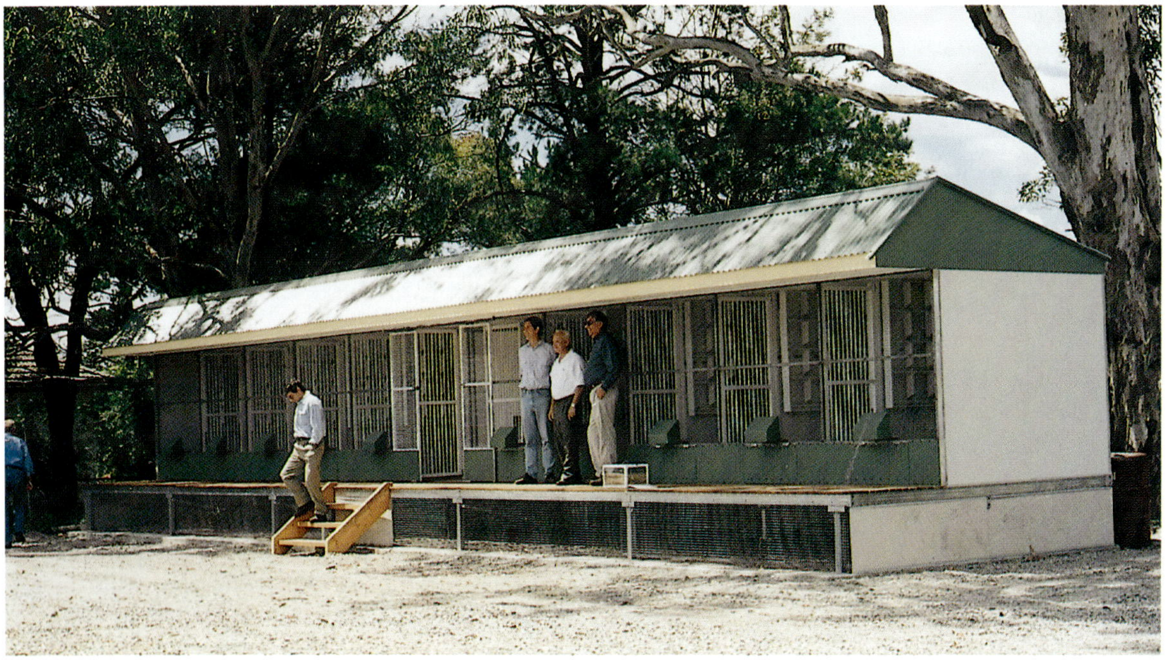

Home of the Sydney Futurity one-loft race, Sydney, Australia.

difficult to build a loft in which the birds can obtain superhealth all year round. Open lofts provide no means of controlling the environment within them and so really only work if located in an environment that is conducive to pigeon health. No area in Australia is perfect all the time, however, most areas are good for certain times, e.g. in Melbourne during September to December when the actual temperature and humidity are ideal for pigeons and so birds can achieve good race form in a relatively poor loft. As modifications are introduced so that the environment within the loft can be kept ideal for longer and longer periods as the weather changes, the design of the loft becomes more and more complex and the potential for mistakes becomes greater.

I find it best to start with a simple box. To this box, openings have to be made to provide ventilation to maintain an ideal temperature. It is important that the provision of ventilation does not create draughts. The design of a successful loft must avoid draughts. The ideal temperature in the loft for a pigeon is approximately 20°C. It is not always possible to attain this, however, and pigeons can race well at temperatures above and below this. Indeed, as mentioned earlier, researchers tell us that the more important parameter is not so much the temperature but rather the variation in temperature over a 24-hour period. Ideally, the temperature in the loft should not change by more than 5°C over a 24-hour period. To achieve this, particularly in colder areas, it is possible to make use of the birds' own body temperature to warm the loft. Overventilated lofts mean that this beneficial heat is lost. It is possible to balance the number of birds in the loft and the degree of ventilation to control temperature swings.

The air in the loft is heated by the birds' bodies and rises. This warmth can be used to advantage to create air exchange without creating a draught. As the air rises, it will carry moisture, dust and unwanted gases with it. This rising warm air must, however, be given an opportunity to escape. In its simplest form, this can be achieved by sloping the roof (usually to the front of the loft) above a false ceiling and having wire between the highest point of the roof and the top of the wall. Alternatively, the roof can be gabled with a capping vent at its highest point. Gabled roofs can be extended beyond the walls so as to create an eave through which fresh air can enter. Any vent in the wall should be just below the roof and well above any areas that the birds might sit. Otherwise, the top perching birds (and these often seem to be the better birds) will be in a draught. 'Chef's hat' vents can be set into the roof, however, as these are wind-driven, the ventilation they offer is variable. Corrugated iron is not a good roofing material as it enables no ventilation and has poor

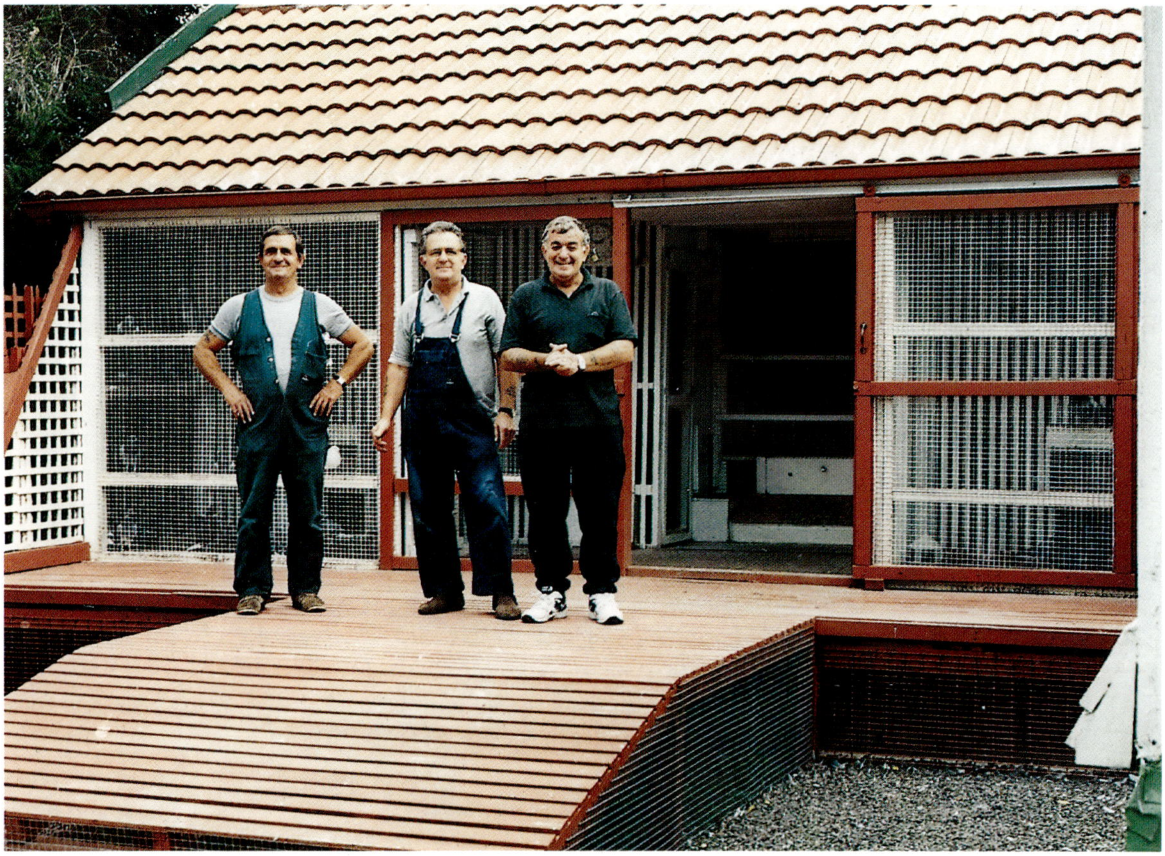

Successful Melbourne fanciers, from left, Barry, Roy and Kevin Harkom, outside their racing loft.

temperature insulation properties. The ideal is a gabled tiled roof where there is considerable tile overlap and vertical space between the tiles that enable free loss of stale air.

Once we have created a situation where stale air can escape without exposing the birds to draughts, openings must be made for fresh air to enter. A loft too closed-in runs the risk of being too hot in hot weather. Openings can be created in the walls until the loft becomes comfortable on a warm day. Permanent openings, however, will mean that the loft is overly temperature-sensitive and will become cold when the weather is cold. Although openings in the loft's walls can create a pleasant environment and prevent high humidity in warm weather, permanent wall openings create several problems. They mean that in cold weather the loft will become cold, particularly when the day is windy. Because they encourage air movement across the loft rather than upwards, they encourage draughts, which are cold streams of air through a warmer environment. They also make it impossible during cold weather to retain the heat generated by the birds, which can be used beneficially to warm the loft. The answer to this problem is to have these openings adjustable. Louvres or hinged or sliding panels can be used to advantage here. The advantage of adjustable openings is that on cold or windy days the loft can be closed. Conversely, on hot days the loft can be opened, always aiming to provide an ideal environment for the birds, all the time making maximal use of the birds' own body heat to aid in temperature control in the loft. Excessive use of glass should be avoided as this has poor insulating properties.

In very windy areas, even in lofts with solid walls, if the ventilation and temperature fluctuation is too high, sliding panels can be inserted below the roof to allow further control of air movement.

For years, the Australian idea of a good loft has been one that has plenty of air. To assess a loft purely on this point is a relic of the past. A resting race bird in a loft that is not overcrowded (i.e. fewer than 25 birds per 2-m x 2-m section) is never going to be short of oxygen where all venting is through the ceiling.

Humidity

The relative humidity refers to the amount of moisture or dampness in the air itself. As air warms, its ability to carry moisture increases. If moisture is available, it will evaporate into and be carried by this warmed air. Air at a particular temperature can only carry so much moisture. If there are still things in the environment that contain moisture, for example, droppings in the loft, they will remain damp.

If the air temperature changes, the air's ability to carry moisture also changes. If it decreases, the moisture it contains will precipitate out, wetting things in the environment.

The air in a pigeon loft should not be moisture-laden, i.e. should not have a high humidity. Moisture-laden air must be given an opportunity to escape, otherwise the loft will be too humid. We all know that in order for its residents to be healthy, a loft must be kept dry, so therefore humidity must be controlled. The ideal humidity within the pigeon loft is 50 – 60%. European writers tell us that, with a humidity greater than 70%, there is clearly a decrease in performance. Over 80%, hardly any birds are in the winning lists, and once over 90%, no prizes are won.

Humidity can be either loft-based or environmental. Although it is not always possible to entirely separate the two of these, as they can both affect each other, it can be a useful way of looking at the control of humidity within the loft.

In loft-based humidity, the dampness comes from the birds themselves. Exhaled air and droppings contain moisture. Loft-based humidity is controlled by two factors: the number of birds in the loft and the amount of ventilation. These in turn affect the temperature in the loft. As the number of birds increases, the temperature within the loft will increase and the ventilation must similarly increase otherwise the humidity may become too high. If loft humidity is high, either the number of birds must decrease or the rate of air exchange must increase. The answer is opening the loft and, as discussed earlier, being able to do this in an adjustable way so that when the weather becomes cold, the loft does not become too cold.

Environmental humidity is associated with the loft's physical location. A pigeon loft might be sited where it is persistently or intermittently damp. As one moves further north in Australia, the weather becomes progressively more and more humid. Lofts near the coast may experience night-time fogs. Lofts near swimming pools are exposed to on-going humidity. Lofts facing south or in shade from trees will stay damp even into a sunny day.

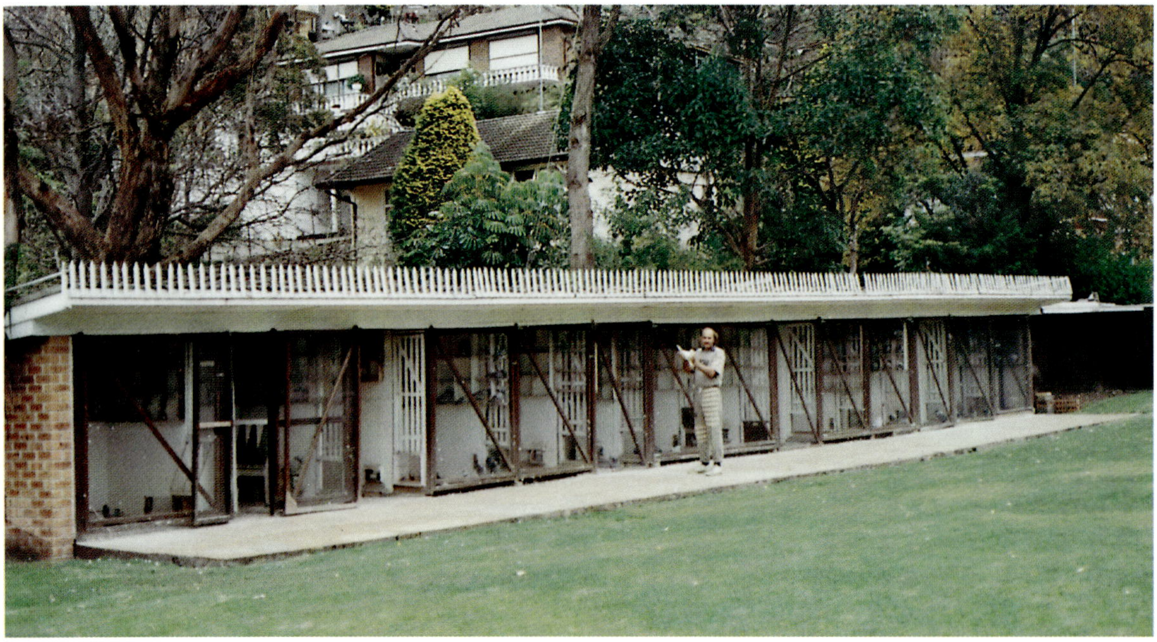

Race loft of Bob Giltinan, Sydney: a common design in the warmer areas of Australia.

Matching loft design to climate

One aim with loft design is to ensure that the loft does not become damp. Dampness in the loft can occur in both low- and high-humidity areas. In cold areas, the air cannot carry very much moisture, so lofts holding too many birds for the level of ventilation will become damp as moisture in the air condenses onto loft surfaces or fails to evaporate from droppings. In hot areas, the warm air may already be saturated with moisture. Dampness is controlled when the air is warm and dry. This occurs when the number of birds and ventilation are correct.

A dry loft can be achieved by different methods in different areas. There are three climate types to be considered:

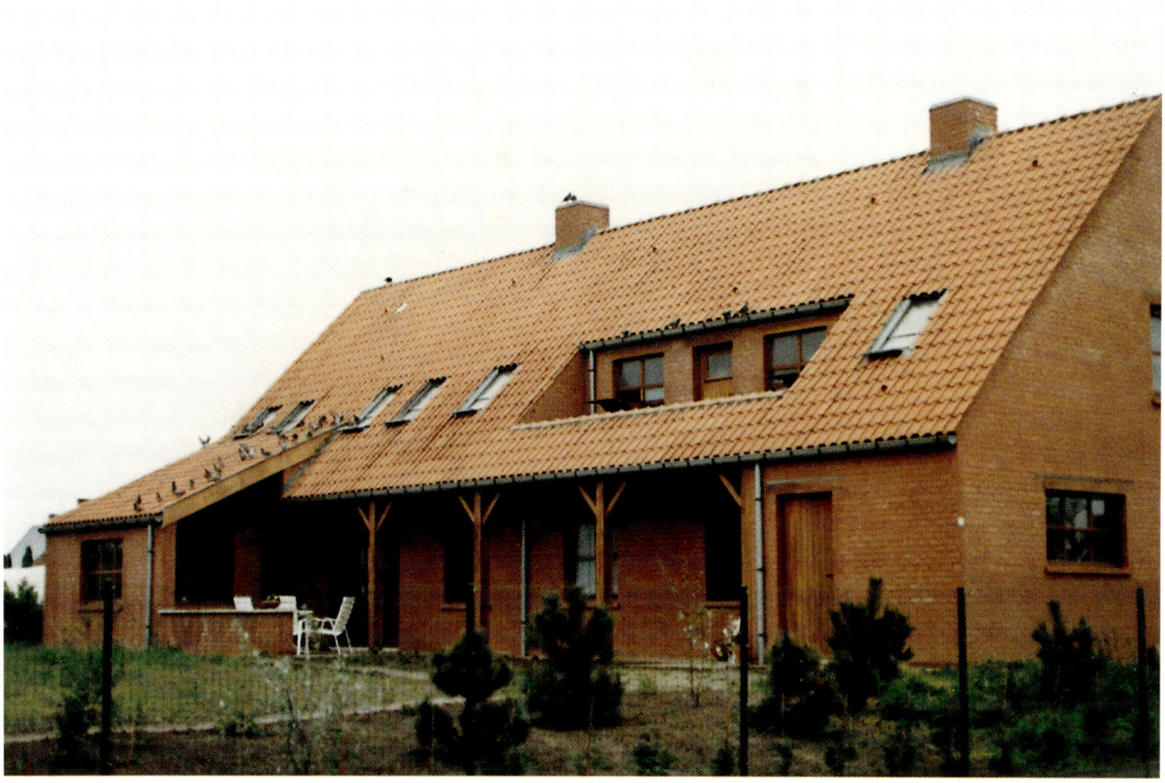

Continental loft in the roof of the owner's house, Bernard Deweerdt, Kortemark, Belgium.

1 **Cold nights and cold days –** Here the persistently cold air cannot carry much moisture and so the droppings will remain damp all day unless removed. Unless the loft is adequately ventilated, exhaled air will condense on the walls and the underside of the roof. The answer is to remove the droppings daily and enclose the loft sufficiently so that it becomes warm through the birds' own body heat. The warm air will rise and must be given an opportunity to escape through the roof or high wall vents. It may be necessary to retain lost heat through sliding roof panels. Low wall vents will mean the loft is impossible to heat and the birds, always being cold, will not become superhealthy. In extremely cold areas, heat pads or heaters may be necessary. The provision of heat pads must, however, be accompanied by appropriate ventilation, otherwise the increase in temperature can lead to increased humidity, leading to a greenhouse-type climate.

2 **Cold nights and warm days –** During the night, the situation described in (1) above essentially applies. The loft should be enclosed so that the birds can keep themselves warm. At night, there should be just enough opening in the roof for rising stale air to escape. As the day temperature rises, the droppings will dry, increasing the humidity in the loft. The sun will increase

the temperature in the loft and this, combined with the birds' body heat, will create a hot humid loft. The loft here must have the facility to open wall vents during the day. Practical things that are commonly used here are louvres and panels that can be hinged and clipped open or slid open. Just how open these need to be depends on the temperature and also the wind. If it is windy, the loft will be better ventilated and the panels will not need to be as open to provide adequate air exchange.

Often with these weather conditions, particular care must be taken in lofts near water. This can include those near the coast but also near backyard swimming pools. Water retains the heat it collects through the day and continues to evaporate into the cool of the evening. I draw the analogy of the way a kettle continues to steam after the stove has been turned off. Lofts built in these areas and also those in areas prone to night-time fogs and frosts are prone to night-time humidity. Such lofts, to be successful, need to be closed off at night so that the birds can keep themselves warm and are not sleeping in dampness.

3 **Warm nights and warm days** – In this situation, quite open lofts can be successful and indeed in some areas the temperatures are so extreme that the lofts need to be open to be successful. Birds cool themselves by evaporation of moisture from their airsacs. When it is hot, a lot of moisture is lost from their system this way and, unless the loft is adequately ventilated, an extremely stuffy humid environment is created. Provided the loft is sufficiently enclosed to protect the birds from the wind and promote a feeling of security under these conditions, quite open lofts can work.

It is in persistently warm and humid areas that the attainment of superform becomes a real challenge. Pigeons did not evolve in a humid environment and so their response mechanisms to humidity are poor. As a result, with persistently high humidity, they become vulnerable to disease. However, it is still possible to keep them healthy, but their management has to be adjusted to cope with this.

Humidity- and temperature-related disease and its control

Failing to control large temperature swings or to keep the humidity low, places stress on the birds, which initiates the disease cascade that has been dealt with earlier. Typically, droppings received at my clinic from lofts with on-going humidity problems contain large numbers of *E. coli* and yeasts and also fungal branches and Coccidia. If these problems are not controlled, the birds break down and go on to develop wet canker and respiratory infection.

Coccidia

Coccidia levels rise in response to stress and, once passed in the droppings into a humid environment, become infective quicker. On-going hygiene is important to minimize exposure. Coccidia can be cleared by a 2-day course of Baycox (1 ml to 2 litres of water). As Baycox (the drug of choice) does not interfere with the developing immunity of the youngster and does not accumulate in the system, it can be used regularly and is best given for 2 days when Coccidia are detected or alternatively for 2 days every 4 weeks until the humidity drops.

Fungi

Fungi, however, are the biggest problem in humid areas. They not only contaminate the seed but will grow (often microscopically) in the loft itself. In the seed, they decrease its nutritional value and some produce toxins that make the birds sick. In the loft, they produce spores that, when inhaled, lead to respiratory disease. Mouldy droppings are a give-away sign that there is a problem with the

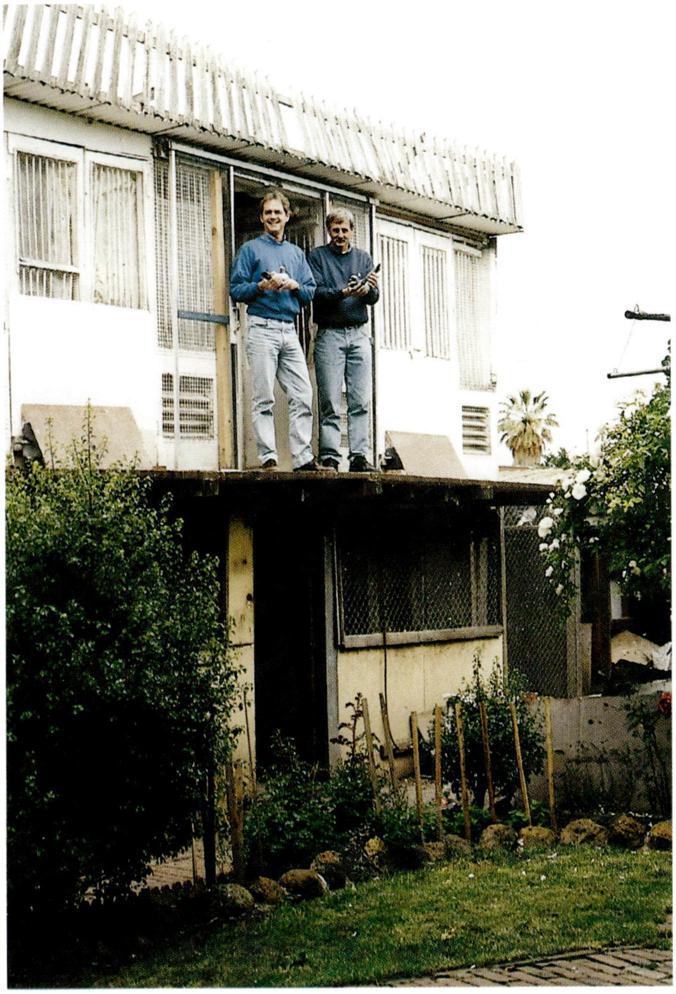

Ken Fawcett and the author in front of Ken's racing loft. The author is holding 1st Federation 700 miles 1999, while Ken is holding 2nd Federation 700 miles 1999.

loft humidity. When the humidity is high, droppings remain moist and provide a substrate for fungi to grow on.

Every effort must be made to decrease exposure to fungi. To achieve this, it is necessary to include measures in the routine management of the birds that are often not necessary in the less-humid southern areas of the country. In addition to regular removal of droppings, lofts should be sprayed regularly (usually weekly) with chloramine. Chloramine is a non-toxic general disinfectant that is effective against fungi. Birds are moved out of the section, which is then scraped clean. The chloramine is misted onto the scraped surface and when the loft is dry, in usually about half an hour, the birds are allowed back into the section. Good seed can be protected from fungal invasion through mixing with monomeric propionic acid (Monoprop, Protonic, etc.).

Because the nose and mouth are continuous in pigeons through the slot (or choana) in the roof of the mouth, inhaled as well as swallowed fungal spores will end up in the droppings. These can be detected in the droppings microscopically where they indicate either fungal contamination of the seed or mould growing in the loft environment. Their presence can be a handy way to detect fungal and therefore humidity problems within a loft without seeing the loft.

Grid floors, in particular, can be a bit of a no-no in high-humidity areas because the accumulation of droppings beneath them remains damp and, as stated above, these provide an ideal base for fungal growth. The droppings should be regularly removed and the area beneath the loft sprayed with chloramine. Grid floors also create problems with loft ventilation and temperature control. I feel also that they are not conducive to a feeling of security in the birds. They can often lead to excessive air movement, leading to a cold and draughty loft. When used in cold areas, it is important that the area between the grid and the ground is boxed in to minimize this problem. Straw can also be risky in humid lofts. Although straw is a good floor covering in many areas, droppings within it remain damp in high-humidity areas. Once contaminated, it cannot be cleaned and provides a base for fungal growth.

E. coli AND YEAST

E. coli and yeast levels rise and fall depending on what stresses the birds are under. With the clearing of Coccidia and fungi, their level will usually decrease. However, if they remain high, the birds will develop green and watery droppings. On days when significant numbers of these are observed, the birds will benefit from treatment with avian probiotics (Probac, 1/2 teaspoon to 2 litres). These

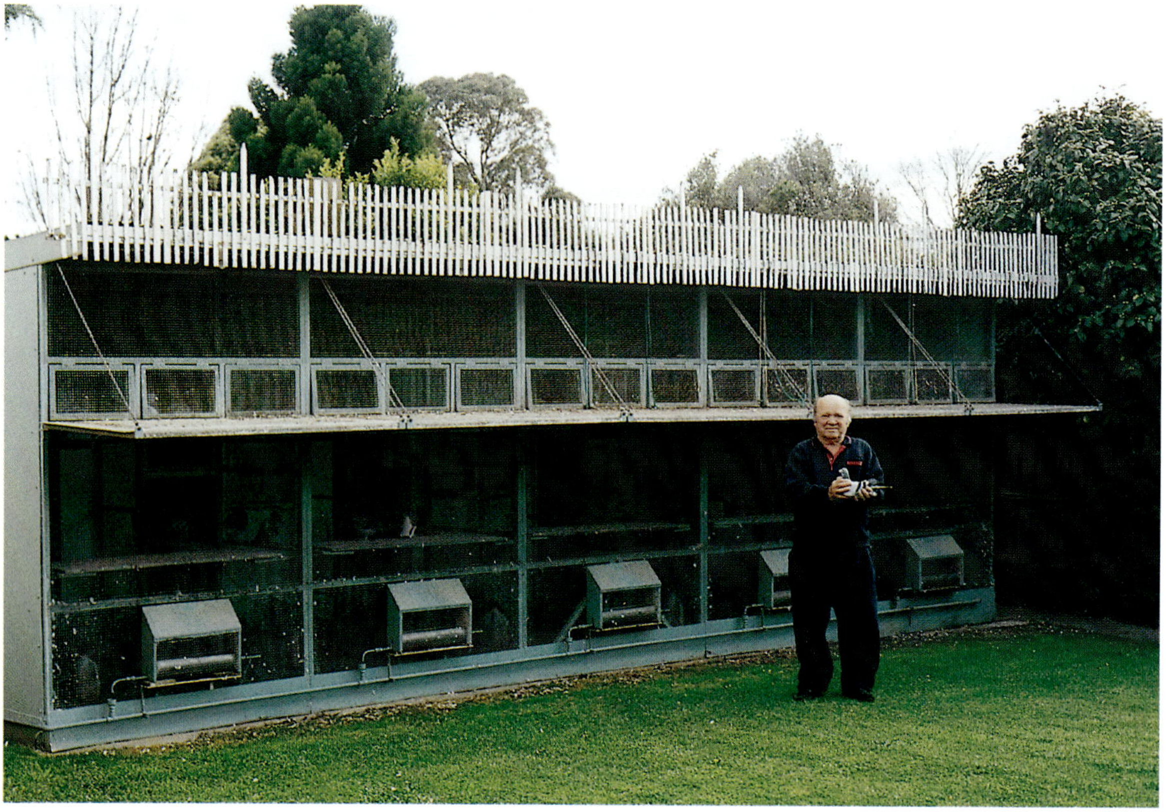

V.H.A. champion for 1996, S. Mazurkewiecz in front of his racing loft, holding his 2-year-old BBC that was 2nd V.H.A. Federation 350 miles and 1st V.H.A. Federation 400 miles.

are continued until the droppings normalize. With on-going stress, probiotics can be used as the need dictates. However, a failure to respond suggests that wet canker or respiratory infection may already be involved.

Program for lofts with humidity problems or in humid areas

- Regular (daily) dropping removal and weekly spray with chloramine.
- Baycox for 2 days every 4 weeks.
- Probac on days when significant numbers of green and watery droppings noticed.
- Monitor for signs of wet canker and respiratory infection.
- Review factors that increase loft-based humidity and modify loft conditions if necessary, i.e. reduce number of birds per section, increase ventilation, increase frequency of dropping removal, insulate roof to keep loft cooler, close loft at night in areas prone to cold nights, etc.
- Consider treating seed with propionic acid.
- Test seed to ensure that it is free of fungi and moulds (see chapter entitled Testing of Bad Food).

Although medication can control any health problem, the longer-term answer is often to modify the loft design or to alter the number of birds kept to improve the loft's temperature and humidity levels so that the birds are under less stress, with the result that the need for medication falls away. However, in areas where extremes of temperature and humidity are unavoidable, with a bit of extra effort and the correct use of medication, winning form can still be attained.

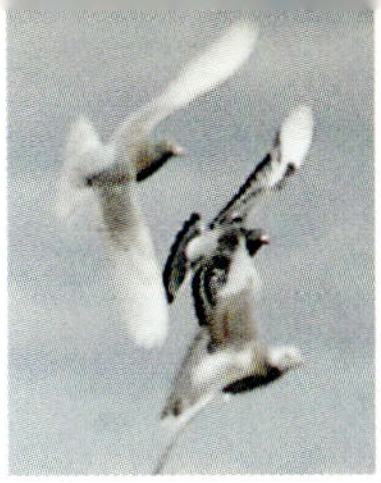

Chapter 33

MOULTING AND RACE PERFORMANCE

It sometimes seems that the most successful fliers are the ones that make the least mistakes. Mistakes with the moult are particularly unforgiving as the new set of feathers must last the bird the full 12 months. Once racing has commenced, good care can minimize damage to feathers. However, unlike other things that can be altered to induce form, if the fancier notices that feather quality is lacking, he can do nothing but learn from his experience to prevent the same thing happening next time. It is therefore important that the fancier has a good understanding of the moulting process so that his birds can have a good set of feathers with which to compete.

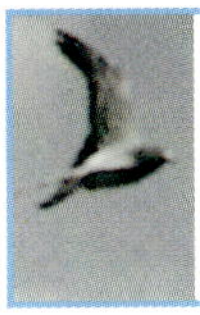

Feather health is vital to the performance of the racing pigeon and a good moult is the basis of the healthy feather.

The feather itself is an amazing structure and performs several roles. A pigeon's normal body temperature is 41.7°C, quite a bit warmer than ourselves, and as a result, pigeons are quite cold-sensitive. The feathers form an effective insulating layer in themselves but, in addition, can be moved away from the body, if necessary, by a set of tiny muscles, each attached to one feather, to trap a further insulating layer of warm, still air against the skin. This is so effective that, from a veterinarian's point of view, it can be frustrating in that they keep the body warm long after death so that decomposition commences within 20 minutes. This means that autopsy opportunities are frequently lost. The feathers similarly shield the bird from heat. They are therefore a movable insulating shield that, incredibly, also gives the bird the power of flight.

The moult

Because of wear and tear, every feather of the pigeon is replaced once a year. The process of old feather loss and the regrowth of new feathers is referred to as 'the moult' and begins after the breeding season and after weaning. Each feather grows from a small structure in the skin called a feather follicle. Several glands are found within each feather follicle and each produces substances essential to the growth of the feather. Blood vessels lead to these and supply them with the nutrients they require. A set of nerves also leads to these. Some act as regulators of the process and at certain times signal the follicles to begin production of a new feather, pushing out the old feather in the process. Other nerves are sensitive to pain and, interestingly, plucking a feather is one of the most painful things that can be done to a bird. This is an evolutionary adaptation to prevent loss of flight, which would make it vulnerable to predation.

The main feathers covering the pigeon's body are called contour feathers. These are divided into flight feathers and body feathers. The flight feathers include the remiges of the wing and the retrices of the tail. There are usually ten primary remiges, numbered one to ten from inside out, and eighteen secondary remiges, numbered one to eighteen from outside in. There are twelve retrices in race birds. Body feathers are contour feathers that cover most of the body. These are all replaced once a year. The old feather is pushed out by the new feather in much the same way that a temporary milk tooth of a mammal is pushed out by the budding permanent tooth beneath it, except that the cycle of moulting is repeated annually throughout the life of the bird. If a feather is plucked, it will be replaced immediately.

Young birds start to moult at the time they get their eye colour (12 weeks). Only the primary feathers moult in a sequence, from the smallest inner flights towards the outside last primary flight. There is no real sequence in the secondaries or tail feathers. Shortly after the fifth primary has been shed, the coverts of the body and throat start loosening and falling out in large numbers. After dropping the sixth primary, the moult of the secondaries begins. The tail feathers usually follow simultaneously with the eighth primary flight.

The body moult is completed usually by May in Victoria, with the final flight dropping in the first round from mid-April to mid-May. This poses problems for fliers in Victoria, where young bird racing is through March and April. When the feather follicle is full of blood, immediately before feather emergence, particularly in the last three flights, the feathers appear painful. Individual birds are reluctant to fly and show signs of discomfort by lifting the wing and repeatedly preening the site after landing. Care must be taken with the racing of these birds. Later-bred youngsters, i.e. weaned after mid-February, will often not complete moulting their flights but will complete their body moult; some late-breds will not drop any flights. Birds that do not complete moulting their flights can be frustrating to race later in the year because when they become fit they will often drop a flight (sometimes two), compromising performance. These then take on average 4 weeks to regrow.

In stock birds, moulting begins when breeding stops. Like the youngsters, they have usually finished their moult in Victoria, Australia, by May. If bred from late, their moult will be particularly heavy to achieve this.

Although contour feathers are replaced once a year, the pigeon does moult continuously throughout the year. Powder down feathers are dropped when the bird is healthy and are replaced. The powder down feather is a specialized down feather which grows and falls out through the entire year (normal down feathers are not common in pigeons). The powder down feathers disintegrate, producing powder as they emerge from the feather follicles. This is spread through the feathers as a preening and waterproofing agent. The vane (extended sides of the feather made up of individual barbs) of the contour feathers can be either pennaceous (compact and closely knit) or plumulaceous (soft and downy). The downy portion produces a fine white waxy powder, which also acts to waterproof and lubricate the contour feathers. Fliers will be familiar with this as a white coating of the outer flights visible in a closed wing.

Powder down feathers are lost all year round. However, the drop of these increases when the health of the bird is increasing, for example, when the weather becomes warm after a cold spell, as the birds recover after a hard fly, or when a higher-energy ration is provided after a poor diet, e.g. all wheat, or a period of starvation. As well, and very importantly, it occurs when birds are coming into race form. Fliers have long associated the appearance of down feathers adhering to droppings in the morning as a good sign, and the appearance of these is a real indicator of the health of the bird. As the drop of feather down feathers increases, more bloom is produced. This means that the feathers are waterproofed and lubricated and are silky and shiny. Feather quality is therefore a reflection of the health of the bird. Conversely, dry brittle feathers are one of the more obvious signs to the fancier that his birds are out of form. When moulting is completed quickly, it indicates that the health and management of the flock are optimal. A slow moult indicates a problem with health or management.

What factors trigger the moult and then the regrowth of feathers?

Hormones

Several of the body's hormones affect the progress of the moult. In young birds, as puberty approaches, a small gland at the base of the brain, called the pituitary, releases increasing amounts of sex hormones. These hormones stimulate the birds' gonads and sexual activity commences. The moult and regrowth of feathers are partially dependent on these. In feeding stock birds, the pituitary also produces a hormone called prolactin. This initiates the production of pigeon milk. Prolactin blocks the production of sex hormones and inhibits the moult. This is an obvious protective mechanism for the birds as both place a big demand on the birds' system and means that the birds' resources are directed towards raising the babies.

A gland at the base of the neck, called the thyroid, produces a hormone called thyroxin. Thyroxin stimulates the moult but its effect is also over-ridden by prolactin during breeding. The production of thyroxin is dependent on adequate levels of dietary iodine and the amino acid tyrosine. If the feed is deficient in either iodine or tyrosine, then the production of thyroxin is inadequate for a normal moult. Some grain-growing areas of Australia are deficient in iodine and there is a possibility of feeding a diet deficient in iodine. Iodine can be added to the diet via commercial additives and indeed the better brands of pink minerals and water-soluble multivitamins contain iodine. Tyrosine levels can be increased by feeding grains high in this amino acid, such as wheat, milo, rice and millet.

The adrenal glands sit in the abdomen near the kidneys, and produce the hormone cortisol. Cortisol production increases in times of stress, and this can stop the moult. Widowhood cocks often moult irregularly and this is thought to be due to fluctuating levels of sex hormones and cortisol. On the Continent, corticosteroids are sometimes given (illegally), usually as an eye drop, to racers to prevent the drop of critical flight feathers when actively racing.

Stress

Stress is essentially any factor that interferes with the birds' physical or mental well-being and includes:

- **Overcrowding,** which leads to physical competition for food, water and perch space, and also decreased rest.
- **Overtraining,** i.e. exercising above the team's level of fitness.
- **Overambitious tossing,** causing anxiety for young inexperienced birds.
- **Incorrect use of medication** – Medication must be used correctly during the moult; antibiotics can upset the normal balance of bacteria in the bowel and therefore affect the absorption of nutrients. In addition, some medications directly interfere with feather formation, causing deformities such as fret marks, e.g. Synanthic.
- **Poor loft design.**
- **Failure to control external parasites** – External parasites adversely affect the moult in two ways. Mites, which predominantly feed on blood, weaken the bird, but also their physical irritation prevents adequate rest. Lice directly damage feathers by feeding on feather debris, interfering with the feathers' insulating property. Lice also eat bloom. This means that instead of the feathers being lubricated and sliding smoothly over each other, they rasp backwards and forwards, creating further wear and tear and increasing the effort necessary for the bird to fly.

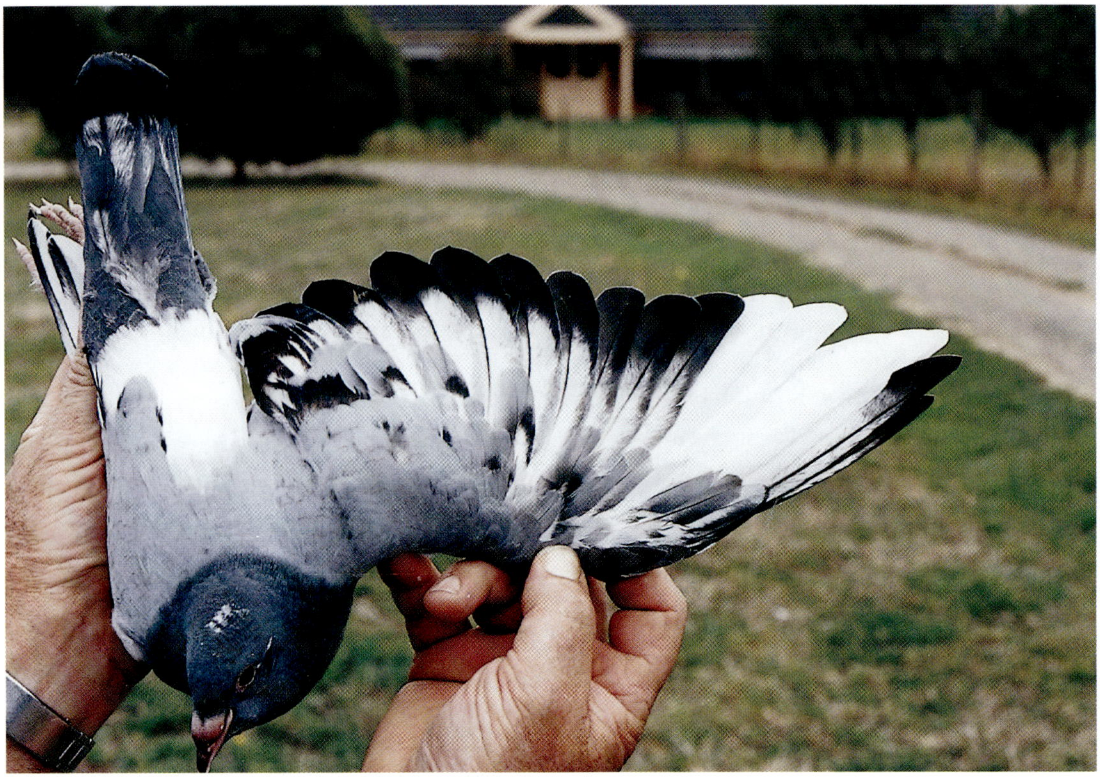

'Grizzling' occurs with anything that interferes with normal deposition of pigment into the growing feather. Possible causes include stress, some medications and certain diseases.

- **Disease –** Sick birds moult slowly and the feathers they grow are of poor quality. In particular, bowel problems such as worms, Coccidia and bacterial infections interfere with the absorption of nutrients into the body, which are essential for feather growth. Any change in the droppings of moulting birds should be investigated promptly before too much damage is done.

Stress causes the body's adrenal gland to produce cortisone, which decreases the activity of the thyroid gland and retards the growth of new feathers, as well as interfering with actual feather development, leading to persistent feather sheaths or fret marks. Fret marks occur as a result of temporary interference with feather follicle function, such as missing a meal or chilling in a youngster, while persistent sheaths, which can give the feather a stalked appearance, indicate a more long-term problem, such as a basic nutritional deficiency. All fanciers can recognize the more severe fret marks, however, I find it of value to open the wing and angle it against a light source, so that the light is reflected off the surface of the quill of each flight. Often both the flier and I are surprised at just how many dints and irregularities become visible using this method. Often, birds that appeared superficially to have moulted well are shown to have many small marks. The feather in this way acts as a diary of the events within the loft, and, as each mark indicates a period when the birds' health was not optimal, gives both the veterinarian and fancier an assessment of just how loft practices during the moult are affecting the birds. To minimize stress, young birds should be kept in a sensible loft routine. A feeling of well-being is created by regular feeding and training regimes. Care must be taken here in Victoria with the early training of young birds so as not to compromise their moult and development. Ideally, the pigeon should complete its moult within 8 weeks of starting the body moult.

Bathing is not necessary for a good moult but it does have psychological benefits, relaxing the birds and assisting with a good moult. Although it is not possible to accelerate the moult in a healthy pigeon, a prolonged moult can be prevented by preventing stress.

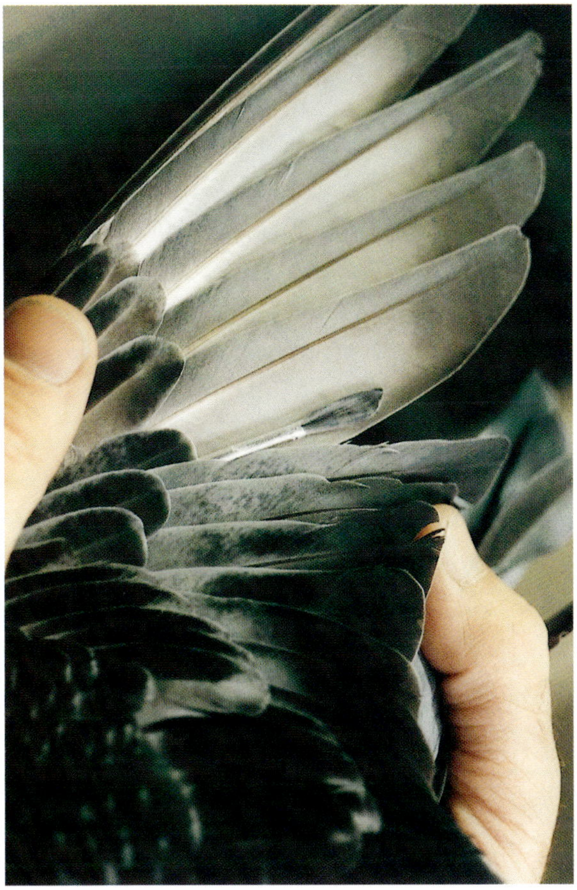

Flight feather with a persistent feather sheath. This bird has come under some form of stress at this stage of its moult.

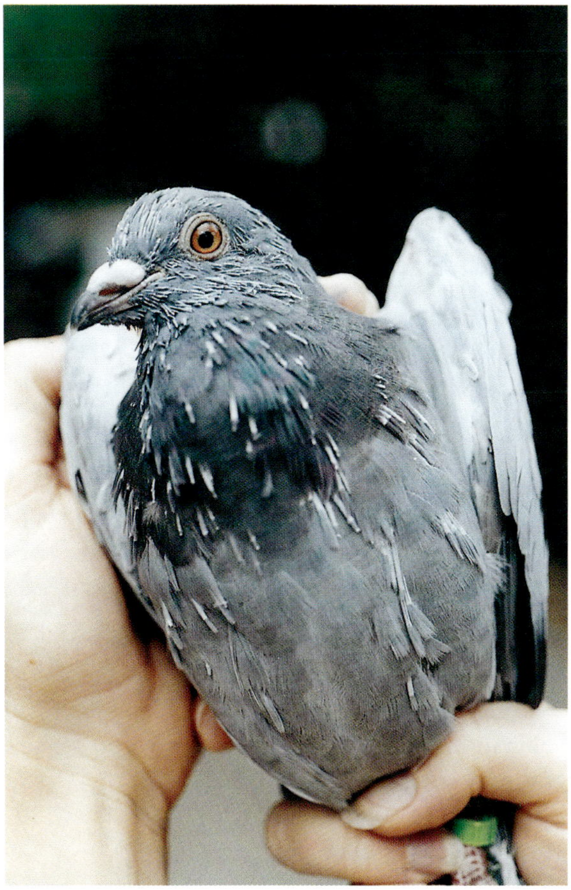

Bird with large number of persistent feather sheaths. Although obviously in general good health, this bird has come under some stress.

Daylength

Shortening daylength stimulates the moult, while increasing daylength retards the moult but only to a point. In fact, it is possible to halt the flight feather moult by providing a constant daylength of 10 hours or less. It is not known exactly how this occurs but it may be due to an effect on the pituitary and resultant sex hormone production.

A good moult is one that is completed within 8 weeks of onset and produces good-quality feathers. For a pigeon to moult well, two basic criteria must be met. Firstly, the pigeon must have at its disposal in its diet the building blocks to produce a good feather, and secondly the bird must be stress-free, which includes being healthy, so that these building blocks can be correctly assembled. Stress relief and good feeding practices are the two most important components of the good moult. Feeding the correct balance of food during the moult is vital to the production of healthy feathers. Any deficiency is reflected in decreased feather quality. This is one of the times when supplementation with vitamins and minerals is of benefit. In addition, because feathers are made of protein, the diet must contain extra levels of protein, which usually means increasing the levels of peas and beans in the seed mix.

Once the birds have had a good moult, the fancier should have in the back of his mind that the feathers do have to last for a full year. As explained, keeping the birds healthy will ensure bloom production and decrease feather wear and tear. Avoiding overcrowding in baskets and minimizing unnecessary basket time will help reduce further mechanical damage. If the quill of a major feather does become bent, it can be straightened by waving it through a jet of steam. Amazingly, the feather will, over a 5 – 20-second period, slowly swing back into its normal position. An on-going program should be set in place for control of external parasites, as outlined in the chapter The Parasitic Diseases.

Program to ensure good feather quality

- Consider feather quality as one of the factors when selecting stock birds. Feather quality is heritable, with certain families having better-quality, silkier feathers. Similarly, feathers of certain colours deteriorate more rapidly, e.g. white.
- A health check before the moult will ensure birds are not carrying any latent disease that affects their health, e.g. canker, or, in particular, bowel problems, such as Coccidia, which will interfere with nutrient absorption. A health check involves a throat swab and dropping analysis.
- Avoid stress during moulting and provide good care to ensure continued bloom production.
- Provide a diet with adequate levels of protein and essential trace elements, such as iodine, during the moult.
- Control external parasites.
- Minimize mechanical feather injury through rough handling and extended basket time.

These points should enable your birds to not only look good but be at their most competitive when in form. However, if feather quality is becoming poor during racing, silkiness can be increased through improving the birds' health, thereby encouraging drop of down feathers and bloom production. This usually involves a health check to identify if there are any disease factors and treating these, together with increasing the energy content of the diet and sometimes decreasing the time the birds spend in the air.

Steaming feathers

It can be very frustrating to find that a race bird has bent one of its primary feathers during the season. A quick and easy solution is to boil a kettle and, while holding the bird, wave the affected flight through the jet of steam. The combination of moisture and heat causes the feather to straighten out in seconds, as if by magic.

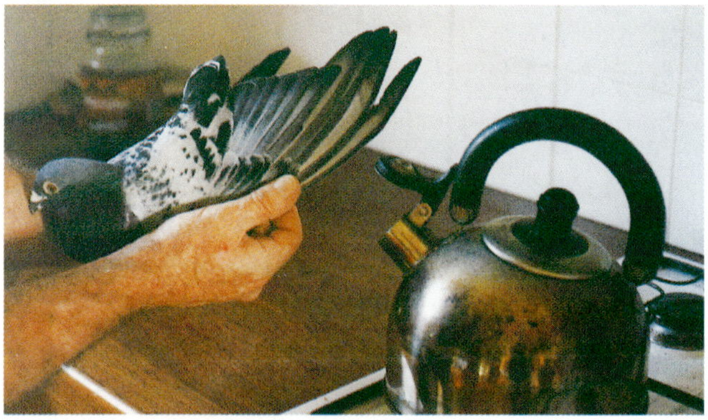

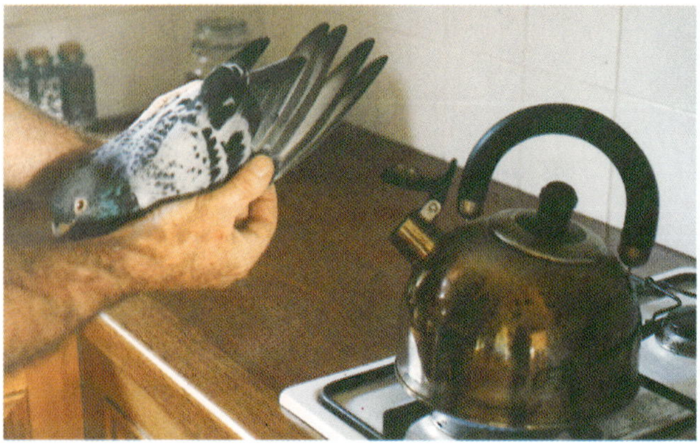

Top right: Race cock with his ninth and tenth flight bent.

Bottom right: Waved through a jet of steam, the two flights snap back into position.

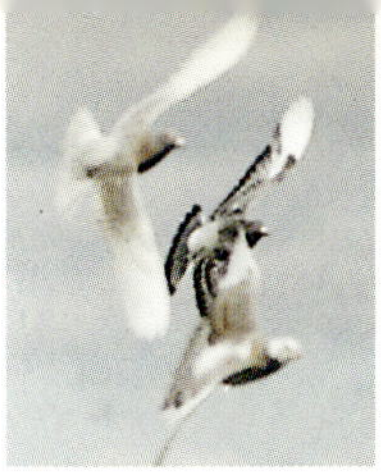

Chapter 34

FOOD FOR THOUGHT –

Snippets from conversations with successful fliers

Over the years, I have had many interesting discussions with fanciers and some of the comments and thoughts of these are fascinating. I thought that others might also find these of interest. One thing I find is that good fliers are often very observant and have the ability to think laterally. Pigeon racing can be much more interesting, I feel, if one can be innovative rather than simply following what everybody else does. After all, this is the way methods that are now regarded as commonplace, such as widowhood, were first developed.

Flock size

Have you ever thought if there is an ideal flock size that birds should train in? Is it best for an individual bird to work in a team of 10 or 15 or a large mob of 200? In large mobs, the birds tend to get in each other's way and perhaps cannot fly as freely. It might be like going for a jog with a dog on a lead, with the dog interrupting your stride. A bird having to lift a wing or jostle to the side in a large mob is perhaps not exercising as well as it might. Yet most people notice how very small mobs of less that 10 pigeons are reluctant to work well, perhaps because they don't have the confidence to range. So what is the ideal size?

Graeme Davison, an extremely successful flier in Wollongong, N.S.W., Australia, feels that about 60 is the best. This is a sufficient number for the pigeons to have confidence to fly but they can still fly tightly as one and

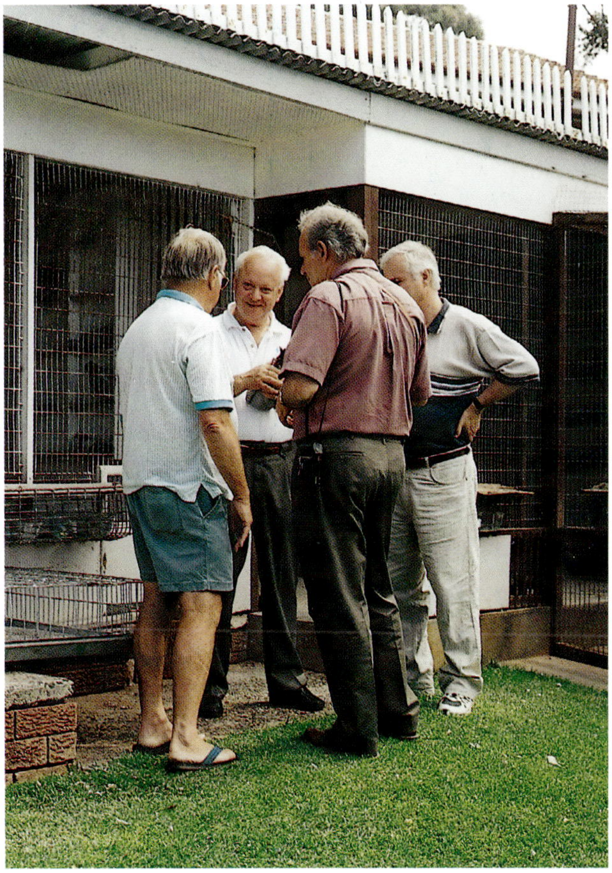

When pigeon fanciers get together, conversation and opinions are never in short supply. From left to right: Graham Davison, Wollongong, Australia, Silvere Toye, Belgium, Tom Wills, secretary of the Australian National Pigeon Association, Sydney, Australia, and Stephen Kearsey, past V.H.A. secretary and successful fancier, Melbourne, Australia.

not get in each other's way, with each bird comfortably stroking the air. In mobs of 60, each bird can see the way ahead as it is not simply looking at the pigeon in front of it. Similarly, birds further back in the flock can't coast in the air stream created by the leading birds (in the way migrating geese do). According to John Pryor, of Adelaide, one of Australia's best fliers, 150 birds is a good size for a working team. He feels that when well, this number of birds can fly in synch and notices that this coordinated flying pattern is lost when a fit team is flying like this and meets a team that is not so well.

Time on the wing

Is time on the wing around the loft just as beneficial as tossing? When birds are flying the roof, they essentially do a variety of circle configurations. It is possible for tired birds to always move to the inside of these circles so that they fly a considerably shorter distance than the other birds. This means that, although the entire team has spent the same time on the wing, the birds flying on the inside of the circle have not flown as far and so must have flown more slowly, spending more time coasting and gliding. One of the benefits of straight-line tossing is that all birds fly the same distance and this distance can be predetermined by the owner.

Training

How much training do birds need to fly a long-distance race? An interesting opinion comes from John Pryor of Adelaide, who states that birds, to fly a long-distance race, need to fly twice the distance in training tosses or shorter races prior to that event. If one of these tosses or races, though, had a tail wind, then its distance should be halved. This would mean that for a bird to fly a 700-mile race, it would need to fly 1400 miles in earlier flights, for example, a 250-, 300- and 350-mile race and ten 50-mile tosses, provided none of them were blow homes. To me, this seems a good yardstick to work by. Doug Ince, a successful flier known for his long-distance achievements in Melbourne, states that it is much better for a pigeon to be slightly 'underdone' than overworked for a long-distance race. It is hard to imagine that a pigeon that has been flattened earlier by overtraining or racing will take on the task of homing well from a long race. However, a fresh pigeon that is prepared to try can make it home because of its blood and fitness.

Assessing winning pigeons

Some interesting thoughts on assessing winning pigeons were provided by Graeme Davison. If a small group of winning pigeons comes into an area and the pigeons break for their lofts, it can end up a bit of a clocking match, but how can one determine the real leader? If the leader was going to the furthest loft, then the velocity of all pigeons will be maintained as he led them over their lofts and they in turn dropped off. If the leader was going to the shortest loft, then suddenly with their leader gone, the others may hesitate and the velocity of the further-flying birds would gradually drop.

Cost of pigeon racing

In Sydney, George Kypreos has some interesting figures that help us decide whether pigeon racing is becoming more expensive. One can compare the cost of a new Holden car, the prize won by the Melbourne Cup winner, the basic wage and the cost of sending a single pigeon to a race in 1965 and in 1995. The cost of the new Holden has increased ten times. The basic wage has increased 13 times. The winner of the Melbourne Cup now receives a prize 11 times higher. Meanwhile, the cost of sending a pigeon to a race in Australia has increased three times. A less quantitative measure, but also of value for comparison, is that the average cost of goods and services has increased ten times. From this, we can only assume that the cost of actually sending pigeons to a race is now relatively much cheaper for fanciers than it was 30 years ago. However, for Federations, the cost of running these races has increased, in keeping with goods and services.

Breeding winners

In Adelaide, John Pryor has some interesting views regarding breeding. He states that 80% of winners are bred from birds where both parents are less than 4 years of age, and that the chance of breeding a winner declines as the birds age, particularly if two older birds are paired together. He states that only 5% of winners are bred from an old hen paired to an old cock. For this reason, he tries to keep the average age of his stock cocks at just over 4 years and the average age of his stock hens at just over $3\frac{1}{2}$ years. If the average age starts to get a little bit high, older birds are replaced deliberately with younger ones to keep the average age down and so try and increase the number of winners bred. Obviously, there are always going to be exceptions but if a fancier wants to have the odds on his side, it seems best to have the age of at least one parent, and preferably both, 4 years or less. Just why this should be so is hard to say as a pigeon's genetic make-up cannot change with age. However, things such as yolk quality are affected by age. John also states that the first pair of eggs from a young hen is of particular value. Although the chance of breeding good race birds from older birds does seem to decline, age doesn't seem to affect the ability of older birds to produce stock pigeons. Perhaps the answer is to breed off your stock birds until 4 – 5 years of age and then breed from the best (i.e. the ones that have bred the winners) to produce stock birds and then replace them with this new stock.

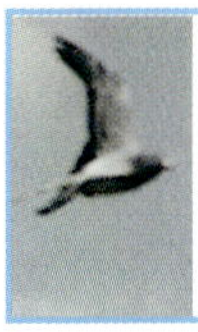

There are always exceptions but racing and breeding programs based on exceptions are statistically less likely to succeed.

But how should these birds be mated to produce stock birds? Silvere Toye of Belgium told me that one of the big advantages that European fanciers had over the British is that many British fanciers still believe in families. What is a family anyway but simply a group of related birds? Fanciers hope that other members of the family carry the winning genes of the famous bird within the family but even though the pigeons may look and handle the same, they may not. Most winners come from crossbreds. This is due to a genetic phenomenon called 'hybrid vigour', which tends to cover up recessive characteristics, which tend to decrease vigour and inhibit performance. Fewer winners are produced if birds from different lines within the same family are mated, and very few race winners are produced if related birds are paired. It is worth noting, however, that if an inbred bird produced in this way does race well, then it is very likely to breed birds as good as itself because it has little genetic variation. On the other hand, crossbred birds that may be excellent racers themselves, often produce youngsters of much more variable quality because of their own greater genetic variation. One should therefore aim to stabilize the required genes through inbreeding to produce stock birds and then cross these to produce the race team.

For example, if one has two cousins or a father and daughter or brother and sister that are independently breeding winners, then mate them together and select the youngsters most like their producing parents to replace them in the stock loft as they age. In this way, an inbred line is created that can then be crossed to another inbred line to produce race birds. If the fancier is keeping the average age of these new stock birds to less than 4 years, he is maximizing his chances statistically of success.

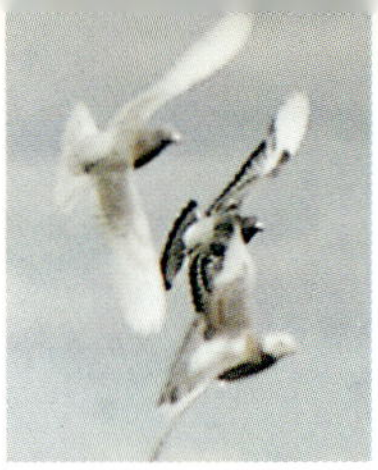

Chapter 35

FUNGI, FEED AND FORM

When feeding methods are discussed by fanciers, emphasis is placed on the type and percentage of various grains in their mixes. It is equally important that the grains used are of high quality. Grain that is dusty, spoiled by insects such as weevils, or visibly mouldy should never be fed to race birds. However, one particular problem is not always visible ... that of fungal toxins. These are a particularly dangerous problem because they can be clear, tasteless and odourless and so the seed can look fine but be contaminated.

Fungal spores are everywhere in the environment. When they get into a situation that is suitable for their growth, they germinate and reproduce. Some grow on seed, spoiling the grain and, in addition, some species during this growth produce substances that are poisonous to our birds. The fungi involved can be divided into two groups – non-toxin producing and toxin producing.

Non-toxin producing

As these non-toxin-producing fungi grow, they progressively spoil the grain. They have the potential to compromise the birds' health in two ways, firstly by robbing the bird of the nutrition found in the grain, and, secondly, in damaging the grain they provide a base for bacterial growth, which is then ingested by the birds. Growing youngsters and competitive birds need the full nutritional benefit of the seed; the ingestion of bacteria and decaying organic matter directly does them harm. Birds weakened by poor nutrition become vulnerable to secondary diseases and mature race birds cannot hold form.

Toxin producing

All fungi as they grow produce by-products of their normal metabolic pathways. In some species, these by-products are poisonous to pigeons (and other animals). These poisons are called mycotoxins, which means poisons of fungal origin. When mycotoxins are inadvertently ingested with contaminated grain, we see a variety of signs, depending on the actual species of fungi and the toxins they produce. Each fungus has its own light, temperature and moisture requirements. Some grow on crops in the field during periods of high moisture content, e.g. *Fusarium* spp. Others grow on foods during storage when moisture contents are relatively low, e.g. *Aspergillus* spp.

The conditions that induce a fungus to produce toxin may be different from those needed for fungal growth. Therefore, the fungus can grow without toxin production. Likewise, the toxin can be present after the fungus has stopped reproducing. Clinically, this means that the presence of a fungus on a seed does not necessarily indicate that a toxin is present nor does its absence mean that food or grain is free of mycotoxins.

The amount of toxin present can vary with any given batch of grain. Depending on the storage methods and size of the stored sample, one area may have no detectable mycotoxin while another may have very large concentrations. This means that a fancier can be unlucky with a single particular bag.

The most common toxins, the fungi that produce them and the problems they cause are set out in the following tabulation.

Fungus	Toxin	Effects
Aspergillus spp.	Aflatoxin	Damage to liver, kidney and bowel; interference with clotting ability; damage to heart; immunosuppression
Fusarium spp.	Trichothecenes	Irritation to mouth, crop, stomach and bowel; damage to liver and kidney
Penicillium spp. (also some *Aspergillus* spp.)	Ochratoxins	Damage to kidney, liver and bowel; airsac inflammation; immunosuppression
Mucor spp. and others	None	General ill thrift; signs associated with poor nutrition and ingestion of bacteria in spoiled seed, e.g. poor growth, reluctance to fly, loss of form, vulnerability to secondary infections

Signs displayed by the birds are affected by the type and amount of toxin ingested and also by the age and general level of health of the birds. Toxins that affect the liver cause the birds to be quiet within the loft, reluctant to fly, lose weight, have a decreased appetite and develop a greenish diarrhoea. Kidney toxins interfere with the kidneys' ability to concentrate urine, leading to watery droppings. Similarly, the kidney loses its ability to excrete the body's wastes, which, again, causes the birds to be quiet, lose weight and be reluctant to fly. Toxins that interfere with the birds' ability to clot blood can lead to the development of large 'blood blisters' under the skin and also, not uncommonly, bleeding from the bowel, with the fancier noticing dried blood in the feathers at the cloaca. Irritant toxins, such as those produced by *Fusarium,* can lead to the development of visible ulcers within the mouth and other signs associated with irritation to the gastrointestinal tract, such as delayed crop emptying and diarrhoea. Other toxins affect other sites, notably the airsacs. In addition, some toxins directly suppress the birds' immune system. However, all toxins generally compromise the birds' health, leading to a vulnerability to secondary infections, such as canker, thrush, Coccidia and respiratory problems. The difficulty comes in that often signs are fairly subtle, particularly in race-age birds, with the fancier feeling that the birds are 'just not right'. Signs displayed by the birds are dose-dependent. Birds that have a lot of toxic grain are obviously unwell. However, those that have had only a small amount may simply lose winning form. Frustrated fliers often wonder why everything seems to be going well but for some reason the birds are just not 'firing'.

Diagnosis

Diagnosis of a fungal problem is based on the signs that the birds are showing, postmortem and microscopic changes and, finally, demonstration of the toxin in the grain. The definitive diagnosis involves the isolation, identification and quantification of the specific toxin. Only certain government laboratories that do a lot of bird work have the capability to perform these complex assays. Diagnosis is not always easy, as the signs shown by the birds are not specific, being similar to those of other more common diseases. Similarly, secondary diseases become involved because of the bird's compromised health, which can complicate and mask the primary problem. Seed is not always available for testing as the contaminated sample may have been completely eaten.

One becomes suspicious of a fungal involvement when signs that may be caused by them correlate with the use of a particular feed. Principal microscopic changes usually involve the liver and kidney as these organs act as the body's 'filters', metabolizing most poisons. More specific confirmatory tests, such as food assays, can then be instigated with some confidence.

If a fancier has birds that are unwell and he is suspicious of a fungal problem, I suggest that the following procedures be adopted :

- Review the use of a particular grain or batch or source of the grain and its correlation with the signs observed.
- Examine the food closely for evidence of spoiling. If either non-toxin- or toxin-producing fungi have grown on the seed, the seed may smell stale or be discoloured. If suspicious, store some grain in an air-tight container at 4°C (i.e. in the fridge) for subsequent testing.
- Submit grain for testing. The submitted grain is initially cultured. If fungi have grown on the grain but are now not visible, the grain may be heavily contaminated with spores. When cultured on a growth medium, usually Saboraud's Agar, these fungi will grow. A detailed outline of available grain tests is given in the following chapter.

Sometimes, bird presentation to an avian veterinarian is of benefit. The birds are clinically assessed and, if warranted, autopsied. Changes visible to the naked eye may be suggestive, However, if necessary, microscopic work can be done on the tissue samples collected during autopsy, looking for changes associated with poisoning. If changes here are also suggestive, toxicity testing on the feed that has been previously stored can then be performed at particular diagnostic laboratories.

Often, however, a loss of form that correlates strongly with use of a particular grain, particularly if the grain is visibly spoiled or positive on culture, is sufficient to make a provisional diagnosis.

Prevention and treatment

There are no specific antidotes for mycotoxins. It is easier to prevent exposure to mycotoxins than to attempt treatment following their ingestion. The quality of grain and the method of storage are therefore very important. The fungal spores, by themselves, do no harm. If a piece of bread or fruit is not eaten for several days, mould will grow from the spores present. If this food had been eaten several days earlier, it would not have caused illness. In the same way, grains contain fungal spores and it is important that they are not given a chance to germinate. Moisture is the one most important factor controlling mould growth. If there is no moisture, then, even though the fungal spores may persist, they cannot germinate. If grain is dried to 13% moisture content, all growth ceases and the fungus becomes dormant, but even a mild increase in humidity can initiate growth and lead to toxin secretion within 6 – 8 hours.

Low temperature also inhibits fungal growth. With increasing temperature, humidity increases, enhancing growth. Interestingly, in some areas of southern U.S.A., where the preferred conditions for mycotoxin production are common (i.e. high temperature and humidity), refrigeration of food is often necessary to prevent mycotoxin production. Grain should be stored in a clean, moisture-proof container at an even temperature, which should be low. Cleaning containers between seed batches is a good idea to minimize contamination from one batch to the next. Similarly, fully use one batch before adding more to the top of the storage bin to prevent the build-up at the base, of older grains, which may harbour spores. Stirring the seed increases ventilation and decreases humidity within the seed itself, further decreasing the chance of mould growth. I believe the famous Janssen Brothers of Arendonk used to stir their seed every day.

If, however, contaminated feed is inadvertently fed, recovery is often rapid after withdrawal. However, this is dependent on the degree of tissue damage that has already occurred. A health profile, i.e. a crop flush and faecal smear, will identify secondary diseases that will need to be treated. In addition, routine stress minimization procedures should be adopted, i.e. no overcrowding, control of parasitic diseases, good hygiene, good-quality foods with a multivitamin supplement, no rationing, and no forced flying, to give the birds the best chance of a full recovery.

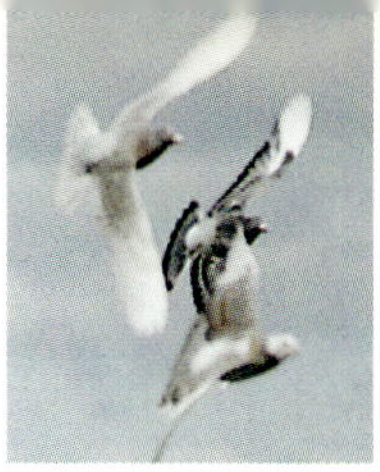

Chapter 36

TESTING OF 'BAD FOOD'

Pigeons relish the taste of good-quality grain. For on-going success, it is important that only the best-quality grain is fed. What is bad food and what is the best way for the fancier to ensure that the grain he uses is good?

It is vital for continued good race performance and the maintenance of form that only good-quality grain is fed. Good-quality grain must not only be nutritious but also free of certain bacteria, moulds, fungi and fungal toxins. Testing is available to the fancier to ensure that the grain he is using is, in fact, good quality. Food hygiene problems for both people and pigeons associated with grain, fruit or vegetables are most likely to be due to fungal growth and the resultant production of toxins by the fungi. These toxins are called mycotoxins. Some of these mycotoxins, e.g. aflatoxins, are amongst the most toxic substances known. Animals and birds are more at risk from fungal toxin poisoning than humans owing to the large proportion of the diet that may come from one batch of feed and because they eat the outer part, i.e. the husk, of the grain where the highest level of toxins can occur.

And so what signs might alert the fancier to problems with the grain that he is using? As mentioned earlier, the degree of problems seen depends on the amount of toxin ingested. Birds that have taken in a high level of toxin are obviously unwell. However, birds that have taken in a lower level of toxin may appear essentially normal around the loft, but during active competition, when the slightest thing can compromise overall performance, signs can be very subtle. In the racing loft, the fancier may notice that his birds are simply a bit quiet or less keen to fly, or that feather down production has decreased. Alternatively, he may have an on-going, low-grade health problem involving wet canker or respiratory infection that is failing to respond to routine medication. In the breeding loft, hens may be late to lay their eggs, youngsters in the nest may be a little underweight and need to be weaned 1 or 2 days later. Despite the best care, feeding stock birds may find raising youngsters excessively draining. In the postweaning time, weaned youngsters may fail to thrive and be especially vulnerable to disease, while during the moult, feather quality will be compromised.

Testing for moulds, fungi and their toxins

By far, the most important thing therefore for the fancier is to ensure that the grain is free of fungal toxins. These damage the bird's liver and kidney and inhibit the ability of the immune system to mount an immune response, creating a vulnerability to infection. In pigeons, the most common secondary infection is respiratory infection. So, what tests are available?

METHOD 1: TESTING FOR FUNGAL TOXINS

Testing for fungal toxins is complex and expensive. Grain needs to be sent to a diagnostic laboratory for this test. The primary function of these labs is to test export grains and oil seeds and food destined for human consumption, such as wheat for bread, fruit, vegetables and fruit juice. There are many different fungal toxins and they can only be tested for one at a time. The cost of testing for each toxin is in the range of AUD$120 – 170. Just because the grain is found to be free of one toxin, other(s) could be there. This form of testing is not recommended. What would be good is an all-encompassing test to see if the grain is contaminated by any fungal toxin. Unfortunately, this is not available as yet. However, there is such a test in the U.S.A. and it is hoped that this will be available more generally soon.

Method 2: Fungal culture and identification

The test that is usually done is a fungal culture. Here, a sample of grain is pulverized and cultured on to a fungal growth medium so that any spores on the grain's surface are given an opportunity to grow. In this way, an estimate of the number of fungal spores per gram can be ascertained. Because grain has to have had a fungus growing on it (which leaves spores behind) to contain toxins, there is a strong correlation between spore numbers and toxin levels. Good-quality grain usually has 80 spores or less per gram, while problem grain will have spore numbers in the thousands per gram. Once fungus, if any, on the grain has grown, then the actual fungus must be identified to see if it is a toxin-producing variety. Not all fungi produce toxins; in fact, only about 1 in 10 do. If a fungus capable of producing toxin is grown, then it is likely that the seed contains some of the toxin that the fungus produces and it is best not to risk feeding that grain to the birds. To culture and identify fungi costs AUD$75 per grain sample. To test each grain in say a five-seed mix becomes too expensive and so what is usually done is the five or so grains that the fancier intends using are submitted for testing mixed as a single sample. Because fungi are often grain-specific, once we know what the fungi are, we usually know which is the problem grain. Interestingly, the fungi that contaminate grain are specific to a geographical area and so a grain that has tested positive should be replaced with grain grown in a different area. In Australia, this is the test that grain merchants that cater specifically for pigeon racers have used. Certification should be available on request.

Method 3: Fungal culture only

A simpler test is available in which grain is inoculated onto a fungal growth medium called Saboraud's Agar and incubated at 25°C for 5 – 7 days. Saboraud's Agar inhibits bacterial growth but promotes fungal growth. This simply gives any fungal spores on the surface of the grain an opportunity to grow. This test has the advantage of being cheap (costing AUD$15) but fails to distinguish between toxin- and non-toxin-producing strains and also makes it difficult to provide an accurate spore count. Non-germinated spores from non-toxin-producing fungi on grain are in themselves no problem and in fact most human food has some on its surface. This test, however, is useful as an initial screening test. If no fungi or an obviously low amount grow, then the sample is fine to use. However, if significant numbers of spores germinate, then the seed can either be rejected or submitted for more thorough testing as outlined in Method 2 above. This test is also useful for fliers who feed a lot of different seed types. Up to 12 different grains can be tested on one plate. Only those that grow fungi then need further testing.

What method is best for the fancier?

I feel the best approach for most fanciers is to go to a grain merchant who has his grain tested. If this is not possible, buy or obtain a sample of seed, ensuring that the merchant has sufficient in stock to last an extended time. Ensure initially that the seed is clean, dust-free, has no water stains, smells fresh and has no sign of weevil damage. Grain husks should adhere tightly to the kernel, particularly with peas, as loose husks can indicate problems with moisture content at the time of harvest. Seed should be hard with a low moisture content. Get this seed sample tested as in Method 2 above. If the test shows the grain to be free of toxin-producing fungi, then buy the batch. Provided the grain is stored well (i.e. at low temperature and low humidity), then the fancier knows that he has good food for his birds. AUD$75 for testing is still quite expensive and so what can be a good idea is to split the cost between three fanciers who then each buy one-third of the batch. For a fancier to spend AUD$25 to ensure that his birds have good-quality feed, to my mind, is money well spent.

Is it really all worthwhile? If you had asked me this question several years ago, I would have said no but I now feel that testing the seed should be incorporated into the annual loft management regime if on-going success is to be enjoyed. Too many times after autopsying birds from teams that are performing poorly and sending samples away to an avian pathologist for analysis, the resultant report states that the birds' tissues have changes indicative of fungal toxin exposure. Fortunately, often the seed that a fancier obtains for use is fine and no problem is experienced but although the gross appearance and smell of grain can give an initial indication of its quality, it is impossible to say whether the seed is free of fungi without testing as fungal toxins are colourless, tasteless and odour-free. 'Bad food' is one of those problems that can eventually catch up with a fancier who does not test. The only sure way to avoid poor race performance due to bad food is to have the seed tested before use. I will relate here an experience from 1998.

A very good flier started the season well, gaining the following Federation positions: 1st followed by a 4th, then a 6th and a 2nd. The food he was using ran out and so he bought additional grain. Over the following weeks his results were 15th, then 48th, then 120th and finally 189th. At this point, having explored other possible causes, grain was submitted for testing. The results showed that two of the grains he used were heavily contaminated with a toxin-producing fungus. He then switched to grain known to be free of contamination and his results over the next 5 weeks were 111th, 89th, 62nd, 25th and 4th.

Bacterial testing

Seed can also be contaminated with a range of bacteria. Here the appearance and odour of the seed do give an indication of the level of contamination. Fortunately, most are not capable of causing disease. The presence of bacteria on the surface of the grain is not necessarily a problem. Human food is not sterile and has bacteria on its surface. The bacteria present on grain can be checked, however, by culturing the grain on media that promote bacterial growth and then identifying what bacteria grow. This involves additional expense and is considered worthwhile only if the birds are having problems with bacterial infection and the fancier is looking for the source of infection.

Gamma irradiation

Fanciers will read in some advertisements that the seed has been gamma irradiated. This involves a process similar to x-raying seed and is sometimes used as an aid in fungal control on grain. The procedure has advantages and disadvantages. Gamma irradiation of grain is good in that it kills any bacteria and fungi growing on the seed's surface, thus preventing their further multiplication. It does not, however, affect the level of any toxin present or reverse any damage to the grain that bacterial or fungal growth may have caused. Irradiation also kills the seed, which means that the seed loses its own innate ability to resist disease. This means that seed after irradiation is more vulnerable to infection and therefore must be particularly well stored.

Testing technique protocol

If a fancier would like his grain tested for fungi, moulds and fungal toxins, he should contact his local avian veterinarian, who should be able to direct him to a testing laboratory or be able to organize the testing for him. Usually a sterile bag will be sent to the fancier. A sample of grain being used or intended to be used is placed inside the bag and the top folded over several times, before sealing the edge with adhesive tape. Because the distribution of fungal toxins through a sample is uneven, it is best to ensure some grains from several points throughout the bag or bags of grain are included so that the sample submitted is truly representative of the grain batch as a whole. In order to avoid contamination, it is best to use a clean dry scoop (e.g. a dessertspoon) to pick up the grain and to place it in the bag. The results of using the recommended technique of Method 2 above are ready in 7 days and the total cost in Australia is AUD$75.

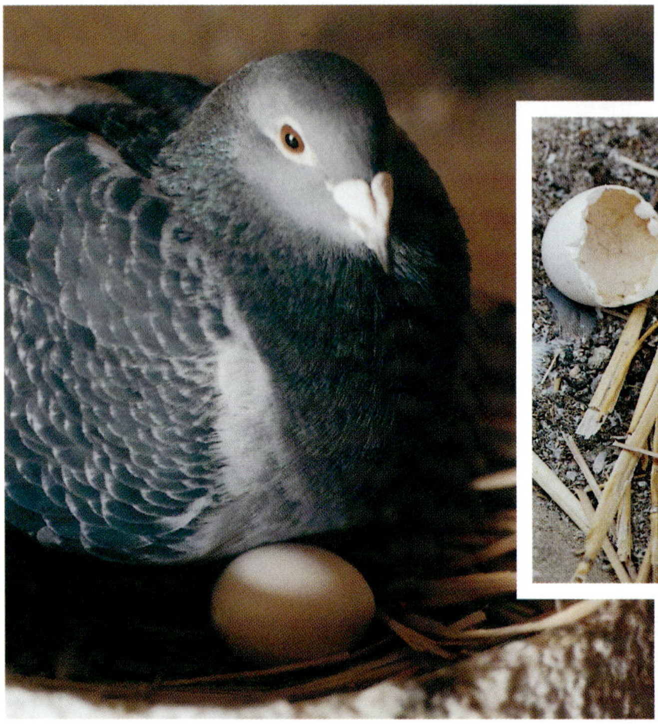

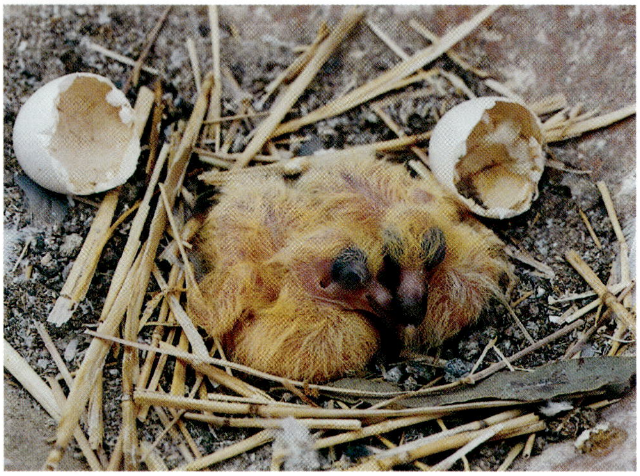

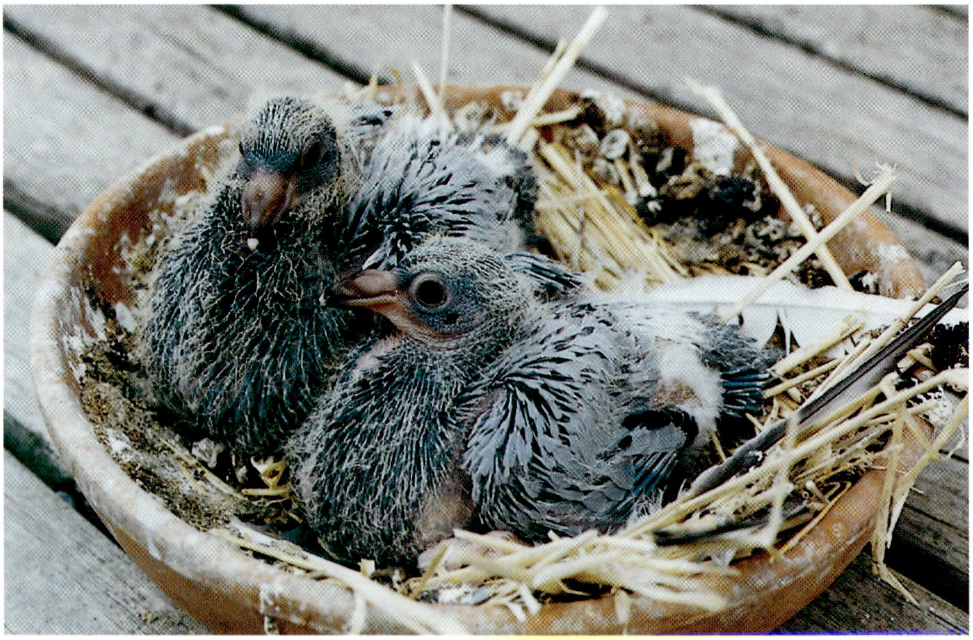

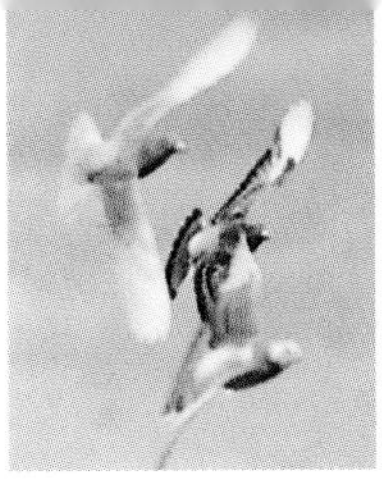

Chapter 37

THE USE OF PROBIOTICS IN RACING PIGEONS*

The bacteria – host relationship

Through evolution, bacteria and warm-blooded animals have closely associated themselves to form a closed system for mutual benefit. Through trial and error, over millennia, populations of bacteria have evolved that are indigenous to their animal host. The animal host receives the benefits of aid in the digestive process, manufacture of essential nutrients, protection against other undesirable bacteria, assistance in control of water in the body and other metabolic advantages. The bacteria in return receive temperatures favourable for their growth, a constant supply of nutrients and essential substances in the form of the body's secretions. Because of the exact nature of this relationship, there are bacterial populations that are the most favourable for the host animal.

Changes

Each member of this mutually beneficial relationship is profoundly influenced by the other. When certain changes occur in the host, corresponding changes are reflected in bacterial populations in the bowel. Bacterial changes may occur as a result of stress, diet change, antibiotic therapy and other factors. Conversely, as the resident bacterial population changes, there are subsequent changes in the animal's activity. These include alterations in the host's ability to digest its food and its ability to protect itself from bowel disease. The animal host then has the problem of getting back to an ideal relationship with its normal resident population of bacteria. Hopefully it can accomplish such a relationship before subsequent challenges again upset the ideal state.

Where animals are not stressed, have an appropriate diet, are not crowded, are not given drugs, do not contract infection or metabolic diseases and live in a clean environment, an ideal level of intestinal bacterial population may be maintained on a rather steady basis. In fact, no differences are generally reported in numerous trials under these ideal conditions.

Imbalance

The conditions described above, however, do not fit the environment under which our pigeons race. Even in the best lofts, under the best managers, birds are subjected to various stresses. This means that disruption of the normal balance of intestinal bacteria can be a common event. If an ideal state is maintained, there is optimal utilization of nutrients and a resistance to harmful organisms. This has been shown in numerous experiments.

What is a probiotic?

The organisms that are normally found in the bowel of healthy non-stressed animals are called probiotics. The probiotic concept involves the refeeding or reintroduction of these bacteria to an animal.

---

* My thanks to PetAg Inc. for much of the scientific data provided for this chapter.

Many studies in many countries have shown that, although these bacteria can control and exclude other harmful bacteria, they are in fact the most likely to be disrupted by stress. Most probiotic products consist of naturally occurring living cultures of specific strains of *Lactobacillus* and enteric *Streptococcus* (*Enterococcus*).

Restoring the balance

Once it was established that the feeding of certain live bacteria to animals has the potential to produce beneficial effects under certain circumstances, i.e. when the normal bacterial balance has been disrupted, the actual delivery of these organisms from the laboratory to the animal became the next hurdle. Pharmaceutical companies have now overcome this. The large Japanese pharmaceutical company Yakult manufactures a human probiotic (*Lactobacillus casei*) as a milk-based drink in Victoria. This is distributed through the eastern States of Australia. One million bottles are consumed by Australians every week. Fourteen million are consumed in Japan every day! Interestingly, in people, studies have shown that individuals who drink 'Yakult' and are exposed to diseases such as *Salmonella* are much less likely to become unwell. Probiotic use in people has also been shown to decrease the chance of bowel cancer. As many of the harmful bacteria produce toxins that are carcinogenic, i.e. can induce cancer, their exclusion can decrease the risk of this disease.

In birds, there are gel preparations of probiotics for individual dosing and also water-soluble powders to treat the flock. These provide selected beneficial live bacteria with excellent stability when protected from extreme heat and moisture. Because of the intimate relationship between the host animal and its bacterial population, it is important that the correct organisms are supplied in probiotic preparation for any given species. Probiotic supplements need to be prepared with a particular species in mind and the more types of normal bacteria that can be provided, the better. For use in pigeons, therefore, multistrain avian-origin probiotic supplements are used.

Mode of action

And so how do they work?

- **Competitive inhibition –** It is known that the beneficial bacteria produce lactic acid, hydrogen peroxide, antibiotic and other substances that help keep potential pathogens under control. As many fanciers are aware, the most likely potential invaders are *E. coli* and *Candida* (yeast or thrush) and in fancy birds, *Salmonella*. These organisms are opportunists, waiting to cause disease whenever pigeons become stressed. Stress causes disruption to the normal bowel bacteria and gives these organisms a chance to invade. The pH in the bowel in health is mildly acidic. With *E. coli* infection, it becomes alkaline. Anything that acidifies the bowel will create a hostile environment for the *E. coli,* thus making it harder for the organisms to survive. This is why the addition of controlled levels of various acids to the drinking water exerts a beneficial effect with these infections and also why the older practice of adding apple cider vinegar (acetic acid) to the water can help. The lactic acid produced by probiotics produces the same result. In addition to weakly acidifying the bowel, probiotics do much more to help the bird in that they produce protective slime layers that coat the bowel lining and also preferentially occupy receptor sites on the bowel wall, in the process excluding bacteria such as *E. coli*. They therefore offer an effective natural way of combating the problem without the need for antibiotics. In addition, there is no risk associated with their use as there can be with acids. By treating the birds, we are simply flooding the bowel with beneficial bacteria, which, through their normal activity, re-establish health.
- **Appetite stimulation –** Probiotics appear to have a strong appetite stimulatory effect. They are known to produce digestive enzymes and B vitamins. These effects help the bird to get the

maximum nutrition from their grain. One recently reported study in America demonstrated that hand-raised cockatiel chicks weaned at 6 weeks of age, supplemented every second day with probiotics, were 14% heavier at weaning than chicks that received no probiotics.

- **Immune stimulation –** Recent work by scientists throughout the world indicates that probiotics stimulate general immunity.

Use of probiotics

So when can the fancier use probiotics to his advantage?

- **After any stress –** It is well known that stress induces a disruption of the normal bowel bacteria and that the beneficial bacteria are the first ones to be lost with stress. Once these beneficial bacteria are removed from their normal environment by stress, many more are lost from the digestive tract and are replaced by an overgrowth of non-beneficial bacteria. This can result in diarrhoea, loss of performance, decreased appetite and, in the stock loft, inhibited growth and limited weight gain in the youngsters. Probiotics restore the balance of beneficial to non-beneficial bacteria. They are best given as soon as possible after the stress or just before the time of the stress. By doing so, disease or performance problems may be avoided.
- **In the stock loft –** Use probiotics regularly in the stock loft as part of routine management, particularly during the breeding season. Use two to three times weekly when the stock birds are feeding youngsters. This helps the birds resist *E. coli* (often associated with wet nests) and ensures that the birds get the maximum nutrition possible out of their seed at a time that often puts real demands on them. Probiotic use will help the parents produce vigorous robust young.
- **In the race loft –** Probiotics can be used in the race loft to both treat and prevent *E. coli* and *Candida* infections. Stress disrupts the bowel bacteria, giving *E. coli* and yeast the opportunity to cause disease. In lofts where these are a problem, probiotics can be used whenever *E. coli* or yeasts are seen under the microscope, when the droppings become green or green and watery, or when there are weather conditions that favour *E. coli*, in particular when the weather is cold and damp or humid. In such lofts, it is a good idea to give probiotics routinely as part of the loft's disease management program, with the focus here being on disease prevention rather than waiting for disease to appear. When *E. coli* and yeast flare-ups are a problem, our challenge is to identify the stress that caused the flare-up while at the same time helping the birds clear the *E. coli* and yeast through use of probiotics. With no on-going stress, the droppings will appear normal within 24 hours of the start of probiotic use. Having said all that, probiotics are not a cure-all. A non-response to probiotics can be expected in one of two situations:
  1. **When the stress is on-going –** It is important to identify and if possible eliminate any predisposing stress to ensure a good response to treatment. I draw the analogy here of trying to dry a floor without turning the tap off. Stress can come from a problem with the loft environment or management or may be associated with one of the more serious diseases such as canker, respiratory infection, Coccidia or worms. With identification and correction of the underlying stress, a good response to probiotics can be expected.
  2. **Severe *E. coli* infection –** Severe infections pass the point where it is possible to treat them successfully with either probiotics or bowel acids and it becomes necessary to use stronger medication such as sulfur-based antibiotics. These actually kill the *E. coli* but they should be used with caution as they also kill many beneficial bacteria, can compromise feather quality and cause nausea in the birds. If given, they should be given for only 1 – 2 days and it is best to use them early in the week so that the birds have a couple of days between their use and basketing. Treating with probiotics can, however, often prevent the infection progressing to the point where these antibiotics need to be used.

- **Postrace –** The stress of racing itself causes disruption to the normal bowel population. Fanciers will have noticed that the droppings of birds that have raced often take 24 – 48 hours to return fully to normal. With my own birds, I find that if they come home to probiotics, then the next morning it is much more likely that the droppings will be normally formed and brown and that the bird will continue with a feather down drop. Probiotics can be combined with electrolytes and vitamins.
- **Postweaning –** At this time, we don't want to use drugs. We want to develop a strong natural immunity. Probiotics specifically stimulate this.
- **Following antibiotic use –** Particularly during racing, probiotic use after antibiotics hastens the re-establishment of the normal bowel population.
- **Moulting –** Maintaining a healthy bowel during moulting aids in on-going nutrient delivery to the developing feather in the feather follicle and decreases the chance of fret marks, etc.
- **In the show loft –** Probiotics can help birds resist *Salmonella.* Although all pigeons are susceptible to *Salmonella,* clinical disease is seen more commonly in fancy breeds rather than racing birds. Certain breeds are particularly susceptible, e.g. Modenas, Show Homers and the high-flying breeds, especially Doneks. The way an outbreak is managed depends on the severity of the problem. Regular probiotics have been shown to help birds resist the disease.

It has become the belief of some fliers lately that fit racing birds should have sterile (i.e. absolutely no bacteria) in their bowels. I can understand how this belief originated in that, with some bacteria, notably *E. coli,* the fewer we can see on faecal smears the better. However, to extend this to all bacteria is a definite mistake. Let me state here that there is absolutely no evidence in the scientific literature to support the belief that a healthy racing pigeon has no bacteria in its bowel. In fact, quite the opposite is the case. What we want is a healthy mixed population of normal bacteria doing their job to help maintain the health of the bird. For many years, I have been examining many droppings every day. Many of these come regularly from top lofts and I have never seen a dropping with no bacteria. Fanciers with their own microscopes will notice that, when their birds are at the peak of fitness, bacteria are visible in their droppings. Closer to home, I have won twelve open V.H.A. Federation races with between 2000 and 9000 birds competing and, despite examining my birds' droppings on a weekly basis, have never found a single sterile dropping. The experts tell us that the only situation in which a pigeon's bowel would become sterile is either through antibiotic abuse or heavy metal poisoning. The last thing you want to do is lose the beneficial population of bacteria in your birds' bowels. I feel that there are already enough theories in pigeon racing, so let's stick to what is known to be fact.

Probac

Probac is a multistrain avian-origin probiotic made specifically for pigeons. It is the probiotic preparation that I recommend. It can be added to the drinking water at the rate of 1 teaspoon to 4 litres or added to the grain (after first moistening with a seed oil, 1/2 – 1 ml per kilogram) at the rate of 1/3 teaspoon (1 gram) to 1 kg.

Note on probiotic use

In some metropolitan areas, the addition of fluoride or chlorine to drinking water may interfere with the action of probiotics. In metropolitan areas, treatment plants are situated throughout the water distribution network. According to Australian authorities, the concentration of fluoride and chlorine throughout most of the network is too low to exert an effect. However, the concentration in the water of fanciers close to a treatment plant may be high enough to kill the probiotics. These substances will, however, evaporate from treated water if it is allowed to stand for 24 hours. Fanciers in any doubt are best to set aside water to be medicated with probiotics for 24 hours before use. Simply standing the required volume of water in several buckets awaiting use is adequate.

Alternatively, most water-soluble probiotic preparations can be added to the seed. Indeed, with some preparations, this ensures a more immediate and effective delivery of the probiotics to the digestive tract.

Probiotic use really is at the forefront of avian veterinary practice. Modern technology involved in probiotic preparation protects the probiotics against stomach acids, bile salts and digestive enzymes so that large numbers of live organisms arrive in the bowel after ingestion to exert their various beneficial effects. Interestingly, human probiotic preparations are being developed to target specific bacterial infections. In man, a bacterium *Bacillus cereus* causes a gastroenteritis. This infection is not fatal but is responsible for many lost days of work annually in the population. Rather than being prescribed antibiotics, patients are prescribed a specific probiotic 'yoghurt' that controls the infection. According to the companies involved, with this technology now in place, more difficult organisms like *E. coli*, which have a large number of strains and mutate more readily, will be tackled. Once available, these preparations will be beneficial and useful to fanciers as they will mean that these infections can be managed without resorting to form-reducing antibiotics.

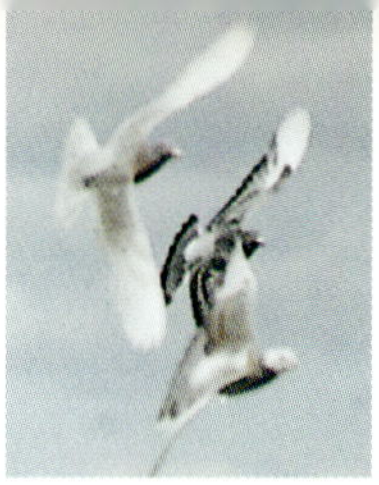

Chapter 38

NATURAL SUPPLEMENTS

The two most commonly used natural supplements are garlic and now also, to some extent, echinacea.

Garlic

Garlic, whose scientific name is *Allium sativum*, is a common plant used world-wide for food. Since ancient times, garlic has been used for a variety of human and animal ailments and problems. Its active agent is allicin, which, with its breakdown products, produces its characteristic odour. When garlic cloves are crushed, allicin is produced by the action of enzymes on a pre-existing chemical known as alliin. The positive effect of the juice of fresh cloves seems fairly certain whereas information from modern commercial preparations such as powders, tablets and oils prepared by heat distillation, etc., is not very convincing. This is because the active ingredient is fragile and is often broken down during processing. It is the breakdown of alliin to allium that produces the characteristic odour and there is a correlation between the odour and the level of active constituent. Potency of garlic to some extent, therefore, depends on pungency. Once garlic is dried into odour-free garlic or pills, it loses many of the properties that make it useful in health promotion. It is best to use either fresh juice from garlic cloves or, if an oil is used, its preparation must not involve any heating process as this will result in loss of potency.

Scientific benefits

Garlic has been used by pigeon fanciers for many decades and there is much anecdotal evidence as to its benefits but what scientific benefits have been attributed to garlic?

Allicin is known to have antibacterial properties. It inhibits the growth of or kills approximately two dozen types of bacteria (including *Samonella*) and at least 60 types of mould and yeast.

It contains the trace elements selenium and germanium. These minerals are important in the normal development of the immune system. It is thought that they boost the immune system of the pigeon to increase its ability to fight disease-producing organisms of many kinds.

Garlic has been shown to have a stimulating effect on certain enzymes that are known to be effective in removing toxic substances from the body. This is why people use the term 'blood purifier' or 'tissue purifier', whatever this means. Both are meaningless expressions that don't explain anything. But that aside, there are chemical compounds in garlic that assist the body to detoxify, neutralize or eliminate poisonous substances. In pigeons, the use of garlic after a race may assist in restoring a bird to normal racing condition. How important lactic acid here is debatable as the major fuel for races is fat, which is broken down aerobically (i.e. with oxygen). Lactic acid is only released when glycogen is broken down anaerobically (i.e. without oxygen). However, lactic acid is produced when pigeons are landing and taking off during the race and would also be involved in birds that sprint during the race and for the loft (if they do this). Pigeons that are not exercised reasonably soon after a tough race will develop hard swollen muscles. It is likely that lactic acid is involved in certain situations and that an early work-out after a race would help eliminate the problem. Garlic at this time provides an added benefit and assists in the return to normal race condition.

Garlic supplementation

There is much still to learn about garlic but based on the knowledge to hand and the anecdotal experience of many fanciers it seems that there is benefit in using garlic in the loft all year round but particularly during weaning and racing. I feel it is of particular benefit in the stressful postweaning period when youngsters are vulnerable to disease. Garlic supplementation is one way of helping them through this time without interfering with their developing natural immunity.

Garlic can be supplemented in two ways:

1 As fresh juice squeezed into the drinker or onto the seed. Whole cloves should not be placed into the drinker as these quickly develop a biofilm over their surface and are then no different from any other decaying plant material in the water.

2 As an oil-based seed additive. Good-quality garlic oil contains the juice of fresh garlic cloves in a base of one or more seed oils. It should not have undergone any heating processes in its preparation that are likely to affect its allicin content. Most garlic oils are added to the seed at the rate of $^1/_2$ – 1 ml per kilogram of grain, which moistens the seed and makes it look clean without it becoming 'gluggy'. This method of supplementation has the advantage that the birds also get some nutritional benefit from the seed-oil base.

There does not appear to be a toxic dose with garlic, i.e. you cannot give too much. However, if it is oversupplemented, the concentration causes palatability problems, with the birds reluctant to take the seed or water.

Echinacea

Echinacea is a derivative of the plant *Augustifolia purpurea*. It is available as a solution designed to be taken orally. This can be added to the water or mixed with a seed oil. It is used as a natural immunostimulant and may speed recovery in some cases of disease and in debilitated birds.

Epsom salts

Epsom salts is the common name for an electrolyte (or salt) combination, magnesium sulfate ($MgSO_4$). It has been used by pigeon fanciers for many years to 'clean the birds out' and in some way promote health. When electrolytes or salts are given orally, fluid moves across the bowel wall to make the concentration of these the same on either side. This natural mechanism is a protective device that re-establishes normal salt concentrations in body fluids if dehydration occurs. With dehydration, body salts become concentrated and so, after drinking, fluid is quickly absorbed from the bowel into the body, diluting the body salts so that normal healthy levels are re-established.

When we give a concentrated salt solution, such as Epsom salts, to a healthy bird, the opposite happens. Fluid rushes from the body into the bowel, attempting to dilute the salts there. As a result, the bowel fills with fluid, in the process dehydrating the bird. The resultant watery dropping is made up of the healthy body's normal fluid. Prolonged supplementation with concentrated salts leads to profound dehydration, irreversible kidney damage and death. This is why people and animals that drink seawater eventually die. It is a myth that the administration of a concentrated salt solution in some way cleans out the birds and, in fact, it moves away from what we are trying to achieve in that it makes the birds deliberately unwell. It is likely that the birds of fanciers who extol its benefits do well despite what their owners have put them through. The use of such salt solutions should be discouraged.

Apple cider vinegar (and other acids)

Adding apple cider vinegar, which is acetic acid, and other acids, such as citric acid, to the water is one of those older practices that at first glance seems like hocus pocus. However, they are of benefit and there is a scientific reason for their use. In health, the bowel is weakly acidic. This is because the normal bacteria found there produce lactic acid as part of their normal metabolism. With stress, these normal bacterial populations are disrupted and the pH within the bowel is altered. Harmful bacteria such as *E. coli* and *Salmonella* do not like acidic conditions and so anything that helps to maintain the weakly acidic environment within the bowel helps to prevent these organisms from becoming established. The usual amount of apple cider vinegar to add is 5 – 10 ml to 1 litre of water, depending on product strength and local water pH.

Interestingly, the commercially available probiotic preparations, because they contain the normal bowel bacteria, produce lactic acid and this is one of the ways they help to maintain bowel health.

Section 8

DIAGNOSIS AND MEDICATIONS

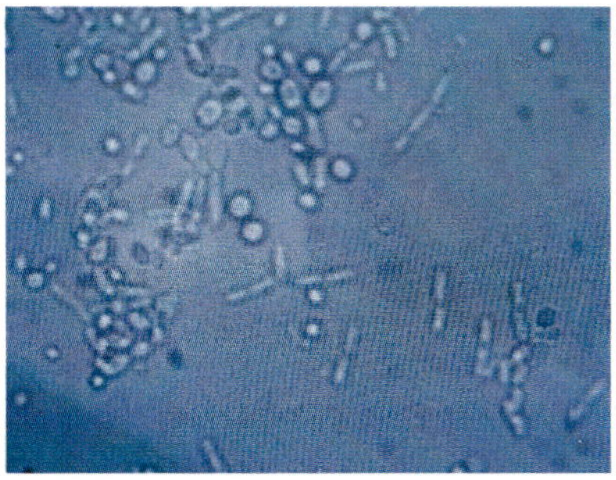

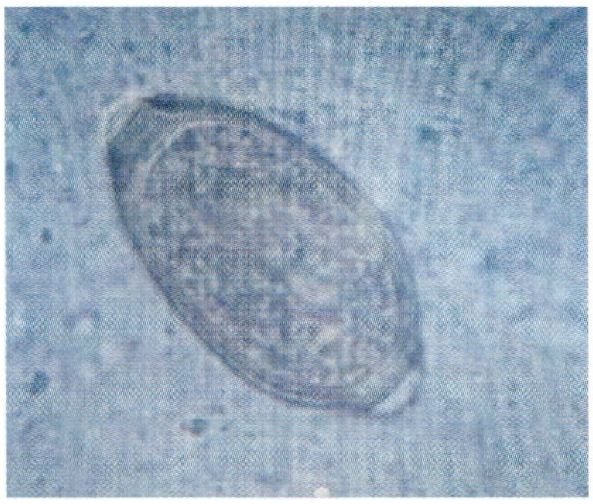

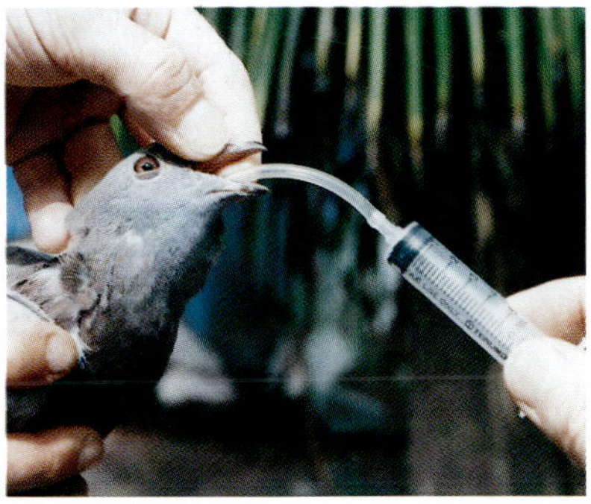

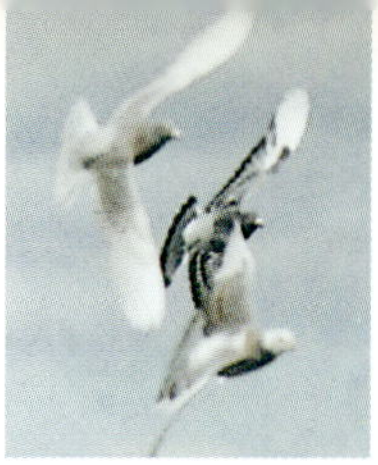

Chapter 39

DIAGNOSIS AT A DISTANCE

Distance and time can sometimes be obstacles for fanciers to get to an avian veterinarian. However, if it is not possible for a fancier to get to a veterinarian, much can still be done. Many of the fliers that seek my advice through the week live a long way from the clinic. Every day there are calls from every State in Australia. The challenge is to diagnose the problem accurately so that effective advice can be given.

In many situations, a detailed description, particularly from an experienced fancier, makes accurate diagnosis possible immediately, for example, description of a canker nodule in the wall of the crop or of a motile tapeworm segment in the bird's dropping. It is, however, very important to interpret observed signs correctly and to place the correct emphasis on these. To use the sign of panting as an example – the temptation is to jump to a diagnosis of respiratory disease because panting is a respiratory act. Although birds with a respiratory infection are more likely to pant, panting is more a reflection on decreased exercise tolerance and can, in fact, occur with any disease that saps energy. The alternatives here include worms, Coccidia, *E. coli*, etc. Panting is also not necessarily associated with disease. The birds may simply be unfit, fat or hot. One must be careful not to jump to a premature diagnosis or place the wrong emphasis on observed signs. Sometimes it is important for the fancier to think laterally. Recently I had a fancier ring and say that his birds' droppings were green and watery. One might think of one of the bowel diseases, such as *E. coli* or coccidiosis, in this situation. It turned out that a hawk was hanging off the wire when the owner was away. The birds could not reach the food, leading to green droppings, and were prematurely emptying their cloaca, leading to watery droppings, when the hawk was there. The dropping change was not associated with disease and no medication would have fixed the birds. At the risk of boring the reader, I relate the following story that illustrates the importance of correctly interpreting the signs seen.

A scientist was conducting an experiment on the ability of frogs to jump. He blew a whistle and the frog jumped 2 m. He recorded this observation. He then cut off one of the frog's legs and blew his whistle again. The frog jumped 1 m. Similarly he recorded this observation. He then cut off the frog's other leg and blew the whistle again. The frog did not move. He made the following conclusion........frogs with no legs are deaf.

Often, however, the problem described by the fancier is non-specific. A fancier, for example, may relate that his birds are reluctant to fly and that his race results are disappointing. This type of problem becomes a bit of a challenge to nut through and may or may not have a health basis. It may relate to a management matter, such as feeding or the level of training, but as often as not, management and health are so integrally related that the solution of a problem involves looking at both aspects. I always try to help with management suggestions where I can but, acting as a diagnosing veterinarian at the distance, I must find out what diseases (if any) are active. Always the initial test is a dropping analysis.

Dropping analysis

Just what problems can we detect from a mailed-in dropping sample? Things that can be very accurately diagnosed are worms and Coccidia. Fungi, yeast, *E. coli* and other bacteria levels change depending on the time since mailing. However, valid conclusions can usually be drawn. Canker and respiratory infection cannot be definitively diagnosed through the droppings. There are, however, changes that alert us to the possibility of these diseases. Canker and the respiratory diseases are primary diseases that stress the birds and so there are changes in the dropping that reflect this stress. These changes are essentially elevated levels of *E. coli* and yeast. These changes are, however, by no means specific, simply telling us that the birds are stressed. This stress could be overtraining, underfeeding, or cold weather, etc. They do, however, alert us to the possibility of one of these primary diseases. Conversely, not all birds with wet canker or respiratory infection will have these changes. Because of the high correlation of exposure to fungal spores with respiratory disease, a lot of germinating fungal spores in the dropping also alert me to the possibility of respiratory disease. Other less common findings in the droppings include airsac mite eggs and red and white blood cells.

The appearance of the dropping upon arrival also gives a lot of information. Bright green small droppings can indicate reduced food intake. Fluorescent green normal-sized droppings can indicate liver problems. Very watery droppings can be associated with wet canker, respiratory infections or indeed a range of other things, as discussed in other chapters.

Once, however, that we have a microscopic dropping result to work with, this points us in the direction that a phone conversation should follow and sometimes tells us what further tests will need to be done to accurately figure out the solution. Continuing with the respiratory example, the most reliable indicator of respiratory infection during racing is sneezing, so if a flier whose droppings contained a lot of *E. coli* said that he had recently started noticing sneezing in the loft, or that one or two birds had a dirty cere, this would be sufficient to make a provisional diagnosis and perhaps warrant a 2 – 3-day trial of medication while monitoring the birds.

Crop flush

The other simple test from which we get a lot of accurate information is the crop flush. It is the definitive test for wet canker because we can actually see the trichomonads present and is a much more diagnostic test for respiratory disease. In the crop flush of a bird with respiratory disease, evidence of the secondary inflammation and infection that occur can be seen. In respiratory infection, mucus is coughed up from the inflamed windpipe lining into the throat or drains through the slot from inflamed sinuses. As it does so, it carries the birds' white blood cells and secondary bacteria (usually *E. coli*) with it, enabling more accurate diagnosis. In crop flushes, we can also find yeasts, bacteria associated with primary crop infections, sometimes crop worm eggs, swallowed mite eggs and red blood cells.

Unfortunately, unlike the droppings, the material aspirated during a crop flush is extremely fragile, being only of diagnostic value for minutes. Questioning of the fancier here again becomes important. I am usually quite comfortable in suggesting a treatment trial with an anticanker drug if there are stress changes in the dropping and the birds are displaying signs of wet canker, such as gulping after eating or displaying a 'penguin posture'. It is here, however, that it is really great that so many fliers now have their own microscopes or have a mate that has one because, to continue with the trichomonad example, it not only allows conclusive diagnosis but can detect a rise in levels before the birds become visibly unwell. It is extremely useful and at times invaluable when fliers ring up and, together with a description of the birds, can describe what is seen down the microscope.

Very often, wandering down the diagnostic pathway of a phone description of what the birds are doing and signs that can be picked up when the bird is handled, coupled with a dropping analysis and, when needed, a crop flush (if possible), enables a good diagnosis to be made.

Treatment trial

The next diagnostic tool available, although I must warn fanciers against jumping to this step a little too quickly, is the treatment trial. Often, based on the above methods, a good provisional diagnosis can be made and I will suggest giving the birds a short treatment trial while monitoring their response. This is quite a reasonable thing to do, particularly as some of the common drugs used in the wrong situation at worst will do nothing, that is they will not do the birds harm. This certainly, however, is not the case with all medications. All too often, I see teams with a minor problem become teams with a major problem through misuse or overuse of medication by an excessively zealous owner.

A treatment trial can be a useful method of diagnosing a problem 'through the back door'. For example, with gulping birds with elevated *E. coli* in the droppings, when it is not possible to organize a crop flush I may suggest a 2-day course of an anticanker medication. If the gulping ceases, and the overall health of the birds visibly lifts, we can make a presumptive diagnosis of wet canker. This can be further reinforced by a dropping test showing resolution of the *E. coli* flare-up.

Autopsy

Sometimes, however, and fortunately this does not happen too often, the birds just do not get better when they should. It is here that I suggest a live bird be submitted for autopsy. This can be expensive and so for this reason must be reserved for those difficult cases. After euthanasia, the autopsy begins. Sometimes, particularly if the bird has been severely ill, changes may be visible to the naked eye, which enable a diagnosis to be made. More commonly, however, it becomes necessary to collect tissue samples during the autopsy and, after fixing these in formalin, to forward them to an avian pathologist for evaluation to reach a diagnosis. Because we are in the realm here of viruses, severe infections and other problems, the news is not always what we want to hear. At least, however, we then do know the exact nature of the problem and the correct therapeutic steps can then be taken, together with the correction of any associated management flaws.

The combination of the fancier in the loft observing his birds and relating information, a dropping analysis and, if needed, a crop flush result, together with a treatment trial or autopsy, tends to solve most lofts' problems.

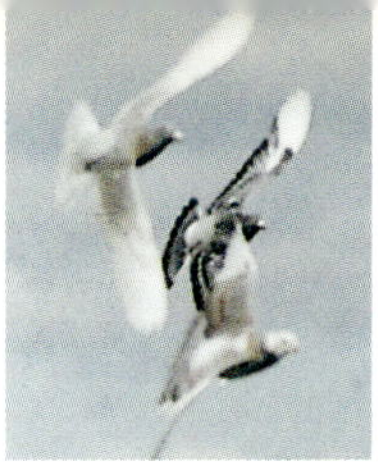

Chapter 40

SUBMISSION OF SAMPLES

As discussed in the previous chapter, the signs observed and described by fanciers to veterinarians often enable a diagnosis to be made. However, it is sometimes necessary for various samples to be taken to a clinic. As many fanciers are at a distance from a clinic, it is not possible always for them to do this personally. It is routine, cheap and easy, however, for droppings, grain and birds to be mailed or sent to a clinic for testing. It is important that fanciers help veterinarians by submitting samples correctly so that they can best help the fanciers.

Droppings

Some things in droppings remain stable for up to 7 days. Worm eggs, Coccidia, yeasts, fungal spores, fungal branches, *E. coli*, other bacteria and *Chlamydia* (with a special test) can all be found by examining droppings. There are, unfortunately, no direct tests for canker or *Mycoplasma* in the droppings but there are sometimes stress changes evident that, when combined with the signs displayed by the birds, allow a diagnosis to be made. *Hexamita* (a canker-like organism that lives in the bowel) dies as the droppings cool and so cannot be detected in mailed samples.

Fresh samples should be collected. The time of day is not important except when the fancier is suspicious of Coccidia as more Coccidia are passed by the birds in the evening. Collect at least 15 droppings from different perches to ensure the less common problems in the birds are not overlooked and that the result is representative of the flock as a whole. All droppings are placed together in a water-tight container. Press-seal plastic bags, such as those used by banks for coins, are ideal, as are freezer bags tied at the top. Alternatively, a small plastic container, e.g. for films, is fine. At many clinics, droppings are processed the day they arrive and results are quickly available.

Grain

Grain is examined visually to assess quality and problems such as weevil contamination. It is then usually tested for fungal and sometimes bacterial contamination.

A teaspoon of each grain (if purchased separately) or a dessertspoon of the mix used should be placed in similar containers to those used for droppings and mailed to the clinic. Some clinics will send out sterile bags to you for this purpose. Depending on the type of test involved, results are usually available in 2 – 7 days (refer to chapter Testing of Bad Food).

Birds

Birds can be sent to clinics either alive or dead. Diagnostically, however, much more information can be obtained from a live bird. Because of the pigeon's high body temperature (41.7°C) and the fact that they are wrapped in very effective insulators (feathers), decomposition starts very quickly. In fact, once they have been dead for more than 20 minutes, much microscope work can no longer be done.

Live birds can be sent by road or rail or to a local airport. It is best to send them in a secure box that does not need to be returned. Live birds can have a health profile (crop flush and dropping analysis) performed in the same way as birds brought to the clinic by local fanciers. A better judgment can be made of the bird's general condition if it is presented alive. If necessary, the bird can be euthanized and suitable samples for bacterial culture and pathology collected.

Birds that die at home are still, however, of diagnostic value. Changes visible grossly, such as internal canker nodules, severe airsac problems, tumours, etc., can still be diagnosed. It is important that they become cool as quickly as possible after death so as to delay the onset of decomposition. This can be achieved by soaking the bird in a bucket of cold soapy water (which penetrates the bloom) for at least 20 minutes, wrapping in Glad Wrap™ or newspaper to keep some of the moisture around the bird, and then placing it in the fridge (not the freezer). The bird should be left in the fridge until being sent. It is best sent in an express package, which usually guarantees overnight delivery.

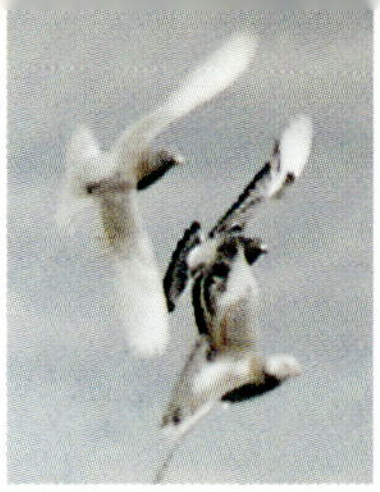

Chapter 41

DROPPING INTERPRETATION

For the fancier, often the first indication that a problem is present in his birds is a change in their droppings. All birds, including pigeons, are able to mask health problems quite well. This allows a problem to progress well into the stage where it can affect race form, with the pigeons still handling normally and looking reasonable. And yet, often with only subtle health changes, the droppings will change. Even if the droppings of only a few birds are affected, they should be investigated as these are often from the first birds 'breaking down' and may represent the 'tip of the ice berg' with some problems going on to affect the team and their form as a whole.

Most pigeon racers like to clean their pigeon loft each morning. In doing so, they are confronted by one of the best things by which to assess the health of their birds – the droppings. By examination of the droppings, the fancier can gather information regarding his birds' appetite, hydration status and gastrointestinal, liver and kidney function. By testing the droppings, the pigeon veterinarian can gather further information.

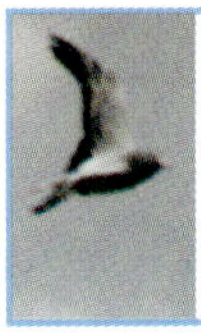

The ideal morning dropping should be a tight brown nut with a distinct white cap and have a down feather stuck to it.

Before being able to interpret the appearance of the droppings, it is important to understand what is normal. Pigeons have a cloaca, which is a bag-shaped structure whose opening the pigeon can relax to empty its contents. Into this bag empties the bowel, the two ureters (tubes that bring waste from the kidneys) and the oviduct leading from the ovary in the hen and the two vas deferens leading from the testicles in the male. Into the bowel open ducts from the liver and pancreas. The appearance of the dropping therefore reflects the function of all of these structures.

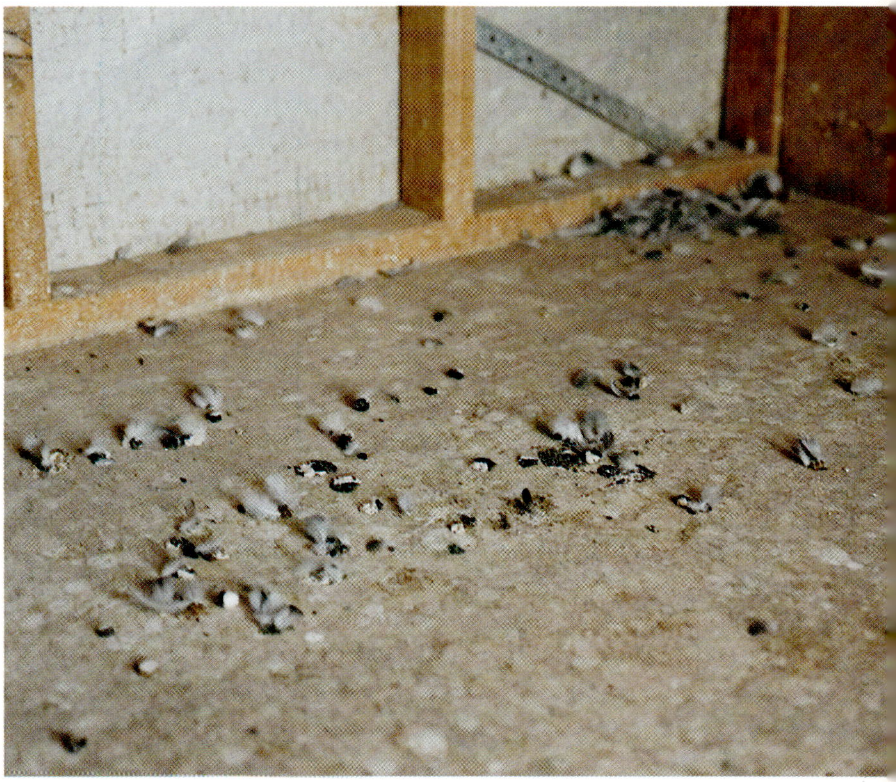

Floor of a loft inhabited by healthy pigeons. Note the tight brown droppings and an abundance of down feathers.

Analysis of organ function

THE KIDNEY

The kidney principally excretes excess water and urea from the system. Unlike mammals, where this is all passed in solution, birds pass the two components separately. In birds, therefore, urinary wastes are passed in two forms:

1 **Solid urine, or urates,** which forms the typical white cap of the dropping, and is made up of uric acid crystals. One of the kidney's jobs is to excrete the body's urea. Urea is the final metabolic product of protein metabolism and, as mentioned, in mammals it is excreted in solution. Birds, however, excrete urea in the form of uric acid crystals.

2 **Liquid urine** – The kidneys' other job is to maintain normal fluid balance in the body. Fluid in excess of the body's requirements is passed in pigeons as a clear liquid. Usually this is absorbed by the wastes from the bowel in the cloaca, and is therefore not visible. However, if the pigeon has not been eating regularly, there may be insufficient faeces to absorb all this fluid, causing the actual dropping to be very watery. To the fancier, this may give the dropping a large wet ring. It is easy to confuse this with diarrhoea. The usual time the fancier sees this kind of dropping is when birds land from races. Once the birds have been home for several hours and have eaten, wastes from the bowel reappear at the cloaca. These wastes absorb the fluid and the droppings again take on their more usual appearance. Interestingly, some water and salts are absorbed from the liquid urine by the wall of the cloaca and also from urine that moves backwards into the large intestine. If a pigeon is scared, it will often jettison its cloacal contents before this process is complete, causing a liquid dropping to be passed. Such droppings should be ignored when assessing the health status of a bird.

A pigeon dropping therefore has three principal components – solid urine, liquid urine and faeces. Watery droppings may be quite normal if food intake has not been constant. More often than not, the amount of urine in these watery droppings is normal; however, in two situations the amount of urine produced can increase:

1 **Disease of the kidney –** If kidney function is compromised, the kidney loses both the ability to excrete solid urine and the ability to concentrate liquid urine. In this situation, the birds are unwell because of the retained urates and produce a lot of dilute liquid urine. Primary kidney problems are rare in pigeons, although they can be associated with some bacterial infections, e.g. *Salmonella*. The kidneys can be damaged in a variety of situations, e.g. overuse of sulfur-based antibiotics, prolonged feeding of pellets made for other species such as chickens, eating toxic plants, or heavy metal poisoning (for example, where drinkers are inadvertently soldered with zinc or where a bird accidentally swallows a small piece of wire etc.).

2 **If the pigeon is drinking more –** Recently weaned youngsters and hens at the time of laying will drink more. A thirst can be created by a dietary component, i.e. an excessive intake of salt or sugar, perhaps from pick stones and grits with salt, or sugar-based medication. Salt and sugar can only be passed from the body at a particular concentration. If there is a lot of these in the diet, then as they are passed, a lot of fluid is lost also. This leads to a lot of urine being produced. The birds risk dehydration unless they compensate by drinking more. Pick stones and grit should be in front of the birds at all times. If access is limited, when reoffered the birds tend to overeat, as they try to obtain the essential minerals they contain. Poor-quality pick stones and grits contain excessive levels of salt. Many antibiotics and multivitamin supplements are sugar-based. The sugar not only causes a thirst but can also predispose the birds to bowel infection, leading to diarrhoea, both of which can dehydrate the bird, leading to a reduction in form. The fancier should be particularly careful of sugar-based water additives. The

sugar can form a substrate for bacterial and fungal growth within the water. Such medication should be frequently changed, particularly on warm days. Similarly, sugar offered in the water to returning race birds, if too strong, can dehydrate them and should therefore be used with caution.

Some diseases can also make the bird thirsty, e.g. wet canker, coccidiosis and *E. coli.* These and other problems can be checked for with simple, quick and cheap tests by a pigeon veterinarian.

Problems in the kidneys can also be reflected in the urates: changes in the colour, consistency and volume are all indicators of health. Volume will increase if birds are fed a high-protein diet (e.g. pea- or bean-based) or also in starvation, when the pigeon is breaking down its own body tissue protein. Viscosity will increase if the bird is becoming dehydrated. The normally white cap of the dropping can become green in liver disease (due to a bile breakdown product accumulating in the blood and being passed through the kidneys as a substance called biliverdin, which is green), bright yellow with vitamin B supplementation, dull yellow with starvation, and red-brown with kidney disease. If the problem is becoming a flock one or if an individual bird of value is affected, an avian veterinarian can check the urine for sugar, blood, protein, pH and specific gravity, and analyse its sediment, which may contain red or white blood cells, epithelial cells, crystals, bacteria, yeasts, fungi, sperm or kidney casts.

The liver

The liver opens via a duct into the upper bowel. It produces an enzyme called bile, which is bright green in colour in pigeons and digests dietary fat. This process is affected by what and when the pigeon eats, but goes on all the time. As the faeces move down the bowel, some bile is reabsorbed back into the system and what is left of the bright green colour becomes non-visible as the bile is absorbed by the other components of the dropping. However, if something has been irritating the bowel, leading to an increased rate of passage, or if the pigeon has been eating a reduced amount, either through being away from the loft or because of disease, this cannot occur and so the dropping becomes bright green. Bright green droppings, therefore, mean that either the pigeon has a problem with its bowel or is not eating properly. If food is available, it is probably not eating because it is sick.

If the liver itself is diseased, it can lose its ability to excrete bile down the bile duct and so the dropping will often become pale. The bile salts then accumulate in the blood stream and eventually are excreted through the kidneys as a substance called biliverdin. This makes the white urate component of the dropping a lime green colour. Common causes of liver disease in pigeons include bacteria such as *Salmonella* and *Streptococcus*, as well as trichomoniasis (the trichomonads gain access via the bile duct from the bowel), *Chlamydia* and Herpes virus. Because the liver is the body's filter, it is vulnerable to damage by toxins. The most common toxins experienced by pigeons are fungal toxins. One of the liver's jobs is to remove old and damaged red blood cells from the circulation. Some of their components become part of the bile. If red-blood-cell breakdown is excessive, even a healthy liver cannot cope with this increased work load and breakdown products will be excreted through the kidneys, giving the urates a reddy brown colour. In Victoria, the usual cause of red-blood-cell damage is, in fact, injury to the pigeon due to attack by a hawk or hitting a wire, etc. However, in other countries, pigeon malaria, caused by a parasite called *Haemoproteus*, which lives within and damages the red blood cell, must be considered.

The pancreas

Like the liver, the pancreas also has a duct that drains into the upper bowel. It produces several enzymes, including lipase and amylase, that digest fats and sugars in the food. Occasionally, in individual birds, the pancreas will fail to produce sufficient levels of these enzymes. This means that the bird cannot digest its food properly. As a result, the droppings are large and pale, and under the microscope a lot of undigested material is visible. Such droppings are sometimes called 'popcorn poos', as a consequence of their appearance. Problems in the pancreas are uncommon but the appearance of the droppings can lead to confusion with bowel or liver problems.

The intestine

The intestine is a muscular tube that pushes food along its length. It is lined by cells that absorb fluid and nutrition into the body. If the bowel lining is inflamed, the rate of progression of food is increased and the bowel's ability to absorb fluids is decreased. These both result in a watery, poorly digested dropping arriving at the cloaca. This is true diarrhoea, and it is important for the fancier not to confuse this with a liquid urine dropping as discussed above.

The increased rate of passage can also affect the colour of the faeces. As mentioned above, bile pigments may have inadequate time to be reabsorbed or mixed with the rest of the dropping, therefore giving the dropping a greenish colour. Diarrhoea, however, is not always green as malabsorption of other faecal components has an effect.

Bowel problems are common in pigeons, and dropping analysis is a useful and often-used diagnostic tool. Common tests include a faecal flotation test, where a measured volume of dropping is placed into a specific gravity medium and disease organisms, with time, separate and rise to the surface. This is then aspirated and prepared as a microscopic slide. This test is used to check for worms, Coccidia, and thrush. Another test, called a wet smear, involves smearing a fresh sample of dropping across a microscope slide with saline. Subsequent examination may reveal protozoans, such as *Hexamita*, or bacteria. Faecal smears can also be stained specifically to reveal bacteria. These bacteria can also be cultured and then tested against a number of antibiotics to see which one is best at killing them. *Chlamydia* is a common cause of respiratory and bowel infection in pigeons. When these organisms increase in number, they are shed through the bowel wall and can be found in the droppings, where a test called a *Chlamydia* antigen test can detect their presence. A sample of droppings is heated to 80°C for 10 minutes in an extraction fluid. This is then cooled and the supernatant placed on a colour-coded, presensitized paper strip. A colour change occurs if *Chlamydia* is present. However, this test does have its drawbacks, as both false positives and false negatives occur.

Many pigments in the grain and grits of a pigeon's diet will pass unaltered through the bowel, so that birds eating a lot of legumes, such as peas, may have slightly green droppings, while grain with a high tannin content, e.g. milo, will cause the droppings to be more reddy brown. When the bowel is inflamed, increased speed of passage of the food leads to less digestion and absorption, and so these colours can be more marked. Undigested food components can be digested by bacteria within the bowel, with resultant gas formation giving the diarrhoea a bubbly appearance.

Practically speaking...

So what does all this mean to the fancier cleaning his loft each morning? Ideally, the dropping should be a shade of green-brown to brown, maintain the shape of the cloaca after being passed and be topped by a cap of white urate. The analogy of a small, snow-capped mountain is apt. The droppings should be uniform throughout the loft. Any divergence from this has happened for a reason and may be associated with an impending loss of form. The fancier should be able to recognize the abnormal and hopefully identify the cause. Similarly, it is important that the fancier realize that some causes can only be identified by testing and that he may need the services of a pigeon veterinarian.

Interpretation of green or watery droppings

The usual changes in droppings that would alert the fancier to a health problem are when they become green or watery or both. However, not all such droppings are associated with disease and I hope the following summary helps fanciers to interpret these two most common changes in the droppings on the perches of their race team.

WATERY DROPPINGS

Ideally we like to see dry, well-formed droppings that are a shade of brown. Not all watery droppings, however, are associated with disease. Watery droppings can appear in the following situations:

1 **Bowel problems –** Watery droppings can be due to a true diarrhoea associated with bowel problems. As discussed above, bowel wall irritation leads to increased rate of passage and decreased fluid absorption. Possible causes can be infective agents such as Coccidia, *Hexamita*, worms or bacteria. Other causes include the incorrect use of medication, e.g. Baycox in extreme overdose, a sudden change of diet, and incorrect use of food supplements (a common example being oil supplements such as cod liver oil that has spoiled).

The flow chart on page 256 is basically designed as the racing fancier's quick guide to possible causes of faecal changes, and is by no means exhaustive. Changes noticed usually involve either the dropping colour, volume or fluid content.

2. **Cloacal emptying –** As mentioned earlier, at the end of the bowel is a structure called the cloaca and material moves from the bowel, kidneys and reproductive organs into this. Mammals do not have an equivalent to the bird's cloaca. Material from the bowel mixes in the cloaca with the bird's urine. As mentioned, birds produce two types of urine, a clear watery fluid like that of mammals and also a solid white material called uric acid. The process of fluid and nutrient absorption is not completed by the time the material reaches the cloaca. Once there, absorption of more fluid from the bowel and also of urine occurs. Some material can even reflux back into the bowel and be absorbed from there. This process is continuous with material being exuded like toothpaste from its tube into the stretching cloacal bag and fluid being resorbed until eventually, in health, the cloaca is full. Once full, the bulging cloaca, with more material coming, becomes uncomfortable. The pigeon then relaxes the cloacal opening and a dropping is passed. This process can be interrupted at any time by the pigeon deliberately opening its cloaca. This is usually in response to the bird being startled or disturbed. If cloacal contents are evacuated before the fluid resorption process is complete, the resultant dropping may be a bit loose (leading to a generally mushy dropping) or visibly contain a lot of clear urine (leading to the so-called 'snake' dropping, which is a firm tube of bowel material lying in a pool of clear urine). Fanciers may mistakenly believe, in this situation, that the birds have a health problem when, in fact, there has just been insufficient time for normal fluid resorption to occur in the cloaca before defaecation. This mechanism can, however, be used to advantage by the astute fancier to evaluate any loft-based stress. Race birds pass most of their droppings through the night. If the fancier finds tight nut-like droppings on his perches in the mornings, this means that the birds have had an uninterrupted night's sleep. Conversely, loose morning droppings that improve through the day indicate a disturbed night. A poor night's sleep inhibits the development of race form and can be caused by things as diverse as:
   - External parasites.
   - Diseases such as respiratory infection (which causes sneezing) and *E. coli* (which causes 'gut ache').
   - Mice, noise and light around the loft.
   - An uncomfortable loft environment, e.g. draughts, a cold loft or high humidity.

   These loose droppings, although not a direct health problem, do indicate the birds are not resting properly and, as we know, inadequate rest is a stress on the birds, which increases their vulnerability to health problems. To maintain race form, the birds must rest well through the night.

Quick-guide flow chart to possible causes of changes in dropping appearance

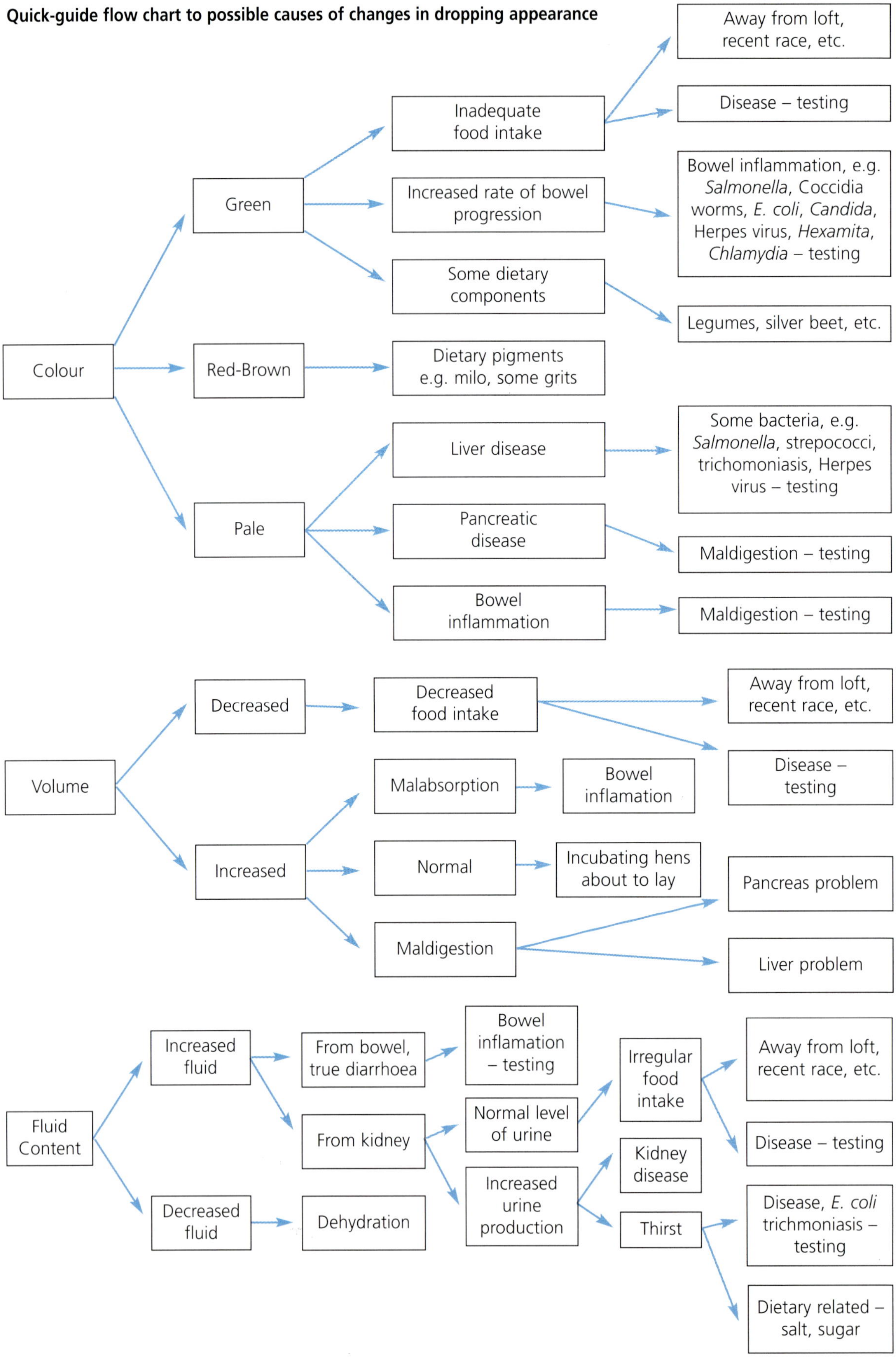

3 **Normal urine production with decreased food intake** – Sometimes fanciers mention that they see wet patches on the floor of the loft. These are usually seen when the birds are due for a feed or have just returned from flying. Urine production is continuous, with bowel content only coming through for a period of time after eating. These wet patches are pools of urine. With feeding, after a few hours, digested food appears at the cloaca, which soaks up the urine like a sponge and normal droppings are produced. The same situation is experienced with returning race birds.

4 **Increased urine production** – Excessive urine production leads to a watery dropping and occurs with:
- Kidney disease, in which the birds cannot concentrate their urine and therefore produce a lot of dilute urine and also need to drink more in order to prevent dehydration,
- The use of excessively salty or sugary medications, grits or pick stones, which either create a thirst or can actually cause fluid to move out of the body into the bowel (e.g. Epsom salts),
- Diseases that create a thirst. The most common one is wet canker, although all diseases that inflame the lining of the digestive tract will cause some increased fluid intake.

Green droppings

Green droppings can be associated with disease but this is not necessarily so. Pigeons digest the green plant pigment (chlorophyll) rather poorly. Green leafy vegetables such as spinach or silver beet, fed to the pigeons will make the droppings green. Similarly, if more than 25% of the grain mix is green dun peas, or the birds are open-lofted and have access to grass, the droppings will become green. Green droppings do, however, alert the fancier to the possibility of a health problem.

Bile is a digestive enzyme produced in the liver. In mammals, it is a yellow-brown colour, which is why mammalian droppings are essentially brown. However, in pigeons it is brilliant green. After production in the liver, it passes down a duct called the bile duct into the stomach and bowel, where it mixes with the food, helping to digest it. Interestingly, unlike mammals, birds do not have a gall bladder. The gall bladder is a sac extending from the bile duct where bile is stored until needed. In pigeons, the bile trickles straight into the digestive system. Once in the bowel, a percentage of the bile is resorbed. The remainder is mixed with the rest of the bowel contents and passed with the dropping. Conditions that irritate the bowel, as mentioned earlier, cause it to contract more quickly, in the process pushing its contents along. This gives the bird less opportunity to absorb the bile, with the result that more is present in the dropping when passed and the dropping is green. Diseases

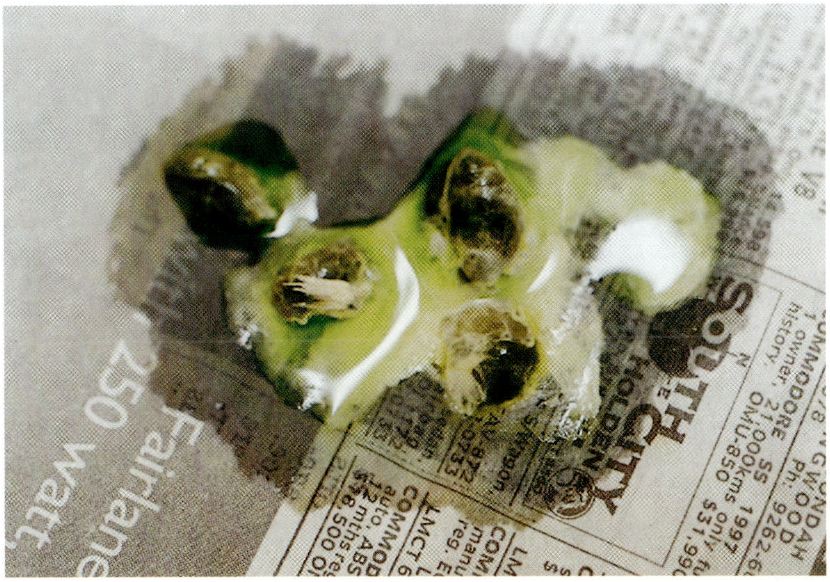

Droppings from an unwell pigeon. Although at first sight it may appear that this bird has diarrhoea, the part of the dropping coming from the bowel is in fact quite normal. This dropping is wet because it contains both an increased amount of liquid urine (which has soaked into a ring around the dropping) and solid urine (with an increased amount of white urate apparent). The urine contains the green bile breakdown pigment biliverdin, and so it is likely that this bird has a problem with its liver or kidneys.

that affect the bowel wall, therefore, cause green droppings. As these diseases usually also interfere with the bowel's ability to absorb fluid, green droppings are often also watery.

Green droppings will also occur if the pigeon's food intake has decreased (whether due to ill health or not). Less food means less volume of dropping, which means that the green bile is less diluted and its green colour more apparent.

This is particularly so in the droppings of recently returned race birds. We have all seen the dropping passed by a newly returned race bird, which is usually just urine with sometimes a green streak of bile through it. As the bird has not been eating, there is no food waste entering the cloaca. Urine and bile production is, however, continuous and it is just these that make up the dropping.

As mentioned earlier, pale green droppings with green urates usually indicate liver problems.

Problem solving

The appearance of watery or green droppings may have a diet- or loft-related cause but can also indicate problems with the bowel, liver or kidneys. The investigative path that I suggest fanciers follow (and this may seem very obvious) is to determine initially whether or not the loose or green dropping is associated with disease. The best initial diagnostic test is the examination of a dropping smear under the microscope. This can be done either by an avian veterinarian or by a fancier with microscope skills. It is here that fanciers or clubs with their own microscope have a big advantage as it is simply a matter of getting the suspect dropping, walking inside, spending a few minutes and having an answer. If a health problem is diagnosed, appropriate medication can be prescribed. As we have a fairly good understanding of what causes various diseases to flare up during racing, once a problem is identified, the longer-term answer may be changes to the loft management or environment to decrease the chance of repeat flare-ups. In the absence of testing, it is tempting to give 1 – 2 days on antibiotics in case the change in dropping is associated with an infection such as *E. coli*, etc. However, antibiotics do have the potential to make matters worse and to some extent distract the fancier from the real issue, which may be to reassess certain management practices and to review loft design. Giving antibiotics as an initial course of action is a bit like calling the fire brigade to stamp out a match. While waiting for a dropping analysis, if there is the need to give anything, give probiotics.

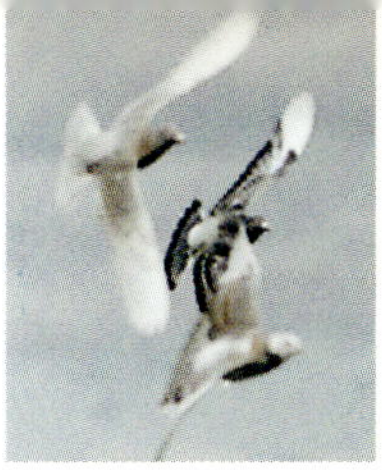

Chapter 42

THE USE OF THE MICROSCOPE BY THE PIGEON FANCIER*

With the competitive nature of modern pigeon racing, many questions arise regarding the flock's health. Some of these can only be answered with the microscope. Regular access to a pigeon veterinarian with his microscope has obvious advantages to the flier. Australia, however, is a big country and, as in other parts of the world, many fanciers are isolated from such services. Similarly, some problems require almost daily maintenance at some times and so, even for city fliers, time and perhaps expense can make the regular use of a pigeon veterinarian difficult. To this end, fanciers are encouraged to learn the use of the microscope so that they can manage the health of their flock on a day-to-day basis or as needed.

Before the knowledge and modern medications that we now have, many fliers would wait until the birds showed signs of illness before seeking a pigeon veterinarian's help. In this situation, the microscope was used for diagnosis and obviously it still has a role to play here. However, once microscopic skills have been acquired, the microscope can also be used to manage the flock by monitoring their health. This is particularly relevant when training or racing. Here, the microscope can be used to select the most healthy birds in the team and can even be used as an aid to pick the pool bird.

The informed use of the microscope by the fancier, acting as a microscope technician, means that illnesses are detected much earlier. This early recognition of illness allows the flock to recover more quickly with no loss of form and without a major interruption to the training or racing schedule.

This chapter describes the equipment and technical skills needed and then continues to explain how to use the microscope to help manage the health of your flock. The purpose of this chapter is not to make you pigeon veterinarians but to train you as skilled technicians. The information you see under the microscope can then be relayed to a veterinarian by a phone call, to enable much more meaningful advice to be given. Veterinarians familiar with pigeons and their diseases have the skill to diagnose most problems from the results of a microscopic examination. A microscope report, together with any other information concerning the birds, enables appropriate advice to be given. There obviously will be times when the problem cannot be diagnosed in this way and further tests on the live bird may be recommended.

Most lofts have a resident health problem, which does not change from year to year. This relates to the loft locality, the training methods, the family of birds, and many other factors, including the fancier himself. For example, an easterly facing loft will receive the morning sun. Droppings produced through the night will therefore dry out more quickly and problems relating to dampness and increased humidity, such as Coccidia and *E. coli*, are less likely to occur. As the wind rarely blows from the east in Australia, it may be possible to have the front of such a loft quite open without exposing the birds to extremes of temperature. A similar open front in a loft facing north would be inappropriate because of the prevalence of strong northerly winds with rain. Similarly, some families of pigeons are more susceptible to particular diseases, such as wet canker. Some families can

* Portions of this chapter were originally published in the *Australian Pigeon Journal* and were co-written with Dr R. Marshall of Sydney. I would like to thank him for his contribution and permission to use this material here.

take, and in fact need, a lot of training to come into form, while others given this amount of work would break down and develop stress-related problems such as thrush. The microscope picture that we develop of a flock and loft over a period of time from phone conversations and dropping analysis will identify the loft's resident problems. Once the resident problems are identified, we know what microscope cues to look for so that, in this way, the fancier is able to manage the flock alone.

The telephone consultation approach, with the fancier fulfilling the role of technician and relaying information to the pigeon veterinarian, is a win – win situation. The pigeon veterinarian is better able to prevent illness in the loft, the fancier is better informed about pigeon health, and the pigeons are healthier because health problems are identified earlier. The fancier becomes a laboratory technician, identifying the microscopic findings of the droppings or crop flush. A pigeon veterinarian then interprets the findings over the phone. Over time, the resident loft health problems are identified and then the fancier is able to monitor and manage the problems more independently.

Technical information

All that is required are a microscope, slides and cover slips, crop needle, syringes and the enthusiasm to learn. This section outlines the diseases that can be identified from the microscopic examination of the droppings and crop wash.

Microscopic requirements

- x10 eyepiece (one or binocular)
- x4, x10, x40 objective lenses – The appropriate lens can be rotated into position as required.
- In-built light source
- Mechanical stage – Enables fine control of slide movement during examination.
- Condenser diaphragm – This can be opened or closed to control the amount of light coming through the sample and also moved up or down to control contrast (down tends to improve contrast).

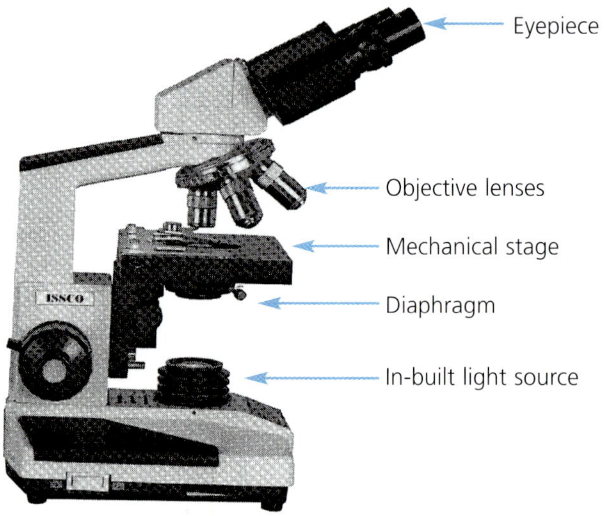

The cost of microscopes with the above features varies from AUD$400 to AUD$2000. The microscope appreciates in value with time and lasts a lifetime. Very little goes wrong with microscopes and secondhand ones are very good value. Look in the *Trading Post* (an Australian newspaper that advertizes secondhand goods) or try the local school or university. New microscopes can be purchased from scientific instrument outlets. Industrial and Scientific in Melbourne, Australia (ph 03 94199191) produces an excellent pigeon diagnostic microscope for AUD$395, which can be sent to most places in Australia for less than AUD$20.

Preparation of the dropping sample into a 'wet smear'

Go through the loft and collect a minimum of five to ten droppings. It is best to collect this sort of number so as to be thorough and avoid overlooking a less common problem in the loft. Be sure to include any droppings that are abnormal in appearance, for example, ones that are green or watery.

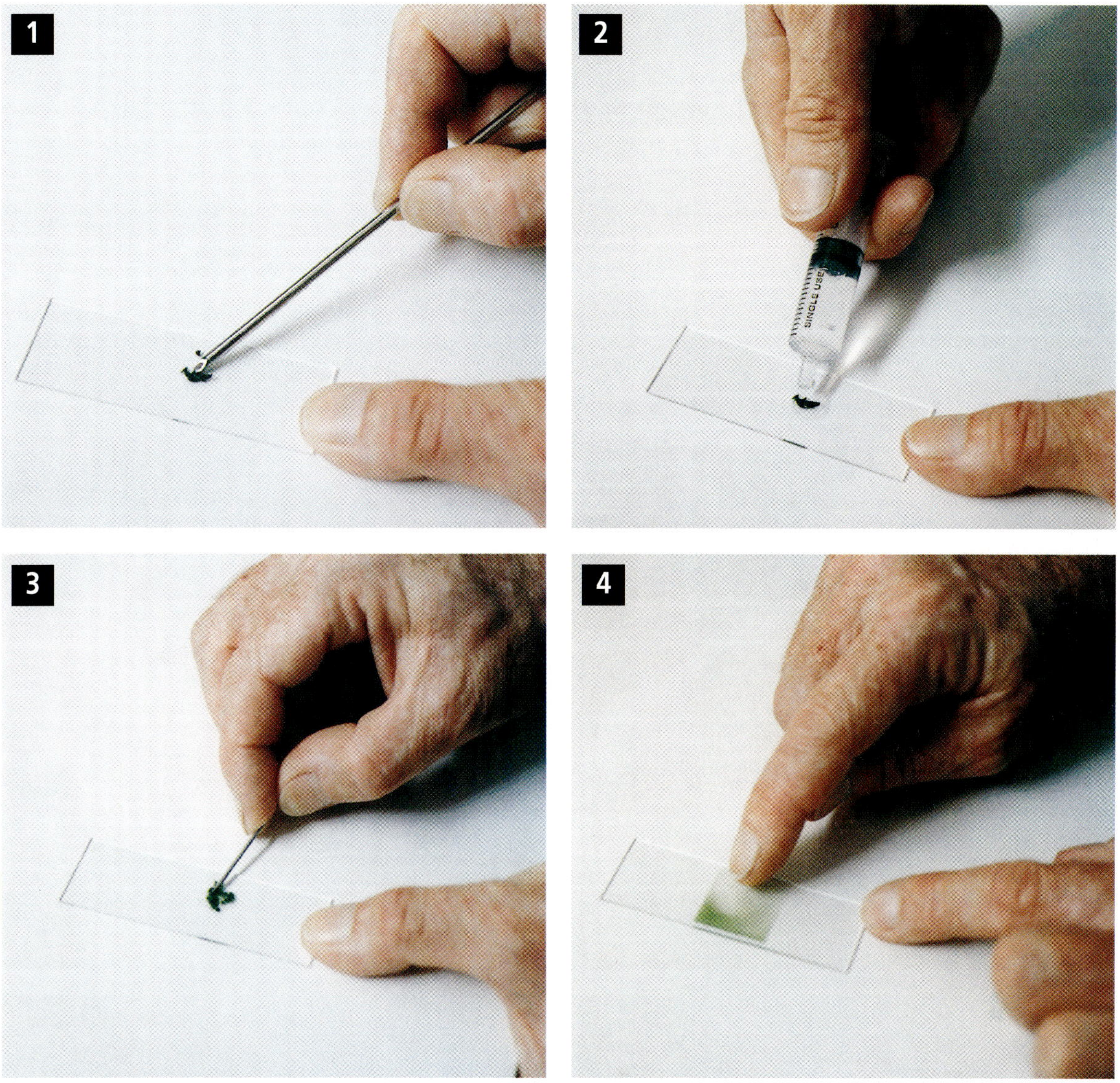

Preparation of a faecal smear.
1: Placing the dropping sample onto a microscope slide.
2: Adding water to the dropping sample.
3: Mixing the dropping sample and fluid.
4: Placing a cover slip on top and gently pushing down while rotating to create a thin dropping film ready for examination.

It is important to include these droppings in the sample because we want to find abnormalities if they are there. Segments from each dropping, approximately half the size of a match head, are placed together in the centre of a microscope slide using a cotton bud or rod. Avoid collecting any of the white (urine) component as this can make subsequent interpretation more difficult. Add one or two drops of saline solution or water and, using a needle or rod, mix into a faecal soup. When the sample is thoroughly mixed, place a cover slip on top. It often helps to push gently down on the cover slip and rotate it slightly, in the process dispersing the sample and making it thinner. The droppings sample must be flattened and spread out thinly onto the microscope slide. Keep pushing down until a fine film of 'soup' is left under the microscope slide. The smear must be thin enough for light to pass through it. Place this onto the microscope deck. Use a x10 eyepiece and a x4 lens on the deck. Looking through the eyepiece, adjust the light so that it easily passes through the sample without being too bright. Focus onto the faecal film. Now swing to the x10 lens on the deck and focus again, then move, if necessary, to the x40 lens.

Crop flush technique and preparation of a 'crop smear'

I use a soft piece of plastic tubing approximately 3 mm across and approximately 7.5 cm long and place this onto the end of a 3- or 5-ml syringe. Holding the bird's beak open, I gently slide this tube over the bird's tongue and the entrance to its windpipe into the back of the bird's mouth and then a further 2.5 – 5 cm into the crop. Gently hold the pigeon's head forward, tenting the skin on the front of the neck over the end of the tube. With moderate negative pressure on the syringe, the crop tube is withdrawn. Try to get the lining of the crop to gently suck onto the end of the tube. As the tube is withdrawn, the tube will then gently 'vacuum' the wall of the crop to collect a sample of crop material. Some fanciers prefer to draw up 1 – 2 ml of water or saline solution into the syringe initially and then, after passing the crop tube, inject this into the crop. Some of this fluid is then sucked back, flushing with it crop material. I personally prefer not to put fluid into the crop first and find it easier to both quantitate and compare samples without putting fluid in first. Try when

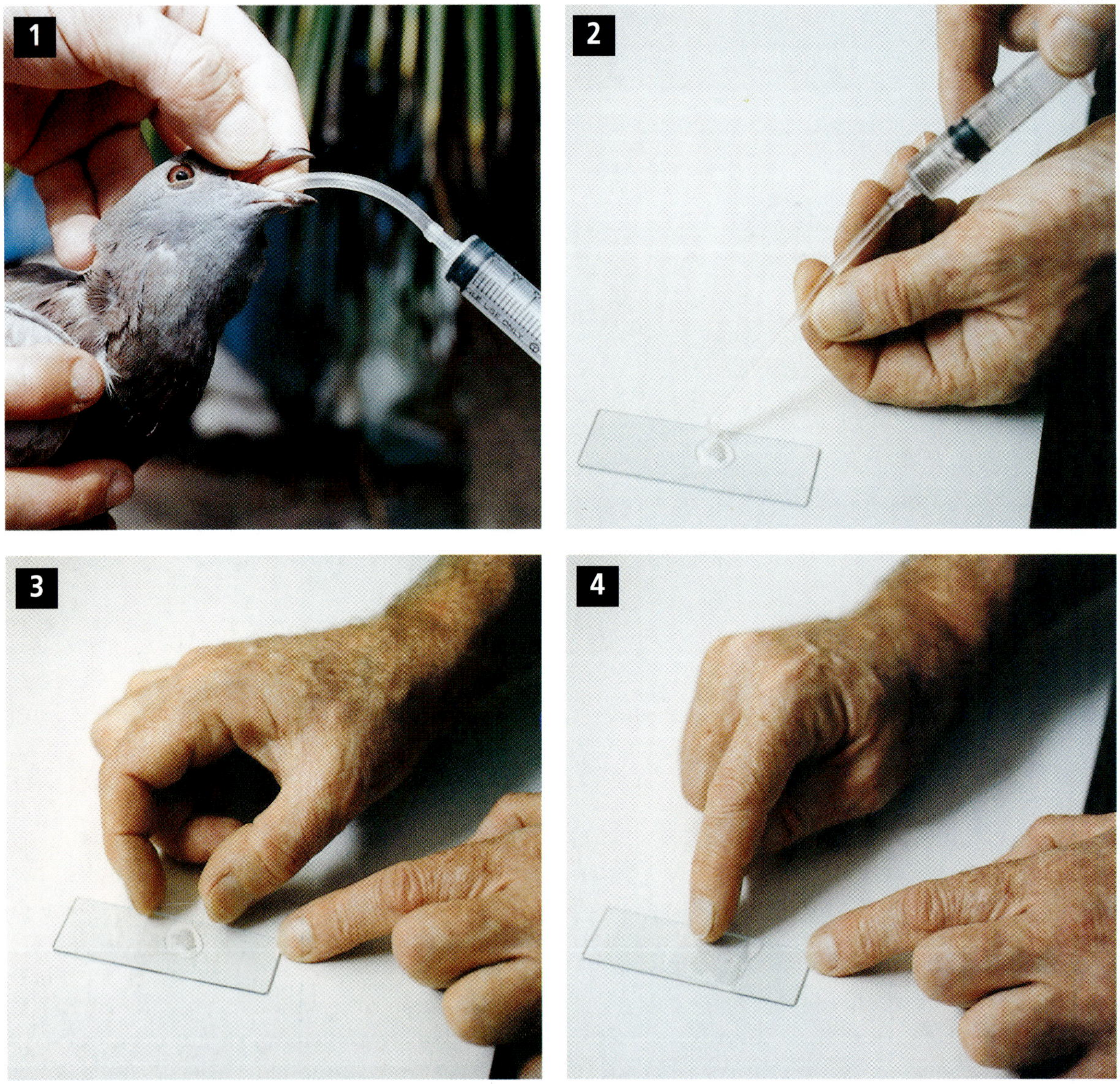

Collection of a crop sample and preparation of a crop smear.
1: Aspiration of material from the crop and throat.
2: After changing syringes, flushing the collected sample onto a microscope slide.
3: Placing a cover slip on top of the sample.
4: Providing downward pressure while gently rotating to create a thin film ready for examination.

vacuuming to get some of the lining cells of the crop as it is here that the canker organisms are in highest numbers. If these cells are not present, the result may be a false negative. Some fanciers use metal crop tubes but as these do not bend it is easier to damage the bird's throat with these. I also personally find it harder to vacuum with a metal tube and therefore to get good samples. Once the tube is removed from the bird's throat, I then take the empty syringe off and attach another syringe prepared in advance containing either warm water or saline solution. Depressing the syringe, I use this to then flush the sample from the end of the tube onto a microscope slide. With some samples, it helps to loosen the sample in the end of the tube with a needle. Try and place a single drop of the crop sample onto the slide and then apply a cover slip. A sample with excessive fluid will be too thick and it will be hard to focus clearly. If necessary, the cover slip can be gently pushed down onto the microscope slide. Focus initially using the x4 objective and from there move to the x10 and x40 objectives.

Information from the dropping wet smear and crop smear

The identification of the various microorganisms (germs) takes time and requires plenty of practice (i.e. practice makes perfect). It is very important that you have an expert check that you are identifying the germs correctly. Often, Coccidia and worm eggs are confused with normal starch granules or air bubbles. The bacteria and thrush identification can be difficult unless the condenser is at the lowest level.

Worms (x10 is best, with condenser lowered to half)

There are three major worms (roundworm, hairworm, cropworm) that can be identified by the microscope. Worm eggs are best seen under the x10 objective lens. Any number of eggs is significant but the whole field must be examined. The healthy pigeon has no eggs visible in a wet smear. Larger samples, where droppings from many birds need to be tested, can be tested simultaneously with a flotation test, where the birds' droppings are mixed and placed in a specific gravity medium for approximately 20 minutes. This allows parasitic eggs present to collect at the top of the medium, which can then be examined. The tapeworm cannot be readily identified by the microscope because it lays eggs in egg packets, which are passed irregularly.

Coccidia (x10 or x40 is best, with condenser down)

Coccidial eggs are best seen from afternoon droppings because the eggs are released more frequently after 2 p.m. The healthy fit pigeon has no coccidial eggs. The number of coccidial eggs per x10 field is helpful in identifying the nature of the problem.

Thrush (x40 is best with condenser down)

The number of thrush germs, and whether they are budding or not, is very important in the final analysis. The in-form pigeon often has no thrush germs present on a dropping or crop smear.

Bacteria (x40, with condenser down)

The number of bacteria, whether they are rods or dots and if they are moving, are all important for analysis.

Fungus (x10, with condenser half-way down)

Fungal hyphae and spores are difficult to detect. Their presence indicates a real problem.

Canker (x40 is best)

Canker organisms may be seen in healthy birds, however, in order to maximize performance it is best that no organisms are present.

The veterinarian, the fancier and the microscope

The microscope is used as a management tool to monitor the health and fitness of the race team. It can be used diagnostically at the first sign of ill health or on a regular basis to manage the health of the flock. To be a good fancier, one must be a good observer of the team. The first indication of ill health in the race team is a change in the droppings. A change in the attitude or demeanour of the team or individual bird should also alert the fancier to a management problem. A microscopic examination of the droppings at this time is the best method of resolving the problem.

The interpretation of the droppings is very difficult, but with time and experience the good fancier can quickly translate what is seen under the microscope into a practical answer for the loft. The answer is not necessarily medicine but may be a change in feeding or training levels, as many times the cause of illness is a management flaw. A knowledge of what is normal is important.

I see my role as one to interpret the fancier's findings under the microscope and to give him guidance. For example, the sudden appearance of thrush may indicate poor loft humidity. The answer to this problem may be to cover the front of the loft at night and to medicate for 1 day with Probac. The influx of thrush in another loft may indicate the beginning of wet canker in a loft with a canker problem. This would then alert the fancier to the need for Turbosole treatment for 1 – 2 days and so on. The appearance of coccidiosis may indicate overtraining and the advice may be to provide Baycox for 2 days, a water-soluble multivitamin in the water for 2 days, and to stop tossing for 4 days. The appearance of fungal branches in the dropping sample a week after the introduction of a new feed may indicate a fungus problem with the food.

As a pigeon veterinarian flying my own team of pigeons, I realize how important it is to have the birds right, and so I am happy to give advice and to interpret loft problems. With veterinary help and the fancier's perseverance, the microscope will become an indispensable part of your racing success.

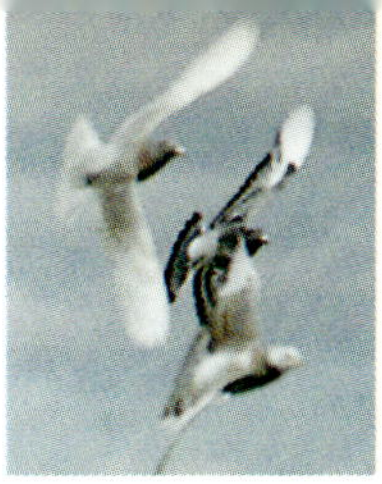

Chapter 43

PRACTICAL MICROSCOPE USE –

Looking for solutions

Examples of situations in which the information gained with a microscope can aid an individual flier to improve his results are given below.

Loss of form

If there are 20 races in a program and a flier is going to do well in, say, six of these, then given the vagaries of wind direction, individual birds becoming fit, etc., one would expect his good results to be scattered through the season. In fact, this is unlikely to be the case. It is more likely that his six good races will occur out of eight starts. Up until recently, this peculiarity was accepted as normal. Such birds were said to have either come into, or alternatively lost, form. Indeed this is the case, but one must ask the question, Why?

When monitoring an in-form team at my clinic, the birds are consistently *Chlamydia*-negative, have no trichomonads in their crop flush and their faecal smears are negative for worms, Coccidia, yeasts and *E. coli*. Most fanciers' tossing, feeding and racing regimes are relatively constant through the season. Given a constant management regime, when form is lost, a health problem is usually detected.

It is unrealistic to think that an individual team is resistant to the factors that lead to loss of form. There is continuous exposure to disease in the race unit and the inherent stress of racing itself leads to disease flare-ups. In the past (pre-1990) when the birds stopped being competitive it was simply agreed, almost as if it was normal, that the birds had lost form. The answer for many fliers was to continue with the same tossing and feeding regimes and hope that form would return or, alternatively, try something different to spark the birds up, e.g. a 'hit out toss' or 'hoppers in, baskets out', etc.

With loss of form, fliers should see if this has a health basis and organize a veterinary check (crop flush and dropping analysis) to identify a problem, which, with correction, will lead to a return of form. More importantly, once a problem (e.g. wet canker) is known to be active in the loft, it can be monitored (through crop flushing) and preventive medication (2 days on an anticanker drug) can be given strategically to prevent further flare-ups.

Unexplained bad year

Even the very best fliers have that occasional bad year that they just want to forget. Even if it is a year that others might consider satisfactory, it may be well below their best. To the concerned, experienced flier standing in his loft, looking over his birds they all seem okay. This year's team is genetically from the same base as in other years, it is in the same loft and under the same management. Then why are the race results just not there? Obviously, in some years breeding produces those one or two exceptional birds, but the overall result should not dramatically change, i.e. in the top 20 in the Federation averages. One factor that can cause a bad year is the birds' health, remembering that most pigeon disease is, in fact, hidden from the naked eye. Problems as diverse as a new strain of *Mycoplasma*, tapeworm infection, a virus, etc., can all appear in a loft, leading to poor results and a frustrated fancier. Straightforward veterinary testing can identify and control such problems.

Resident diseases

Resident diseases take several forms. They can either be loft-based or relate to the birds themselves. When a fancier persistently fails to achieve good results at a particular time of year, this is suggestive of a loft-based health problem. Closed-in lofts give the fancier control of the birds' environment and enable the fancier to create the ideal temperature and humidity conditions for health all year round. In open lofts when the weather gets cold, the birds get cold and form is lost. Pigeons can always handle a single stress but when stresses start overlapping their health breaks down. If the birds are stressed, e.g. by a hard race, and we then superimpose cold, high humidity or draughts, then the birds will break down.

A good example of a loft-based resident disease is *E. coli* infection. *E. coli* is a bacterium that is found in the bowel of pigeons almost always, but usually in low numbers. Its level fluctuates over a 24 – 48-hour period, depending on what stresses the birds are under. When levels are high, they cause a low-grade enteritis, interfering with nutrient and electrolyte metabolism and, in the process, lead to the birds developing green droppings or, with on-going stress, green and watery droppings. The problem is managed by identifying and correcting, if possible, any predisposing stress and, on days when significant numbers of green droppings are noticed, by treating the birds with probiotics. A common stress associated with *E. coli* is cold, damp conditions and so we see it as an intermittent but persistent problem in certain lofts, for example, open lofts, lofts facing south, lofts overshadowed by trees or in particular geographical locations. Some avian veterinarians state that mild *E. coli* is worth 10 minutes in a normal 200-mile race. Once veterinary checks identify this as a problem, longer-term steps can be taken to control the problem, which may involve structural changes to the loft. However, if predisposing factors cannot be avoided, e.g. high-humidity areas, fanciers aware of the problem when alerted to a flare-up by the presence of green droppings can effectively minimize any loss of form through the use of probiotics.

Also as mentioned, some resident diseases relate to the birds themselves. Some strains of pigeons under particular management regimes are more susceptible to particular diseases. A well-known example here is wet canker and respiratory infection in some strains of European birds, particularly when in full training. Wet canker and respiratory infection have an enormous effect on results but only if not identified. Once these diseases are identified and correctly managed, the birds can win and win well.

The microscope as a management tool

Traditionally, the microscope has only been used to diagnose a problem when the birds appear unhealthy, and yet the microscope, just like the perch scraper, can be used to manage the birds. Many organisms that cause disease in pigeons are always present in low numbers and their levels fluctuate, depending on what stress the birds are under. Regular checks can monitor these levels and can be used as a guide to modify the birds' training regime. For example, when pigeons are stressed for any reason, initially the *E. coli* level but later also the level of yeasts in the droppings start to increase. A common stress for a race team is overtraining, i.e. too much tossing. If a flier wants to check whether his current level of tossing is excessive, he can check the droppings microscopically to see if the *E. coli* is elevated or if yeasts are starting to appear. If they are present, he knows it is best to cut back on the team's tossing for a while. If they are not present he knows he can continue.

Interestingly, in winning teams it is not unusual to find elevated yeasts in individual birds. Fliers that are not doing well often do not toss their birds much and give their birds, perhaps, too much to eat. These birds are not under stress, no stress changes (i.e. elevated *E. coli* and yeasts) are detectable in their droppings but they are not winning either. Fliers with currently winning teams exercise and work their birds to create a race fitness and trim out excess fat while, at the same time, monitoring both the quantity of grain and energy content of the feed mix. These birds, once right, are fit and can win but are being pushed close to the edge and can therefore more easily break down. If training is overdone, *E. coli* and yeasts will start to increase in individual birds. The astute flier can learn to monitor these changes microscopically and use this to help manage his birds' training.

Healthier individual teams improve the quality of racing for everyone. With individual fliers ensuring that their birds' health problems are controlled, not only is racing better for the individual bird but the general level of health of the entire race contingent is higher. This not only improves the quality of racing but makes racing more enjoyable and obviously benefits the sport in general.

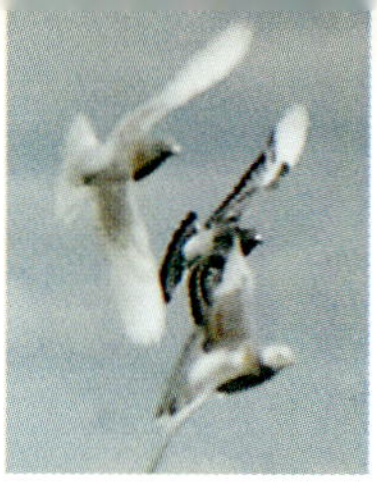

Chapter 44

A PICTORIAL GUIDE TO MICROSCOPE USE FOR THE FANCIER

I receive many calls from fanciers with microscopes with queries regarding identification of what they are seeing down their microscopes. The microscope can only be of real diagnostic value if fanciers are able to identify confidently what they are seeing. Verbal descriptions and drawings are only of certain value and so what is needed is a series of photos. These photos need to be not only of the disease-causing agents but also of the normal things in the dropping, some of which look quite similar to, and are therefore easy to confuse with, pathogens.

In this chapter, I want to develop a pictorial guide so that fanciers looking down a microscope can flick through and find a photo illustrating what they are seeing at that moment. The two common tests that are done using the microscope are the faecal smear and the crop flush.

Faecal smear

The faecal smear involves the preparation of a fine film of dropping onto a microscope slide. The technique involved in preparing a faecal smear is outlined in the chapter The Use of the Microscope By the Pigeon Fancier. This simple diagnostic test enables the birds to be examined for many things. Most commonly, the test is used to check for roundworm, hairworm and Coccidia infection. However, problems such as yeast, *Hexamita,* filamentous fungi and airsac mites can also be evaluated. Relative bacterial populations can be assessed. Occasionally, red and white blood cells are seen. And so what do these things look like?

The larger something is, the easier it is to visualize clearly under the microscope and therefore the easier it is to identify, and so I feel it is best to start with the group of largest infective agents, namely the worm eggs.

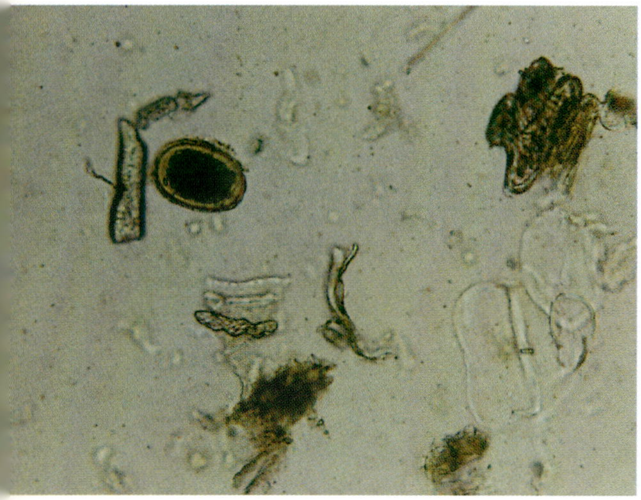

Roundworms

Roundworm infection is usually diagnosed by microscopic examination of a faecal smear. Usually, a x10 eyepiece is used with initially a x10 lens on the deck and sometimes later the x40 lens. The condensor is best in the middle position (half up / half down).

If present they will look like photos 1 and 2.

Roundworm eggs are comparatively large. Their size and shape are always the same, but their appearance under the microscope can vary. This is because they are shaped like an AFL or rugby football, and in the same

Photo 1: Roundworm egg at x100 magnification (i.e. x10 eye piece, x10 lens on deck).

way that a football can roll through the air, roundworm eggs can swing through the fluid of the faecal smear and stop in a variety of positions. They can, therefore, sometimes look almost circular. They do, however, usually lie on their side and so appear elliptical under the microscope.

Roundworm eggs have a capsule that is thick, readily visible and of uniform width all the way around. The developing larva inside the egg has a granular appearance and fills the entire egg, right up to the capsule. The main distinguishing characteristics of the roundworm egg are its size, thick even wall capsule and its usual elliptical shape.

Roundworm eggs can usually be readily diagnosed when magnified 100 times, but to see more detail, swing the x40 lens onto the deck to see the egg at x400 magnification. At this magnification, they look like photo 3.

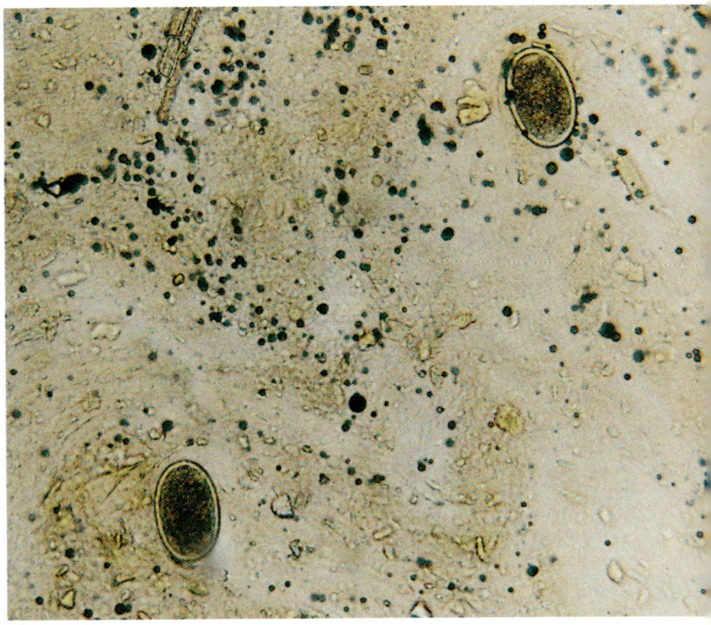

Photo 2: Two roundworm eggs at x100 magnification.

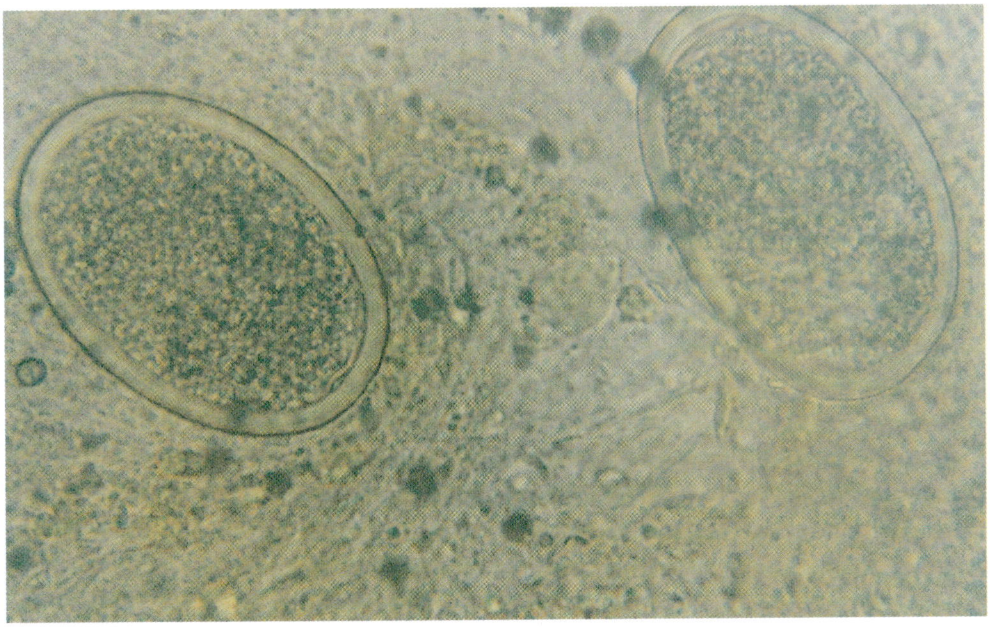

Photo 3: Two roundworm eggs at x400 magnification (i.e. x10 eye piece, x40 lens on deck).

There are things within the faecal smear that can be confused with roundworm eggs. These are:

- **Plant cells –** Plants (like us) are made up of lots of individual structures called cells. These are all stuck together like tiles in a mosaic. Unlike in animals, the walls of cells in plants are made up principally of a substance called cellulose, which birds cannot digest. This means that sheets of these undigested cell walls, which are really 'cellulose chambers' or 'cell skeletons', are passed in the droppings. An example is shown in photo 4 on page 270.

  Different plants and their seeds, e.g. peas, corn, etc., have a myriad of different cell types that vary in both their shape and their size. These sheets of 'cellulose chambers' can therefore vary in appearance under the microscope. During digestion, these sheets of cell remnants are ripped into pieces of different sizes. As the sheets of cell remnants are ripped into pieces, some as small as three, two or even one cell, some pieces, if about the same size as a roundworm egg, can look like a roundworm egg. They do, however, as they rip away from the adjacent

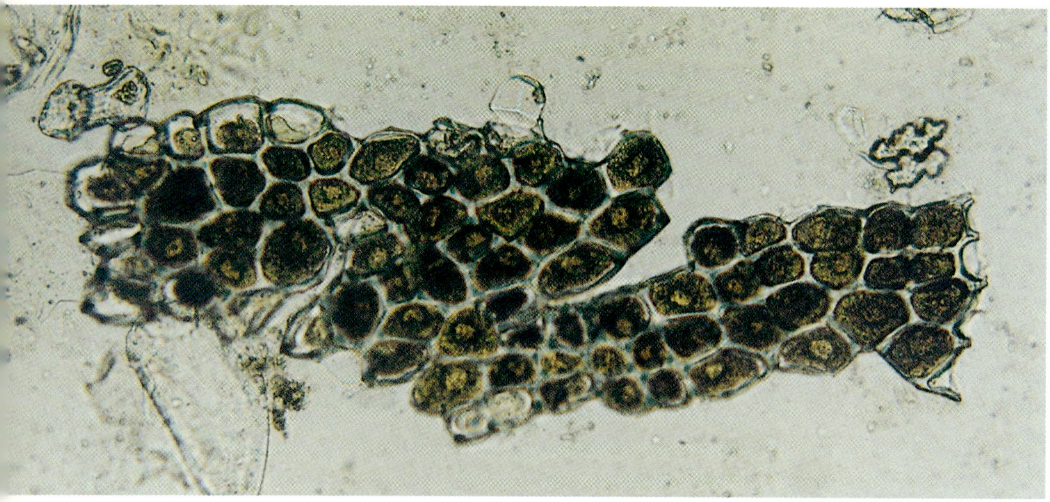

Photo 4:
Sheet of digested plant cells, showing cellulose chambers under x100 magnification.

cells, tend to carry bits of the adjacent cell wall with them and so they do not have a uniform capsule as does a roundworm egg. In plant cells that are about the same size as a roundworm egg, look for the slightly irregular shape and thickness of the wall to distinguish them from a roundworm egg. Sometimes material will partially overlap a roundworm egg, altering its appearance. If there is any doubt, it is best to continue examining the microscope slide for further eggs as they rarely occur singly.

To further complicate things, not only are the sheets of cell remnants ripped into pieces of different sizes during digestion but also their contents are broken down to different extents. This can give the internal structure of a plant cell a varied appearance under the microscope.

One of the things that plant cells contain is a complex sugar called starch. This is the energy that the plant contains and it is one of the reasons why birds eat seed and we eat fruit and vegetables. Because digestion is never 100% efficient, cells will often contain some undigested starch granules when passed in the droppings. These are visible and shown in photos 5 and 6. If a structure looking like a roundworm egg contains a starch granule, we know that it must, in fact, be a plant cell. Sometimes the outer wall of the plant cell can be broken and starch granules can float free. These can be confused with both Coccidia and thrush and will be discussed later.

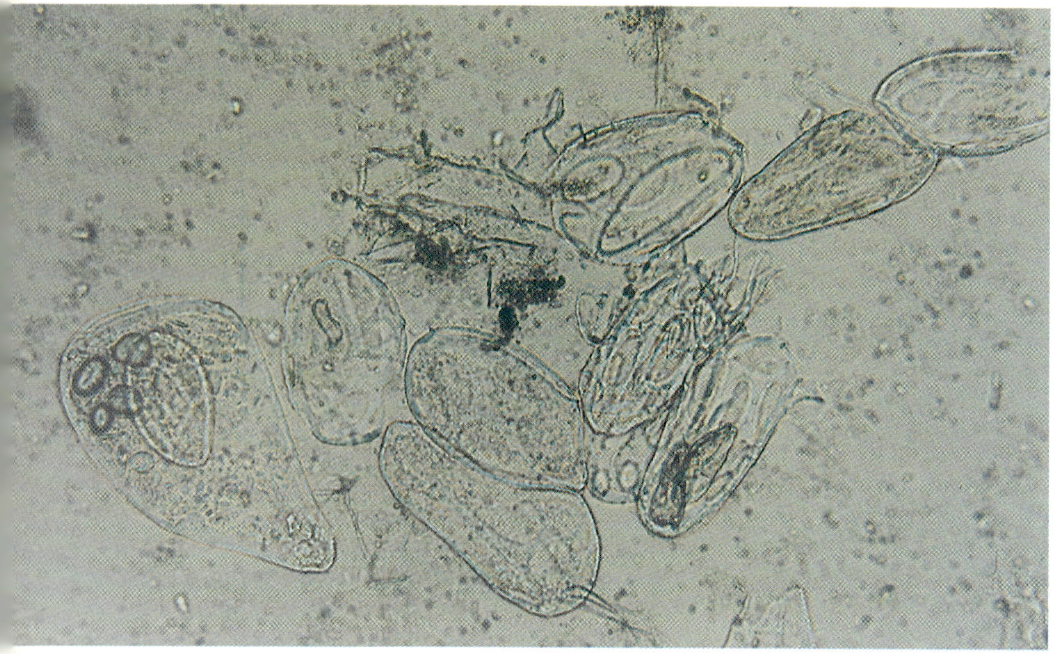

Photo 5:
Empty cell chambers except for one containing four starch granules, x100 magnification.

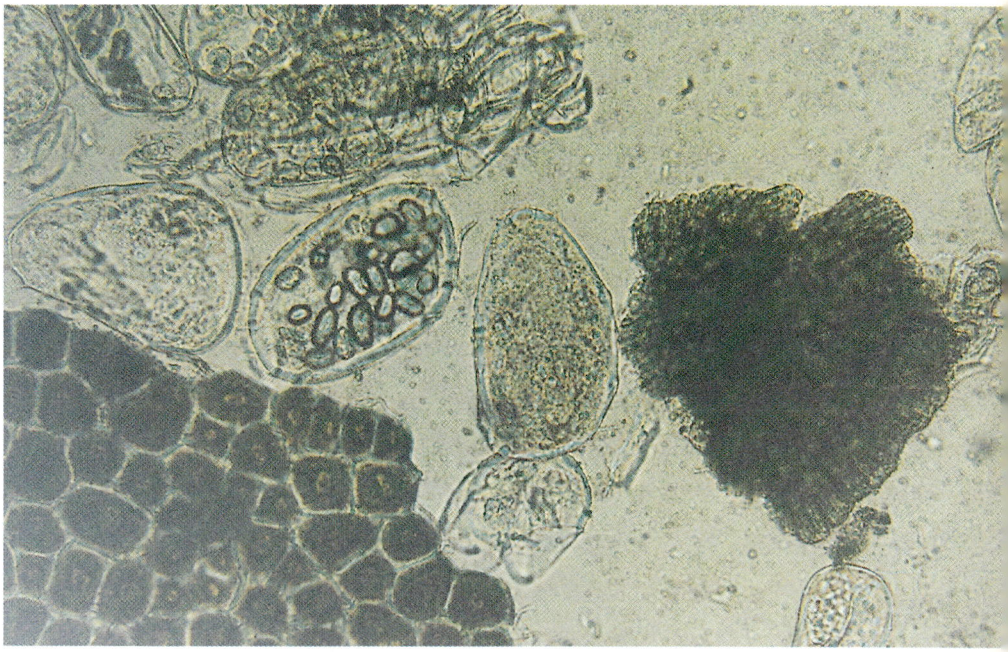

Photo 6:
Plant debris. Sheet of plant cells, bottom left; several cell chambers in centre and top left, one just left of centre packed with starch granules; denser sheet of plant cells to right. x100 magnification.

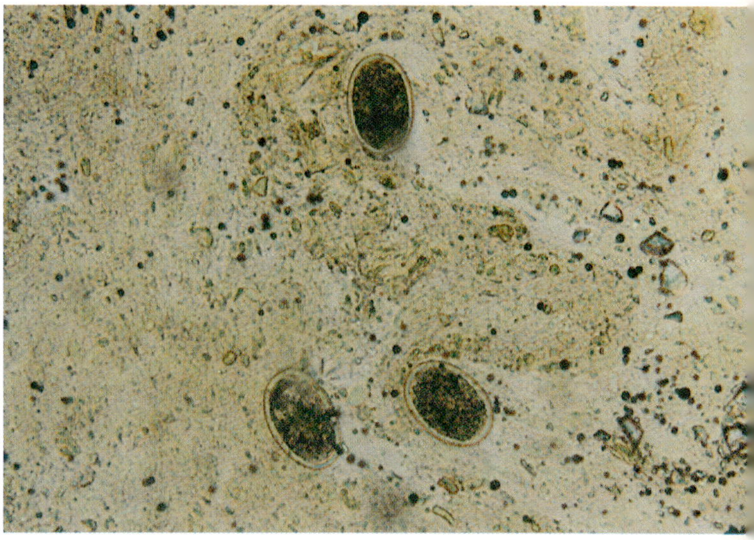

Photo 7:
Three roundworm eggs. The lower one on the left is superimposed with debris, thereby altering its appearance. x100 magnification.

- **Air Bubbles –** Pockets of air frequently become trapped under the microscope slide. These vary in size, are always circular, have a uniform black outer ring and a white centre. Their shape and clear centre distinguish them from a roundworm egg. When magnified 100 times, they look like photo 8.

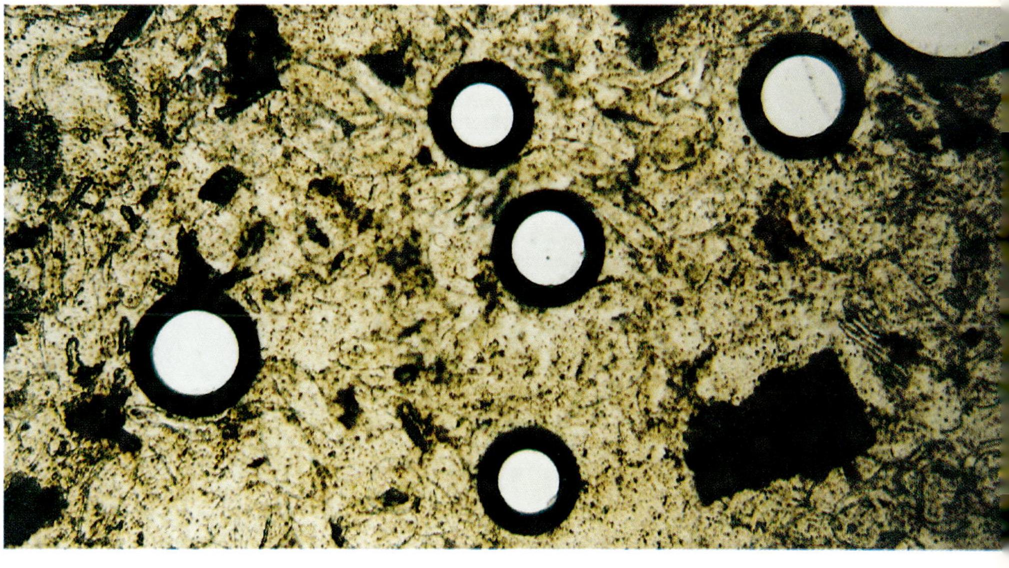

Photo 8:
Air bubbles of different sizes, x100 magnification.

And so for comparison, let's look at a number of things on the one slide (see photo 9).

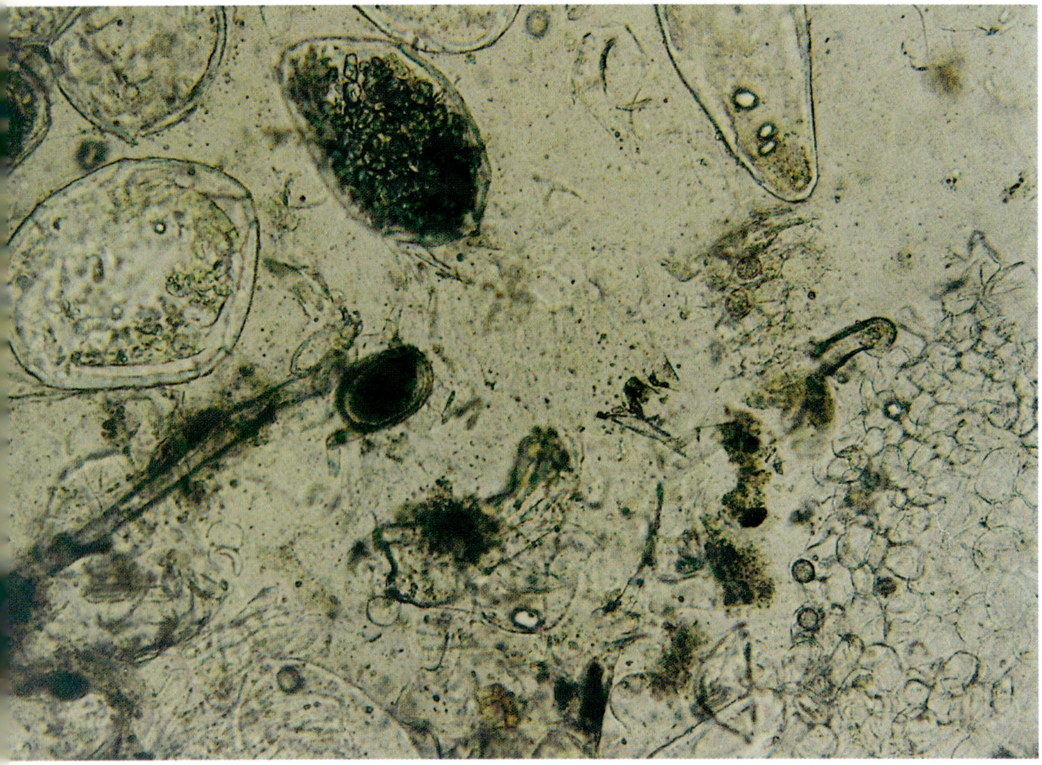

Photo 9:
Roundworm egg, left of centre; small empty cell chambers, bottom right; large cell chamber containing three starch granules, top right; cell chamber packed with starch granules above roundworm egg; large empty cell chamber, left of roundworm egg; all superimposed on well-digested plant debris. x100 magnification.

Hairworm Eggs

The technique for setting up the faecal smear for examination is exactly the same as for roundworm. Hairworms are not as prolific egg layers as roundworms so their eggs can be harder to find in that the number to look for is less.

Hairworm eggs are about half to two-thirds the size of a roundworm egg. They always lie on their side and so their shape and size are always the same. They are usually brownish in colour but may have a greenish tinge. Their capsule is very different from that of the roundworm and incorporates two thickened bubble-like areas at the egg's two 'ends', which are called bipolar plugs. This feature is characteristic and only displayed by worms of the hairworm family. When magnified 100 times, they look like photo 10.

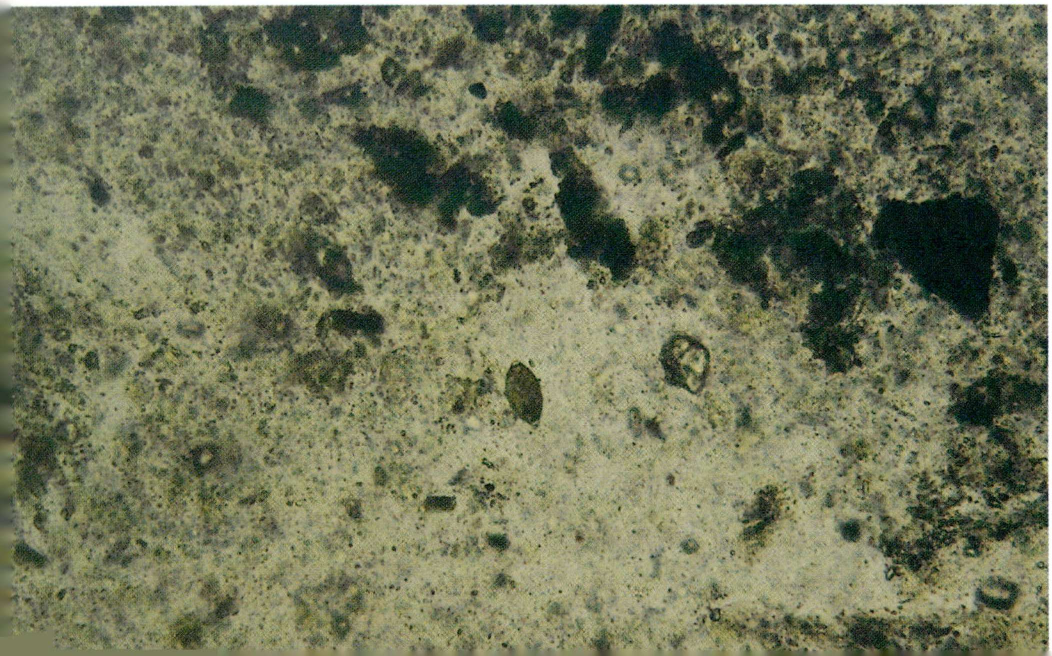

Photo 10:
Hairworm egg (in centre of photo), magnified x100.

Like the roundworm egg, they can be confidently diagnosed when magnified 100 times, but can also be examined under x400 magnification, when they look like photo 11.

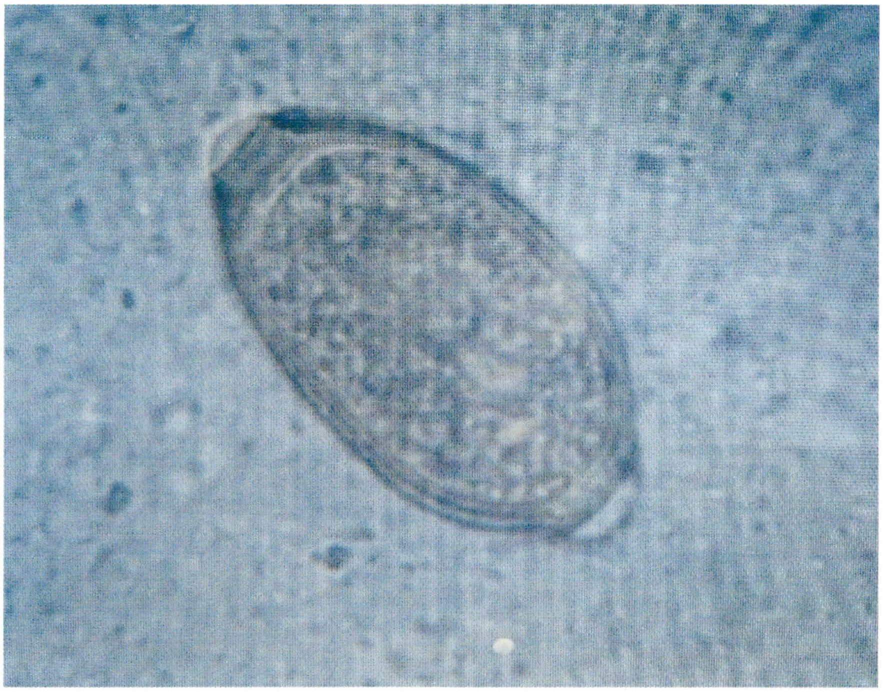

Photo 11: Hairworm egg, magnified x400.

Tapeworm Eggs

Tapeworms are not diagnosed with the microscope. Their eggs are usually released in packets called proglottids, which are visible to the naked eye. They have a fascinating lifecycle. The worms grow in the pigeon's bowel, burying their head deeply in the bowel lining. Maturing proglottids develop behind the worm's head to form a ribbon with the oldest, most mature proglottid at the end of this ribbon. Within each proglottid are both male and female genitals, which release, through pores on the proglottid surface, the tapeworm equivalent of sperm and eggs. These run the risk of being lost in the bowel and so the pores are in close proximity, usually leading to the sperm fertilizing the eggs within the same proglottid. In this way, the proglottid becomes a bag containing fertilized eggs. When this process is complete, the mature proglottid or 'egg packet' snaps from the end of the worm and is passed in the dropping. These vary in size from 1 cm x 0.5 cm down to the size of a match head. They are usually creamy white and when passed in the dropping are initially capable of moving. They are readily visible to the naked eye and can usually be seen as light-coloured 'grains of rice' or 'maggots' either on the dropping or sometimes sludged to a stop on the perch around the dropping.

Occasionally, egg packets break open inside the bowel and the microscopic eggs they contain will be passed in the droppings. The identification of these can be tricky but as the larger egg packets will also be found in the dropping it is easier for the fancier to simply look for these. As fanciers would be aware, these egg packets are not directly infectious to other pigeons, but rather need to be eaten by an intermediate host, usually an insect such as a beetle or weevil. Once in the insect, the tapeworm eggs hatch and undergo several lifecycle stages to become infective larvae. Pigeons become infected by eating insects containing these larvae.

Coccidia

Coccidia infection is usually diagnosed by preparing a wet smear of the droppings and examining this microscopically, looking for the parasite's eggs. As they have not been in the environment for long, they have not become infective (i.e. have not sporulated, see the chapter The Parasitic Diseases) and so, as described earlier, are thin-walled with a single roughly circular granular blob inside. In pigeons, coccidial eggs are usually round or slightly ovoid.

Preparation of the wet smear is the same as for roundworm eggs. After focusing onto the faecal film with the x4 lens, swing to the x10 lens on the deck and look for Coccidia eggs.

If present, the Coccidia eggs will look like photo 12.

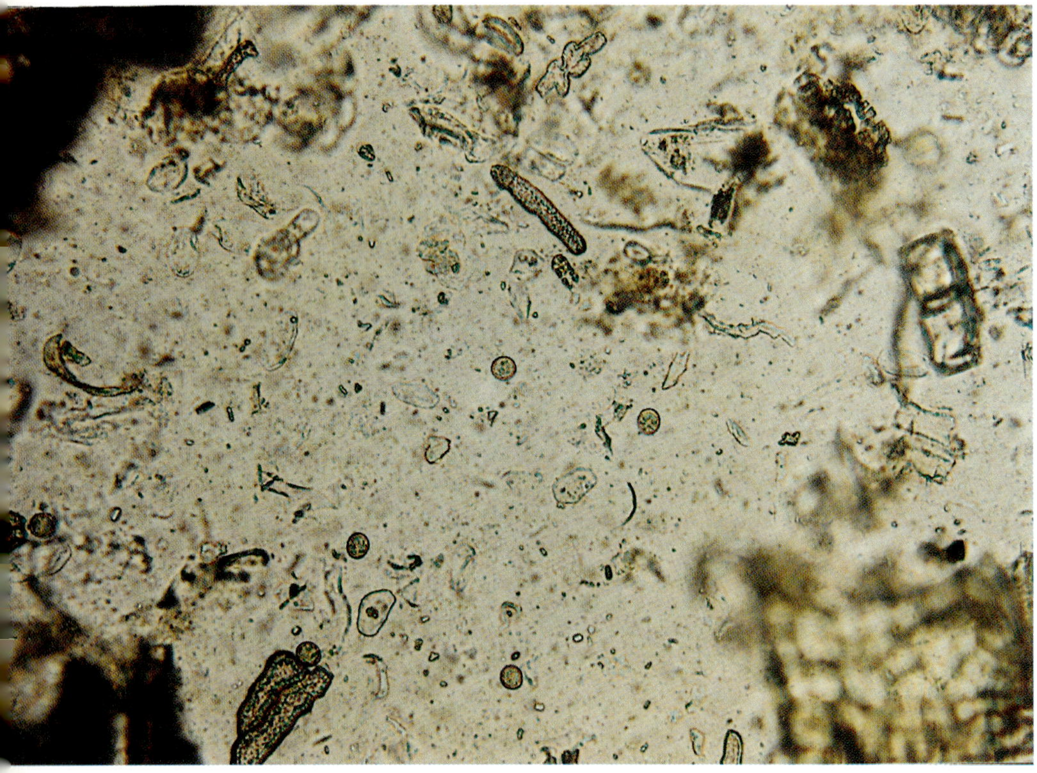

Photo 12:
Five Coccidia eggs at x100 magnification. One is in the centre of the photograph. After identifying this, look for the other four eggs, which are identical. All other material visible is partially digested plant debris.

Coccidia eggs can usually be diagnosed when magnified 100 times (i.e. x10 eyepiece and x10 lens on the deck) but, if there is any doubt, swing the x40 lens onto the deck to see them at x400 magnification. At this magnification, they look like photo 13.

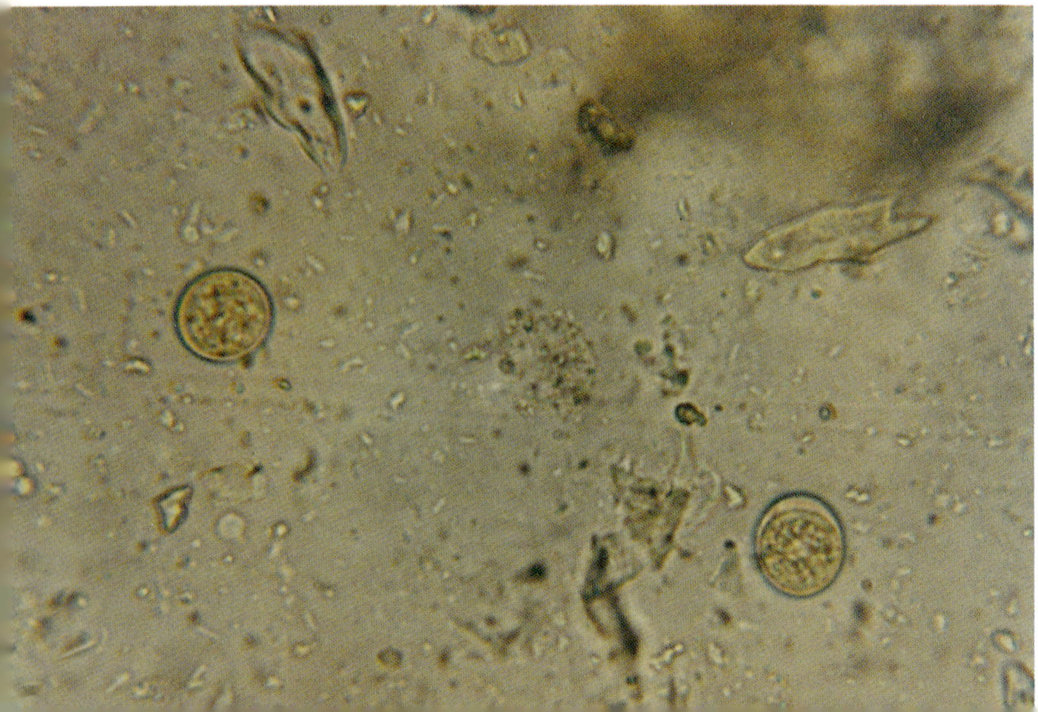

Photo 13:
Two coccidial eggs, magnified 400 times. The other structures of similar size are plant debris, while the smaller light-coloured dots and lines (rods) are bacteria.

Coccidia are about one-twentieth the size of a roundworm egg but are about the same size as the starch granules described in the previous section on roundworm egg identification. They are much bigger than yeasts, which can only confidently be identified under 400 times magnification. A handy diagnostic feature is that many Coccidia (depending on their orientation towards the microscope lens) have what appears as a clear lunette filling the rest of the egg on top of the sporoblast. The egg to the right on photo 13 demonstrates this.

Things that resemble Coccidia and can confuse particularly the microscope beginner are:

- **Starch granules –** These are the complex sugars stored within plant cells, which are often passed undigested in the pigeons' droppings. They appear in photo 5. Although about the same size as Coccidia, they are irregular in shape, have no internal structure and usually, but not always, are found within plant cells.
- **Uric acid crystals –** These make up the solid urine or white material in the pigeon's dropping. These are always circular but variable in size, with the biggest ones only being about one-tenth the size of a Coccidia. They often appear a greenish brown colour microscopically. When viewed under x400 magnification, they appear to have little lines and crosses in their centre, which is the effect given when looking down on top of any crystal. If you are confused, deliberately make a wet smear of only the white part of a pigeon's dropping and all you will see are these. Under x400 magnification, they look like photo 14.

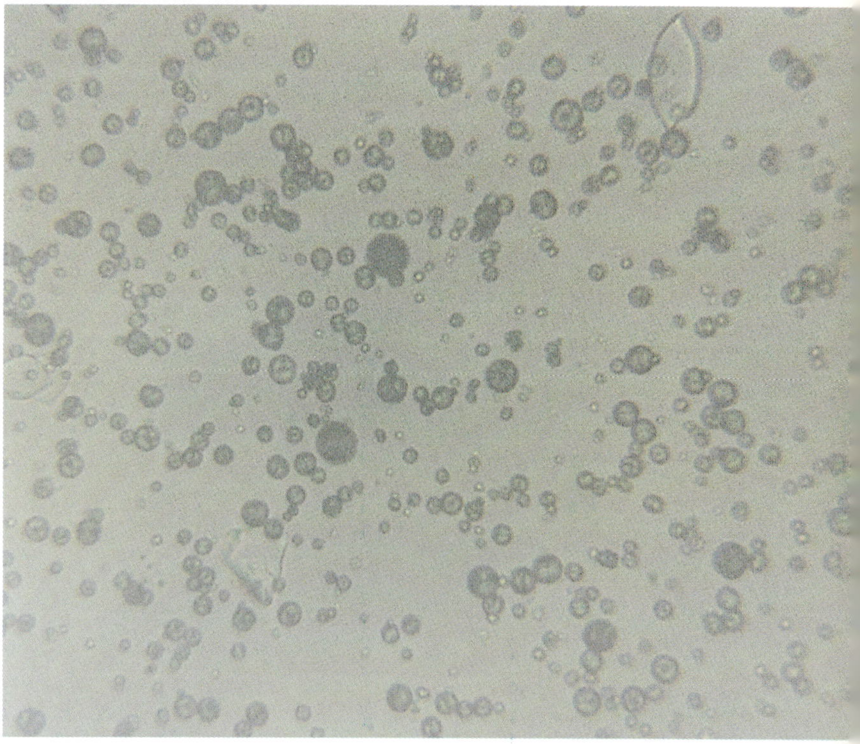

Photo 14:
Uric acid crystals, magnified 400 times.

- **'Thrush' –** Animals infected with yeasts, which are a type of fungi, are said to have 'thrush'. They are only about one-twentieth the size of Coccidia, are circular to elliptical, appear to have no internal structure, and when reproducing have little nipples, called buds, growing from their surface. They look like photos 15 and 16.

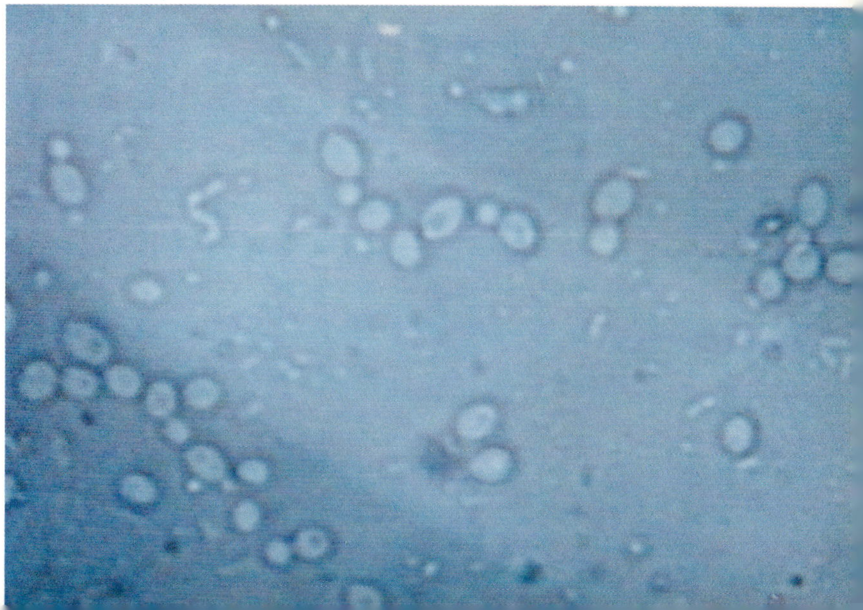

Photo 15:
Yeast organisms, magnified 400 times.

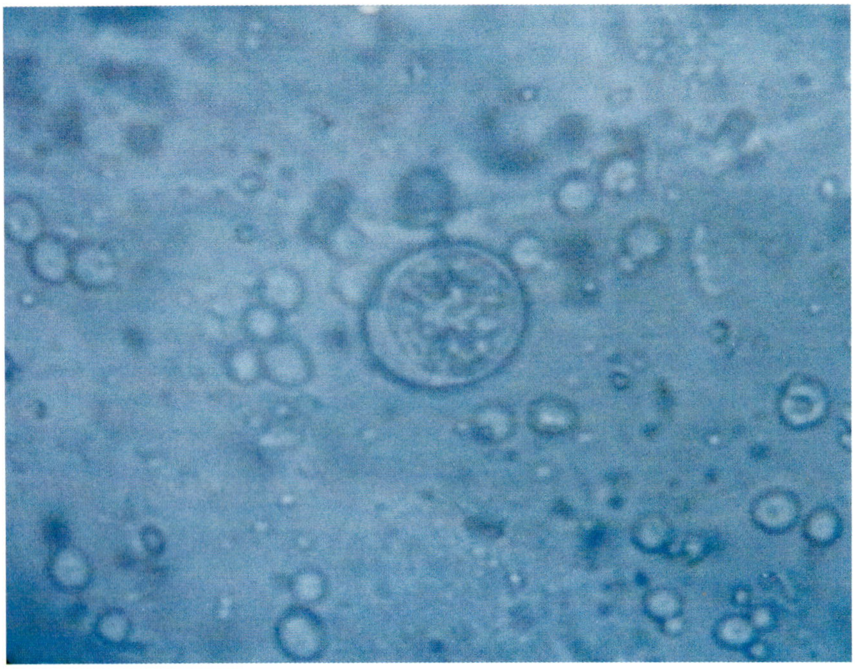

Photo 16:
A single Coccidia egg and yeast organisms, magnified 400 times.

- **Some plant cells –** Some single plant cells can look superficially like Coccidia, particularly if their contents have not been digested. They are, however, usually much larger than Coccidia and their walls are of irregular width and angular rather than circular, as in Coccidia.

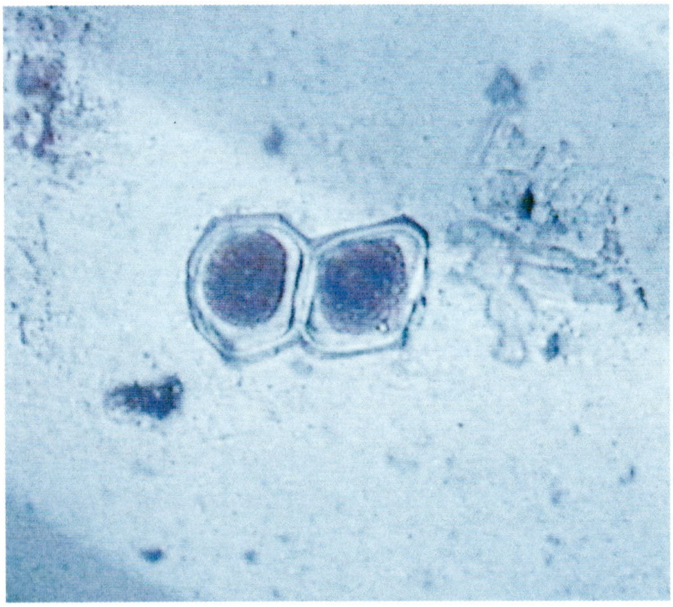

Photo 17:
Two plant cells, magnified 100 times.

Remember that if you do find some Coccidia eggs in the birds' droppings out of the race season, then provided that the birds are well otherwise, it is usually best not to treat. This level of infection is necessary and beneficial, tending to reinforce the birds' natural immunity. However, once racing, we don't want to see any Coccidia in the faecal smear and so usually the finding of any is an indication for treatment. Their sudden appearance can, however, indicate that something else is running the birds down (in many lofts, there is a high correlation between wet canker in the crop flushes and Coccidia in the droppings) and, to ensure a good response to treatment, these will have to be identified and corrected too. Often, low levels in a good loft during racing will respond well to rest and 1 or 2 days on energy (seed oil and yeast) and multivitamin supplements.

If lots of Coccidia are found when examining birds with diarrhoea, this is likely to be the cause but the diarrhoea can sometimes precede the output of eggs by 1 – 2 days or persist for several days after successful treatment. Eggs are also shed in higher numbers in late afternoon. Therefore, it is not always possible to find eggs in a single dropping sample; multiple examinations are sometimes required.

Hexamita

Hexamita are discussed in the parasitic section in the chapter The Common Diseases. They are approximately the same size as trichomonads (canker organisms) and so are therefore just visible when magnified 100 times and are clearly visible when magnified 400 times. Like canker organisms, they are motile. However, they tend to move about faster and with a more direct movement. They quickly lose their motility and die as the droppings cool and, as it is this motility that enables easy recognition, they can only be reliably diagnosed in a fresh dropping sample that is still warm. When magnified 400 times, they look like photo 18.

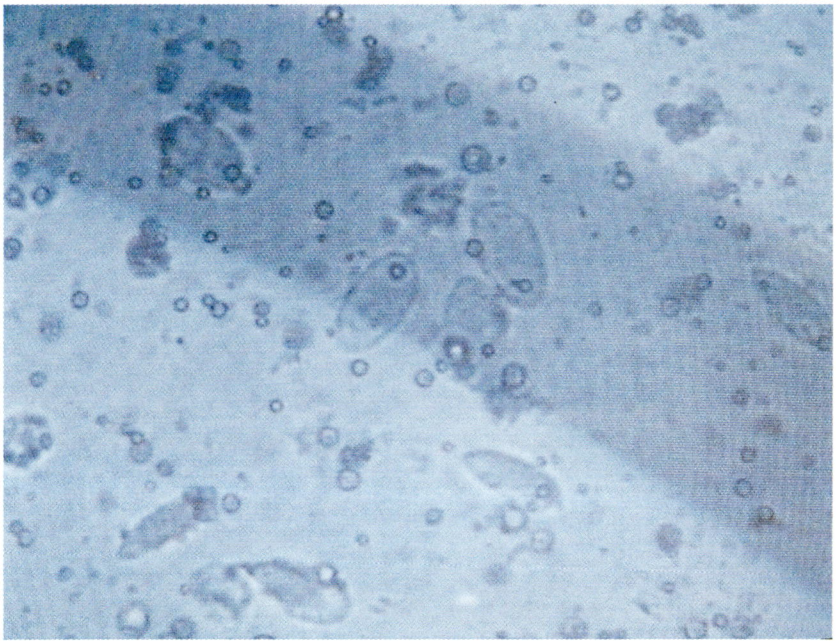

Photo 18:
Hexamita organisms in a faecal smear, magnified 400 times.

The crop flush

The crop flush involves the aspiration of material from the back of the bird's throat and crop. As discussed earlier, it is a necessary procedure to diagnose wet canker and can give an indication of respiratory infection in birds that may still look normal on the perch. How are these diagnoses made, and once a crop flush is prepared as a microscopic slide, what is the fancier likely to see?

For the technique involved in doing a crop flush, refer to the chapter The Use of the Microscope by the Pigeon Fancier.

The fancier is likely to see epithelial cells, mucus, food, trichomonads, heterophils, yeasts, bacteria, worm eggs and airsac mite eggs.

Epithelial cells

Easily visible when magnified 100 times, these are the large plate-like cells that normally line the crop. During collection of the crop flush, they often crinkle up, looking a bit like a sheet that someone has slept on. They are very loosely attached so their aspiration is in no way painful, in fact fanciers can look at some of their own epithelial cells by gently rolling a dry cotton bud on the inside of their cheek and then rolling this onto a microscope slide. As stated above, when looking for wet canker, I feel that it is important to have these in the sample so as to ensure that no trichomonads are overlooked. At x100 magnification, they are shown in photo 19 on page 278.

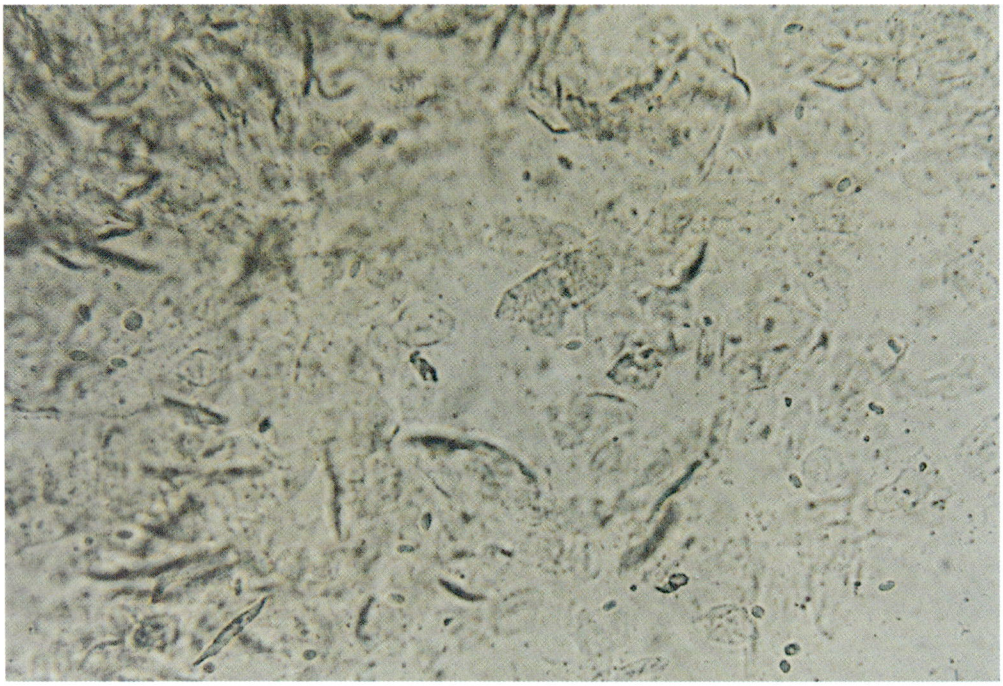

Photo 19:
Epithelial cells.

Mucus

Mucus is an amorphous material that often appears as a series of swirly grey lines. As some mucus is always present, its appearance does not indicate a problem.

Food

It does not really matter whether the birds have been fed or not before a crop flush as disease organisms are either going to be there or not. However, for the beginner, it may be best to do crop flushes when the crop is empty. Food takes on a variety of appearances depending on how long it has been in the crop. With recent feeding, large visible pieces may suck into the crop tube. However, if the food has been in the crop for some time, it becomes softened and sheets of plant cells similar to those found in droppings (illustrated earlier) can be found.

Trichomonads

Trichomonads are the organism that cause canker and their detection is the main reason for doing any crop flush. I feel that if the only thing a fancier can confidently diagnose with his microscope is wet canker, then this in itself justifies the expense of the microscope. Trichomonads can just be seen when magnified 100 times and look like photo 20 when present in large numbers. In lower numbers, they look like photo 21.

However, they are easier to identify when magnified 400 times. Often it is their movement that attracts one's eye. If, however, the water used on the microscope slide is either too hot or too cold, they will lose their motility. Similarly, if the birds have been treated with an anticanker drug in the previous 24 hours, the trichomonads may not move. They have several whip-like tails that enable them to move and it is usually possible to see these when magnified 400 times. They occur either singly or in clumps (usually attached to an epithelial cell) but can occur in vast sheets filling the whole microscope field. Different strains vary in their shape, some being circular while others are more elliptical to bullet-shaped. Whether the fancier uses saline solution or water as a diluent also affects the shape. Saline solution enables the trichomonads to keep their shape, whereas they absorb water, which tends to make them swell and assume a more rounded appearance.

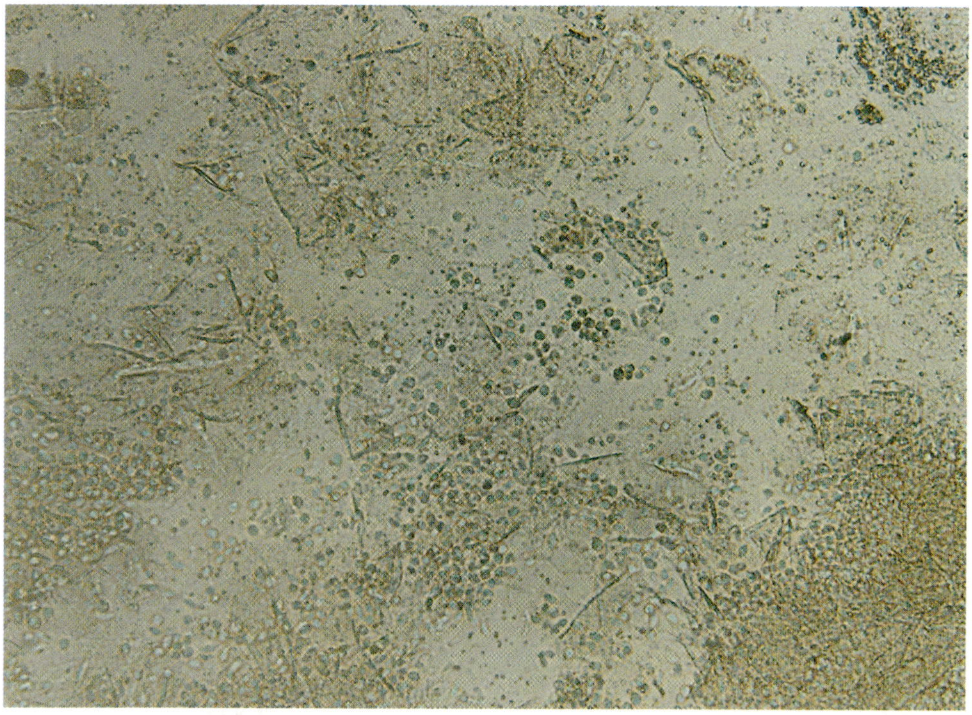

Photo 20: Trichomonads, magnified 100 times.

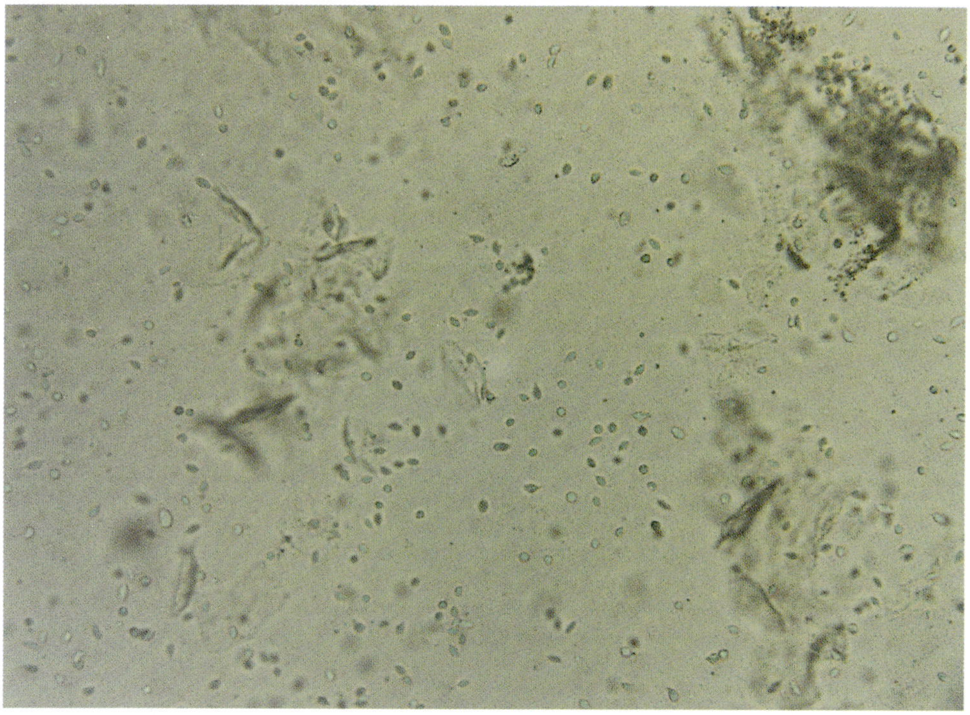

Photo 21: Trichomonads, magnified 100 times.

Remember that, out of the race season, the detection of trichomonads in birds that are otherwise well is not an indication for treatment. Their presence simply acts like a vaccination, strengthening the bird's developing natural immunity. However, once racing starts, we do not want to find any trichomonads on the crop flush. As trichomonad numbers rise, performance falls. After a 2-day course of an antitrichomonad drug, in most race lofts no trichomonads will be present. With the on-going stress of racing, trichomonads will gradually re-establish. How quickly depends on the level of natural immunity formed by the birds before racing. With regular crop flushes, the fancier can determine how long they take to reappear in his team and treat accordingly.

HETEROPHILS

Pigeons have five common types of white blood cell in their circulation. Heterophils are the most common one, being involved in the bird's initial response to infection and inflammation. When membrane surfaces become inflamed, heterophils will be lost in the resultant discharge. This occurs with inflammation at any site. However, as inflammation of the respiratory system can lead to the accumulation of heterophils in the throat, their appearance can be a useful indicator of respiratory infection. With one-eye colds and sinus inflammation, they drain through the slot in the roof of the mouth into the back of the throat. With inflammation in the windpipe, they are coughed up into the throat.

Finding the odd heterophil in a crop flush is of no concern. However, when large numbers are detected, they alert the microscope user to the possibility of respiratory infection. It is then important to relate their detection to what the birds are doing clinically. If the birds are reluctant to fly, panting readily and, in particular, sneezing, the appearance of heterophils lends weight to the diagnosis of respiratory infection. During racing, a good indicator of respiratory infection is sneezing. If a fancier wants to know whether the sneezing is due to respiratory infection or not, he can crop flush several of his birds and look for heterophils.

Heterophils are the same size as trichomonads. However, they are invariably circular. Some are degenerate, i.e. in the process of breaking down, and so their appearance can vary. A fresh heterophil has a distinct cell membrane (outline). Each one has several internal nuclei that are joined by strands called spindles. This gives them a granular appearance and the description of 'little pizzas' is apt. To definitively see heterophils, all a fancier has to do is crop flush a bird with an obvious respiratory infection, e.g. an eye cold or dirty cere. The real benefit of their recognition is the monitoring of respiratory infection during racing in birds that may, in fact, look quite normal on the perch. When magnified 100 times, they look like photo 22.

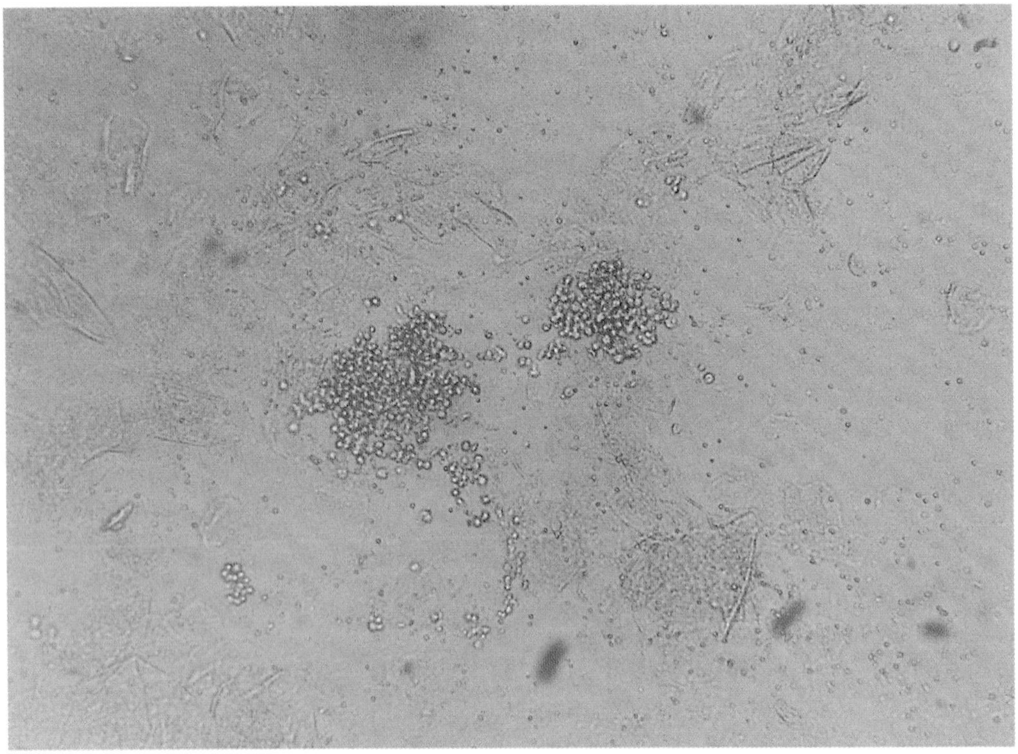

Photo 22: Heterophils magnified 100 times.

At x400 magnification, they look like photo 23.

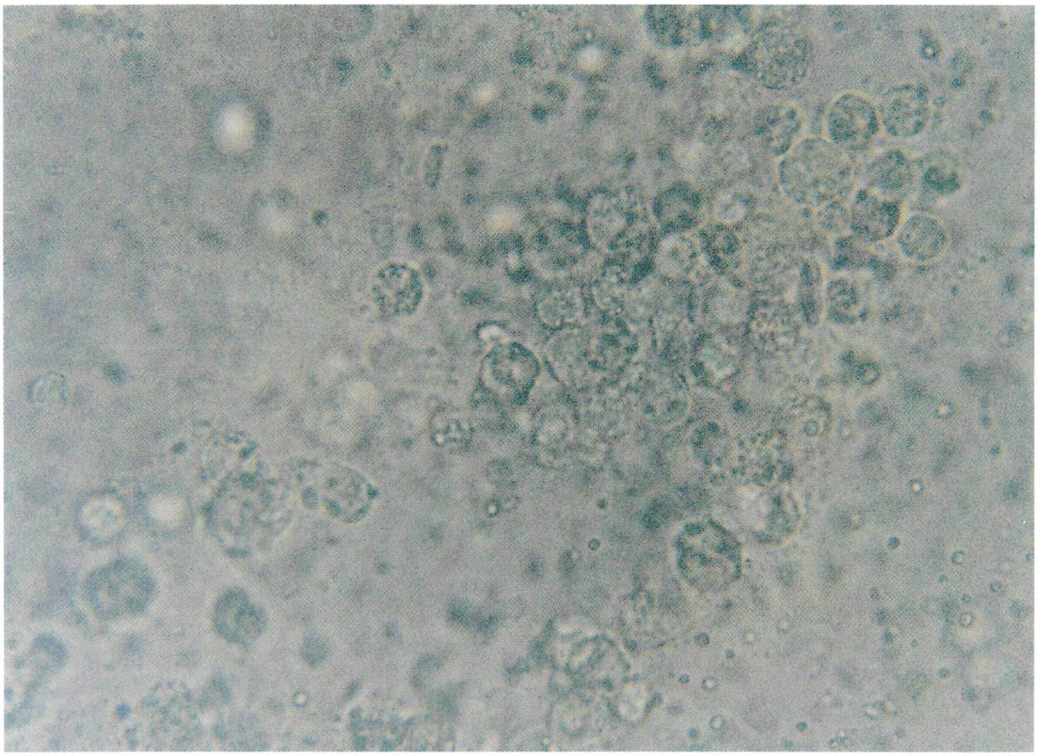

Photo 23: Heterophils magnified 400 times.

Red blood cells

The appearance of red blood cells in the crop flush means that the lining of the crop, throat or sinus has been broken and bleeding has occurred. They will therefore appear as a result of injury or disease, such as a bleeding canker nodule. However, the fancier must ensure that he has not, through poor technique, been rough and caused superficial injury to the throat or crop with the crop tube. Crop walls and throats that are already inflamed can be quite fragile. However, improved technique comes with practice. Red blood cells can be seen when magnified 100 times but are easier to recognize definitively when magnified 400 times. They are about the same size as a trichomonad and heterophil but are elliptical in shape and contain a single large nucleus, which is also elliptical in shape. In fact, they look like a small AFL football inside a slightly larger AFL football and usually occur in groups.

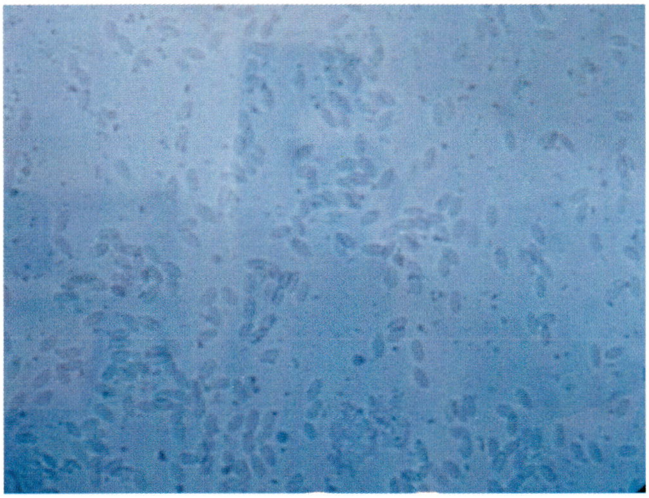

Photo 24: Red blood cells, magnified 100 times.

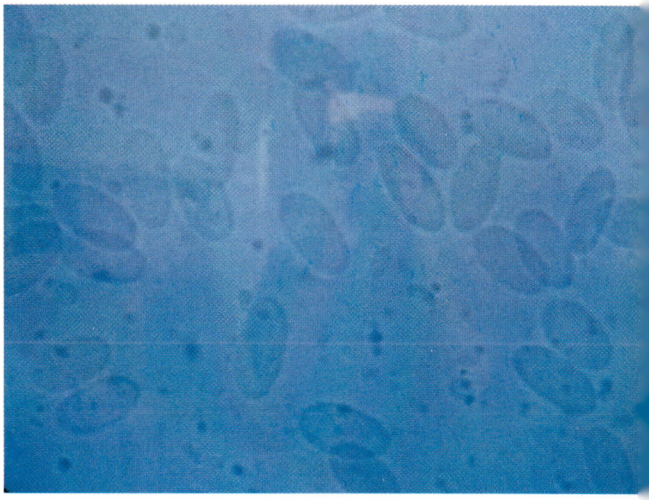

Photo 25: Red blood cells, magnified 400 times.

Yeasts

Yeasts and their appearance under the microscope are discussed in more detail under the section Fungi in this chapter. Their appearance in the crop is identical to their appearance in the dropping. Healthy pigeons never have reproducing yeasts in their crop. Their appearance usually indicates that the pigeons have become very run down. They will appear with any condition that interferes with crop emptying and also sometimes for 1 – 2 days after an antibiotic course. They will also appear after the use of feed supplement yeasts such as Brewer's Yeast and ID Yeast for a short time until the crop pushes them into the stomach where these yeasts are digested. These look identical to the yeasts that are capable of infecting the crop but are obviously not a problem. The appearance of reproducing (i.e. budding) yeasts indicates a serious health problem that needs attention.

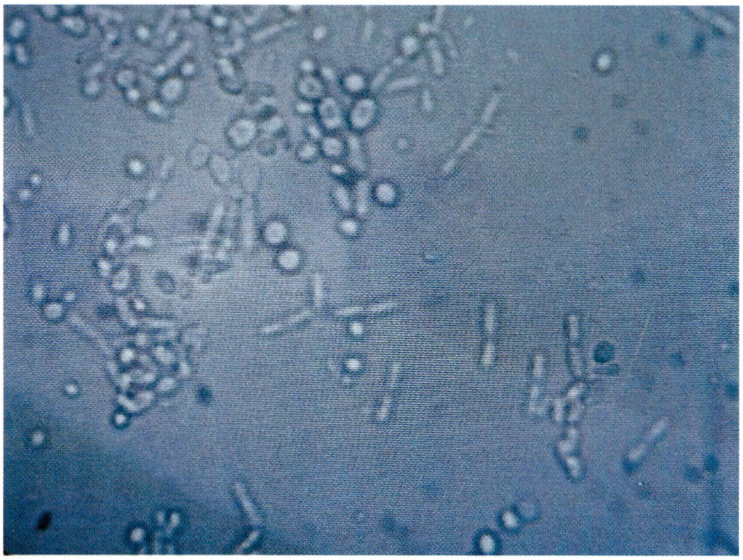

Photo 26:
Yeasts and early fungal branches in a crop flush, magnified 400 times.

Bacteria

It is not normal to see large numbers of bacteria of any description in a pigeon's crop and, in fact, their presence can be hard to detect in in-form teams. Elevated levels of bacteria will occur with contaminated food and water, delayed crop emptying, inadequate hygiene with drinkers, poor feeding technique, deep vomiting, primary bacterial infections of the crop wall and secondary to respiratory infection and wet canker. It may, however, be normal to see small numbers of cocci (i.e. the dot-shaped bacteria). From a veterinary point of view, we like to see fewer than 5% of the bacteria being what we call gram-negative, with no single bacterial type predominating. If needed, swabs can be taken, which are then grown on special media (McConkey/BAP) for identification. The microscopic appearance of bacteria in the crop is the same as in the droppings. This is dealt with in more detail later.

Worm eggs

Several types of worms can infect the crop, namely *Capillaria* (hairworm) and *Ornithostrongylus* (large roundworm). Sometimes their eggs will appear on crop flushes. Photos of these appear earlier.

Airsac mite eggs

Two types of mite actually live within the cere, sinuses, windpipe and airsacs of pigeons. They should always be thought of when there are on-going signs of respiratory infection that do not respond to antibiotics. The adults are just visible to the naked eye and sometimes one can be lucky enough, when opening the pigeon's mouth, to see one run across the floor of the mouth into the windpipe or alternatively disappear up into the slot. The eggs that they lay are coughed into the throat and so therefore can be found in the crop flush and later the droppings. However, they are not prolific egg layers and so diagnosis is not easy. Their eggs are similar in appearance to roundworm eggs but are a bit bigger and have a slightly thinner capsule ('shell').

Fungi

Fungi can be detected in both the crop flush and faecal smear on occasion and their appearance cannot only indicate a health problem but they can also be used to assess the quality of the birds' food and the loft environment and also to evaluate training regimes.

Fungi are a type of plant. In the same way that there are lots of other types of plants, there are lots of different types of fungi and also in the same way that each type of plant will only grow under certain situations, this is also true for fungi. The fungi that are important to the fancier with his microscope fall into two types, the yeasts and filamentous fungi.

Yeasts

Some yeasts live in the environment, usually on organic matter (e.g. Baker's and Brewer's Yeasts), while other types can live within animals. These types are usually found within the digestive tract. However, one thing they all have in common is that they reproduce in a process called budding. In this process, a small lump or nipple appears on the surface of the yeast. This gets bigger and bigger. As it grows, its point of attachment to its 'parent' gets thinner and thinner, forming a 'neck', until finally, when this bud is almost as big as the original, it breaks free to produce a new yeast. Budding is a very handy diagnostic feature and it is what we look for to recognize the yeasts against the backdrop of dropping debris under the microscope.

There are lots of different types of yeast and not all have the potential to infect pigeons. In fact, some can be beneficial. Those that grow on grain such as Brewer's Yeast and Baker's Yeast are a valuable and useful food source for birds, being high in both protein and vitamin B. The yeasts of concern regarding the birds' health belong to a genus called *Candida* and they live in the digestive tract of pigeons. They are almost always present but usually in low numbers. Their numbers are kept in check by the normal beneficial population of bacteria in the bowel, which are in competition with them. If anything gets rid of these bacteria, then the yeasts are free to multiply and cause disease. These bacteria are eliminated in one of two ways, either through the use of antibiotics, which kill them, or through stress, which alters the environment within the bowel, favouring the growth of harmful organisms. *Candida* is what we call an opportunist, in that as soon as the good bacteria are gone, they will opportunistically multiply and increase. Pigeons with a large number of yeasts causing disease are said to have 'thrush'.

Diagnosis of thrush

Yeasts can be found in both the faecal smear and also the crop flush. The techniques for making a faecal smear and a crop flush have already been discussed. When magnified, yeasts appear to have a dark outline and a clear white centre. They can be circular to elliptical in shape and it is important to look for some with buds as these are their principal diagnostic feature. They are just visible when magnified 100 times (i.e. x10 eye piece, x10 lens on microscope deck) and look like photo 27.

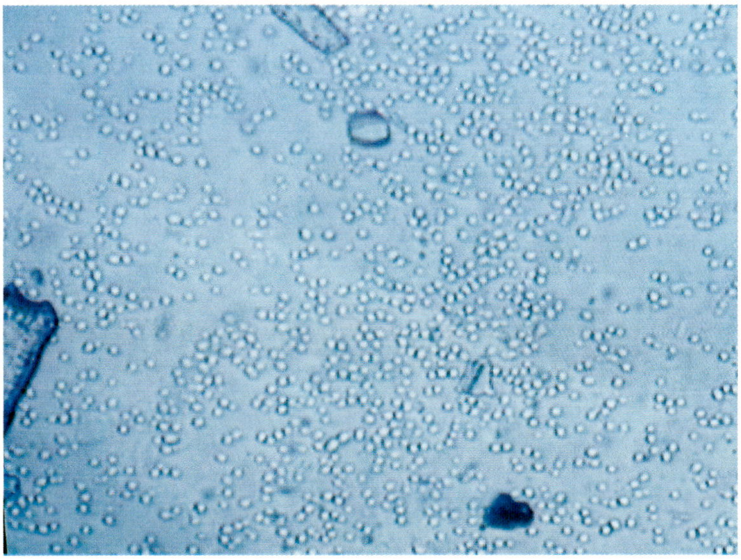

Photo 27: Yeast organisms, magnified 100 times.

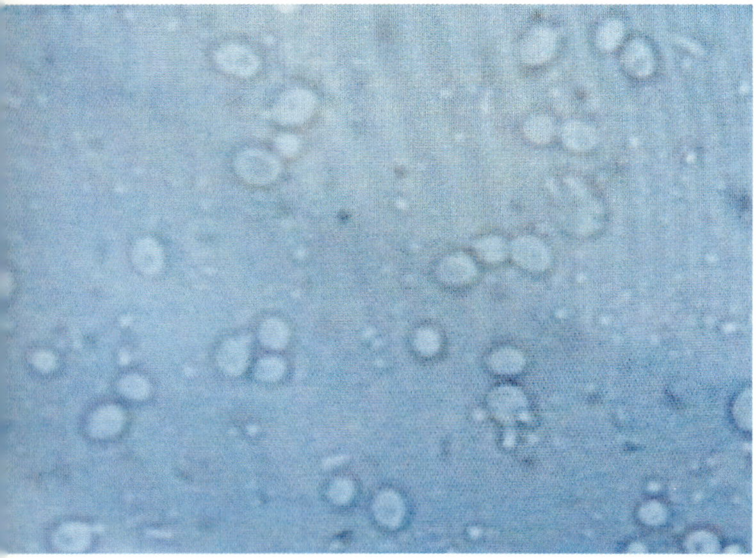

Photo 28:
Yeast organisms, magnified 400 times.

However, to differentiate for sure, swing the x40 lens onto the deck to magnify the field 400 times and look for the tell-tale buds. When magnified 400 times, they look like photo 28.

Once the yeast is recognized, it is important that the fancier interprets his finding correctly. If there are only three or four per x100 microscope field, they are probably of no concern and the best thing is to do nothing for the time being but monitor the situation and recheck the droppings in 24 hours. If levels higher than this are encountered, and indeed sometimes yeasts can be jostling for space with each other, then their presence is significant. If an antibiotic course has just been completed, then this will be the cause. A 24 – 48-hour course of probiotics and all should be fine. If the birds have not had antibiotics, then the appearance of the yeasts is likely to be associated with stress. The fancier must identify anything about his loft and management that may be stressing the birds. At times this can be very hard to put a finger on. Check on the same faecal smear and a crop flush for evidence of a concurrent disease that may be weakening them. Often the cause in a good loft is overtraining. In this case, rest (i.e. no tossing), good food and 1 day on a multivitamin or probiotic will do the trick. Persistent high levels of yeast indicate a serious on-going stress that may be associated with the loft, training, feeding, or another disease. Feed supplement yeasts (such as those found in ID Yeast) do not live in the bird and therefore do not confuse results as they are digested.

Yeasts are never found in the crop flush of a healthy bird. They appear in the crop flush for the same reasons that they appear in the bowel, however, the birds have to be considerably sicker for them to do so.

Things that look like yeasts include:

- **Dot-shaped bacteria –** These are much smaller, being only about one-fiftieth the size.
- **Uric acid crystals –** Discussed earlier, some are about the same size as yeasts but are usually smaller and have the characteristic 'star' in their centre due to looking at the crystal end-on, while yeasts appear to have no internal structure.
- **Coccidia –** Much larger with an internal granular blob (the blastospore). See photo 16, which compares yeasts with Coccidia.
- **Starch granules –** Much larger. Similar dark outline and clear centre but are irregular in shape.
- **Trichomonads** (canker organisms) and **heterophils** (white blood cells), which are both found in a crop flush. Photos appear on pages 279 – 281.

Filamentous fungi

Like yeasts, filamentous fungi can grow either in the environment or in an animal. They do not, however, reproduce by budding in the same way as yeasts and so their appearance is very different under the microscope. Filamentous fungi produce the fungal equivalent of a flower called a fruiting

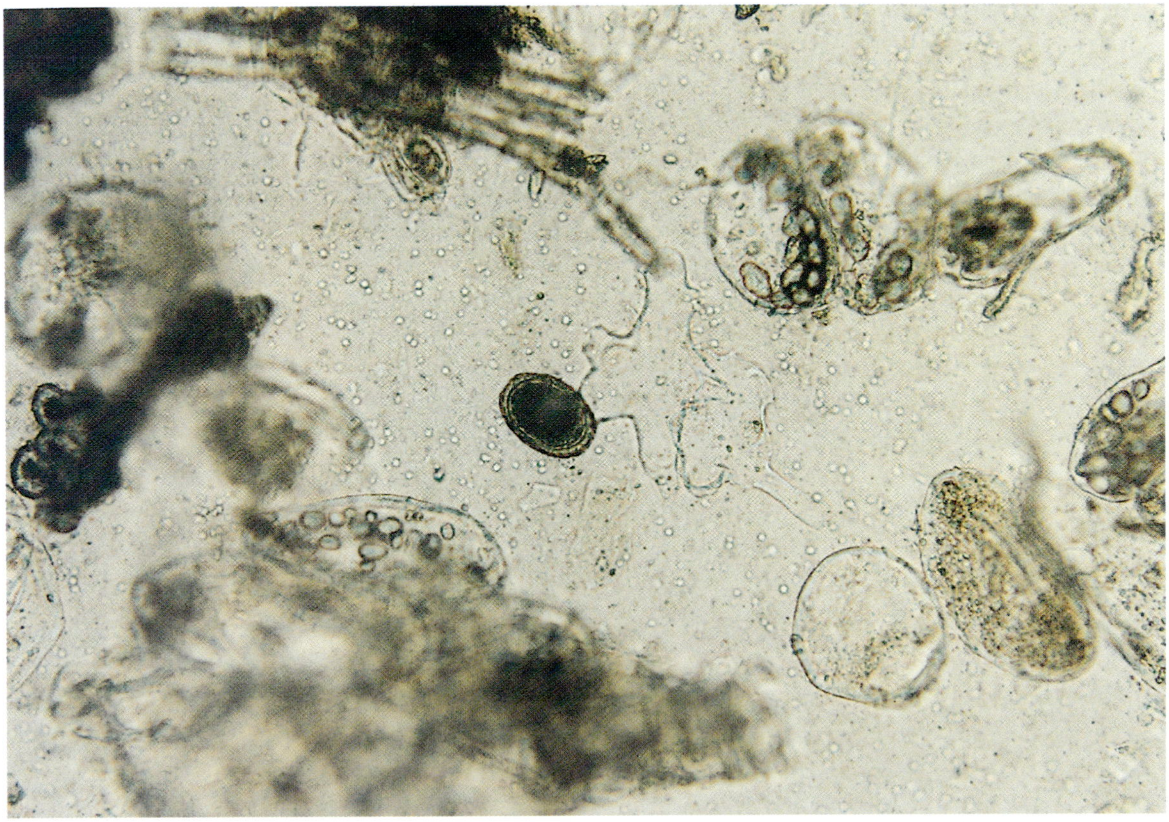

Photo 29: For size comparison, compare the roundworm egg in the centre to the yeasts. Yeasts are the small white dots scattered in the background.

body. This in turn produces fungal seeds called spores. These are released into the environment and, when they land on a suitable substrate, they germinate, producing fungal roots or branches, called hyphae. What we look for in a faecal smear are germinating fungal spores and fungal branches.

Fungal spores are difficult to differentiate microscopically from yeasts until they start to grow. As they grow, the root (branch or hyphae) 'sprouts' from the spore, giving it a tubular appearance. This continues to extend, becoming thicker and wider before bifurcating. Growth continues with further divisions until eventually a dense network of filaments is formed. Microscopic appearance will depend on the time between germination and examination.

Germinating fungal spores are best examined under x400 magnification, and they look like photo 30.

Interpretation is very important. Droppings, once passed, will eventually be colonized by fungal spores blowing free in the breeze if they remain moist in the environment. The appearance of mouldy droppings in itself therefore does not represent a problem. What it does tell us though is that the droppings have remained

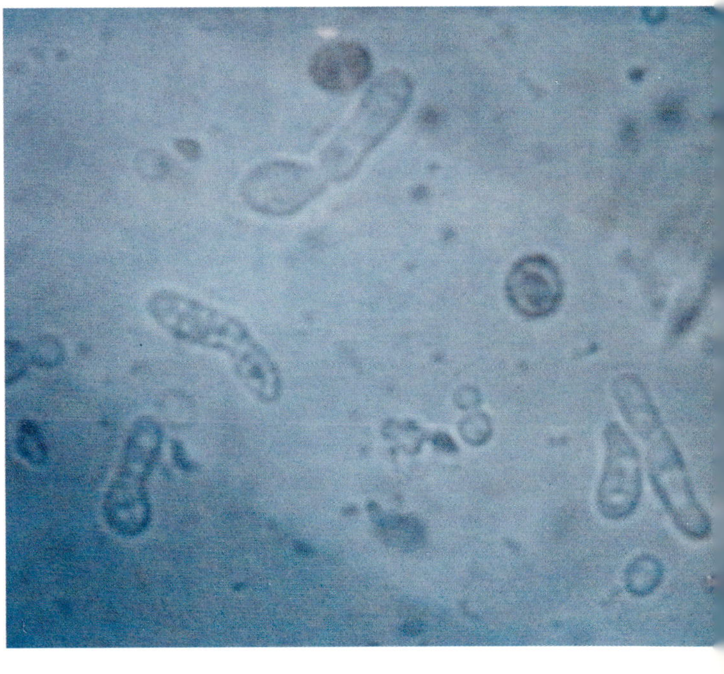

Photo 30:
Germinating fungal spores, magnified 400 times.

damp in the loft, which does tell us that the loft is too humid and this may be a problem. Except in the humid north of Australia, droppings that are not removed will be dry by mid-morning and resistant to fungal growth in a correctly ventilated loft. In the same way, if there is a delay in examination of droppings that remain moist, such as in mailed-in droppings, the appearance of fungi may simply indicate contamination by environmental fungal spores, which take advantage of the time in transit to germinate. The finding of fungi in such droppings does not have any relevance to the birds' health.

What we want to know is if the dropping contained fungi when it was passed. If fungi are passed in the dropping, this means the bird must either have swallowed or breathed them in (because the nose and mouth in birds are continuous through the slot in the roof of the mouth). If fungi have been swallowed, this points the finger at the quality of the grain. If they have been inhaled, this means fungal moulds are growing in the birds' environment, e.g. on straw, accumulated droppings, or, in the humid north, the loft itself. As inhaling fungal spores predisposes the bird to respiratory problems and as seed contaminated with spores may also contain fungal poisons, it is important that both possible scenarios are investigated, otherwise the birds will not be able to perform.

Fungal branches can easily be seen when magnified 100 times, and eventually, as the plant matures into a mould, it can be seen with the naked eye.

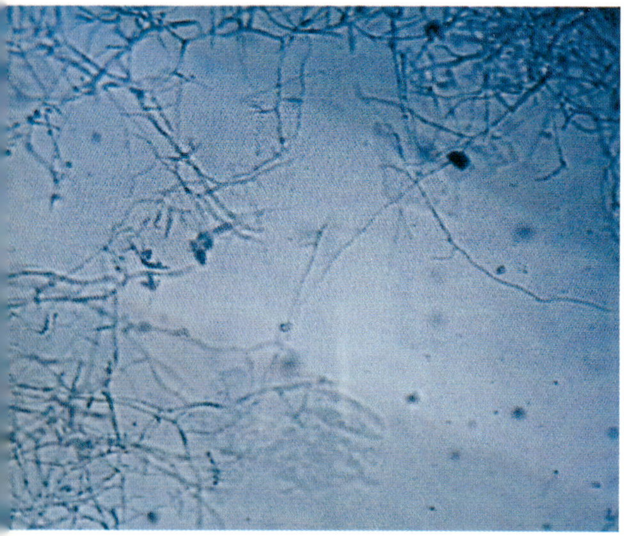

Photo 31: Fungal branches, magnified 100 times.

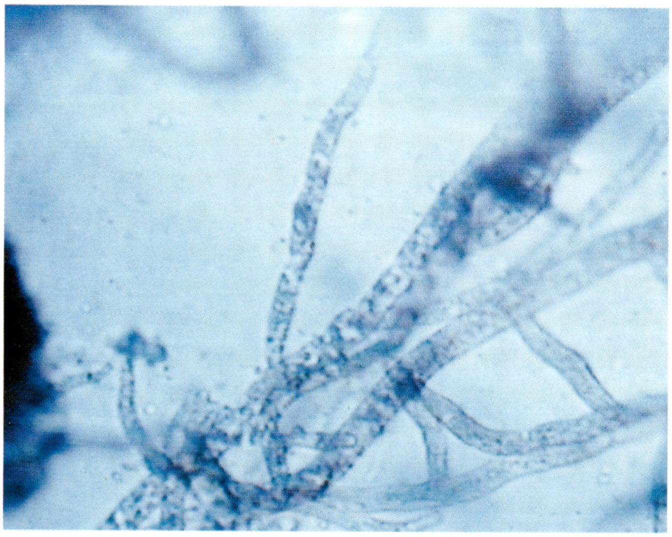

Photo 32: Fungal branches, magnified 400 times.

There is no routine effective flock medical treatment for fungi! If fungi are identified in the droppings, it is a matter of determining the source and preventing further exposure. If contaminated seed is the problem, swallowed fungal spores rarely grow in the bowel and damage caused by possible concurrent toxin exposure heals once exposure ceases. If spores are inhaled, these can germinate in the airsacs but there is no water-soluble drug that is absorbed from the bowel to act on fungal respiratory infections that is practicable to treat large numbers of birds. There are some drugs, however, e.g. ketoconazole, available to treat smaller numbers of birds. If fungi are identified in the droppings, management focuses on identifying and eliminating their possible source, i.e. the seed or environment, and therefore avoiding further exposure.

Bacteria

Bacteria are extremely small, and it is not possible to see them when magnified 100 times. It is only when the x40 lens is swung into position, so that the contents of the microscope slide are magnified 400 times, that they become visible. Even at this magnification, they are still much smaller than anything described earlier, most being only one-hundredth the size of a yeast ('thrush' organism). Bacteria can be seen in the samples obtained from both a crop flush and a faecal smear. Interpretation of their appearance in a crop flush has been discussed. Preparation of a wet smear for bacterial examination is the same as that discussed earlier.

The interpretation and identification of any bacteria seen on a faecal smear is the most difficult of all things attempted by a fancier with his microscope. Some fanciers may choose not to use their microscope for bacterial identification but rather leave it to the experts. This is quite reasonable for, as mentioned earlier, the ability to recognize Coccidia, worm eggs and, in particular, trichomonads (canker organisms) would justify a fancier having his own microscope. Indeed, the identification of bacteria in a faecal smear at times can be difficult for even the experts.

All animals and birds have a resident population of bacteria in the bowel, which is not only normal but, in fact, essential for health. These bacteria aid in protecting the bowel from disease and are necessary for normal digestion to occur. The microscope user must be able to recognize what is normal and what is abnormal, but at the same time recognize the limitations of trying to identify bacteria purely from a faecal smear.

What information about bacteria cannot be obtained from a faecal smear

Bacteria are identified by their appearance, their ability to take up certain stains and also their growth characteristics when cultured on media in the laboratory. On the faecal smear, all we can see is their appearance, i.e. size, shape and motility of the bacteria. This, although helpful, is not sufficient information to definitively type the bacteria. An analogy might be that a sheep and pig, when recognized with this criteria, being about the same size and shape and moving in the same way, would be classified as the same animal when obviously they are different. It is therefore not possible, just by looking at bacteria on a faecal smear, to tell what type they are with certainty. To type them for sure requires the additional laboratory tests of staining and culture.

Similarly, it is not possible to accurately estimate their numbers. To accurately estimate numbers requires a number of special calibration techniques, e.g. the use of a calibration chamber in the laboratory. Bacteria on a faecal smear can appear in large numbers but, by pushing and rotating the cover slip, the dropping film becomes thinner and the bacteria more dispersed, giving the impression that the bacteria are in lower numbers.

What information about bacteria can be obtained from a faecal smear

The most important thing that a fancier at home with his microscope examining his birds' droppings for bacteria can assess is bacterial ratios. It is often not necessary to know the actual type of bacteria present. In the healthy bowel, no single bacterial type dominates. There are a range of bacterial forms. Most bacteria occur in two basic types, dots (cocci) and rods (bacilli). The dots and rods vary in size and motility depending on the actual type of bacteria involved. In the healthy pigeon's dropping, most bacteria are different types of dot-shaped bacteria that vary in size. There will also, however, be some rods and these will also vary in their size and motility. In health, therefore, there is a mixture of these bacterial types, the normal pattern of which can be recognized by the regular examination of healthy birds' droppings microscopically. The fancier is alerted to a problem when there is a divergence from this normal pattern. With infection, a particular bacterial type increases in number. Similarly with stress, certain types of bacteria will die off. Both processes lead to one type of bacteria increasing in number and starting to dominate the faecal film.

The bacterial type that is most likely to increase in number as a result of stress is *E. coli*. *E. coli* is a mid-size, motile rod and it is the only bacterium with this appearance occurring commonly in the droppings of a pigeon. There are, however, other bacteria that do look like this (e.g. *Pseudomonas, Klebsiella, Citrobacter, Enterobacter*) but an increase in the proportion of mid-size motile rods visible alerts us to the possibility of an *E. coli* problem.

Most of the small dots seen are part of the normal bacterial population of the bowel and are called enterococci (which literally means dot-shaped bacteria living in the bowel). There are, however, a variety of others, e.g. *Streptococcus* and *Staphylococcus*.

Usually in the healthy dropping, one will also see rods that are about twice the size of *E. coli*. Many of these are bacteria called *Lactobacillus* and they are also part of the normal bacterial population of the bowel. In fact, these are often the first ones to disappear as a result of stress and so it is always good to see some of these present. Some fanciers say to me they can see large numbers of mid-sized motile rods, which can often be assumed to be *E. coli* and say that they are very active, referring to how much they move. There is, however, no correlation between motility and the potential to cause disease. We must always get back to the ratios. A low number of rods, even if they are motile, is likely to be normal.

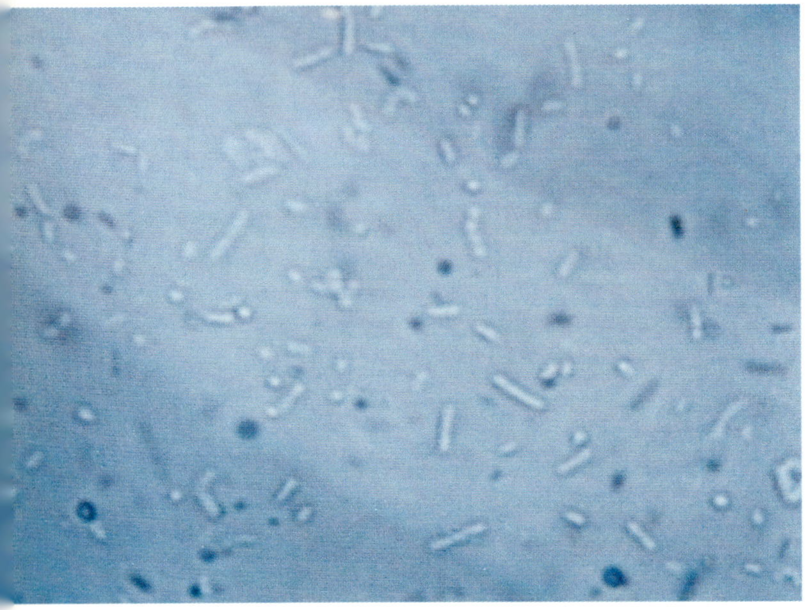

Photo 33:
A mixture of dot (cocci) and rod (bacilli) bacteria, magnified 400 times.

A very important factor to consider when assessing the appearance of the droppings under the microscope is the appearance of the droppings on the perch. Don't create a problem when one isn't there. When the birds look well and the droppings are brown and tight, the bacterial population seen must be normal. A fancier here may see droppings containing a number of different types of rod bacteria, each about the same size, and may assume that these are all the same type, in particular *E. coli,* and feel that he has a problem when, in fact, he doesn't. If the droppings become green and watery, this immediately alerts the fancier to a possible bacterial problem within the bowel. If microscopic examination reveals a divergence from the bacterial pattern that he normally sees in his birds' droppings, in particular, if there is one type of bacteria that now predominates, it is likely that there is, in fact, a problem. Do remember, however, that all green droppings are not necessarily a bacterial bowel problem. Droppings will become green with decreased food intake, wet canker, some forms of respiratory infection and the ingestion of foods containing the green plant pigment called chlorophyll, e.g. dun peas, silver beet and grass. This is one of the big advantages that the fancier with a microscope has in that, if his birds' droppings become green, he can immediately get some of these green droppings and examine them to see if a bacterial bowel problem is a possibility or not.

If either the droppings themselves look different or their microscopic appearance changes in a way that suggests a problem, probiotics are fast becoming the drug of choice because of their 'no harm' effect. The quicker the fancier can normalize any bacterial disruption by flooding the bowel with the normal beneficial bacteria found in probiotic preparations, the quicker health is re-established. Antibiotics are best reserved for use following the additional diagnostic steps of staining and culture to confirm that the loft does have a problem with a particular bacterial type.

Remember that it is not possible to control *E. coli* with antibiotics. *E. coli* at a low level is part of the normal bacterial population and therefore will quickly re-establish once antibiotics are withdrawn. An imbalance in the levels of the various bacterial types found in the bowel during racing usually occurs as a result of stress. This allows opportunistic bacteria, such as *E. coli* and others, to increase in number and dominate the microscope field. Usually the best approach to handling this problem is rest, time, probiotic use and identification and correction of the underlying stress. If despite these measures the droppings are persistently green and watery or it appears that one particular bacterial type is still predominating or the birds are unwell, it is time to see a veterinarian. Special stains and culturing will show whether there is a problem or not by identifying specifically the bacteria present. Once the laboratory can put a name to the bacteria, we then know whether it is capable of causing a problem, which is the best antibiotic to use, the biology of the organism and with this its likely origin, e.g. one bacterial type, *Citrobacter,* is often associated with contaminated water, all of which helps in the overall control of a problem in the loft.

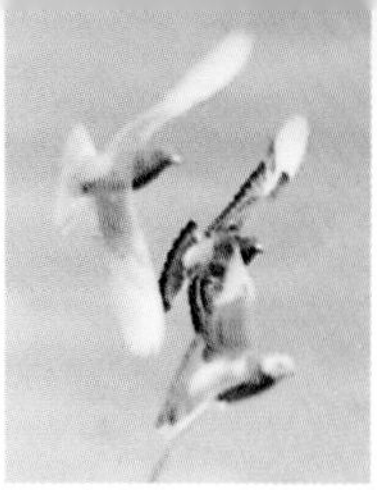

Chapter 45

PIGEON QUERIES, A – Z

Air under skin – Indicates a ruptured airsac. Like ourselves, birds inhale air through a windpipe into a set of lungs. In addition, birds have a number of sacs that lead from the lungs. If one of these ruptures, air will percolate through this tear and accumulate under the skin. The tear is usually a result of injury, often hitting something hard during flight, but can occur secondary to respiratory airsac infection. Air is removed from under the skin with a hypodermic syringe and needle twice daily and the bird confined and sometimes placed on antibiotics until healing occurs (usually 3 – 10 days).

Appetite

Decreased – Usually idicates poor health, although the food intake of teams as they come into form may marginally decrease.

Increased – Can indicate good health, however, food intake will increase with parasitic disease, in particular wet canker.

Beak

Soft base – Seen in youngsters at weaning with calcium or vitamin D deficiency.

Pale base – A genetic characteristic, normal in many families, e.g. slatey Janssens.

Yellow nodule in or on beak – Mucosal pox. If an imaginary line is drawn through the base of the beak, any 'canker-like' lesions in front of this are likely to be pox because this area is just too exposed for the fragile trichomonad organism to survive.

Slightly open when bird held – Associated with conditions that interfere with full distension of airsacs, e.g. egg laying, fat and respiratory infection. Distress in a bird when its beak is held closed can indicate sinusitis associated with respiratory infection.

Cere

Chalky – The way it should be in health.

Discoloured – With the pigeon equivalent of a runny nose, nasal material will stain the cere a green-brown colour. Often associated with respiratory infection.

Pink – Seen particularly in young hens following billing and in birds exercised in rain.

Swollen at base – Sinusitis associated with respiratory infection or extension of trichomonad nodule into sinus.

Feather loss at base of cere – A sign seen in certain race birds towards the end of the season, indicating chronic fatigue, overtraining or poor health management.

'Cocky comb' – Refers to the way the feathers immediately behind the cere stand upright. Will occur in healthy birds when they are cold, tired or hungry, but also occurs in birds that are sick for any reason.

Delayed crop emptying – Occurs with either primary disease of the crop, in particular wet canker, but also when the birds are run down for any reason (postrace fatigue, systemic disease).

Droppings

Abnormal colour

Green – Caused by some dietary components (silver beet, dun peas, etc.), inadequate food intake (due to time away from the loft or disease), diseases that irritate the bowel wall, liver infection.

Red/brown – Caused by dietary components, e.g. some grits, milo.

Pale – Indicates internal disease, e.g. liver and pancreas.

Volume

Increased – Indicates malabsorption, maldigestion problems associated with bowel, pancreas or liver disease; sometimes normal, e.g. hens about to lay, pairs bred in small individual runs.

Decreased – Caused by decreased food intake, either due to time away from the loft or disease. In birds that are approaching true form, droppings will often become a bit smaller, tight and nut-like.

Fluid content

Increased – May be associated with the bowel and be true diarrhoea or alternatively associated with the kidney and be urine. Urine will be more visible if the bowel content of the dropping is decreased, e.g. recent return from a race or due for feeding. Such droppings will quickly become normal with a meal. Increased urine will be produced with conditions that make the birds thirsty, e.g. supplements that contain salt, medications that contain excessive sugar, kidney disease, wet canker and respiratory infection.

Decreased – Dehydration.

Mould on droppings – Occurs either in humid conditions when non-removed damp droppings provide a base for fungal spores, which are everywhere in the air, to land and germinate. More likely to appear quickly when the dropping contains a lot of fungal spores when passed, as occurs when the birds are fed seed contaminated with fungal spores or alternatively inhale high levels of fungal spores (e.g. from contaminated straw or an accumulation of mouldy droppings under a grid floor).

Mushy droppings in morning – Indicate a restless night's sleep. Seen with mites, mice, noise around the loft, etc., or with an unhealthy loft environment that is not conducive to sleep (high humidity, cold and windy).

Droppings on tail – With decreased bloom production, feathers can become soiled more readily and droppings are more likely to stick to them.

Eye

'Glass' – Used to describe the eye of a very fit bird. The eye appears wet, translucent and has a brilliantly clear iris.

Watery – Occurs in only one of two situations, either when something irritates the eye, causing more tears to be produced (e.g. respiratory infection, foreign body, injury, eyelid lesion) or when the tear duct is obstructed, preventing tear drainage from the eye through the duct into the roof of the mouth (e.g. respiratory infection, mouth lesion, scarring left from an injury or earlier infection).

Pale –

One eye – Birds with a pale iris are said to have a uveitis, which is an inflammation of the iris and its support structures. This can result from a blow to the eye, which bruises the iris within the eyeball, or from a blood-borne disease that is capable of inflaming the iris, such as respiratory infection due to *Chlamydia* or pigeon pox.

Two eyes – Usually associated with severe internal disease, leading to anaemia or a drop in peripheral blood pressure.

Cluster – A term to describe a persistent pupillary membrane. The embryo has no pupil. As development proceeds, the centre of the iris disintegrates, forming a hole, which is called the pupil. If this fails to happen correctly, residual persistent strands of membrane are left behind, leading to interference with vision. Sometimes associated with other eye deformities. Some fanciers claim it is associated with enhanced breeding potential but this is unlikely.

Pupil – The pupil of the healthy bird should constrict quickly when exposed to light. A slow constriction indicates fatigue, ill health or primary disease of the eye.

Eyelid

Lump on eyelid – Pox lesion, U.V.-induced tumour, particularly in pieds and reds, accumulated inflammatory tissue due to repeated rubbing (this is often associated with older birds with poorly fitting or overdeveloped eyelids), poorly healed eyelid injury, Goblet cell cyst (Goblet cells within the eyelid produce a mucus that enables the bird's tears to adhere to the eyeball, keeping the bird's eye surface wet even in windy conditions and when flying at speed).

Prominent third eyelid – Pigeons have a third eyelid covered by a membrane called the conjunctiva. With respiratory infection or other irritation, the conjunctiva swells, making it difficult for the third eyelid to be withdrawn behind the two main lids. Can take several weeks to resolve, even after successful treatment. Some fanciers report that the third eyelid quivers in certain birds when they are very fit.

Sluggish blink – Seen with fatigue and dehydration, particularly in recently weaned youngsters.

Feathers

Dry – Associated with poor health. All feathers on the body except down feathers are moulted once per year. Down feathers, which occur mainly over the side of the bird's body and tops of the thighs, are lost whenever the birds are well. Disintegrating down feathers form part of the bird's bloom, which lubricates and softens the feather. When birds fail to produce bloom, the feathering becomes dry and harsh.

Fret – A defect across the quill and sometimes also the vane of the feather, indicating that there has been interference with nutrient supply to the feather follicle at this stage of feather growth. Associated with inadequate nutrition, exertion, drugs, e.g. some antibiotics and wormers, and in nestlings, chilling.

Grizzling – Describes white and red pigments being visible in the vane of the feather in birds not this colour. May be genetic but may be associated with medication or other factors interfering with nutrient delivery to the feather follicle during feather growth.

Wing coverts pinched up – Usually genetic.

Persistent feather sheaths – Usually indicate that something is 'not quite right' with the birds' management, in particular associated with Circo virus infection; however, may in some birds be heritable.

Pin holes – A row of lines in the vane of the feather due to feather flies inserting their probosci in the growing feather follicle to drink blood.

Bald area – Patchy bald areas over the entire body are usually due to mite infections. A patchy bald area in the centre of the chest, although sometimes due to mites, is most commonly caused by repeated rubbing, e.g. on the edge of a hopper. Was at one time thought to be associated with fungal infections.

White lines on flight feathers – Marks made by bloom on the feathers during flight, called friction rubs, and often seen in a fit bird.

Fluffed up – An attempt by the bird to trap a layer of warm air around its body. More likely to occur when the bird is fatigued, sick or hungry.

Frayed end – Due to damage to developing feather follicle. Seen in particular in the end flights of youngsters that are forced to fly when the feather is emerging from the tip of the follicle.

Failure to moult particular feather – Associated with injury or infection of the feather follicle, which damages it. If this feather is pulled, the new feather may also be deformed due to this damage.

Flight

Wobbly – Birds that can still fly but in an asymmetric way usually have a minor wing injury, often associated with damage to the ptagial ligament. This ligament runs along the leading edge of the wing web and is stretched or torn when the extended wing is physically forced back against the side of the bird, e.g. when a bird at speed hits a wire or branch. Also seen in birds with the joint form of paratyphoid.

Forceful and fast – A sign of health.

Floating and slow – The way tired or unwell birds fly when forced.

Gulping – Often associated with the penguin posture. May indicate that the bird has a sore throat and is often associated with wet canker. Also seen when large-diameter seeds, such as corn or peanuts, or abrasive seeds, such as barley, are fed.

Handling

Leady – A heaviness to the bird when handled. Often the result of an unwell bird flying less and eating more when compared with other members of the team. Often associated with wet canker.

Buoyant – Power without weight. A bird whose pectoral muscle bulk is full but actually is quite light in the hand. Associated with race fitness; some strains are easier to make buoyant than others.

Keel

Condition spot – A red spot or short line that appears on the keel. Not necessarily associated with fitness but does indicate that the birds are healthy and stress-free.

White – Health.

Pink – Often associated with myositis (muscle inflammation) due to overwork.

Bent – Can have a genetic basis but also associated with calcium or vitamin D deficiency during growth or inappropriate nesting material.

Leg

Splay – Nestling deformity in which one or both legs develop abnormally so that the bird is unable to bring them under its body and support its weight. Can have a genetic and nutritional basis but is usually associated with failure to provide adequate support within the nest bowl for the developing youngster.

Flaky skin – Can indicate infection with the scaly mite *Cnemidocoptes*.

Horny growths on toes – Usually age-related.

Warm and clean – The way a race bird's feet are when fit, even in wet or cold conditions.

Yellow swelling on ball of foot – Foot abscess, usually associated with staphylococci infection and more likely to occur with hard or irregular flooring.

White nodules under skin – 'Gout', accumulation of uric acid under the skin, which may be associated with high-protein diets, kidney disease or spontaneously in the well bird, particularly with age.

Lumps

At cloaca – A firm mass under the skin at the cloaca in prepubertal birds is an infection in the Bursa of Fabricius (an area of tonsil-like tissues in the floor of the cloaca), usually due to canker. A pink fleshy mass here will be a cloacal prolapse, in which the cloaca everts due to repeated straining associated with diarrhoea or egg binding.

At navel – A red/yellow firm swelling here indicates a navel infection, often associated with canker.

Under the skin of the throat – Mobile firm masses of various sizes here are usually canker nodules.

In the skin over the abdomen – Masses here are usually benign fat-based tumours called fibrolipomas. These are straightforward to remove surgically but this should be done as soon as they are noticed and still small so as to avoid a bigger operation later on. Navel hernias can also occur, particularly in older hens, where the muscles in the abdominal walls tear, allowing abdominal contents to move through this tear under the skin.

In the 'small of the back' – May be an infection, cyst or tumour of the preen gland.

At the wing butt – Another common site for fibrolipomas to occur.

Swellings in the joint – Either on the wing or leg. Can occur with bacterial infection, in particular with *Salmonella* species (paratyphoid).

Muscles – Pectoral (flight)

Colour

Pink – Healthy.

Blue – Occurs in three situations: 1. Birds that have difficulty breathing or oxygenating their blood, which with exertion due to its low oxygen content becomes a bluish colour. This colour is reflected in the muscles, which remain bluish for a short time after exertion before becoming pink as the birds catch their breath. 2. Birds that are exercised beyond their fitness capability develop myositis (muscle inflammation) or cramping, which also turns the muscles a bluish colour. This discolouration is persistent until the muscles have healed, which may take several days. 3. Associated with poor health or management practices, which inhibit the development of fitness. (Refer to Blue Muscle Syndrome in the chapter Exercise, Diet and Electrolytes)

Soft – Lack of fitness.

Hard – Associated with myositis and cramping. Occurs if birds are exercised beyond their current fitness. Accumulated lactic acid and other muscle metabolites lead to a localized chemical 'burn', which makes the muscles inflamed, swollen and hard. A trap for beginners, with such birds feeling superfit. These birds should not be forced to fly until the muscles have once again become normally toned, at which point they can gradually be reintroduced to work. In birds with myositis, the muscles become painful and so they often resent handling and wriggle during palpation of their muscles.

Pliable – In the fit bird, the flight muscles (pectoral) are pain-free, toned and resilient without being either hard or soft.

Flaky skin over the pectoral muscles – As the muscles increase in size due to fitness, the skin breaks into large segments and superficial pieces may break away. A good sign if the muscles are also pink and toned.

Small – Reduced muscle size occurs with decreased calorie intake associated either with time away from the loft or disease. As overweight birds come into race fitness, their muscles will also decrease in size. It is important to remember that not all birds when fit will handle the same and that certain birds, and indeed strains, will handle 'thinner' when fit than others.

Panting – Birds with respiratory infection are more likely to pant but it is more a sign of decreased exercise tolerance. It is more likely to be seen when the weather is hot, when birds are fat, when they are unfit, when birds have been forced to fly hard for a short period of time, such as to avoid a falcon attack, during certain stages of the moult, during infections that sap energy, e.g. parasites, and conditions that prevent full distension of the airsacs, e.g. ovulation in hens.

Poor race results – If one race only, review management, feeding, training and preventive health measures over the previous week. If longer term, review loft environment, bird genetics, motivation systems and overall management; seek advice from successful fanciers and pigeon veterinarians.

Posture

Penguin – Where the pigeon leans back on its tail, arching its head backwards. Associated with low crop or proventricular (first stomach compartment) pain, an attempt by the bird to get comfortable; often associated with wet canker.

Horizontal – Where the bird's back is parallel to the ground. Usually due to abdominal pain. Often associated with other signs, such as feathers over the abdomen fluffed out. Seen in conditions such as *E. coli* and worms.

Race losses

Minor – Think of fitness, grain or grit problems or minor resident diseases, e.g. *E. coli* or thrush.

Major – Think of serious diseases. Compare percentage of late and non-arrivals with other (honest) fanciers.

Reluctance to fly – Fit healthy birds should explode from the loft for exercise. Reluctance to fly indicates a problem with the loft environment or management or alternatively disease or fatigue.

Slot – Refers to the birds' choana or longitudinal opening in the roof of the mouth. May be open or closed in individual birds. However, edge of slot can become red and swollen in respiratory infection, so a decrease in its opening in an individual bird can be an indication of this problem.

Slow to leave tossing point – May indicate inexperience or alternatively overtraining or a health problem. Birds are usually slower to leave both training and race points in adverse weather conditions.

Smells in loft

'Chook' – A fowl smell coming from the droppings, which is often associated with *E. coli* or yeast infection.

Health – When the birds are in form, some fanciers describe an odour that appears in the loft as clean and sweet.

Wet – Birds that are either wet or have worked hard on a hot day release characteristic odours.

Sneezing – Indicates nasal or sinus irritation. May be due to respiratory infection, airsac mites, dust or irritant fumes. Often seen in conjunction with other behaviour such as scratching at the nose and wiping the nose on the wing butt.

Swollen abdomen

Fluid – The abdomen will distend with fluid with inflammatory conditions within the abdomen, liver disease, cancer and heart disease.

Mass – Solid masses in the abdomen can enlarge it, e.g. tumours, normal eggs or retained soft-shelled eggs.

Fat – Some birds retain a lot of fat in the abdomen, particularly out-of-breeding-season stock hens fed either too much food or a mix that has too high a calorie content. Barley has a real use here.

Tail trembling – Fit birds often display this characteristic.

Throat

Pale pink – Health.

Red – Indicates dehydration or inflammation, usually associated with wet canker or respiratory infection.

Grey – Indicates longer-term health problem, e.g. unmanaged wet canker or more serious internal disease.

Mucus in throat – May be normal. Pigeons quite normally have up to 1.5 ml of mucus in their throat. Mucus levels increase with inflammatory throat conditions. Clear mucus is less likely to be associated with a problem than white or coloured mucus. More mucus is visible in the throat after feeding or exercise.

Yellow spots in soft palate – Usually microscopic pockets of inflammation (microabscesses) that appear with active disease, often associated with wet canker or respiratory infection, can take weeks or months to disappear after successful treatment. Also associated with vitamin A deficiency and inflammation of the salivary ducts.

Yellow spots on floor of windpipe – Microscopic pockets of inflammation in tonsil tissue, which appear during active respiratory infection, are sometimes the only outward sign of *Chlamydia* or wet canker in nestlings or recently weaned youngsters. Can take weeks to disappear after successful treatment.

Large yellow nodule – Trichomonad nodule, 'dry canker'.

Tongue

Pale tip – A pale pink tip is seen in the healthy bird. A white tip may mean slight anaemia or low blood pressure with disease.

Blue or black tip – Sometimes seen with severe respiratory infection, however, some birds do have pigmented tongue tips and are therefore always like this.

Tongue tip missing – Earlier injury or pigeon pox infection.

Position – In health, the tongue should lie flat on the floor of the mouth. As the windpipe opening becomes round, the tongue tip elevates and so this may be associated with difficulty breathing.

Vomiting – Associated with either irritation to the lining of the crop or stomach (seen with wet canker, some forms of respiratory infection, bacterial or fungal infections of the crop wall and following ingestion of toxic or irritant substances) or alternatively severe internal disease.

Windpipe

Opening elongated and still – The way it should be in health.

Opening round – Making the windpipe round enhances air movement, increasing ease of breathing. A round windpipe is therefore associated with shortness of breath. This may be due to fatness or masses in the abdominal cavity, which prevent distension of the airsacs (e.g. an egg or tumour) or alternatively respiratory infection.

Wing

Dropped – Indicates severe injury, usually a fracture.

'Kicked up' – Also indicates major injury (fracture or dislocation) but involving either the shoulder or top of the first wing bone (humerus).

Tips folded out – 'Angel wing' deformity in nestlings. (Refer to Angel Wing section in chapter Problems of the Breeding Season).

Yawning – Seen in birds attempting to relieve throat or sinus irritation; may be associated with wet canker or respiratory infection, including airsac mite infection. Sometimes seen after feeding small seeds, in particular linseed, which can become stuck in the throat.

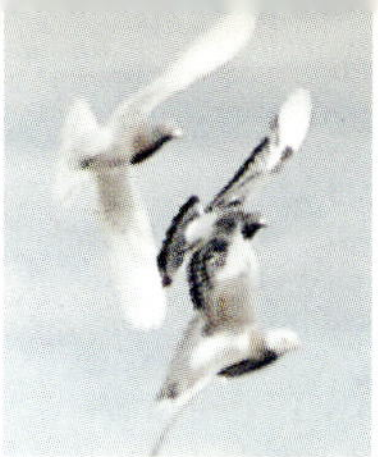

Chapter 46

MEDICATION GUIDE

In this chapter, I will discuss various medications and supplements used in pigeons. They are not discussed with the veterinarian in mind but rather the pigeon fancier. Instead of providing an exhaustive list of medications and go into a lot of medical detail, I aim to provide practical, usable information for the fancier. I have listed the current medications under the names that are most likely to be encountered by the fancier and have indicated which medications are considered to be most suitable for each condition.

Amprolium – Used to treat Coccidia. Has the disadvantage that treatment needs to be continued for 5 days to be effective.

Aureomycin – Brand name of chlortetracycline. See Chlortetracycline.

Avermectins – Group of medications used in the treatment of roundworms, hairworms and mites. See Ivermec, Ivomec, Moxidectin.

Baycox – Current drug of choice to treat coccidiosis in pigeons. The dose is 1 ml to 2 litres of water and the usual treatment time is 48 hours. It is poorly absorbed from the bowel, making it ideal for use during both racing and breeding. Other medications, once swallowed, are absorbed into the system before passing back into the bowel and treating the Coccidia. Coccidia live in the wall of the bowel and Baycox effectively flushes through, in the process clearing the Coccidia. Because of this unique mode of action, it cannot affect race form. Baycox does not affect the immune system, which means it is safe to use in birds of any age, including youngsters, and because it does not accumulate in the system, it can be used repeatedly. It does not affect the moult and can safely be used during breeding. During the race season, it is best given early in the week so that the birds' health has an opportunity to lift following clearing of any Coccidia present, before basketing. It is safe to use in a routine preventive race program, with the recommendation being that it is given for 2 days every 4 weeks.

Baytril – Common brand name of enrofloxacin. Available in a variety of forms including a clear water-soluble liquid. It can be added to the drinking water at the rate of 1 ml to 1 litre of water for flock treatment and can also be used to treat individual birds at the dose of 3 drops twice daily. It is very useful in several situations, including treating individual birds with respiratory infection, e.g. a youngster with one-eye cold. Here, response to treatment is very rapid with often only one or two doses being required. It can also be used to treat respiratory infection in a team during racing. However, regular use in such a situation should be discouraged as, being broad spectrum, it also kills many of the normal bacteria of the bowel and there can be a transient loss of form until these are re-established. If used during racing for more than 3 days, the birds are predisposed to a secondary thrush (*Candida* infection), leading to green droppings through loss of normal bowel bacteria. It is useful to treat individual unwell birds where the exact cause is as yet unknown but an infection is suspected, and as stated earlier it is the treatment of choice in an outbreak of paratyphoid (*Salmonella* infection). Its use during breeding should be avoided as it has been associated with embryonic death and abnormalities of cartilage deposition in joints of chicks. However, these are dose-dependent side effects. See Enrofloxacin.

Calcium – Mineral that is essential for health and, in fact, normal breeding cannot occur unless this is supplied at adequate levels. Available in the form of grits, pink minerals, pick stones, water-soluble liquids and a variety of commercially available supplements. It is the job of the fancier to ensure that sufficient of these are made available to the birds.

Carnidazole – Anticanker medication, with a wide safety margin. Safe to use during racing, breeding and moulting. Available only in tablet form under the brand name Spartrix. See Spartrix.

Chloramine – Effective non-toxic general disinfectant suitable for use in lofts and also to clean hoppers and drinkers. Odourless and non-staining. Available under a number of brand names, including Halamid, Halasept.

Chlorhexidine – An effective non-toxic general disinfectant suitable for use in lofts and also to clean hoppers and drinkers. Odourless but can stain slightly pink. Available under a number of brand names, which vary in strength, including Chlorhex, Aviclens.

Chlortetracycline – A tetracycline antibiotic in the same group as doxycycline. Replaced therapeutically by the newer doxycycline, which has advantages in treatment.

Ciprofloxacin – A fluoroquinolone antibiotic. See Enrofloxacin.

Dimetradazole – Anticanker medication. Available as a water-soluble powder called Emtryl. The drug has a narrow safety margin, with overdose leading to a reversible loss of balance and coordination and, with on-going intake, death. Can interfere with sperm production in cocks, leading to a temporary infertility, and so is not recommended for use during breeding. Lower dose rate is used during hot weather and in stock birds feeding youngsters due to an anticipated greater water intake. See Emtryl.

Doxycycline – An antibiotic. World-wide veterinary therapeutic agent of choice for the treatment of *Chlamydia*, a principal cause of respiratory infection. Available under a wide variety of brand names as tablets and water-soluble powders. One of a group of antibiotics called tetracyclines including oxytetracycline (common brand name Terramycin) and chlortetracycline (common brand name Tricon). Doxycycline has several advantages: greater activity, providing effective blood levels for up to 20 hours after a single dose compared to 4 hours for older tetracyclines; causes less disruption to the normal bowel bacteria; has less detrimental effect on the immune system; and is less affected by calcium and other minerals. The effectiveness of all tetracyclines is decreased by calcium and other minerals such as iron, magnesium and zinc. A lower dose rate can therefore be used if grit, sand and other sources of minerals are removed during use. The oral dose with grit available is 75 mg per day, while the oral dose with mineral sources, including grit, removed is 12 mg per day. Not only has activity against *Chlamydia* but also *Mycoplasma* and a range of bacteria. As with Ronidazole, water-soluble preparations contain the active constituent at various strengths. The more concentrated the preparation, the shorter is the treatment time. However, the drug is bitter and once concentrations of over 10 – 12% are offered, palatability problems are encountered. A common preparation used during racing is doxycycline 12%, where the dose is 1/2 teaspoon to 1 litre of water. During racing, treatment time is based on the severity of the problem but is usually 2 – 5 days. The drug can be used at all times of the pigeon year but is best given under veterinary supervision. Doxycycline is commonly combined with other antimicrobials, in particular tylosin and spiramycin. In areas with hard water, medicated water will become brown/pink. This can also happen with exposure to sunlight and indicates that the drug has lost its effectiveness. Common tablet brand name is Vibravet 50 mg; dose is 1/2 tablet once a day.

Doxy -T – Brand name of antibiotic preparation containing doxycycline and tylosin. Used to treat respiratory infection. Dose is 1/2 teaspoon per litre of water; usual treatment time 2 – 5 days. See Doxycycline, Tylan, Tylosin.

Droncit – Tablet containing praziquantel, used to treat tapeworm. See Praziquantel.

Dynamutilin – Brand name of tiamulin, an antibiotic effective against *Mycoplasma*. See Tiamulin.

Echinacea – Available as a solution (a derivative of *Augustifolia purpurea*) for oral use. Used as an immunostimulant. Useful supplement in the postweaning time and in birds recovering from disease.

Electrolytes – Salts that occur naturally in the body and are lost from the system during exertion. Used as a water additive for birds returning from long races, particularly on hot days, with the aim of speeding recovery. Also of benefit following extended periods of diarrhoea. Wide variety of brand names available. Manufacturing dosage instructions must be followed as, if used in too strong a concentration, can cause dehydration.

Emtryl – Brand name of dimetradazole. Used to treat canker. Available as a water-soluble powder. Dose is 3 g (approximately 1 level teaspoon) to 4.5 – 7 litres, based on anticipated water intake. See Dimetradazole.

Enrofloxacin – A fluoroquinolone antibiotic. Fluoroquinolones have a broad spectrum of activity, being effective against *Chlamydia* and *Mycoplasma* (associated with respiratory infection), *E. coli* (involved with bowel infection) and *Salmonella*. They are the antibiotic of choice to treat *Salmonella*. The usual brand name is Baytril 2.5%. See Baytril.

Flagyl – Brand name of metronidazole, used to treat canker. Available as a 200-mg tablet, dose 1/4 of a tablet per bird once daily, and as a water-soluble syrup, which has a strength of 200 mg/ml. The dose is 5 – 10 ml per litre of water. This syrup has a high sugar content and is rather unpalatable to the birds. See Metronidazole.

Furacin – Brand name of nitrofurazone. See Nitrofurazone.

Furazolidone – An antibacterial drug. An older drug used at one time to treat coccidiosis and some bacterial bowel infections such as those caused by *Salmonella*. Its use has been associated with deaths in young birds.

Garlic – Derivative of *Allium sativum*. Widely used pigeon supplement. Much anecdotal and some scientific evidence of benefit. Contains an immunostimulant, allicin, which may be of use, particularly in the postweaning time and in birds recovering from disease. Often combined with a variety of oils, which are then added to the birds' seed, thereby concurrently providing birds with a nutrient source. The juice can be placed in the drinking water. However, the cloves should not be used in water as they quickly become covered in a biofilm.

Gonadotrophin – Group of hormones that act on the testicles and ovary. Used to stimulate follicle formation and ovulation in hens and sperm production in cocks. Usually given as weekly injections for 2 – 4 weeks. See Hormones.

Hormones – Natural regulators of bodily processes that are now available synthetically. The only hormones used with any frequency in pigeons are the sex hormones, or gonadotrophins. See Gonadotrophin.

Hydrochloric Acid – Can be used as a bowel acidifier with extreme care, as an aid in the prevention or treatment of *E. coli* infection. A 1 molar per litre solution is mixed at the rate of 60 ml per litre of drinking water.

ID Yeast – Common brand name of yeast feed supplement. See Yeasts.

Iodine – Component of many essential amino acids for birds, some of which are incorporated in the proteins that make feathers. Due to the loss of all feathers annually and other metabolic needs, birds have higher requirements for iodine than mammals. In the past, fanciers have added iodine to the water of their birds. However, such practices are not without their risk as excessive supplementation can be harmful. Iodine is best provided as a component of a balanced supplement that not only supplies iodine but other essential nutrients. It is found at adequate levels in the better brands of pink minerals and pick stones.

Ivermec – One of a group of drugs called avermectins. Available under a wide number of brand names of various strengths, the most readily available being Ivomec. Used in a similar way to Moxidectin. See Moxidectin.

Ivomec – A brand name of ivermec. See Ivermec.

Ketoconazole – An antimicrobial used to treat thrush and fungal infections. One of the few fungal drugs that is absorbed from the bowel and can therefore be used to treat fungal airsac infections.

Levamisole – Wormer, used to treat roundworm and hairworm. At one time popular but has now been supplanted by the avermectins, its main disadvantage being that food needed to be removed for 12 – 24 hours before use and for approximately 6 hours after use, making the drug hard to use during both racing and breeding. If the birds are fed during use, they almost invariably vomit and many still vomit despite removal of food. Available in both tablet and water-soluble liquid form under a wide variety of brand names, including Avitrol tablets, Spartakon tablets, Vital tablets and Nilverm liquid.

Lincomycin – An antibiotic sometimes combined with spectinomycin. May be effective in treating respiratory infections caused by *Mycoplasma*.

Maldison – An organophosphate that is the active constituent in many insecticidal preparations, such as Malawash and Malaban. Its use is definitely not recommended in pigeons as even slightly elevated absorption can cause death. The drug is absorbed through the skin after spraying or dipping as long as the skin is wet. When used on warm days, when the birds quickly dry, results may be satisfactory. However, when used on cold days or at even slightly elevated doses, fatal levels can be reached. In case of overdose, seek immediate veterinary assistance as injectable antidotes are available.

Metronidazole – Anticanker medication. Wide safety margin, safe to use during breeding, moulting and racing. Available as a tablet and water-soluble syrup under the brand name Flagyl. See Flagyl.

Moxidectin – One of a group of drugs called avermectins. Currently the world-wide veterinary medication of choice to treat roundworm and hairworm in pigeons. Wide safety margin. Safe to use during breeding, racing and moulting. Also kills any external parasite that feeds off body fluid and therefore kills all mites, including airsac mite. Limited activity against lice as these primarily feed off feather debris and skin dander. A clear water-soluble palatable liquid that is available in a variety of strengths. Usual strength available is 2 mg/ml and the dose rate is 5 ml to 1 litre of water. Usual treatment time is 24 hours. However, if the weather is cool and the birds' water intake is down, the drug is safe enough to use for 48 hours. The drug is well tolerated, with the birds showing no sign of nausea. They can be loft-flown, exercised and fed normally during treatment.

Nitrofurazone – Antimicrobial that has action against *E. coli*, *Salmonella* and Coccidia. An older drug no longer recommended. Common brand name is Furacin. Not as effective as more recent medications such as Baytril and Baycox. Overdose may cause nervous signs or death.

Nystatin – Antimicrobial that is used to treat thrush and fungal infections. Nystatin must come in contact with these organisms to be effective and as it is not absorbed from the digestive tract, can only treat infections here.

Oils **–** Seed oils are useful grain additives as they provide the unsaturated fatty acids necessary for a lustrous moult, increase the energy and calorie content of the seed mix and, as many oil seeds are prone to fungal contamination, represent a safe way of providing much of the nutrition that these seeds contain. Single oils can be added, such as peanut oil or wheatgerm oil, or alternatively there is a range of commercially available oil blends, e.g. Polyseed Oil. Usual addition rate is 1/2 – 1 ml per kilogram of grain, which tends to make the seed look clean without making it unduly sticky. Animal-origin oils, in particular cod liver oil, should not be used as pigeons cannot digest these as well as seed oils. See Polyseed Oil.

Oxfendazole **–** Palatable liquid medication with the advantage of being effective against roundworm, hairworm and tapeworm. It has three disadvantages for use in pigeons: it needs to be given for 5 days straight, it is poorly water-soluble, with the water needing to be agitated every few hours to keep the medication in suspension, and it causes fret marks and so cannot be used during moulting. Most common brand name is Synanthic. See Synanthic.

Oxytetracycline **–** Tetracycline antibiotic in the same group as doxycycline. Replaced therapeutically by the newer doxycycline, which has advantages in treatment. Common brand name is Terramycin.

Permethrin **–** Synthetic pyrethrin used to control external parasites on birds and to control insects within the loft. Available as water-soluble powders and water-soluble liquids. See Pyrethrins.

Pick Stones **–** Various blends of both hard and soft grits suspended in a variety of mineral or clay bases. Aim to provide the grits necessary for health in a palatable form. Wide variety on the market, with big range of quality. Good-quality pick stones should provide numerous different types of both hard and soft grits that have been graded to the correct size for ingestion by pigeons. They need to be sufficiently hard to hold their shape but soft enough for the pigeons to easily break apart. Reputable companies will list the mineral content on the packet and have specific trace elements such as sulfur added to create a nutritionally balanced supplement. They should not contain an excessive level of salt, with approximately 1 gram of salt per kilogram being regarded as adequate.

Pink Minerals **–** Palatable powder preparations containing vitamins and minerals made specifically for pigeons. Wide variety of brand names available, of similar price, varying slightly in the level of vitamins and minerals they contain. Look at list of components on package to compare levels and to decide which is best value. Pink colour comes from the vitamin B_1 and iron oxides they contain. Useful and efficient supplements, widely used by fanciers world-wide. Common brand names include Vitamineral, PVM Powder, Vitacalc.

Piperazine **–** Older worming preparation now replaced by the avermectins. Does not kill worms but rather paralyses them and then relies on the muscles of the bowel to expel the paralysed worms before they revive and can maintain their position in the bowel. As a result, is not 100% effective. Only has action against roundworms and many of these are resistant. Available in a range of liquids and tablets. See Avermectins.

Polyseed Oil **–** Brand name of a blend of eight seed oils used as a feed additive. See Oils.

Praziquantel **–** Treatment of choice for tapeworm. Dose is 5 mg per pigeon as a single dose. Available as tablets and water-soluble liquids. Its advantage over older tapeworm preparations is that it can be used during the moult, the liquids are fully water-soluble and treatment times are short, with only a single dose being required if tablets are used or, in the case of liquids, only needing to be available for 24 hours. The drug is well tolerated, with the birds showing no sign of nausea. They can be loft-flown, exercised and fed normally during treatment. A common tablet brand name is Droncit, which contains 40 mg of praziquantel. The dose is 1/8 – 1/4 tablet once per bird. The brand name of a water-soluble liquid is Prazivet (25mg/ml), the dose rate of which is 5 ml per litre of water for 24 (– 48, if cool) hours or 1/4 ml per bird single dose. See Droncit, Prazivet.

Prazivet – Water-soluble preparation of praziquantel. For the treatment of tapeworms. See Praziquantel.

Probac – Avian-origin multiorganism probiotic. Can be added to the water at the rate of 1/4 teaspoon per litre or to the seed at the rate of 1/3 teaspoon per kilogram (following moistening with a seed oil). See Probiotic.

Probiotic – Term to describe a preparation of living organisms similar to those that inhabit the bowel of healthy animals. Disruption of normal bowel organisms occurs with stress and following antibiotic use. Maintenance of the normal bowel population aids in nutrient absorption and digestion and helps protect the bowel from disease. Becoming increasingly popular as fanciers realize the benefits of their use. Probiotics specifically made for birds are now available. Common brand name is Probac. See Probac.

PVM Powder – Pigeon Vitamin Mineral Powder. Brand name of a pink mineral, a vitamin/mineral supplement. See Pink Minerals.

Pyrethrins – Preferred insecticidal agents for use in birds. Much safer than the organophosphates and hydrocarbons that have been used in the past. Principal use to control lice but also effective against mites and insects generally. Usually type used is a synthetic pyrethrin called Permethrin. See Permethrin.

Reosole – Brand name of antimicrobial preparation containing ronidazole and doxycycline. Useful preparation to treat wet canker and *Chlamydia* infection simultaneously, both of which often occur together in young pigeons.

Resfite – Brand name of antibiotic preparation containing doxycycline and spiramycin, used in the treatment of respiratory infection. Dose rate 1/2 teaspoon per litre; usual treatment time 2 – 5 days. See Doxycycline, Spiramycin.

Ronidazole – Currently the world-wide veterinary choice as the best medication to manage canker. Wide safety margin. Safe to use during racing, breeding and moulting. Available under a variety of brand names around the world, including Ridsol-S, Turbosole, Tricho-Plus, Ronivet 4 Pigeons, which contain the active constituent at various strengths. The more concentrated the preparation, the shorter is the treatment time. However, the drug is bitter and once concentrations of over 10 – 12% are offered, palatability problems are encountered.

Spartrix – 10-mg Carnidazole tablet, used to treat canker. Dose 1 tablet per adult pigeon daily until well. Youngsters can be effectively medicated in the nest by comparing their size with that of an adult and giving the appropriate proportion of the tablet. See Carnidazole.

Spectinomycin – An antibiotic often combined with lincomycin, which has action against a range of bacteria, including *E. coli.*

Spiramycin – Antibiotic used in combination with other antibiotics, usually doxycycline, in the treatment of respiratory infection. Common brand name is Suanovil and, in combination with doxycycline, Resfite. See Doxycycline, Resfite, Suanovil.

Suanovil – Brand name of spiramycin, an antibiotic, used to treat respiratory infection. See Spiramycin.

Sulfa AVS – Brand name of a potentiated sulfonamide antibiotic. See Sulfonamides.

Sulfonamides – Group of antibiotics that may either be used by themselves or potentiated with other drugs to enhance their action, the most common combination being trimethoprim and sulfadiazine. Many sulfonamides are poorly absorbed from the bowel but are effective against organisms capable of infecting the bowel. They are used to treat *E. coli* and *Salmonella* infection and they also have some action against Coccidia. Main disadvantage for treatment of *Coccidia* is that treatment often needs to be extended for 7 or 10 days to be effective. Their tissue-penetrating properties are fairly poor and so their effect in the non-bowel forms of *Salmonella* is fairly limited. They also kill many of the normal bacteria of the bowel and so, if used during moulting, because of the interference with nutrient delivery to the feather follicle, can result in feathering abnormalities, including depigmentation. They do, however, have their uses in pigeons and can be used for 2 or 3 days to treat *E. coli* if diagnosed during racing. However, their use does seem to cause some nausea and so they should be used 3 or more days before basketing. Common brand names include Trimsul, Tribrissen, Sulfa AVS. See Trimsul, Sulfa AVS.

Synanthic – Brand name of oxfendazole, a wormer. Usual strength used contains 18 mg/ml and the dose is 5 ml per litre for 5 days. See Oxfendazole.

Terramycin – Brand name of oxytetracycline. See Oxytetracycline.

Tiamulin – Effective against *Mycoplasma* spp. However, less effective generally at clearing these organisms than tylosin. Narrow safety margin. Can cause feather abnormalities and death at elevated dosage rates. Common brand name is Dynamutilin. See Dynamutilin, Tylosin.

Toltrazuril – Active ingredient of Baycox. See Baycox.

Tricon – Brand name of chlortetracycline. See Chlortetracycline.

Trimsul – Brand name of a potentiated sulfonamide antibiotic. See Sulfonamides.

Turbosole – 10% Ronidazole, water-soluble powder. See Ronidazole.

Tylan – Brand name of tylosin, an antibiotic used to treat *Mycoplasma*. See Tylosin.

Tylosin – Antibiotic with good activity against *Mycoplasma* and some bacteria. When combined with doxycycline, it is the current choice for treatment of respiratory airsac infection during racing. Less effective when given by itself because *Mycoplasma*, although often being the primary agent of airsac infection, usually occurs concurrently with secondary agents such as *Chlamydia* and *E. coli*. The combination of Tylan and doxycycline treats all infective agents involved. Common brand name is Doxy-T. See Doxycycline, Doxy-T, Tylan.

Vibravet – Brand name of a doxycycline tablet. Usual strength used is 50 mg; dose is 1/2 tablet per adult bird per day. See Doxycycline.

Vitamineral – Brand name of a pink mineral, a vitamin/mineral supplement. See Pink Minerals.

Vitamins – Supplementation of pigeons with vitamins is regarded as a contentious issue by some fanciers. Non-stressed birds being fed a complete diet, including a wide variety of grains, may receive little benefit from an additional multivitamin supplement. However, when birds have been away from the loft racing, which often involves missed or irregular meals, or when high demands are being made on their system, such as towards the end of breeding for stock pigeons and during the heavy body moult of youngsters, multivitamin supplementation does have its benefits. Multivitamin supplements developed for use in other species should not be adapted for use in pigeons as their requirements are specific. Birds require higher levels of vitamin B and iodine, for example, than mammals, but produce their own vitamin C. Provided they are eating, there is no benefit in a multivitamin containing vitamin C. Multivitamin preparations should contain concentrated vitamins to allow a low dose rate as various forms of sugar are used as bulking agents in some preparations. Drinking a sugary solution can create a thirst and predispose the birds to bowel problems, neither of which are conducive to the development of form. Excessive sugar in the drinker with the vitamins also provides a greater opportunity for bacterial multiplication.

Yeasts – Common and useful feed supplement in pigeons. Yeasts such as those used to make beer and breads are a natural palatable food source of vitamin B and protein. Usually added to the seed with a seed oil such as wheatgerm oil or Polyseed Oil, which act as 'sticking' agents. Used during breeding to increase the percentage of protein in the diet and as a conditioning agent at other times to put weight on the birds. Sterile, killed yeasts, which lack the contaminants of Brewer's Yeast, etc., are now commercially available. Common brand name is ID Yeast (inactivated dried yeast), added to the seed at the rate of 3 teaspoons per kilogram. See ID Yeast.

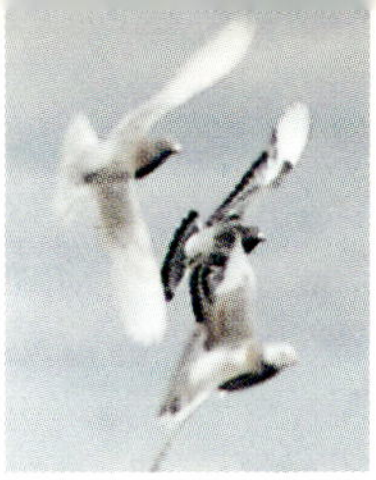

Chapter 47

DR COLIN WALKER'S AUSTRALIAN PIGEON COMPANY

Quality products that prevent disease by promoting health

Dr Colin Walker established the Australian Pigeon Company in 1994, to develop, manufacture and distribute a range of veterinary health supplements for pigeons. Dr Walker's veterinary expertise, together with his knowledge of the requirements of pigeon fanciers, gathered through experience of his own race team, place him in the unique situation to develop such products. The result is a small range of quality products made for the pigeon fancier and based on sound veterinary knowledge. The aim of these products is to prevent diseases by promoting health. Most fanciers realize the tremendous importance that health has to play in the performance of their birds and yet prefer not to use prescription medicines on their birds, if possible. These supplements are made from natural ingredients and it is hoped that, combined with a good loft environment and common-sense management, these products will help the birds grow, develop and form a strong natural immunity to disease. Through the application of modern veterinary knowledge and the utmost care in manufacture, the following products are now available.

Pick stones

MINERAL BLOCK

A pick stone that provides a range of hard and soft grits in a mineral matrix, which the birds enjoy eating

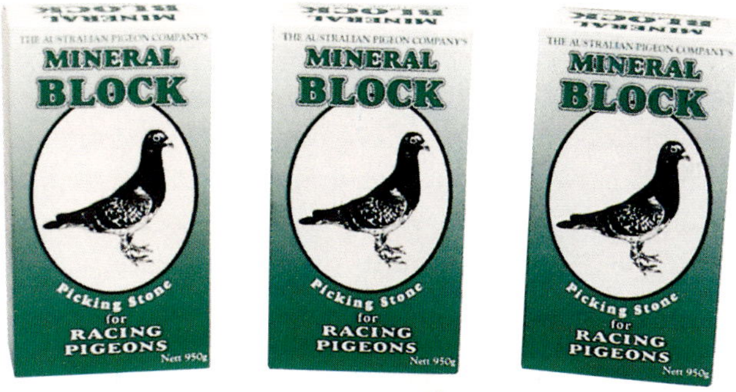

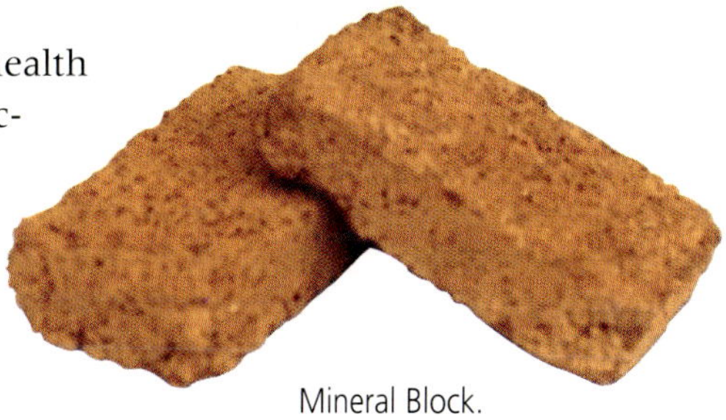

Mineral Block.

The Australian Pigeon Company's Mineral Block is a complete and balanced mineral supplement that can be used as a grit substitute. It has been developed under veterinary supervision specifically for pigeons. It brings natural grits, trace elements and minerals necessary for health into the loft in an hygienic, palatable form, reproducing the selection available to free-ranging birds.

Pick stones fulfill two vital nutritional functions. They provide hard grits, which act as digestive stones, grinding down swallowed grain, releasing the contained nutrition, and also soft grits, which slowly dissolve, releasing minerals and trace elements necessary for health. Hard grits describe material that is either not or only partially digested and include small stones such as granite and quartz. Unlike other birds such as parrots, pigeons swallow their grain whole. Because of the tough nature of the fibrous coating of these seeds, a small supply of digestive stones is kept in the pigeon's stomach. As the muscular stomach wall contracts, the hard grit acts like a mini-grinding mill, pulverizing the seed, making the nutrition they contain available to the bird. The Australian Pigeon Company's Mineral Block contains three different hard grits. Soft grits are also retained in the stomach but gradually dissolve, releasing the minerals and trace elements they contain. The pick stone made by the Australian Pigeon Company contains four soft grits, namely sterile egg shells, sterile sea shells, calcite and charcoal. Egg shells, sea shells and calcite are rich sources of the calcium that is so necessary during breeding to ensure good-quality crop milk, well-formed egg shells, decreased difficulty with egg laying, and strong bones in the nestlings.

One has to be careful, however, when using sea shells as a calcium source. If the shell is recently collected, the decomposing mollusc may still be inside. This small section of decomposing meat can contain bacteria that can make the bird sick. Some bacteria also produce toxins that can poison the birds. One of note here is called *Clostridium*, which produces a toxin that affects the nervous system, leading to a condition called botulism. Interestingly, in Victoria in 1992, we had 10 lofts all develop birds with botulism over a short period, which were all able to be traced back to a single load of contaminated grit. The sea shells and also the egg shells contained in the Australian Pigeon Company's Mineral Block have been sterilized. Shells from the sea can also contain a lot of salt, which, if the birds are deprived of water, can also cause problems. The level of salt in this block has been chemically analysed and is at the correct level for the racing pigeon. Shell sections can be too large and have sharp edges that can damage the throat, predisposing the bird to canker. The shells in the Australian Pigeon Company's block have been graded to avoid this problem.

Charcoal is a natural bowel astringent, actually absorbing many toxins from the bird's system, in the process contributing to health. The charcoal in the Australian Pigeon Company's Mineral Block has been made from non-treated timber. Many of the substances used to treat timber are poisonous and can survive the charcoal-making process. It is important that the birds are not exposed to these toxins.

Confined birds, which include most stock birds, are totally dependent on their owners to provide everything that they need nutritionally. A nutritional deficiency in the short term will cause no problem, however, even a subtle deficiency over an extended time will compromise health. This shows as a lack of vitality, decreased reproductive performance, and a poor moult. It is well known that the nutritional demand of the pigeon cannot be met by a grain diet alone. Access to a grit or pick stone is necessary for health. We have all seen the keenness with which birds allowed outside the loft examine areas such as the garden, incinerator, and gravelled surfaces. They are looking for the substances that a balanced mineral block contains. The practice of open lofting, although giving the birds the opportunity to find these things, is not without its risks. If health problems such as worms and Coccidia are present, then the droppings around the loft will contain infective eggs, which serve to reinfect the birds following effective treatments. The birds are also exposed to harmful fungi and bacteria. Many of the insects, such as slaters, around the loft can carry tapeworms. The Australian Pigeon Company's Mineral Block brings the minerals and trace elements that birds try and obtain from the loft environment into the loft in an hygienic form. The Mineral Block is palatable to the birds, which means that it is not only something that is good for them but something that they enjoy eating.

In summary, the block contains four soft grits – calcite, charcoal (from non-treated timber), sterile egg shells and sterile sea shells – together with three hard grits in two pure clays. To this have been added specific trace elements, in particular iron, sulfur and iodine, to create a balanced mineral supplement. The block's contents have been chemically analysed and adjusted to ensure that the minerals and trace elements it contains are at the correct levels and proportions for optimal health. No salt has been added. All grits have been graded to be of an appropriate size for the pigeon. All blocks are baked so that they hold their shape but can easily be broken down with the pecking action of the birds. The result is a pick stone that is not only good for the birds but is something they enjoy eating. Its use has been shown to decrease disease problems and to produce tight brown droppings, robust quick-growing youngster and good-quality feathers. It should be made available to the birds at all times.

Each pick stone, with a minimum weight of 600 grams, comes individually wrapped in its own packet. Available singly or in cartons of twenty four.

CALCIUM CAKE

A calcium-rich pick stone

Calcium Cake is a calcium-based pick stone. It is made from 100% Australian ingredients and is a blend of five calcium-based grits suspended in a mineral and clay matrix. The cakes are oven-cooked to remove all bacterial and fungal contamination. The cooking also makes them hold their shape but when pecked they easily break into nutritious bite-sized pieces. Although recommended for year-round use, Calcium Cake was developed with the breeding stock bird in mind. During breeding, pigeons have particularly high requirements for calcium, with calcium deficiency leading to soft-shelled eggs, poor-quality egg shells, difficulty with egg laying, poor-quality crop milk, and runting and deformity in babies. The cake is extremely palatable to the birds, in particular, stock birds feeding babies will devour it with gusto.

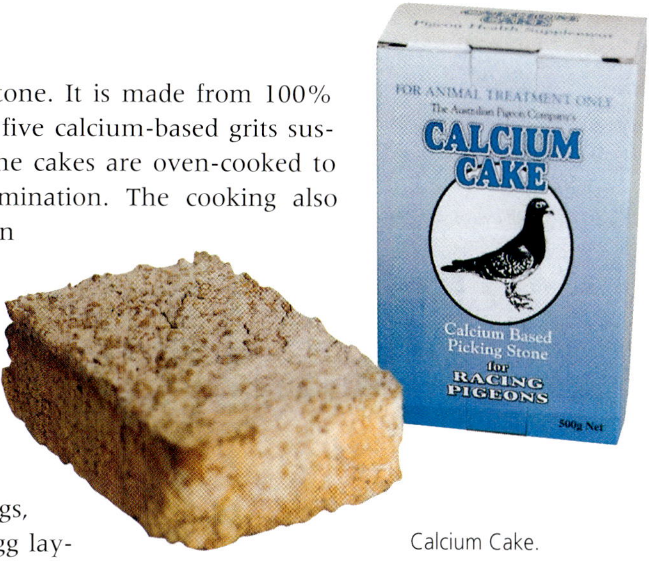

Calcium Cake.

Each 500-gram Calcium Cake comes individually wrapped in its own packet.

Mineral/vitamin powders

PVM POWDER

A highly palatable Australian-made pink vitamin and mineral powder

PVM Powder (pigeon vitamin/mineral powder) is a highly palatable Australian-made pink mineral powder packed with vitamins and minerals. This is an extremely popular product that is familiar to most Australian pigeon fanciers. To make it, it was essentially a matter of scanning the available veterinary texts to find out what were the optimal levels of the various vitamins and minerals for pigeons and then producing them in a balanced form that the pigeons would enjoy eating. PVM Powder contains all the minerals necessary for a balanced diet in pigeons, in particular calcium, iron and iodine, and also the vitamins that can be kept stable in this form, namely vitamins A, B, D, E and K. PVM Powder contains on average 20% higher levels of these vitamins than other similar brands of pink minerals and in addition also contains iodine. The pigeons seem to realize that it is good for them, with the birds eating it greedily, with some birds trying to snatch it from the air as it falls from the packet into the food tray. It is best supplied in a clean, dry bowl that cannot be tipped over or soiled by the birds, which is then placed on the loft floor in the same manner as a grit bowl. It can be made available to the birds at all times.

In the race loft, all birds will routinely eat a small amount. Fanciers will notice that birds coming from hard races and any young

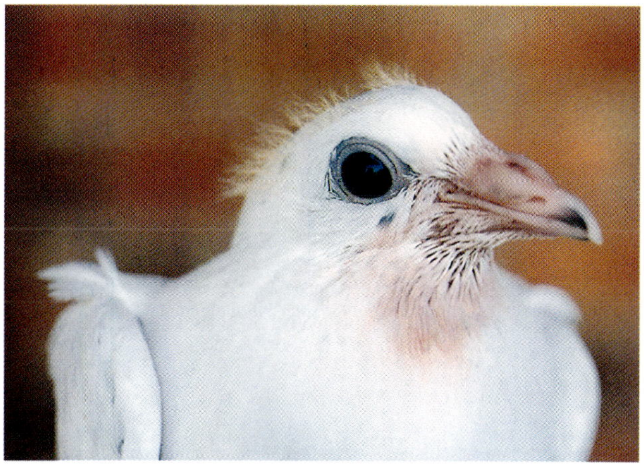

A PVM baby.

hen about to lay will eat substantially more, in the process replacing lost mineral salts. However, it is in the stock loft that PVM Powder is of particular benefit. Feeding stock birds, particularly those with rapidly growing (10 – 20 days old) youngsters, will eat large amounts and their youngsters will thrive. Being so palatable, it ensures that the birds eat the calcium and other nutrients it contains so necessary at this time. Eight pairs of feeding stock birds will eat up to one 600-gram packet per week. Feeding stock birds will pump it directly into their youngsters, leaving them with pale pink rims around the base of their beaks. It aids in the production of strong chubby youngsters ready for weaning at 26 – 28 days. Birds fed PVM Powder will no longer have the same grit requirement. Non-balanced grits force the birds to scratch through, looking for what they need. This leads to scatter and wastage. Because PVM Powder is balanced, the birds eat the lot, actually licking the bowl clean if it is not topped up.

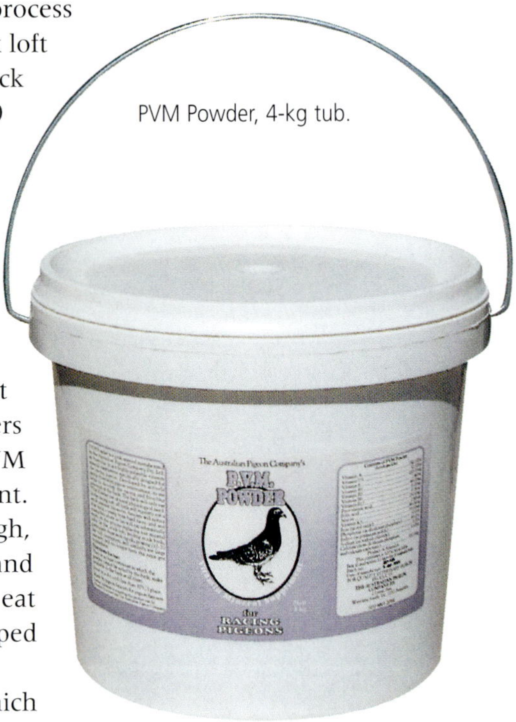

PVM Powder, 4-kg tub.

PVM Powder is available in 600-gram packets, which are heat-sealed to ensure freshness, and in 2-kg and 4-kg resealable buckets.

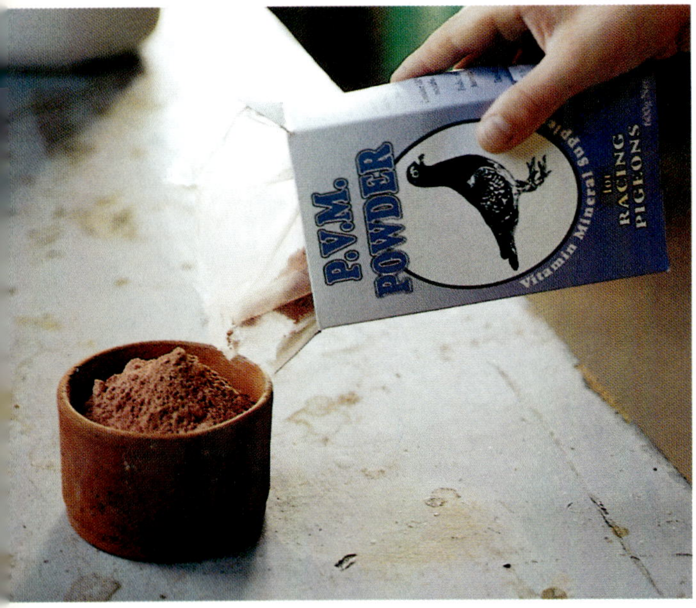

PVM powder, 600-g pack.

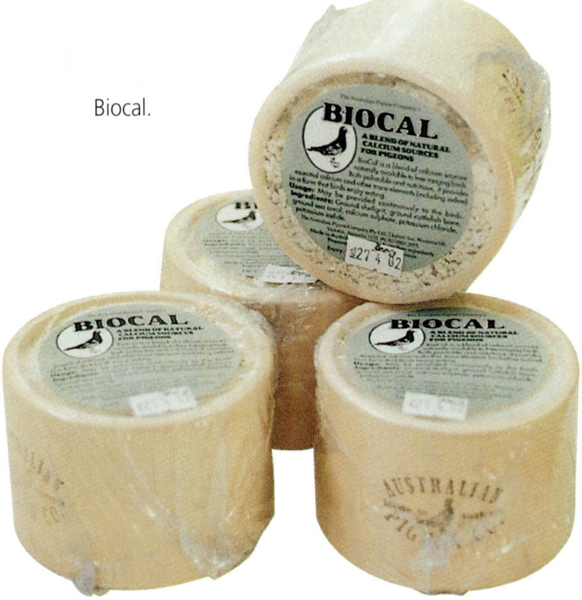

Biocal.

BIOCAL

Biocal is a fine white grit that is a blend of naturally occurring sources of calcium. It comes in its own reusable pick pot and is provided *ad lib.* Biocal is made from 100% Australian ingredients and contains ground shell grit, ground cuttle fish bone, ground sea coral and calcite. It is naturally rich in calcium and iodine. The result is a totally natural beneficial supplement, which the birds enjoy eating.

Available in a 500-gram reusable, pigeon-embossed terracotta pot. Each terracotta pot is individually shrink-wrapped to ensure freshness.

Conditioning oils

POLYSEED OIL

A high-energy, high-calorie feed additive that is a blend of eight seed oils

Polyseed Oil is a unique blend of eight seed oils (including peanut) with a natural preservative. Adding seed oils to the birds' grain mix is advantageous because the oil contains much of the nutrition available in the seed as a whole, including the fatty acids essential to growth, general vitality and the formation of healthy silky feathers. Highly palatable to the birds, Polyseed Oil is an efficient way of providing the birds with the energy and nutrition these seeds contain with no risk of fungal contamination to which all oil-based grains are prone. Added to the seed at the rate of 1/2 – 1 ml per kilogram, Polyseed Oil increases the calorie, nutrient and energy level of the seed mix and is used when increased demands are being made on the birds. It is quickly digested and provides fast energy release. It is useful when the stock birds are feeding young and in the postweaning time when the youngsters are developing. It is useful during moulting because it contains many of the unsaturated fatty acids necessary for lustrous feathers. Polyseed Oil, however, is of particular value during the exertion of the racing season when it can be added to the birds' seed to produce an especially nutritious meal after a hard race or toss or during cold weather.

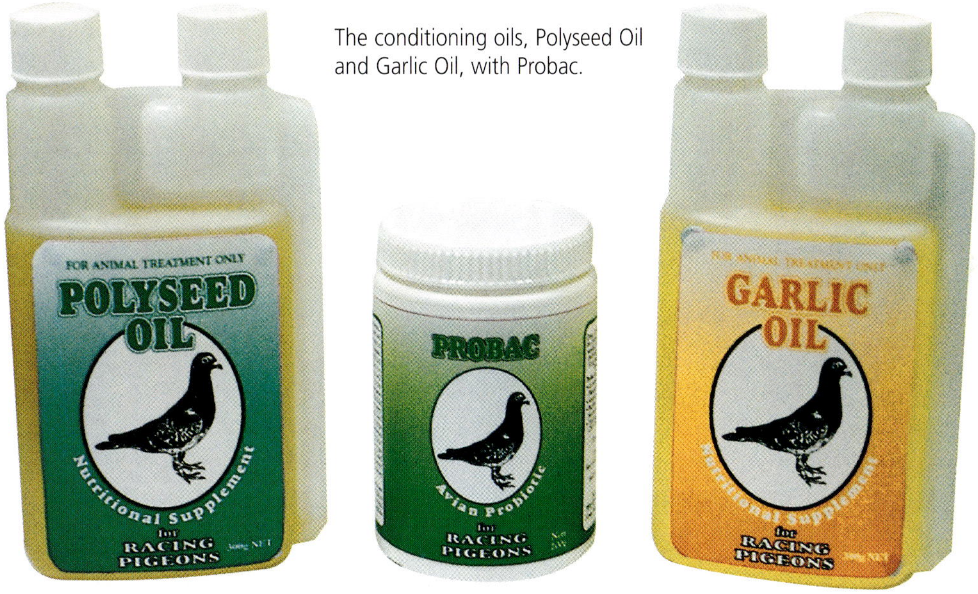

The conditioning oils, Polyseed Oil and Garlic Oil, with Probac.

Available in a 250-ml bottle with a 10-ml measuring chamber in the neck. Simply squeeze the bottle until the chamber fills to the desired level and then add to the seed.

TURBOVITE OIL

Turbovite Oil is a yeast-based energy oil that is added to the grain. It contains essential oils, yeast and a range of vitamins. It is a completely natural product with no artificial additives. Yeasts contain high levels of protein and vitamin B. The yeasts are in an unsaturated fatty acid base, which includes wheatgerm oil (itself a rich source of the vitamin B group and vitamin E). Unsaturated fatty acids are a high-energy, high-calorie food source. To this are added calcium, copper, zinc, iron, manganese and magnesium to further increase its nutrient value. Turbovite Oil contains the vitamins thiamine, riboflavin, pyridoxine, niacin, pantothenic acid, folic acid, vitamin B_{12}, choline and vitamin E and the natural amino acids arginine, glycine, glutamic acid, histidine, lysine, methionine and tryptophan.

Turbovite Oil is added to the seed at the rate of 10 ml to the seed of 50 birds (approx. 2 kg) to create an especially nutritious meal. It can be used after any stress, e.g. a hard toss, hard race, following medication, during recovery from disease or during cold weather, to help lift the birds and speed the return of form.

During the race season, for birds in full training, it can be used every day. However, because it is so nutritious, the birds' buoyancy should be monitored otherwise they can become overweight. It is ideal to put condition on birds that are handling a bit light.

Turbovite Oil used during breeding helps keep the stock birds in condition and helps provide many essential amino acids necessary for growth and development in the youngster. Many flyers have commented on the quality of feather produced in youngsters supplemented with Turbovite Oil. This is as would be expected as the amino acids it contains are needed for new feather production and the fatty acids produce an extremely silky feather. Good health leads to bloom production and accentuates the silkiness of the feathers. During breeding and the postweaning time, Turbovite Oil is good to use every 2 – 3 days.

Turbovite Oil is available in 250-ml resealable bottles with a measuring chamber in the neck.

GARLIC OIL

As discussed in the chapter Natural Supplements, pigeons have been supplemented with garlic to their benefit for decades. The Australian Pigeon Company's Garlic Oil contains the juice of fresh Australian garlic in a seed-oil base. Particular care has been taken not to use any chemical or heat process in its preparation that would decrease its effectiveness. It is added to the seed at the rate of 1/2 – 1 ml per kilogram of seed before feeding.

Available in a 250-ml bottle with a 10-ml measuring chamber in the neck. Simply squeeze the bottle until the chamber fills to the desired level and then add to the seed.

Grits

HEALTH GRIT

Health Grit is a premium-quality grit. It is a blend of nine different hard grits, each in the right proportion to provide the correct levels of calcium, iodine, iron and other essential minerals. It is also a source of digestive stones and contains charcoal. It is made from 100% Australian ingredients with the shells it contains being harvested from the pollution-free tropical beaches of Western Australia. It is non-moisture-absorbing, free of bacterial and fungal contamination, double graded to remove all large and small pieces, dust-free and contains no added salt. It is a highly palatable health promotant for the competitive bird and is designed for the actively competing race team for which everything to enhance health needs to be done to achieve top form.

Available in heat-sealed 5- and 10-kg bags.

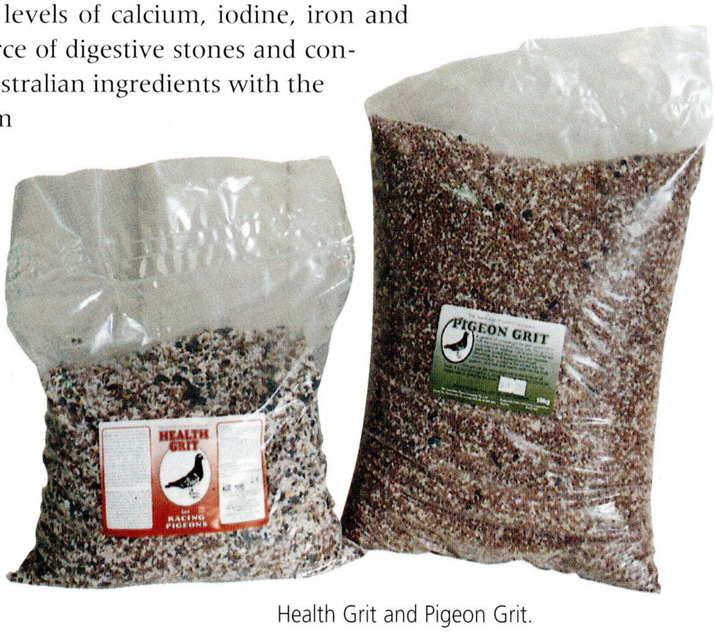

Health Grit and Pigeon Grit.

PIGEON GRIT

Pigeon Grit is an economical general all-purpose grit for year-round use in both the breeding and racing lofts. It is a triple blend of red stone, calcite and crushed sea shells from Western Australia with added charcoal. Like Health Grit, it is non-moisture-absorbing, free of bacterial and fungal contamination, double graded to remove all large and small pieces, dust-free and contains no added salt.

Available in heat-sealed 10-kg bags.

Health promotants

MULTIVITE PLUS – *'The Golden Boost'*

A water-soluble vitamin/mineral powder

Multivite Plus is a water-soluble vitamin/mineral powder that represents tremendous value for the pigeon fancier. It is complete, containing 13 vitamins and six trace elements (including iodine). At the same time, it is concentrated and economical, with only $^{1}/_{3}$ of a teaspoon being required for each 5 litres of drinking water. Nicknamed 'The Golden Boost' in Australia because of the way it turns the water a light golden colour and seems to give the birds a lift, it is readily taken by the birds. Multivite Plus can be given routinely as part of a health management program for 1 or 2 days per week or as required. It can be used to assist in recovery following any stress and to promote natural health during breeding, weaning, moulting and racing. Multivite Plus is sugar-free.

I feel that it is good to incorporate a complete multivitamin into the routine health management of the loft. Given 1 or 2 days per week, it helps to ensure that the birds are not lacking anything in their diet. This is particularly important during racing when birds either miss meals while away in units or eat irregularly, arriving late from races.

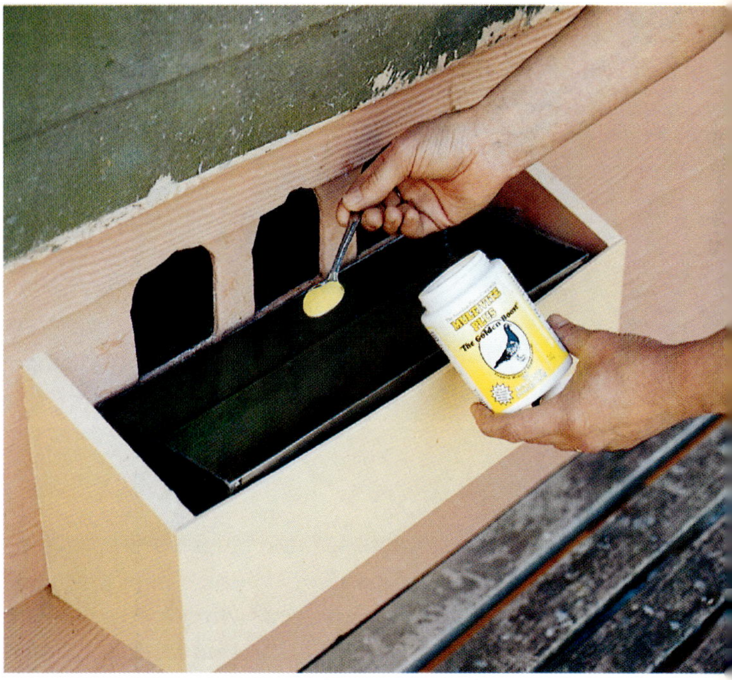

Multivite Plus.

Vitamins are fragile molecules: their effectiveness is decreased by heat, U.V. light and contact with organic materials such as droppings and seed. To ensure the birds get the full benefit of Multivite Plus, it should therefore be mixed fresh immediately before use and is best prepared just before feeding the birds. Once it is mixed, ensure that it is out of the sun and that it cannot become soiled. A fresh solution is best mixed every 12 hours. Containers made of stainless steel, glass or glazed pottery are preferred because they can be thoroughly cleaned. Glass or plastic containers should preferably be opaque. Containers should be cleaned before and after use to remove any persistent biofilm.

Specifically formulated for pigeons, Multivite Plus is a balanced, fully water-soluble preparation that the birds enjoy drinking. It is available in 200-gram plastic jars with a screw-top resealable lid; a measuring spoon is enclosed.

NUTRIBLOOM

Nutribloom is a vitamin, mineral and trace element feed supplement. It is balanced, palatable and nutritious. Grain is first moistened with a seed oil such as wheatgerm oil or Polyseed Oil at the rate of $^{1}/_{2}$ – 1 ml per kilogram before adding the Nutribloom at the rate of one measure (5 g) to the seed of 100 birds (approx. 4 kg). It can also be made available *ad lib* in a picking pot.

Nutribloom can be used during breeding, young bird development, the moult and racing. Its regular use during breeding helps the stock birds remain healthy and produce robust young. Weaned youngsters develop well and are better able to resist disease. During the moult, Nutribloom assists in the production of strong silky feathers, while its use during racing helps the birds maintain their fitness and vitality.

CALCIUM/VITAMIN D_3 SYRUP

Despite free access to calcium supplements such as pink minerals and pick stones, some birds will not voluntarily eat sufficient levels to meet their requirements. This is particularly so in recently weaned babies and some individual breeding stock birds. Adding a calcium supplement to the water helps ensure that all birds get what they need. The usual recommendation is that Calcium/Vitamin D_3 Syrup is added to the drinking water of breeding stock birds 2 – 3 days per week once paired and particularly towards the end of breeding, and to the water of weaned babies for 2 – 3 days in the first 10 days after weaning until the youngsters are settled and eating properly. The Australian Pigeon Company's Calcium/Vitamin D_3 Syrup is a clear water-soluble palatable solution that is sugar-free. It is added to the water at the rate of 10 ml to 1 litre. The vitamin D_3 it contains helps with absorption of the calcium from the bowel into the body.

Available in a 250-ml bottle with a 10-ml measuring chamber in the neck. Simply squeeze the bottle until the chamber fills to the desired level and then add to the water.

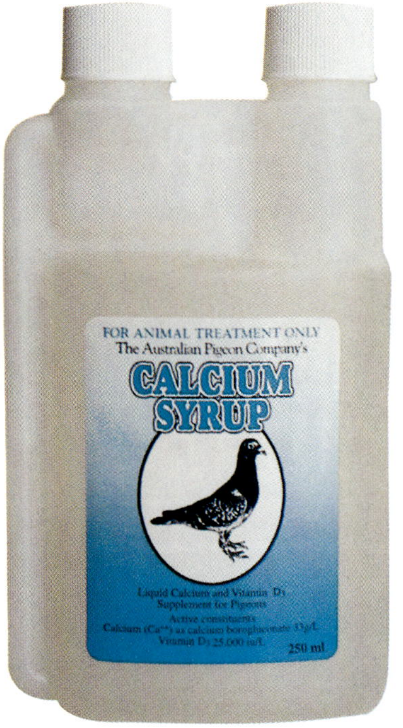

Calcium Syrup.

BATH SALTS

This is a blend of salts with added natural herb oils that has both antiseptic and feather-conditioning properties. Regular use helps in the maintenance of a lustrous plumage and will assist in skin health.

Available in a 700-gram resealable jar. 1½ tablespoons are diluted in 10 litres of lukewarm water.

BIO PIGEON TEA

The Australian Pigeon Company's Bio Pigeon Tea is a herbal tea that is a natural tonic. It is a dry blend of natural herbs that, when brewed, creates a refreshing drink. It is made from 100% Australian ingredients and contains echinacea, marigold, yarrow, peppermint, meadowsweet, alfalfa, caraway seeds, nettle and dandelion.

The tea is available in 150-gram resealable plastic jars. 1 tablespoon is added to 2 litres of just-boiled water. After standing for 15 minutes, it is strained and allowed to cool before being offered to the birds.

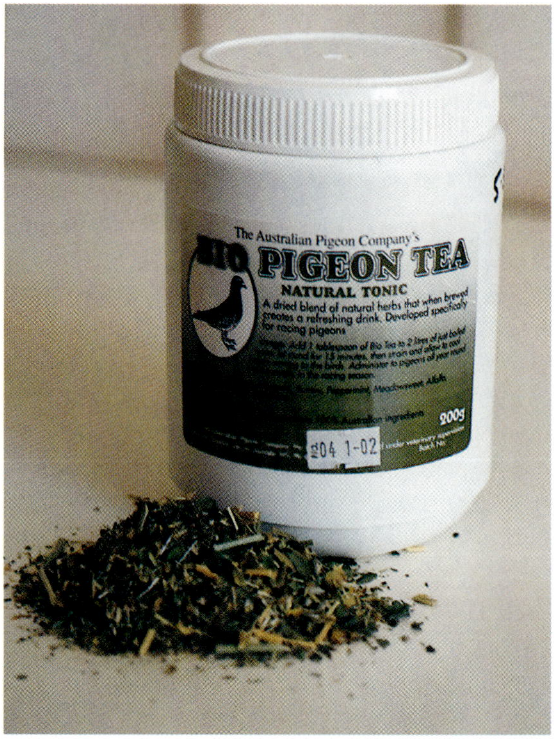

Bio Pigeon Tea.

ID YEAST

A natural yeast feed additive that is rich in vitamin B and high in protein

For many years, the benefits of yeast supplements have been known to fanciers world-wide. De Scheemaecker Brothers (the owners of the Natural Company of Belgium) recommend the birds receive them weekly during moulting for good feather development. Dr D. Marx, the noted American pigeon veterinarian, states that, although the supplement can be given continuously, he feels that it is best given sporadically and suggests that two to three times per week is adequate. He feels that it is good for both racers and breeders, creating a good appetite.

Essentially, yeasts are a natural food that is high in protein and rich in vitamin B. The level of protein required in the diet of a pigeon when not breeding, moulting or racing is approximately 11%. This can be achieved by feeding a grain mix that contains approximately 40% peas or beans (which are 20 – 25% protein) or other protein-based grains such as vetches (which are approximately 35% protein). Higher levels of protein are required during breeding, growth, disease, exertion, moulting and stress, generally. Failure to provide adequate protein levels during breeding results in slow-growing, underweight youngsters, which have to be weaned later than 28 days. Failure to provide adequate protein during moulting results in poor-quality feathers. ID Yeast is an ideal way of increasing the protein level of a basic grain mix and is very tasty for the birds.

The B-group vitamins are fairly common in food sources but generally at only low concentrations. Many forms found in grain are not readily available for digestion. Pigeons have high requirements for vitamin B; they are essential for health.

ID Yeast is an inactive, dry yeast. It is a fine yellow powder with a sweet smell. It is produced by non-alcoholic propagation and therefore contains none of the impurities that may be found in Brewer's Yeast. It has been sterilized to remove bacterial contaminants. It is extremely nutritious, containing 45 – 50% protein and approximately 70 mg per 100 gram of vitamin B. Its use during breeding helps in the production of robust young, which are ready for weaning at 26 – 28 days. If used during breeding, it helps in the production of lustrous feathers, while if used during racing, it leads to a quicker recovery following a hard fly. Mix with the grain immediately before feeding at the rate of 1 soupspoon per kilogram of seed, following moistening of the grain initially with a vegetable oil. It is ideal to use in combination with Garlic Oil or Polyseed Oil.

ID Yeast is available in a 400-gram resealable screw jar. A measure is included.

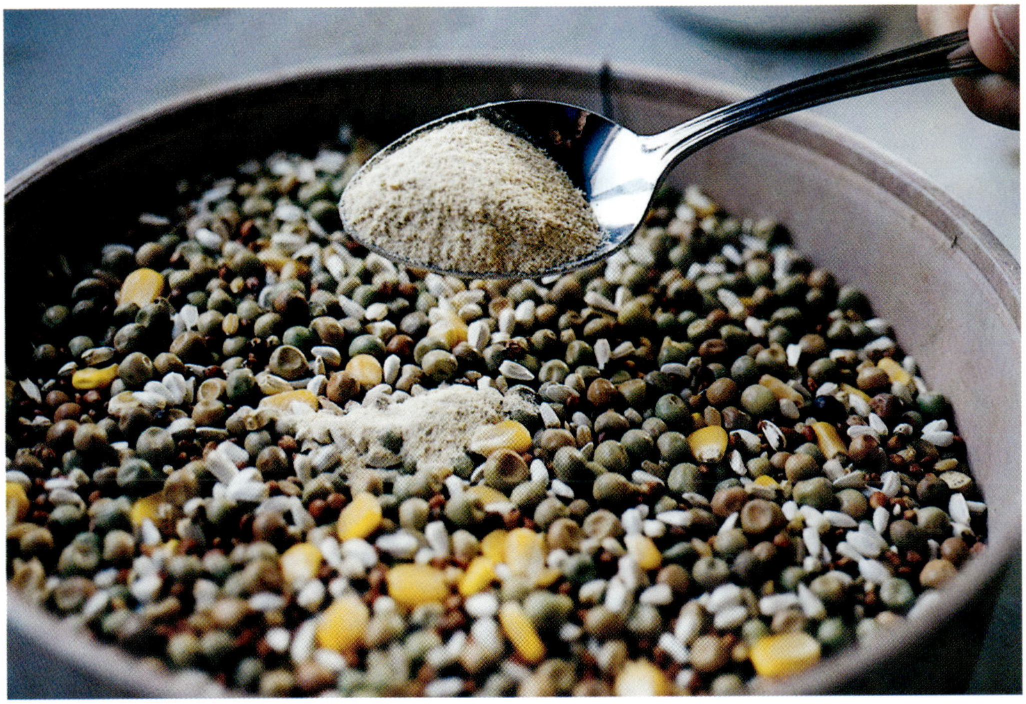

Yeast being added to the grain.

Section 9

MANAGEMENT DIARY

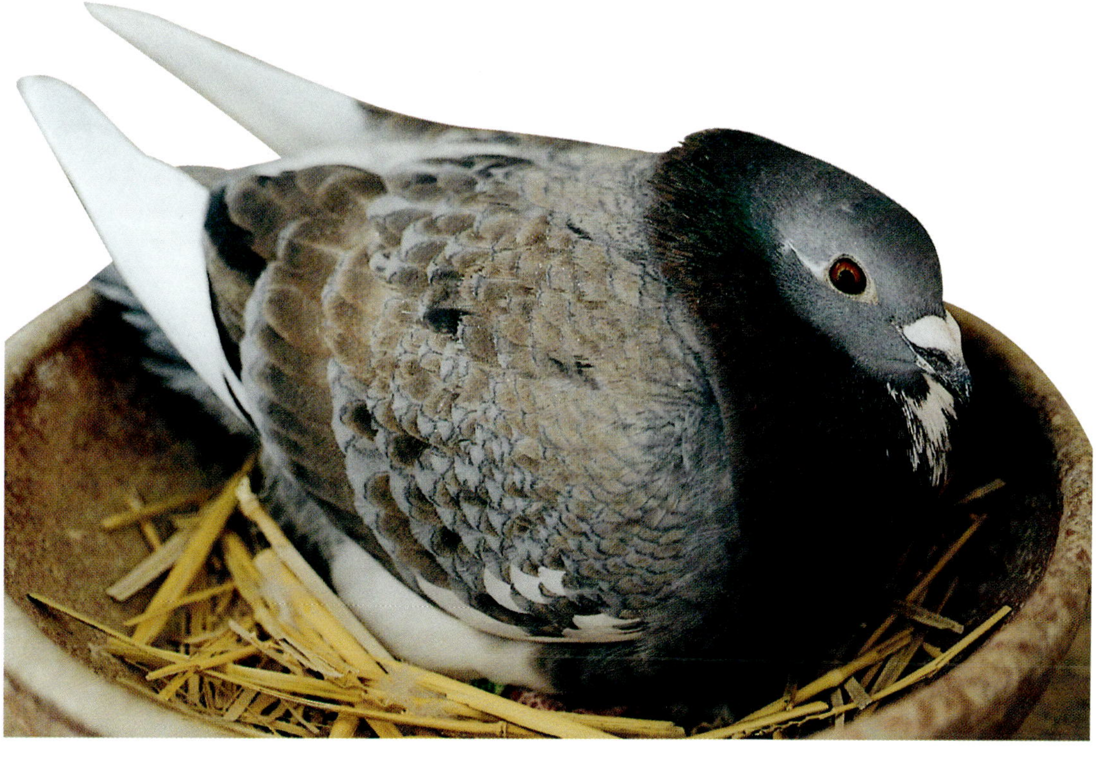

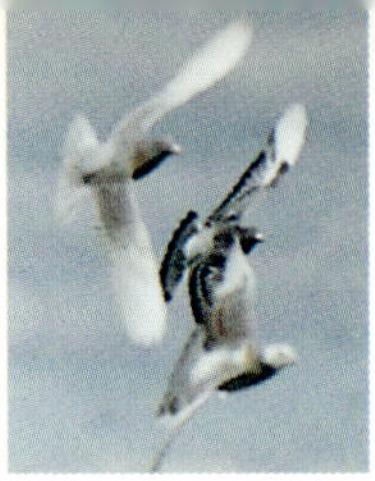

Chapter 48

THE PIGEON YEAR –

A management diary for the Southern Hemisphere

The successful racing loft can be viewed as an enterprise, where the produce is pigeons that can win and whose business it is to win races. A successful year does not occur by accident but is the result of plans put into action, which hopefully have developed from the experience of previous years. The year planner below is based on Victorian conditions in Australia. It is hoped that the basic principles, however, can be more widely applied. In Victoria, the racing season is divided in two. It consists of an eight-race program from 80 to 250 miles for young birds. This runs from the first weekend in March to the last weekend in April. No racing is conducted through winter, with the second season beginning mid-July and finishing in the end of November. In this second series of races, birds of any age may compete. The Victorian Homing Association program is very distance-orientated, with eight races 300 miles or less and 14 races ranging from 350 to 730 miles to the longest fliers. Racing finishes in November because, although it is still cool in Victoria, high temperatures are encountered at the race points hundreds of miles north of Melbourne, through western New South Wales and southern Queensland. This planner is by no means exhaustive, and ideally should be read in conjunction with the other chapters discussing management.

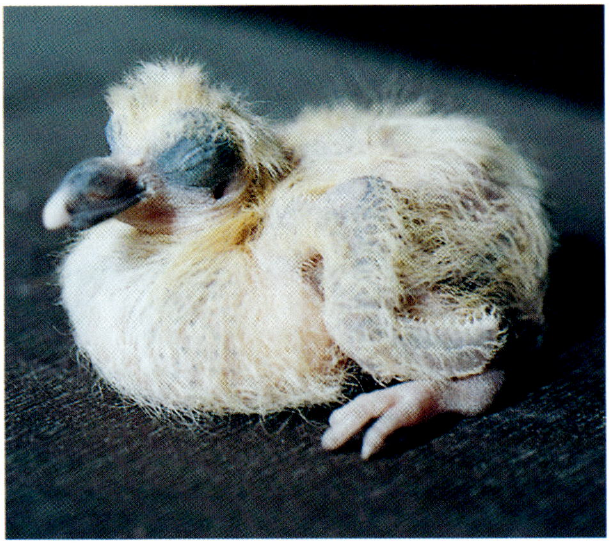

The raw material.

January

The loft is progressively filling with youngsters. From now until May, there are multiple stresses on these youngsters, notably the moult, training, establishing themselves within the loft, which involves some competition for food, water and perch space, possibly overcrowding, and disease. In addition, at this time of year, the weather is changeable, from dry and warm to wet and cool, with variations in temperature and humidity, particularly with an open loft design. Hawk activity is also high during this period, keeping the birds flying and causing psychological stress.

The main aim during this time is to keep stresses low and to allow the young birds to develop a natural immunity to the common diseases. Keeping stresses low minimizes the chance of disease and enables the birds to develop as well as they can. At the same time, to develop a natural immunity, controlled exposure to these diseases is necessary. It is important that medication, if required, is used correctly. This involves treating unwell birds if they occur but at the same time avoiding overuse of medication.

The principle disease from now until May is respiratory infection. Most respiratory disease in pigeons is due to a combination of *Chlamydia*, *Mycoplasma*, bacteria (in particular *E. coli)*, and stress. *Chlamydia* is found within the system of approximately 75% of pigeons all the time. With stress, the organisms are able to increase in number and cause clinical disease, in particular in the respiratory system. Most commonly they cause a conjunctivitis, that is the classic 'one-eye cold', dirty ceres, sneezing and a reluctance to fly. Birds with infection deeper in their airsacs may pant, but I regard this as a poor indicator of problems as this is affected by other variables including the birds' level of fitness, stage of moult, and environmental temperature. The disease is managed initially by identifying any obvious stress and correcting this. Assess the number of birds in the loft. Reappraise the loft design. Consider using a multivitamin supplement and decreasing their exercise. If the birds are unwell, there should be no rationing. Similarly, a health check to rule out primary parasitic diseases, such as worms and wet canker, is a good idea. These diseases often decrease the vitality of the young ones, enabling secondary problems, such as respiratory infection, to occur. Respiratory infection cannot be controlled unless these problems are also controlled. In addition, drugs can be sensibly used to lower the *Chlamydia* level. Response to any medication will be poor if any underlying stress fails to be identified and corrected. The best medications are Baytril and doxycycline. Both have side-effects in the growing youngsters and should be used under veterinary supervision. Well birds should not be treated so as not to interfere with their developing natural immunity. If only a few birds are affected, treat these individually with Vibravet (doxycycline), ½ a 50-mg tablet once daily until well (usually 3 – 5 days). There is no need to separate unwell youngsters as once on medication the birds stop shedding the organism. However, if the problem is becoming a flock one, all birds may be dosed for 3 – 5 days with water-soluble doxycycline 12% powder (1 teaspoon to 2 litres). The aim of treatment is not to eradicate the organism but rather to reduce it to a level where it is not causing harm.

February

Keep an eye open for other young bird diseases. As discussed in the chapter Medical Problems In Young Pigeons, I find it easiest to divide these into four groups: respiratory signs, bowel signs, canker and others. Most can be handled by stress reduction measures and hygiene. At this stage, the young birds have not had sufficient controlled exposure to disease to have developed the natural immunity of an adult, and also do not have the energy reserves in the form of body fat of the adult. As a result, they quickly succumb to illness. If you are suspicious of problems, prompt attention is necessary. A health profile, which involves a faecal examination and a crop flush, will normally identify the problem and correct treatment can be commenced.

In Australia, the moult begins in earnest in February. Young bird racing begins in March, and February is therefore the time of tossing. Now is a good opportunity to do a health check on the young bird team so that problems can be managed before racing commences. It is important to ensure that the team is ranging around the loft before the first toss. I feel that, for young birds, tossing on-line is important. My team's first toss is usually 7 – 10 miles, and I find that they do better at this distance. Any closer and they just range as they would if released at home. Take them several times to this point until they leave quickly and know the routine, and then gradually increase to 25 – 30 miles. This is all young birds need if the first race is 70 miles. Approximately 15 tosses should be adequate to educate them before the first race. Remember, they are still growing, so be careful to not overdo it. Each bird can race for several years; don't throw away a whole race career for the sake of half a dozen young bird races.

March

Daylength is decreasing. Breeding is over or finishing. The old birds are now moulting heavily. Ensure good diet and control of external parasites for a good moult, as discussed in the section The Parasitic Diseases. Moxidectin (2 mg/ml) may be added to the drinking water at the rate of 5 ml to 1 litre for 24 hours, or alternatively, the birds may be dipped in or sprayed safely with Permethrin. The first and second rounders are now over most of their stress, their body moult is almost finished and they have approximately one-third to two-thirds of their flights to go. The third rounders are in their body moult and may be struggling in an overcrowded loft.

Late March is the start of the cold, wet weather, and is the time we start to see Coccidia problems. Monitor the birds' droppings closely, and if suspicious of problems, submit a faecal sample for testing. If Coccidia becomes a problem, it can be controlled through regular cleaning, faecal monitoring and, if necessary, medication. The drug of choice is Baycox (1 ml to 2 litres of water for 2 days). Coccidia and other bowel problems are particularly relevant during moulting. Enteritis leads to diarrhoea, dehydration and interference with digestion and assimilation of nutrients, resulting in a poor moult. If possible, medication should be avoided during moulting as some, e.g. Synanthic, directly affect feather quality, while others, such as the tetracyclines and sulfur-based antibiotics, interfere with the normal bacteria in the bowel and, as a result, digestion, leading to poor availability of nutrients.

In March and early April, there are cold nights and sometimes very warm days. As discussed in Loft Design, a wide temperature variation within the loft over a 24-hour period is not conducive to form. It is important to have a loft design in which temperature can be controlled to maintain form in the young bird team.

April

During this month, fogs begin, resulting in increased humidity. It is important to monitor droppings, particularly after rain. In Victoria, the final young bird races are on. Members of the young bird team are usually dropping their final three flights. There are many theories as to when and when not to race young birds with regard to their flights. With my own team, I take particular note of them during their training session on the morning of basketing. If a bird is keen to fly and shows no signs of wing soreness when landing, it is sent that night. Alternatively, if an individual bird is reluctant to fly, pulls out of the bunch and lands prematurely or shows signs of wing soreness when landing, such as holding the wing out from the body, repeatedly preening at a particular site, etc., then no matter what its flight condition, it stays at home. There does seem to be some correlation with soreness when the follicle is at the blood-filled stage immediately before the follicle dries and the feather curls from its end. Once the level of blood in the follicle is reducing and the new feather is longer than 1 cm, the level of soreness seems to decrease daily. Snipping 0.5 – 1 cm from the tip of the tenth flight after the ninth flight has been dropped does seem to delay its drop. I sceptically started doing this to my own young bird team several years ago in order to prevent individual birds casting this flight in the days leading up to the last one or two young bird races. It does seem to work, but the exact mechanism is unknown.

May

Daylength is now becoming shorter and shorter and passes the threshold where there is no longer sufficient daylight hours for moulting to continue. Moulting therefore ceases. The first, second and some of the third rounders will have finished their moult, but some of the third rounders and the late-breds will not have finished and will fly the long races on varying numbers of nest flights. In May the weather is more stable, the birds are older, fitter, are getting used to the loft routine and should by now have developed a natural immunity to the common diseases. This, together with the end of moulting, means that disease problems in the youngsters are essentially over.

In Victoria, young bird racing is now over and it is a good time to vaccinate against pigeon pox and paratyphoid, if appropriate (refer to the sections Pigeon Pox and Paratyphoid).

June

In Victoria, breeding will begin in 2 months time, and as discussed in Problems of the Breeding Season, disease, if it appears once the stock birds are mated, is difficult to manage. It is important that any diseases present in the stock birds are identified now so that there is time to control them before pairing. A health check for the stock birds is a good idea. In the absence of testing, an eradication program may be followed as in the chapter Health Management Programs for All Stages of the Pigeon Year.

Old bird racing starts in 4 weeks, and the race birds are receiving longer tosses now. A health check is a good idea on the race team before racing.

July

This is the start of the main racing season in Victoria. Once racing starts, not only does the level of stress that the birds are under increase but also the exposure to disease, particularly with the commencement of Thursday night basketing. It is here that the understanding of pigeon diseases has changed dramatically in the last decade (refer to Health and Its Effect on Race Form). Fanciers are familiar with the clinical signs exhibited by youngsters with Coccidia, canker and *Chlamydia* infections. However, in race-age birds, although no sign of disease may be visible to the fancier other than poor returns or poor performance, the same diseases are at work. The diseases appear differently because the birds are older, have developed some natural immunity and, as a result, their response to infective organisms is modified. The levels of Coccidia, *Chlamydia* and trichomonads rise and fall in teams through the race season, depending on other stresses in their lives. Over the last few years, where we have been monitoring teams through the season, the correlation between test results and race performance is phenomenal. Usually, by midseason, I can tell which teams definitely will not get in the result that week and which teams, because of their negative results, may. Dr A. Scheers, the Dutch veterinarian, in his video 'Healthy Pigeons', summarizes the situation. He feels that birds that are extremely good can win with a trichomonad level of 10%, but no matter how good the breeding or the training of a team is, once the trichomonad level is 25% they cannot win. At my clinic, rather than estimate a percentage, we do straight counts. Once there are more than five trichomonads in a x100 microscope field, performance starts to drop. In some teams, there can be literally hundreds of trichomonads jostling for space under the microscope, and there can be no obvious sign in the hand other than they are just 'not right'. One factor affecting canker in race birds in particular is the genetic make-up of the birds, and it seems that particular strains are more susceptible to canker than others. Factors such as this, explain, I feel, why some fanciers speaking from experience with their own birds say that birds should only be raced every 3 weeks, while others disagree and say racing the same birds several weeks in a row is better. Both fanciers are probably right, for their teams of birds, but without testing don't know all the reasons why. Interestingly, with monitoring, teams of susceptible pigeons can have their trichomonad highs identified, be managed medically to bring the trichomonad count down more quickly and, as a result, return to race form quicker.

Consider this. If a loft is going to get six prizes out of 18 starts through a season, then given the random nature of wind direction and the condition of individual good birds within the team, one would expect the six good results to be scattered through the 18 starts. This is in fact usually not the case. The six good results are more likely to be grouped together and occur out of seven or eight starts. This is because the birds have come into form. Obviously, many things affect race form, but when in-form teams are checked their test results are always negative. When results become positive, form is lost. Many fanciers have known this for years, and it is the job of the astute fancier, through testing, to identify and head problems off before they have a chance to affect form. Testing from one year to the next identifies problems within that loft so that recognized treatment regimes can be adapted to that particular situation. For example, in cold open lofts or damp humid lofts, Coccidia can be a problem and we use Baycox for 2 days every 4 weeks. Similarly, wet canker (elevated trichomonads) in lofts needs to be managed. Dr Stosskopf, in charge of the Natural Breeding Station in Holland for De Scheemaecker Brothers, states that no drug keeps the trichomonads out of the crop for longer than 5 – 6 weeks, and only the drug ronidazole 10% has the potential to keep them free for this period. Depending on loft factors, the trichomonads will return at different times. Once the fancier knows this for his own loft, he has a basis for effective ronidazole use. *Chlamydia* acts in a similar way. Once racing commences, disease monitoring through regular checks is therefore of value.

All problems except canker and respiratory infection can be monitored through faecal testing, and some of the things we are looking for remain stable for up to 7 days. This allows the mailing of samples to racing pigeon veterinary clinics. Trichomonads are detected in a throat swab. They are fragile and only remain active outside the bird for several minutes. Although transport kits are available, their use makes interpretation of levels difficult. For this test, it is best if birds are presented live at a clinic.

August

The stock birds are paired. The actual time to pair the stock birds is determined by the need to have youngsters of sufficient maturity to compete in the early races the next year, but at the same time not have large numbers of youngsters weaned into race sections before completion of the current season in lofts with limited space. Depending on the loft accommodation available, any youngster weaned will not only get in the way of the distance teams training but will also be intimidated by the older birds present. I therefore aim to wean the youngsters on the weekend of the last race. Allowing 10 days from pairing to laying, 18 days incubation and weaning at 28 days, means pairing the birds 8 weeks before this. As racing finishes late November, my stock birds are paired late August. Our young bird program starts in the beginning of March and over the years, having kept records of all youngsters' weaning dates, I have found that youngsters weaned after 5 December are more likely to be lost and less likely to do well in the young bird series. Interestingly, older youngsters, weaned before the start of October, also seem to do less well. There are always exceptions, but programs based on exceptions are statistically less likely to succeed. Weaning the first round at this time means that they have 2 months to become familiar with the loft and loft routine before tossing commences, which ideally should be 4 weeks before the first race. In the absence of any set-backs, this time appears sufficient.

The middle-distance races are now in progress in Victoria.

September

The late-breds in the race team are now starting to go through puberty. In Victoria, this is the time of our 350- and 400-mile races. The late-breds have not had the physiological drain of a whole moult and have the vigour and keenness for flying of youth, but are mature enough to navigate the long races. Once motivated by their developing libido, good results can now be achieved by these younger birds in the team. In my own team, I always aim to wean some nice young hens off the distance pairs into the race loft during February for this reason.

The stock birds are incubating the first round. If canker has been a problem in the previous year's breeding season, now is the time to start a canker preventive program (refer to the chapter Canker).

October

Long-distance racing is now in progress. It is here that the fitness, motivation and genetic make-up of the birds are put to the ultimate test. It is important that tossing and feeding are matched to the birds' level of fitness (refer to the chapters Developing Race Fitness and Winning).

November

The race program is finishing, and first-rounders are being weaned into the racing loft (refer to the chapters Weaning and Medical Problems in Young Pigeons). High-quality food is needed for stock birds, with free access to shell grit and preferably a pick stone and pink minerals at all times (refer to the chapter Problems of the Breeding Season).

December

Birds in the first round have dropped their first and second flights by the end of December, and they should be ranging now. The stock birds are incubating the third round of eggs and will be showing signs of stress. Beware, in particular, of canker and, if it appears, manage as discussed in the chapter Canker. It is important at this time that the stock birds are well fed and there are particular advantages in calcium supplementation. I use and recommend that calcium syrup be placed in the water several days per week, particularly towards the end of breeding. In the coming months, as a normal feature of their existence, the young birds will come under much stress. A big factor in the birds' ability to manage this is their level of parasitism, which ideally should be zero. At this time of year, youngsters are straying from other lofts and race birds lost in the distance events may return. Both serve as sources of infection. Parasites, in particular, are of concern and there are those of the bowel, i.e. worms, the crop, i.e. trichomonads, and the skin and feathers, i.e. mites and lice. All not only cause disease directly but also weaken the birds generally. They increase the birds' vulnerability to secondary diseases, in particular respiratory infection, in the coming months and therefore need to be correctly controlled as outlined in earlier chapters.

Summary

- **June**
  Health check for stock birds before pairing; treatment if necessary. In absence of testing, start of prebreeding preventive program. Longer training tosses now for old bird race team. Health check for race team before start of racing season.
- **July**
  Start of main racing season. Disease monitoring every 1 – 3 weeks during race program.
- **August**
  Stock birds paired. Commence canker prevention program, if canker was a problem in previous year. Start of distance races.
- **October**
  Distance races now on. Tossing and feeding regimes to match work done by teams. Stock birds feeding first round.

- **November**
  Completion of race program. First-rounders weaning into race loft.
- **December**
  First round ranging. Stock birds showing some stress. Monitor youngsters in nest, in particular for canker now. Calcium supplementation for stock birds. Control of parasites in race loft.
- **January**
  Loft filling with young birds. Keep stresses low. Allow development of natural immunity. Monitor closely, in particular for respiratory infection, and treat as is necessary.
- **February**
  Moult begins in earnest, contributing to stress, therefore monitor young birds closely for disease. Tossing for young bird racing. Health check for race team before commencement of young bird racing; treatment if necessary.
- **March**
  Start of cold wet weather. Breeding over. Heavy body moult for old birds. Young bird racing in progress. Third round now weaned, therefore monitor closely.
- **April**
  Final young bird races. Monitor droppings, particularly after rain Coccidia may be a problem.
- **May**
  Moult finishes. End of most young bird disease problems. Vaccinations, if appropriate.